SPORTS MEDICINE:
CORE KNOWLEDGE
IN ORTHOPAEDICS

SPORTS MEDICINE: CORE KNOWLEDGE IN ORTHOPAEDICS

MARK D. MILLER, MD

Professor of Orthopaedic Surgery
Head of the Division of Sports Medicine
University of Virginia
Charlottesville, VA
Team Physician
James Madison University
Harrisonburg, VA

JON K. SEKIYA, MD

Assistant Professor of Orthopaedic Surgery
Center for Sports Medicine
University of Pittsburgh Medical Center
Pittsburgh, PA

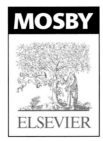

MOSBY

ELSEVIER

MOSBY
ELSEVIER

1600 John F. Kennedy Blvd.
Ste 1800
Philadelphia, PA 19103-2899

SPORTS MEDICINE: CORE KNOWLEDGE IN ORTHOPAEDICS   ISBN-13: 978-0-323-03138-7
Copyright © 2006, Mosby Inc.   ISBN-10: 0-323-03138-2

Notice

Knowledge and best practice in this field are constantly changing. As new research and experience broaden our knowledge, changes in practice, treatment, and drug therapy may become necessary or appropriate. Readers are advised to check the most current information provided (i) on procedures featured or (ii) by the manufacturer of each product to be administered, to verify the recommended dose or formula, the method and duration of administration, and contraindications. It is the responsibility of the practitioner, relying on his or her own experience and knowledge of the patient, to make diagnoses, to determine dosages and the best treatment for each individual patient, and to take all appropriate safety precautions. To the fullest extent of the law, neither the Publisher nor the authors assume any liability for any injury and/or damage to persons or property arising out or related to any use of the material contained in this book.

The Publisher

Library of Congress Cataloging-in-Publication Data

Sports medicine : core knowledge in orthopaedics / editors, Mark D. Miller, Jon K. Sekiya;
   associate editors, Jennifer Hart ... [et al].—1st ed.
     p. ; cm. — (Core knowledge in orthopaedics series)
   ISBN 0-323-03138-2
    1. Sports injuries—Surgery. 2. Orthopaedic surgery, 3. Sports medicine I. Miller, Mark D. II. Sekiya, Jon K.
III. Series.
  [DNLM: 1. Athletic Injuries. 2. Orthopedics—methods. 3. Sports Medicine—methods.
QT 261 S76498 2006]
RD97.S66 2006
617.1'027—dc22   2005053448

Publishing Director: Kim Murphy
Developmental Editor: Anne Snyder
Project Manager: David Saltzberg
Design Direction: Gene Harris

Printed in China

Last digit is the print number: 9   8   7   6   5   4   3   2   1

Working together to grow
libraries in developing countries

www.elsevier.com | www.bookaid.org | www.sabre.org

ELSEVIER   BOOK AID International   Sabre Foundation

Associate Editors

JENNIFER HART, MPAS, PA-C,
Department of Orthopaedic Surgery, University of Virginia, Charlottesville, VA

J. SCOTT QUINBY, MD,
Sports Medicine Fellow, University of Virginia, Charlottesville, VA

Associate Editors—Elbow, Wrist, and Hand

MICHAEL E. PANNUNZIO, MD,
Associate Professor of Orthopaedics, University of Virginia, Charlottesville, VA

SCOTT M. WEIN, MD,
Resident, Department of Orthopaedic Surgery, University of Virginia, Charlottesville, VA

LANCE M. BRUNTON, MD,
Resident, Department of Orthopaedic Surgery, University of Virginia, Charlottesville, VA

Associate Editors—Head and Spine

FRANCIS H. SHEN, MD,
Assistant Professor, Department of Orthopaedic Surgery, Division of Spine Surgery, University of Virginia, Charlottesville, VA

DINO SAMARTZIS, BS, DIP. EBHC,
Graduate Division, Harvard University, Cambridge, MA; Division of Health Sciences, University of Oxford, Oxford, England; London School of Economics and Political Science, University of London, London, England

To my friends and associates who helped me with this book—Jen, Q, Mike, Frank, and all others—thank you; I literally couldn't have done it without you! And, of course, to my family, who allow me to take on these projects—I wouldn't want to do it without you!

MDM

To my parents, Fred and Pat—thanks for your love and support through the years, as well as for instilling in me the importance of a good work ethic.
To my wife, Jennie—thanks for your enduring support and love through this "project." You are truly my life and the "wind beneath my wings."

JKS

Contents

Preface   xiii

Section 1   Knee

1. **Knee Anatomy and Biomechanics**   1

2. **Knee History, Physical Examination, and Imaging**   8

3. **Knee Arthroscopy**   22

4. **Meniscal Pathology**   27

5. **Osteochondral Injuries to the Knee**   42

6. **Synovial Lesions**   51

7. **Anterior Cruciate Ligament Injuries**   55

8. **Medial Collateral Ligament Injuries**   62

9. **Posterior Cruciate Ligament Injuries**   69

10. **Lateral Collateral Ligament and Posterolateral Corner Injuries**   76

11. **Multiple Ligament Injuries**   90

12. **Patellofemoral Disorders**   96

13. **Arthrofibrosis of the Knee**   109

14. **Pediatric Knee Injuries**   113

Section 2   Hip and Thigh

15. **Hip Anatomy and Biomechanics**   121

16. **Hip Arthroscopy**   127

17. **Groin Pain** 134

18. **Hip Overuse Syndromes** 140

19. **Snapping Hip** 143

20. **Hip and Thigh Muscle Strains and Contusions** 150

21. **Nerve Entrapment Syndromes of the Hip and Knee** 157

Section 3 Leg, Ankle, and Foot

22. **Leg, Ankle, and Foot Anatomy and Biomechanics (Including Gait)** 162

23. **Ankle Arthroscopy** 181

24. **Leg, Ankle, and Foot Overuse Syndromes** 187

25. **Exertional Compartment Syndrome** 206

26. **Ankle Instability** 209

27. **Lower Extremity Fractures** 220

28. **Leg, Ankle, and Foot Nerve Entrapment Syndromes** 226

29. **Toe Injuries/Disorders** 234

Section 4 Shoulder

30. **Shoulder Anatomy and Biomechanics** 239

31. **Shoulder History, Physical Examination, and Imaging** 252

32. **Shoulder Arthroscopy** 263

33. **Anterior Shoulder Instability** 270

34. **Posterior Shoulder Instability** 276

35. **SLAP Tears and Internal Impingement** 285

36. **Rotator Cuff Injuries** 293

37. **Muscle Ruptures of the Shoulder** 313

38. **Shoulder Loss of Motion** 319

39. **Nerve Entrapment at the Shoulder** 328

40. **Upper Extremity Fractures** 331

41. **Acromioclavicular, Sternoclavicular, and Clavicle Injuries** 342

Section 5   Elbow

42. Elbow Anatomy and Biomechanics   350

43. Elbow History, Physical Examination, and Imaging   363

44. Elbow Arthroscopy   367

45. Elbow Instability   370

46. Tendon Injuries about the Elbow   372

47. Nerve Entrapment   375

48. Elbow Overuse Injuries   378

49. Elbow Loss of Motion   381

Section 6   Wrist and Hand

50. Wrist and Hand Anatomy and Biomechanics   383

51. Wrist and Hand History, Physical Examination, and Imaging   389

52. Wrist Arthroscopy   393

53. Carpal Instability   396

54. Ulnar-Sided Wrist Pain   399

55. Wrist and Hand Overuse Injuries   404

56. Finger Injuries   406

Section 7   Head and Spine

57. Concussion in Sport   413

58. Basic Anatomy of the Spinal Column   419

59. Cervical Spine Injuries   423

60. Disc Disease   431

61. Dealing with Low Back Pain   437

62. Spondylolysis/Spondylolisthesis   445

Section 8   Sports Medicine/Team Coverage

63. Preparticipation Evaluation   449

64. Team Medical Coverage   462

65. Drug Use/Abuse/Ergogenic Aids/Supplements/Nutrition   466

66. The Female Athlete   476

67. Medical Conditions   481

68. Ethical and Legal Issues   491

69. Research Principles   493

Index   499

Preface

Several years ago the publishers at Elsevier envisioned a series of orthopaedic textbooks that would cover all of the subspecialties in orthopaedic surgery. The Core Knowledge in Orthopaedics series is a culmination of this idea. We are proud to have been chosen to develop *Sports Medicine: Core Knowledge in Orthopaedics*. Our field has blossomed over the past several years, and even academic guys like us have a hard time keeping up. This book has given us a chance to catch up with our ever-expanding field, and more importantly, it will give YOU a chance to catch up as well! The timing couldn't have been better. Orthopaedic sports medicine has recently been awarded the opportunity for subspecialty certification. Efforts are under way to develop an examination for this purpose—in fact, questions for this examination were being written at the same time that we were writing this text. So, not only does this text serve an important position in the Core Knowledge in Orthopaedics series, but it also represents THE core knowledge necessary to prepare for this examination! And . . . because we all want to pass that examination, we will stop here and allow you to turn the page and begin your preparation.

With sincere best wishes—good luck!

Mark D. Miller, MD
Jon K. Sekiya, MD

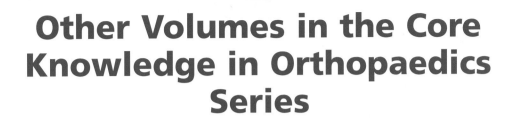

Other Volumes in the Core Knowledge in Orthopaedics Series

Spine

Pediatric Orthopaedics

Hand, Elbow & Shoulder

Trauma

Adult Reconstruction and Arthroplasty

Foot and Ankle

CHAPTER 1

Knee Anatomy and Biomechanics

Introduction

- The primary joint of the knee is the tibiofemoral joint. This joint is composed of two femoral condyles (medial and lateral) and two corresponding tibial plateaus (medial and lateral).
- The medial femoral condyle is longer and larger than the lateral femoral condyle.
- The lateral femoral condyle has a notch, or sulcus, between the anterior one third and posterior two thirds.
- The medial tibial plateau is concave and wide, whereas the lateral tibial plateau is convex and smaller (Figure 1–1).
- The proximal tibiofibular joint is distal to the primary joint and is a gliding joint.
- The patellofemoral joint is discussed later.

Ligaments

- There are four ligaments and two "corners" in the knee (Figure 1–2).
- The anterior cruciate ligament (ACL) runs from the area between the two tibial eminences up to the lateral femoral condyle.
  - It is approximately 3 cm long and 1 cm in diameter.
  - It has two bundles: an anteromedial bundle, which is tight in flexion, and a posterolateral bundle, which is tight in extension.
  - The ACL is the primary restraint to anterior translation and functions with the knee in slight flexion (30 degrees).
  - The middle geniculate artery is the primary blood supply for both the ACL and the posterior cruciate ligament (PCL).
  - The ultimate strength of the ACL is approximately 2200 Newtons (Figure 1–3).
- The PCL runs from the posterior tibia (midline, below the joint surface) to the medial femoral condyle.
  - It is almost 4 cm long and 1.3 cm in diameter.
  - It also has two bundles: an anterolateral bundle, which is tight in flexion, and a smaller posteromedial bundle, which is tight in extension.

- It also has variable meniscofemoral ligaments that run from the posterior horn of the lateral meniscus to the front (Humphry) and back (Wrisberg) of the PCL.
- The PCL is the primary restraint to posterior translation of the tibia and functions with the knee in 70- to 90-degrees flexion.
- The ultimate strength of the PCL is approximately 2500 Newtons.
- The medial collateral ligament (MCL) has both a superficial and deep component.
  - It runs from the medial epicondyle (adductor tubercle) to the proximal tibia and inserts along an extended area.
  - It is the primary restraint to valgus stress for the knee.
  - The ultimate strength of the MCL is approximately 4000 Newtons.
- The lateral collateral ligament (LCL) is a cordlike ligament that runs from the lateral femoral epicondyle to the posterior tip of the fibula.
  - It is tight in extension.
  - It is the primary restraint to varus stress for the knee.
  - The ultimate strength of the LCL is approximately 750 Newtons.
- The "posteromedial corner" of the knee includes the MCL; the posterior oblique ligament; the semimembranosis attachment; and, more superficially, the sartorial fascia. It prevents excessive internal rotation of the knee.
- The "posterolateral corner" of the knee includes the LCL; the popliteus; the popliteofibular ligament; the posterolateral capsule; and, more superficially, the biceps and iliotibial band tendons. It prevents excessive external rotation of the knee (Figure 1–4).

Patellofemoral Joint (Figure 1–5)

- The patella is a sesamoid bone that serves as a fulcrum for the knee extensors (quadriceps muscles), increasing their moment arm (Figure 1–6).
- The patellofemoral joint is fully engaged at approximately 40 degrees of knee flexion.

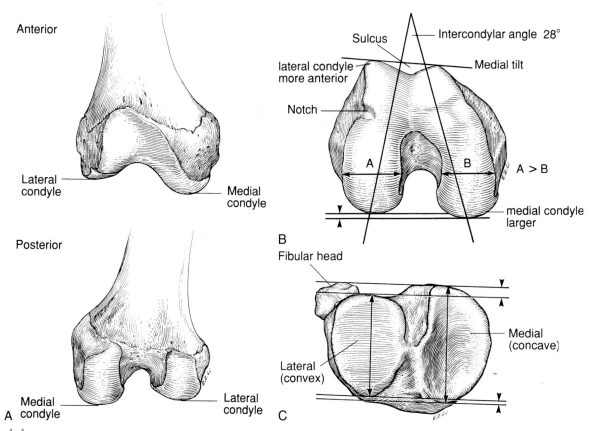

Figure 1–1:
A, Anterior and posterior view of the right distal femur. **B,** Flexion view of the distal aspect of the right femur. **C,** Superior view of the right tibial plateau. (From Tria AJ Jr, Klein KS: *An illustrated guide to the knee.* New York, 1992, Churchill Livingstone.)

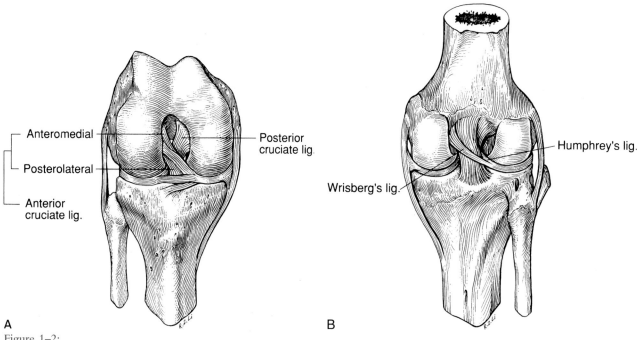

Figure 1–2:
A-E, Ligaments of the knee, **A,** Anterior view. **B,** Posterior view (deep).

(continued)

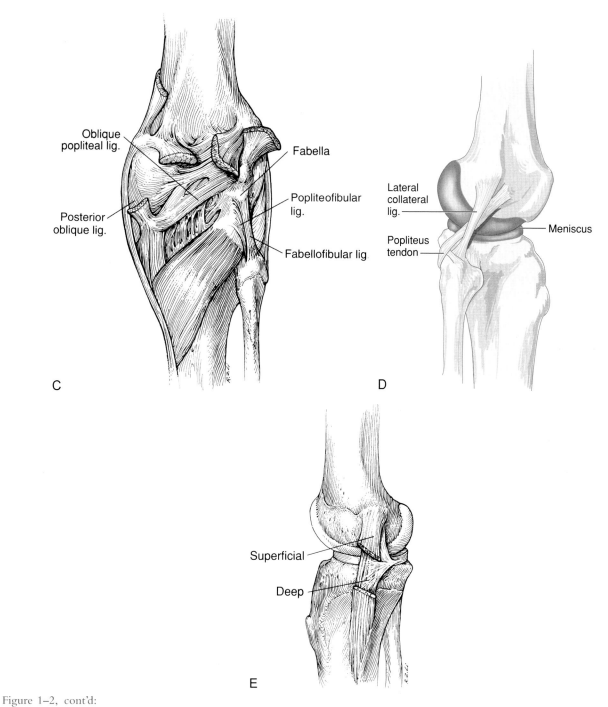

Figure 1–2, cont'd:
C, Posterior view (superficial), **D,** Lateral view, **E,** Medial view. (From Tria AJ Jr, Klein KS: *An illustrated guide to the knee.* New York, 1992, Churchill Livingstone.)

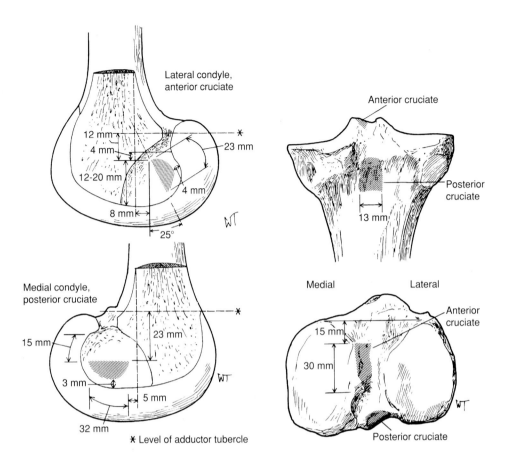

Figure 1–3:
Origins and insertions of the anterior cruciate ligament (ACL) and posterior cruciate ligament (PCL). (From Girgis FJ, Marxhall JL, Al Monajem ARS: *Clin Orthop* 106:216-231, 1975.)

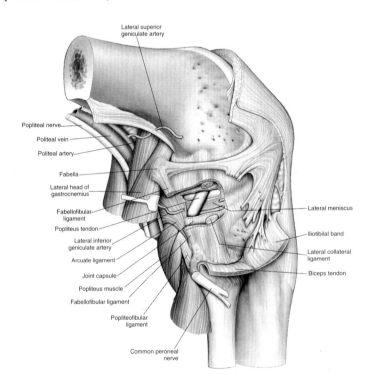

Figure 1–4:
Anatomy of the posterolateral corner of the knee. (From MacGillivray JD, Warren RF: *Op Tech Orthop* 9:309-317, 1999.)

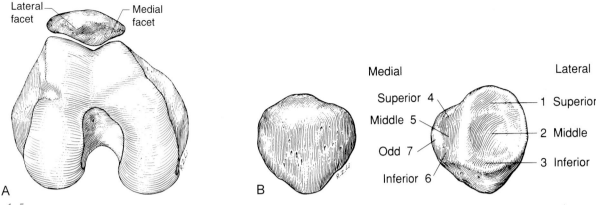

Figure 1–5:

A, Anatomy of the patellofemoral joint. **B,** Anterior and posterior view of the patella. (From Tria AJ Jr, Klein KS: *An illustrated guide to the knee.* New York, 1992, Churchill Livingstone.)

- The articular cartilage covering the patella is the thickest in the body—5-mm thick in some places.
- The patella must withstand forces in excess of three to five times body weight.
- The patella has two main surfaces (facets): a smaller medial and a larger lateral facet.
- The medial patellofemoral ligament (MPFL) is the key restraint to lateral displacement of the patella (Figure 1–7).

Menisci

- Menisci are crescent-shaped fibrocartilage structures that protect the articular surfaces of the knee.
- The menisci are composed of important longitudinal (circumferential) type I collagen fibers and radial (tie) fibers (Figure 1–8).

- Only the peripheral 25% to 30% of the menisci are vascularized (medial and lateral genicular arteries) (Figure 1–9).
- The medial meniscus is more C-shaped and the lateral meniscus is more semicircular (Figure 1–10).
- The medial meniscus has insertions that are much farther apart than the lateral meniscus.
- The posterior horn of the medial meniscus is an important secondary stabilizer to anterior translation of the tibia.
- The lateral meniscus has two times the excursion with knee motion as the medial meniscus.

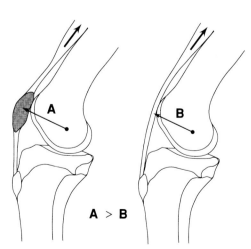

Figure 1–6:

The patella as a fulcrum to improve quadriceps function. (From Tria AJ Jr, Klein KS: *An illustrated guide to the knee.* New York, 1992, Churchill Livingstone.)

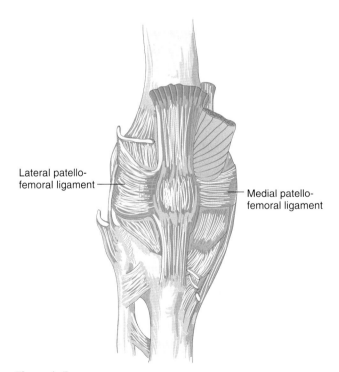

Figure 1–7:

The medial patellofemoral ligament (MPFL) is the primary restraint to lateral displacement of the patella.

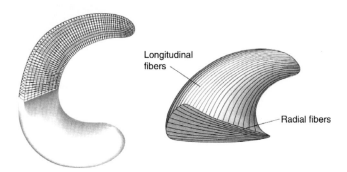

Figure 1–8:
Radial and longitudinal fibers of the menisci. (From Tria AJ Jr, Klein KS: *An illustrated guide to the knee.* New York, 1992, Churchill Livingstone.)

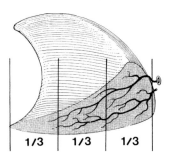

Figure 1–9:
The vascularity of the meniscus. (From Tria AJ Jr, Klein KS: *An illustrated guide to the knee.* New York, 1992, Churchill Livingstone.)

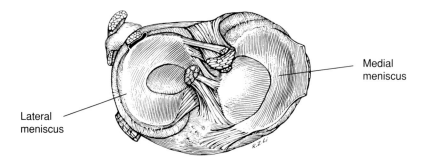

Figure 1–10:
Superior view of a right proximal tibia demonstrating the menisci. (From Tria AJ Jr, Klein KS: *An illustrated guide to the knee.* New York, 1992, Churchill Livingstone.)

References

Berlet GC, Fowler PJ: The anterior horn of the medial meniscus: an anatomic study of its insertion. *Am J Sports Med* 26:540-543, 1998.

This is an anatomic study of cadaveric knees that describes the incidence of four tibial insertion sites for the anterior horn of the medial meniscus. Type I (in the "flat intercondylar region") is found in 59% of knees. Type II ("on the downward slope from the medial articular plateau to the intercondylar region") is found in 24% of cases. Type III (on the anterior slope of the plateau) is found in 15% of knees. Type IV (no attachment) is seen 3% of the time.

Fuss FK: Anatomy of the cruciate ligaments and their function in extension and flexion of the human knee joint. *Am J Anat* 184: 165-176, 1989.

Using cadaver dissection along with radiography, the change in tension of the cruciate ligament can be accurately observed. The author uses the term "guiding bundles" to describe the few fibers of both the anterior and posterior cruciate ligament that remain taut throughout the normal arc of motion. Fibers of the ACL are predominantly taut in extension, whereas the PCL is more taut in extreme flexion.

Fuss FK: Principles and mechanisms of automatic rotation during terminal extension of the human knee joint. *J Anat* 180:297-304, 1992.

The author describes three mechanisms for automatic knee rotation during terminal extension. The first mechanism is oblique torque produced by the taut fibers of the PCL. The second is described as the ACL becoming "too short" as the knee moves into terminal extension. Finally, the third mechanism is the deflection of the medial femoral condyle by the tibial eminence.

Gupte CM, Bull AM, Thomas RD, Amis AA: A review of the function and biomechanics of the meniscofemoral ligaments. *Arthroscopy* 19:161-171, 2003.

An anatomic review of 1022 cadaveric knees shows that 91% had at least one meniscofemoral ligament, 48% had an anterior meniscofemoral ligament, and 70% had a posterior meniscofemoral ligament. Thirty-one percent had both an anterior and posterior meniscofemoral ligament. Theories about the function of these ligaments include a possible role as a secondary stabilizer for the PCL.

Komistek RD, Dennis DA, Mabe JA, Walker SA: An in vivo determination of patellofemoral contact positions. *Clin Biomech* 15:29-36, 2000.

Fluoroscopy and video imaging show that the contact position starts on the inferior aspect of the patella in full extension and progresses superiorly as the knee is actively flexed. In addition, patellar tilt increases with increased knee flexion.

Matsumoto H: Mechanism of the pivot shift. *J Bone Joint Surg Br* 72:816-821, 1990.

Performing pivot shift testing on cadaveric knees shows that sectioning the iliotibial tract in addition to the ACL stopped the pivot shift that is observed when only the ACL was sectioned. The MCL serves as the axis of rotation of the pivot point.

McLeod WD, Moschi A, Andrews JR, Hughston JC: Tibial plateau topography. *Am J Sports Med* 5:13-18, 1977.

Cadaver examination shows that the shape of the tibial plateau plays a significant role in normal knee biomechanics. The shape of the lateral tibial plateau allows for less bony congruency on that side and plays a role in determining the path taken by the lateral femoral condyle during terminal extension.

Shim SS, Leung G: Blood supply of the knee joint: a microangiographic study in children and adults. *Clin Orthop* 208:119-125, 1986.

The anastomosis that supplies the knee joint is formed by the genicular arteries including the superior medial and lateral, middle (posterior), and inferior medial and lateral genicular arteries. The predominant difference between the vascularization of the knee in the child versus the adult is the separation of vessels to supply the epiphyseal plate in children.

Terry GC, LaPrade RF: The posterolateral aspect of the knee: anatomy and surgical approach. *Am J Sports Med* 24:732-739, 1996.

Identification of anatomic structures most at risk during a posterolateral approach to the knee is crucial to a satisfactory outcome. Aside from the neurovascular structures in this area other structures of concern include the iliotibial (IT) band, hamstring tendons, LCL, posterolateral capsule, and popliteus.

Van Dommelen BA, Fowler PJ: Anatomy of the posterior cruciate ligament. *Am J Sports Med* 17:24-29, 1989.

The anatomy of the PCL is important to understand to restore function with reconstruction. The variation of PCL tension from flexion to extension and the close anatomical relationship among the PCL, popliteus, and lateral meniscus are important considerations during reconstruction.

Wretenberg P, Ramsey DK, Nemeth G: Tibiofemoral contact points relative to flexion angle measured with MRI. *Clin Biomech* 17:477-485, 2002.

Three-dimensional measurements of knee flexion using magnetic resonance imaging show that the area of greatest tibiofemoral contact moves anteriorly, superiorly, and laterally as the knee goes into flexion. The greatest amount of displacement occurs in the lateral compartment. Three to five degrees of tibial rotation also occurs as the flexion angle continues.

CHAPTER 2

Knee History, Physical Examination, and Imaging

Knee History

- Age can help narrow the differential diagnosis of knee injuries.
- Young patients, especially adolescent females, with atraumatic symptoms commonly complain of anterior knee pain.
- Older patients may present with degenerative arthritis or meniscal tears without history of trauma.
- A well-documented history can often direct the diagnosis (Box 2–1).
- Anterior cruciate ligament (ACL) tear—traumatic episode, significant swelling, twisting injury, associated noncontact injury with "pop," feeling of "giving way."
- Ligamentous injuries or meniscal tears (in younger patients) usually require a significant traumatic episode.
- History of significant swelling within several hours of injury suggests an ACL tear, osteochondral or intraarticular fracture, extensor mechanism rupture, or a patellar dislocation.
- Twisting injuries or noncontact pivoting injuries with a "pop" and immediate swelling are suggestive of ACL tear.
- Dashboard injuries or direct posterior directed blows to the anterior tibia are suggestive of posterior cruciate ligament (PCL) tears.
- Mechanical symptoms, reported pain on the medial or lateral knee, delayed swelling, and locking or catching symptoms of the knee are suggestive of meniscal tears or loose bodies.
- Patients complaining of symptoms of "giving way" should be carefully questioned to elucidate the exact meaning of this phrase—often, this complaint does not represent true knee instability but rather quadriceps inhibition or patellar instability.
- Symptoms of "giving way," typically associated with ACL tears, may also be found in patients with patellar subluxation or dislocation or chondral flap tears.

- Pain without an associated traumatic injury often suggests overuse injuries such as tendinitis/tendinosis or lateral patellar compression syndrome and not ligament or meniscal tears (except in older patients).
- Injuries with the knee in varus, hyperextension, and tibia in external rotation may result in posterolateral corner pathology.
- Multiple ligament injuries are most commonly associated with high-impact trauma such as motor vehicle accidents.
- Determining what previous treatment has been received (including previous surgery) may help narrow down the differential diagnosis and guide further treatment.

Box 2–1 History and Likely Associated Pathology

- Anterior knee pain—tendinitis, extensor mechanism injury, bipartite patella, patellofemoral syndrome
- Medial knee pain—medial collateral ligament (MCL) or meniscal injury, arthritis, pes anserinus
- Lateral knee pain—lateral meniscus injury, iliotibial band syndrome, arthritis
- Posterior knee pain—posterolateral corner (PLC) or meniscal injury
- Acute swelling—anterior cruciate ligament (ACL) tear, acute peripheral meniscal tear, intraarticular fracture, patellar dislocation, extensor mechanism disruption.
- Noncontact injury with "pop"—ACL tear, patellar dislocation
- Contact injury with "pop"—collateral ligament, meniscal tear, fracture
- Twisting injury—ACL or meniscal tear
- Locking, pain with squatting—meniscal tear
- "Giving way," "buckling"—ACL tear, patellar instability, extensor mechanism weakness or disruption
- Dashboard injury—posterior cruciate ligament (PCL) tear, patellar injury
- Pain after sitting or when climbing stairs—patellofemoral pathology
- Stiffness—arthritis, traumatic effusion

Physical Examination

- Physical examination findings can assist in defining possible underlying pathology (Table 2–1).
- Observation—gross swelling or deformity may suggest a significant traumatic event resulting in multiple ligament injuries and/or fractures. An assessment of standing alignment (varus/valgus) is also important (Figure 2–1).
- Gait—a varus dynamic thrust or standing alignment suggests posterolateral corner injuries; walking with a bent-knee gait may suggest a flexion contracture (Figure 2–2).
- Pes planus can be associated with chronic anterior knee pain.
- Painful squatting at the joint line may indicate meniscal pathology (Figure 2–3).

- Range of motion is determined and compared with the contralateral normal knee (normal 0 to 135 degrees ±5 degrees) (Figure 2–4).
- Active extension is always tested to verify an intact extensor mechanism (quad or patellar tendon rupture) or an extension lag.
- Meniscal injury is determined by a number of clinical tests including an evaluation of medial or lateral joint line tenderness (Figure 2–5A and B); the presence of a small effusion; pain with squatting or duck walking on the medial or lateral compartment; a positive Apley grind test; and a positive McMurray's test, which involves pain or a palpable click on the affected compartment joint line with knee flexion while rotating the tibia internally and externally and applying a valgus and varus stress (Figure 2–5C and D).

Table 2–1: Physical Examination Assessment and Associated Pathology

EXAMINATION	METHOD	SIGNIFICANCE
Standing/gait	Observe gait	Based on pathology
Deformity	Observe patient standing	Based on pathology
Effusion	Patella: ballot/milk	Ligament/meniscus injury (acute), arthritis (chronic)
Point of maximum tenderness	Palpate for tenderness	Based on location (joint line tenderness = meniscus tear)
Range of motion	Active and passive	Block = meniscus injury (bucket handle), loose body; ACL tear impinging
Patella crepitus	With passive ROM	Patellofemoral pathology
Patella grind	Push patella with quadriceps contraction	Patellofemoral pathology
Patella apprehension	Push patella lat. at 20–30° flexion	Patella subluxation/dislocation
Q angle	ASIS-patella-tibial tubercle	Increased with patella malalignment
Flexion Q angle	ASIS-patella-tibial tubercle	Increased with patella malalignment
J sign	Lateral deviation of the patella in extension	
Ext rotation recurvatum	Pick up great toes; knee-varus and hyperextension	
Patella tilt	Tilt up laterally	>15° = Lax <0° = tight lateral constraint
Patella glide	Like apprehension	>50° = Incr. medical const laxity
Active glide	Lat. excursion with quad, contraction	Lat. > prox. excursion = incr. functional Q angle quadriceps
Quadriceps circumference	10 cm (VMO), 15 cm (quad.)	Atrophy from inactivity
Symmetric extension	Back of knee from ground or prone heel height difference	Contracture, displaced meniscal tear, or other mechanical block
Varus/valgus stress	30°	MCL/LCL laxity (grade I-III)
Varus/valgus stress	0°	MCL/LCL and PCL
Apley's	Prone-flexion compression	DJD, meniscal pathology
Lachman	Tibia forward at 30° flexion	ACL injury (most sensitive)
Finacetto	Lachman with tibia subluxing beyond post. horns of menisci	ACL injury (severe)
Ant. drawer	Tibia forward at 90° flexion	ACL injury
Int. rotation drawer	Foot int. rotated with drawer	Tighter = (normal), looser = ACL injury
Ext. rotation drawer	Foot ext. rotation with drawer	Loose (normal), looser = ACL/MCL injury
Pivot shift	Flexion with int. rotation and valgus	ACL injury (EUA)
Pivot jerk	Extension with int. rotation and valgus	ACL injury (EUA)
Posterior drawer	Tibia backward at 90° flexion	PCL Injury
Tibia sag.	Flex 90° observe	PCL
90° quad. act	Extend flexed knee	PCL
Asymmetric external rotation	"Dial" feet externally at 30° and 90° flexion	Asymmetric increased external rotation > 10°-15° = posterolateral corner (PLC) injury. If asymmetric at both 30° and 90° = PCL + PLC
Ext. rotation recurvatum	Pick up great toes	PLC injury
Reversed pivot	Extension with ext. rotation and valgus	PLC injury
Posterolateral drawer	Post, drawer, lat. > med.	PLC injury

From Miller MD: *Review of orthopaedics*, 4th ed. Philadelphia, 2004, Saunders.

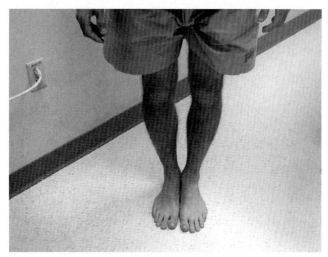

Figure 2–1:
Assessment of standing alignment. This patient has bilateral genu varus.

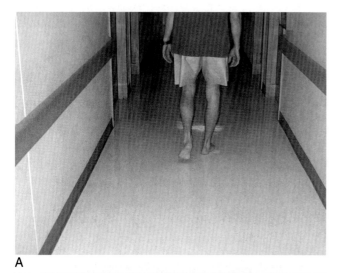

A

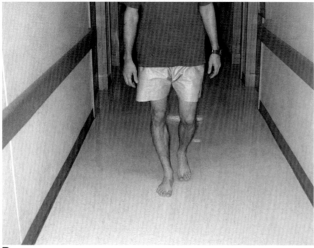

B

Figure 2–2:
Gait assessment from the back (A) and front (B). This is useful for diagnosing dynamic instability patterns such as a varus thrust or antalgic, painful gait patterns.

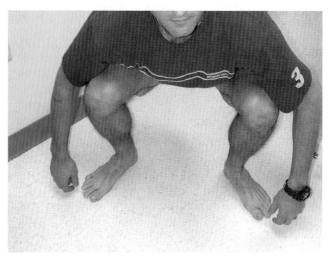

Figure 2–3:
Squatting can elicit painful medial or lateral joint line pain from a meniscus tear or anterior pain from chronic patellofemoral chondrosis.

- Swelling is differentiated between intraarticular swelling (intraarticular pathology present) or soft tissue swelling (medial collateral ligament [MCL] or posterolateral injury) (Figure 2–6).
- The physical examination should be performed in a systemic, familiar manner to ensure a complete evaluation in a timely fashion and supplemented with special tests according to the history and differential diagnosis.
- Patellofemoral examination includes an assessment of alignment, patellar tilts (Figure 2–7A), the presence of patellofemoral crepitation with range of motion and grind test, presence of patellar apprehension (Figure 2–7B) or subluxation, medial and lateral glides (Figure 2–7C), and medial or lateral patellar facet tenderness.
- Pain at the inferior pole of the patella with the knee in extension that improves in flexion is suggestive of patellar tendinosis.
- Quadriceps (Q) angle is the angle between the anterior superior iliac spine, the patella, and the tibial tubercle with the patient in the supine position—an angle of 10 to 15 degrees for males and 15 to 18 degrees for females is generally considered normal. Abnormal angles imply an increase in the lateral force imposed by the quadriceps, which can result in lateral subluxation of the patella. Quadriceps angle can also be measured with the knee flexed at 90 degrees. Angles greater than 8 to 10 degrees are considered abnormal.
- Assessment of patellar tracking during knee extension may reveal a J sign—this is the patella subluxating laterally out of the femoral trochlea as the knee is extended.
- Ligamentous testing involves an assessment of the integrity of the ACL, PCL, MCL, lateral collateral ligament (LCL), and posterolateral corner (PLC) of the knee. This may be difficult to perform in the acute setting and can be delayed until the pain is better controlled.

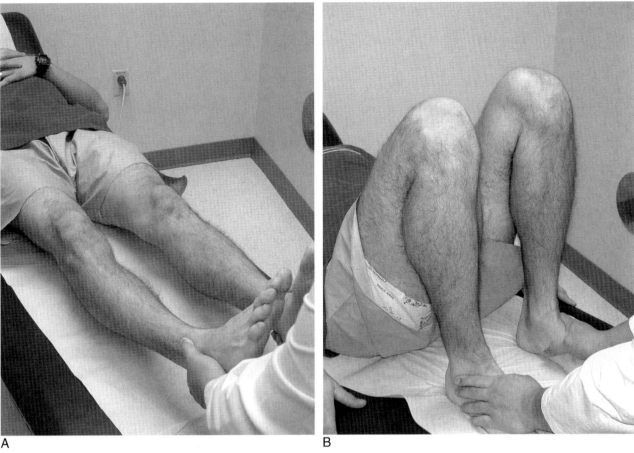

Figure 2–4:
A and **B,** Range of motion is assessed and compared with the contralateral normal extremity to be used as a control.

- Anterior drawer testing is performed with the knee in 70 to 90 degrees of flexion and an anteriorly directed force on the tibia—in general, with ACL injuries, the anterior drawer exhibits less anterior translation than the Lachman's test because of the stabilizing effect of the iliotibial band and the posterior horn of the medial meniscus (Figure 2–8*A*).
- Lachman's test is the most sensitive and specific test for ACL deficiency and involves anteriorly translating the tibia with the femur stabilized at approximately 20 to 30 degrees of flexion—this is compared with the contralateral normal knee (Figure 2–8*B*).
  - Grading is determined as follows according to the International Knee Documentation Committee: normal or grade 0: 0 to 3 mm of translation, grade I: 3 to 5 mm, grade II: 5 to 10 mm, and grade III: greater than 10 mm.
- The pivot shift test is performed with the knee placed in internal rotation, valgus, and an axial-directed load with the knee in full extension (anterior translated) (Figure 2–8*C*). When the knee is carefully flexed to 20 to 30 degrees, the tibia, which is anteriorly translated, suddenly reduces posteriorly (secondary to the pull of the iliotibial band), giving the sensation of a pivot or shift. This test is

very specific but less sensitive for ACL tears and is difficult to perform in the acute injury setting. This test is best appreciated under anesthesia.
- The pivot jerk test is performed similar to the pivot shift except the knee is extended from a flexed position, observing for subluxation of the tibia anteriorly.
- Posterior drawer testing evaluates (and is the most sensitive test) for PCL injury—this is determined by the anterior medial tibial stepoff (approximately 10 mm with intact PCL) in reference to the medial femoral condyle with the knee in 90 degrees of flexion. This is compared with the contralateral knee.
  - A slight decrease in the stepoff but not flush with the medial femoral condyle is a grade I injury (approximately 3 to 5 mm), flush with the medial femoral condyle is grade II (5 to 10 mm), and behind the medial femoral condyle is grade III (greater than 10 mm).
- In chronic PCL injury, the tibia sags posteriorly, so care must be taken to reduce the tibia anteriorly to a normal tibial stepoff before determining the degree of posterior translation. This posterior sag sign is used to diagnose PCL (and PLC) injuries and is best appreciated by

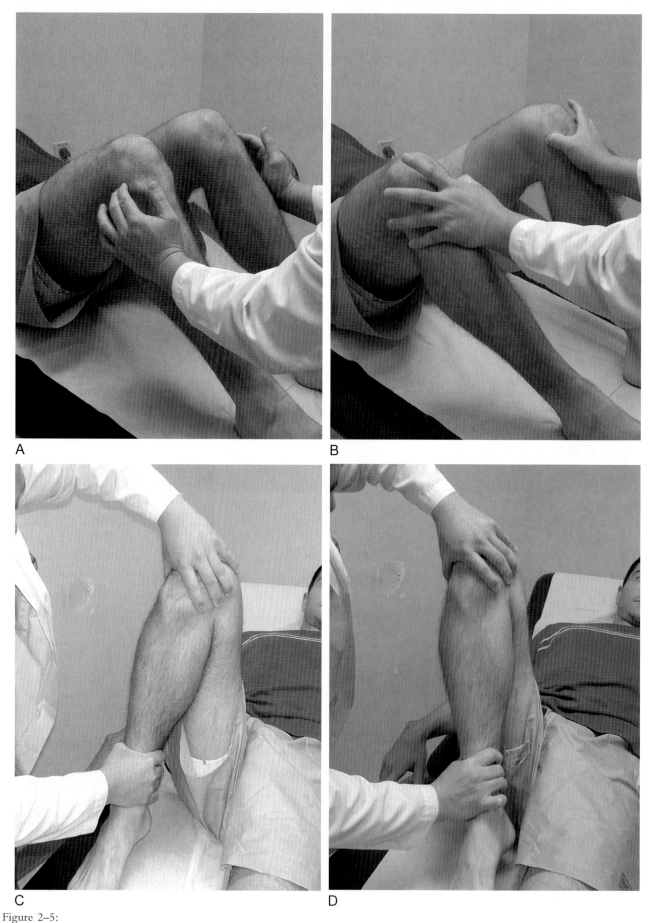

Figure 2–5:
Lateral **(A)** and medial **(B)** joint line tenderness is determined with the knees in 90 degrees of flexion and compared with the contralateral normal knee. **C** and **D,** McMurray's testing is determined with hyperflexion of the knee and internally and externally rotating the tibia on the femur. Pain with a palpable catch along the joint line is considered a positive sign.

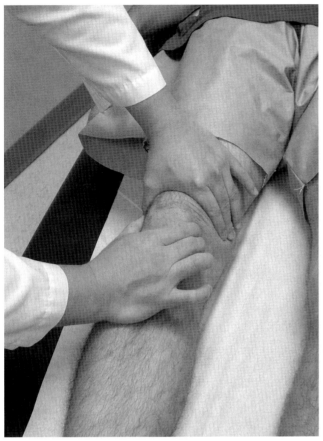

Figure 2–6:
Assessment of an intraarticular effusion. The left hand milks the suprapatellar pouch distally and the right hand palpates the medial and lateral parapatellar gutter to assess for an effusion.

looking at the leg from the side with the hip and knee flexed to 90 degrees (Figure 2–8D).

- Because of the posterior sag that is commonly involved with PCL injuries, the quadriceps active test must first be performed between 70 and 90 degrees of flexion to "reduce" the tibia anteriorly to a normal stepoff. Once reduced, the posterior stress can be applied and measurement made of posterior translation.
- KT-1000 or KT-2000 arthrometry can also be used for PCL injuries but is more difficult.
- MCL injury is determined with medial joint opening with a valgus force applied with the knee tested at 0 and 30 degrees. Opening at 30 degrees may suggest an MCL injury, whereas opening at 0 degrees may suggest a combined MCL/bicruciate ligament injury.
- LCL injury is determined with lateral joint opening with a varus force applied with the knee tested at 0 and 30 degrees. Opening at 30 degrees may suggest an LCL injury, whereas opening at 0 degrees may suggest a combined LCL/bicruciate ligament injury.
- Testing of the MCL and LCL can be graded similar to other ligaments with grade I (1 to 5 mm) denoting a minimal tear, grade II (6 to 10 mm) associated with

a moderate tear, and grade III (greater than 10 mm) suggesting a complete tear of the collateral ligament.
- PLC injuries are evaluated with a number of tests, including an evaluation of injuries to the LCL.
- The external rotation dial test, performed in either the supine or prone position (preferred), is tested at 30 (Figure 2–8F) and 90 degrees (Figure 2–8G) and compared with the contralateral knee. Increases in external rotation as little as 10 degrees can be significant. Increases at 30 degrees that improve at 90 degrees suggest involvement of the posterolateral corner, whereas increases at 90 degrees with improvement at 30 degrees suggest involvement of the PCL. Increases at both 30 and 90 degrees suggest a combined PCL and PLC injury.
- The external rotation recurvatum test is performed by lifting both extremities by the feet. An appreciation of varus angulation, hyperextension, and external rotation of the tibia of the affected limb in comparison with the normal contralateral leg suggests injury to the PLC.
- The reverse pivot shift test is performed with the knee in 20 to 30 degrees of flexion, external rotation, valgus, and an axial load (posterolaterally displaced). As the knee is extended, the tibia suddenly reduces anteriorly and is felt as a pivot or shift. This test, when positive, signals a posterolateral corner injury, although it is not very specific.
- A dynamic varus thrust or lateral thrust during gait assessment is pathognomic for a PLC injury.
- Instrumented arthrometer testing with a KT-1000 or KT-2000 (Medmetric Corporation, San Diego, CA) provides an objective measure of anterior translation in millimeters and can be compared with the contralateral knee (Figure 2–8H).

Imaging

- Plain radiographs should be obtained for all knee complaints as a basic screening tool.
- A standard four-view series should include an anteroposterior (AP), 45-degree flexion weight-bearing posteroanterior (PA), lateral, and patellar views.
- AP views may reveal several characteristic radiographic changes associated with underlying pathology (Figure 2–9 and Table 2–2).
  - Fairbank changes defined by squaring of the condyle, joint space narrowing, and ridging are suggestive of degenerative changes postmeniscectomy.
  - A Segund fracture is characterized by an avulsion fracture of the proximal lateral tibia and is often associated with an ACL tear.
  - The Pellegrini-Stieda lesion demonstrates calcification of the MCL, usually near the femoral insertion site, and is consistent with chronic injury to the ligament.
- The 45-degree flexion weight-bearing view allows the best evaluation of the posterior condyles and can

Text continued on p. 18

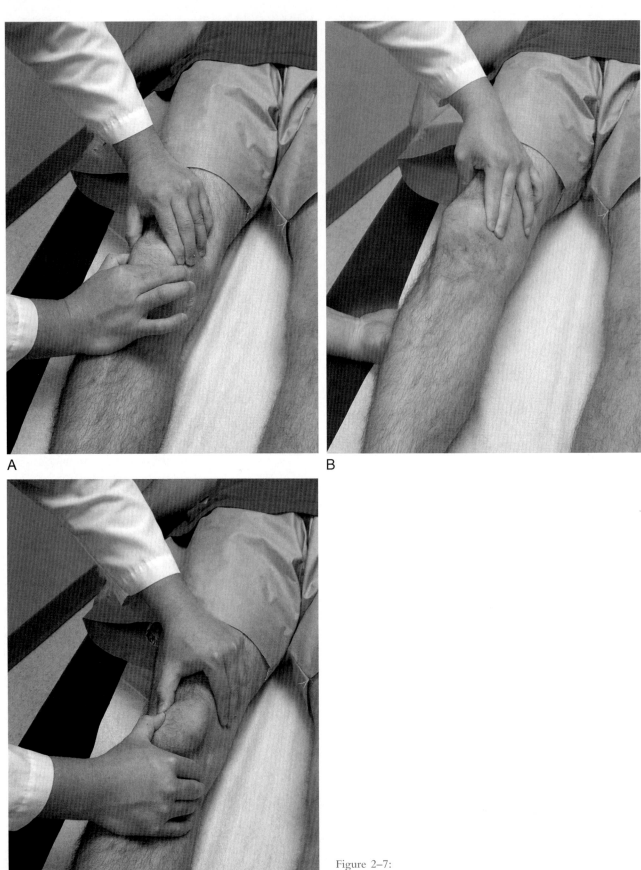

Figure 2–7:
Patellofemoral examination. **A,** Patellar tilt is determined.
B, Lateral patellar apprehension is testing with the knee in
30 degrees of flexion. **C,** Medial and lateral patellar glide
testing.

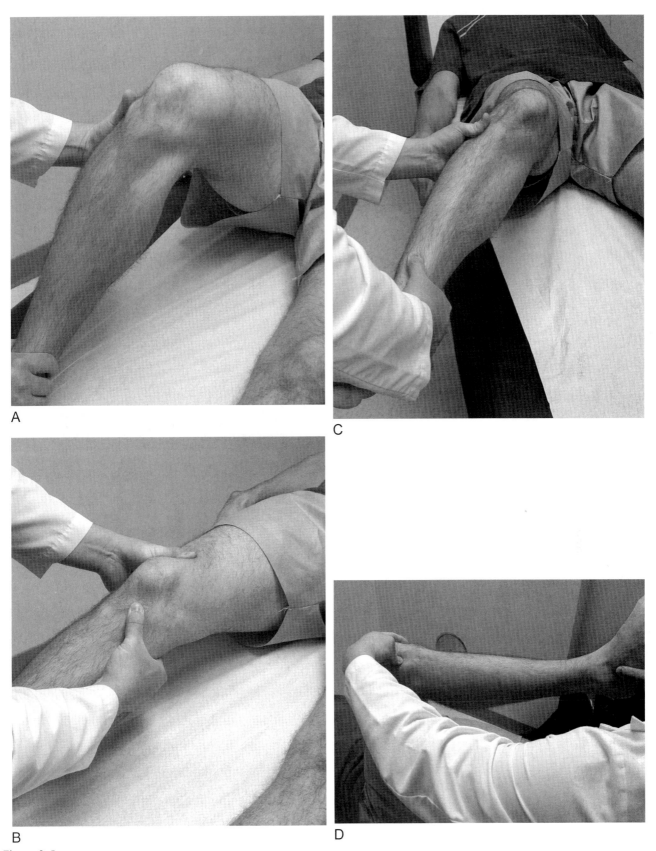

Figure 2–8:

Knee ligament testing. **A,** Anterior drawer testing with the knee in 90 degrees of flexion. **B,** Lachman's testing with the knee in 30 degrees of flexion. **C,** Pivot shift testing. **D,** Posterior sag.

(continued)

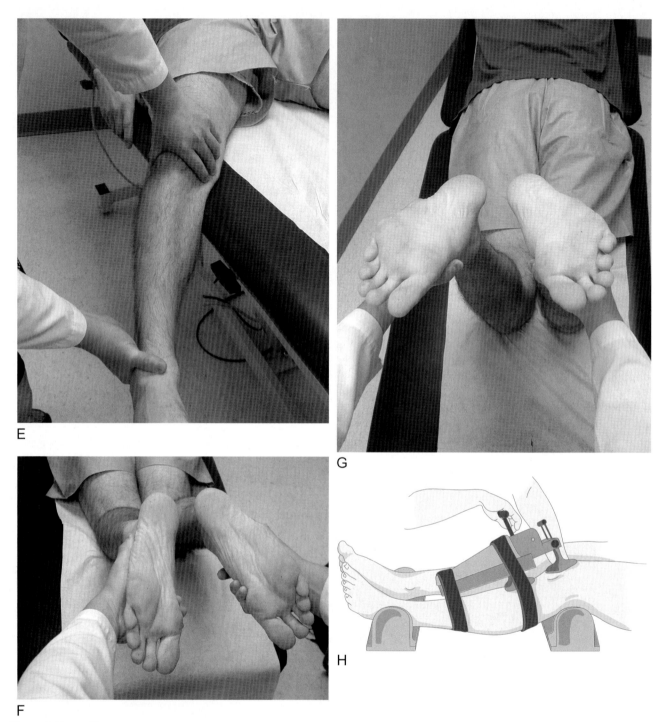

Figure 2–8, cont'd:

E, Varus/valgus testing with the knee in 30 degrees of flexion. Prone external rotation testing at 30 **(F)** and 90 degrees. **(G). H,** Instrument testing of the anterior cruciate ligament (ACL) using the KT-1000 arthrometer. (H from Daniels DM, Stone ML: KT-1000 anterior-posterior displacement measurements. In Daniels DM, Akeson WY, O'Connor JJ, editors: *Knee ligaments: structure, function, injury, and repair.* New York, 1990, Raven Press.)

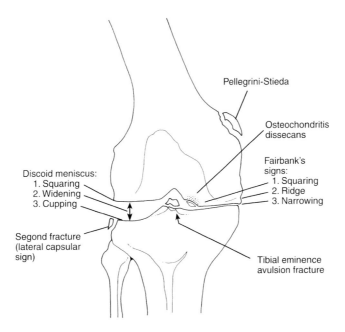

Figure 2–9:
Schematic of an anteroposterior (AP) radiograph showing various characteristic findings of diagnostic importance. (From Brinker MR, Miller MD: *Fundamentals of orthopaedics.* Philadelphia, 1999, Saunders; Maseur MD: *Primary care orthopaedics.* Philadelphia, 1996, Saunders.)

Table 2–2:   Radiographic Findings and Associated Pathology

VIEW/SIGN	FINDING	SIGNIFICANCE
Lateral-high patella	Patella alta	Patellofemoral pathology
Congruence angle	$\mu = -6°$ $SD = 11°$	Patellofemoral pathology
Tooth sign	Irregular ant patella	Patellofemoral chondrosis
Varus/valgus stress view	Opening	Collateral ligament injury; Salter-Harris fracture
Lateral capsule (Segund) sign	Small tibial avulsion off lateral tibia	ACL tear
Pellegrini-Stieda lesion	Med. femoral condyle avulsion	Chronic MCL injury
Lateral stress view—Stress to anterior tibia with knee 70° flexed	Asymmetric posterior tibial displacement	PCL injury
PA flexion weight-bearing		Early DJD, OCD, notch evaluation
Fairbank's changes	Square condyle, peak eminences, ridging, narrowing	*Early DJD* (postmeniscectomy)
Square lateral condyle	Thick joint space	Discoid meniscus
Arthrogram	Dye outline	Meniscal tear
MRI	Intraarticular path	Specific for lesion
Bone scan		Stress fractures, early DJD, RSD
CT		Tibial plateau fractures, patellar tilt

From Miller MD: *Review of orthopaedics*, 4th ed. Philadelphia, 2004, Saunders.

reveal joint space narrowing when AP views are normal. It can also serve as a notch view and identify loose bodies, osteochondritis dissecans, osteonecrosis, and osteoarthritis.

- Lateral views are useful in calculating several patellar height measurements (Figure 2–10).
  - Blumensaat line—a line drawn anteriorly extending from the superior aspect of the intercondylar notch with the knee flexed at 30 degrees. Normally, the inferior pole of the patella should sit on the line.
  - Insall-Salvati index—the ratio of patella tendon length to patella length is normally 1.0. Patella alta and baja are considered when the ratio is greater than 1.2 or less than 0.8, respectively.
  - Blackburne-Peel index—ratio of the distance from the tibial plateau to the inferior articular surface of the patella to the length of the articular surface of the patella (determined arbitrarily) is normally 0.8. An index greater than 1 may suggest patella alta.
- Patellar views include the Merchant, Sunrise, and Laurin views, which are tangential views of the patella at various degrees of knee flexion. These views allow an assessment of patellar subluxation, joint space narrowing, osteochondral injuries, and patellar tilt.
- Several angle measurements are available to assess patellar alignment, subluxation, and dislocation using the Merchant view (Figure 2–11).
  - Sulcus angle—angle produced by drawing lines from the deepest section of the intercondylar sulcus to the highest points of the lateral and medial femoral condyles. Angles above the normal range (126 to 150 degrees) suggest patellar subluxation or dislocation.
  - Congruence angle—angle formed by a line drawn from the apex of the sulcus angle through the lowest ridge of the patella and a line that bisects the sulcus angle. Angles greater than 15 degrees are considered abnormal.
  - Laurin's angle—angle constructed from a line drawn from the medial and femoral condyles and a line running parallel to the lateral surface of the patella. Recurrent subluxation of the patella is considered when the lines are parallel or the angle opens up medially.

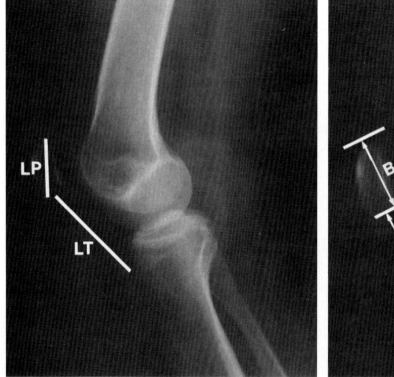
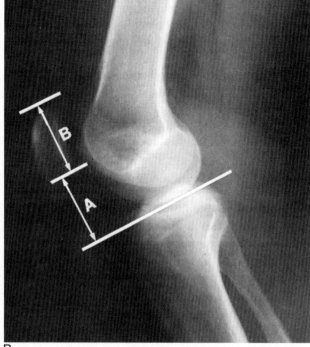

A   B

Figure 2–10:

Radiographic evaluation of patellar height. A, Insall-Salvati index: the normal ratio of patella tendon length (LT) to patella length (LP) is 1. An index greater than 1.2 or less than 0.8 is consistent with patella alta or baja, respectively. **B,** Blackburne-Peel index: The normal ratio of the distance from the tibial plateau to the inferior articular surface of the patella *(A)* to the length of the patella articular surface *(B)* is 0.8. An index greater than 1 is consistent with patella alta. (From DeLee JC, Drez D Jr, Miller MD, editors: *DeLee and Drez's orthopaedic sports medicine: principles and practice,* 2nd ed. Philadelphia, 2003, Saunders.)

- AP internal and external rotation views can be helpful for tibial plateau fractures.
- Long cassette lower extremity views from hip to ankle allow an assessment of lower extremity alignment and are crucial determining factors in cases of knee realignment procedures such as a high tibial osteotomy. One line is drawn from the center of the femoral head to the center of the ankle joint, and where the line passes through the tibial plateau is where the weight-bearing center is for that knee. This is always compared with the contralateral lower extremity. A second line is drawn from the center of the femoral head to the center of the distal femur, and a third line is drawn from the center of the femur to the center of the ankle. The angle between the second and third lines is the mechanical alignment angle. This angle is in varus if the weight-bearing line passes medial to the center of the tibia or is in valgus if the line passes lateral to the center of the tibia (Figure 2–12).
- Stress radiography is an objective means to determine the amount of posterior tibial translation in response to a 20-pound posterior tibial load compared with the contralateral knee (Figure 2–13). This may be more sensitive than KT-1000 or KT-2000 arthrometry, which tends to underrepresent the degree of posterior laxity.

- Stress views may also be helpful in demonstrating occult physeal injuries.
- Technetium-99m bone scanning can be helpful to evaluate stress fractures and increased overload suggestive of early arthritis and pain. This is particularly useful in chronic PCL injuries to determine if the patellofemoral and/or medial compartments have increased signal or in meniscal deficiency to evaluate whether transplantation may be indicated.
- Computed tomography (CT) scanning is particularly useful when the bony architecture needs particular scrutiny. It is recommended for evaluation of tibial plateau fractures and certain osteochondral injuries or osteochondritis desiccans and assessment of patellar tracking.
- Magnetic resonance imaging (MRI) is an extremely useful tool for evaluating soft tissue injuries to the knee joint including the ACL, PCL, MCL, LCL, menisci, and chondral surfaces of the knee.
- A grading system to describe meniscal changes on MRI has been devised, but only grade III lesions, which demonstrate extension to the articular surface, truly represent meniscal tears (Figure 2–14).
- MRI is also useful for looking at bone bruise patterns (which, before MRI, were undiagnosed),

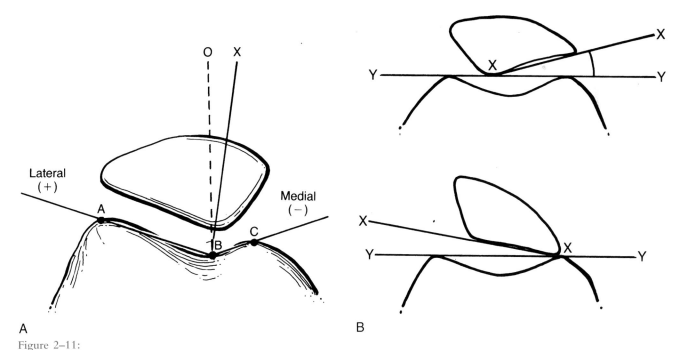

A

B

Figure 2–11:

Radiographic evaluation of patellar alignment: **A,** Using the Merchant view, line BO intersects the angle ABC (sulcus angle). Line BX passes through the lowest point on the median ridge of the patella. Angle OBX is known as the congruence angle. When BX falls medial to the line BO, the angle is expressed in negative degrees (normal values are approximately −6 degrees in males and −10 in females). When line BX falls lateral to line BO, the angle is a positive value. **B,** Laurin's angle is formed by line YY drawn across the anterior portions of the femoral condyles and line XX that follows the edge of the posterior edge of the lateral facet. Parallel lines or an angle that opens medially are considered abnormal. (From DeLee JC, Drez D Jr, Miller MD, editors: *DeLee and Drez's orthopaedic sports medicine: principles and practice,* 2nd ed. Philadelphia, 2003, Saunders.)

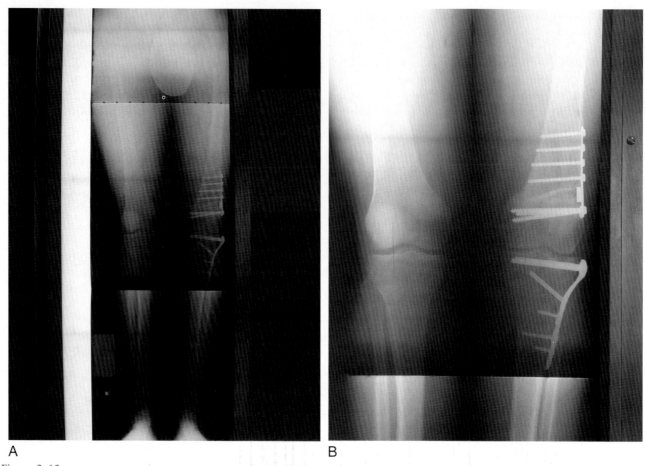

A   B

Figure 2–12:
Long leg alignment assessment. **A,** Long leg alignment films from center of the femoral head to the center portion of the tibiotalar joint. **B,** Close-up showing the right leg in valgus and the left leg in varus after undergoing a distal femoral opening wedge osteotomy to correct valgus malalignment from posttraumatic arthritis of the lateral knee compartment following a plateau fracture.

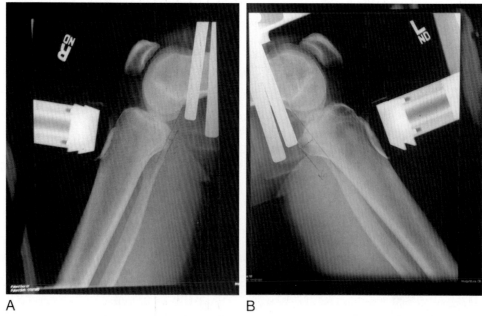

A   B

Figure 2–13:
Stress radiography for posterior cruciate ligament (PCL) insufficiency. **A,** Normal PCL with mild posterior tibial dropback following a 20-Newton stress. **B,** Grade III PCL injury with 16 mm of posterior tibial dropback following a 20-Newton stress.

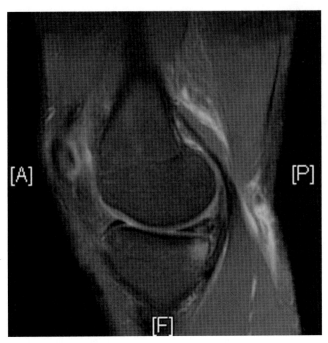

Figure 2–14:
Magnetic resonance imaging (MRI) of the medial meniscus with grade III signal representing a meniscus tear.

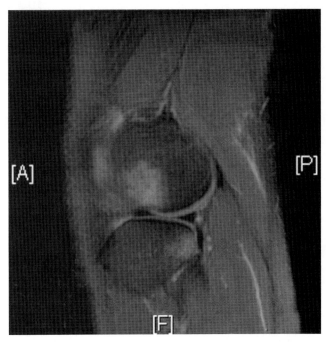

Figure 2–15:
Magnetic resonance imaging (MRI) of the lateral knee compartment in a patient with an anterior cruciate ligament (ACL) tear. Note the classic bone bruises seen in this injury.

osteonecrosis, occult fractures, and stress fractures (Figure 2–15).

- Ultrasonography is a tool more commonly used in Europe for the diagnosis of knee injuries, but a few centers have had success in the United States. Indications are few but include soft tissue masses and evaluation of popliteal cysts and PLC injuries.

References

Baugher WH, White GM: Primary evaluation and management of knee injuries. *Emerg Med Clin North Am* 2:347-359, 1984.
> *Authors review important anatomic structures about the knee and a general approach to evaluate patients with knee injury. Authors define and stress a systematic approach to the physical examination with key points, beginning with an assessment of the patient's overall condition. An algorithm for the initial evaluation and treatment of knee injuries is provided.*

Eren OT: The accuracy of joint line tenderness by physical examination in the diagnosis of meniscal tears. *Arthroscopy* 19:850-854, 2003.
> *Prospective cohort study using 104 young male patients with suspected meniscal lesions. Accuracy of medial or lateral joint line tenderness on examination was evaluated with final arthroscopic diagnosis. Of 54 knees suspected with medial meniscal tears, 32 were confirmed at arthroscopy. Lateral meniscal tears were suspected in 27 patients and confirmed by arthroscopy in 25 cases. Five medial and two lateral meniscal tears were identified at arthroscopy that were not suspected on examination. Results demonstrated greater accuracy (96% vs. 74%), sensitivity (92% vs. 86%), and specificity (97% vs. 67%) of joint line tenderness as a test for lateral meniscal tears compared with medial meniscal tears.*

Hak DJ, Gautsch TL: A review of radiographic lines and angles used in orthopedics. *Am J Orthop* 24:590-601, 1995.
> *Review of commonly used radiographic lines and angles in orthopaedic evaluations with their associated methods and significance.*

Hoppenfeld S: Physical examination of the knee. In *Physical examination of the spine and extremities*. Norwalk, CT, 1976, Appleton & Lange.
> *Thorough step-by-step physical examination about the knee is described with several illustrations and discussions of findings.*

Malanga GA, Andrus S, Nadler SF, McLean J: Physical examination of the knee: a review of the original test description and scientific validity of common orthopedic tests. *Arch Phys Med Rehabil* 84:592-603, 2003.
> *Comprehensive description and review of orthopaedic physical examination tests and maneuvers, including referenced sensitivities and specificities from literature review.*

Ritchie JR, Miller MD, Harner CD: History and physical evaluation. In Fu FH, Harner CD, Vince KG, editors: *Knee surgery*. Baltimore, 1994, Willams & Wilkins.
> *Comprehensive review of the history and physical examination of the knee. Discussion primarily focuses on ligament, meniscal and extensor mechanism injuries, and knee instability and associated findings during evaluation.*

Stabler A, Glaser C, Reiser M: Musculoskeletal MR: knee. *Eur Radiol* 10:230-241, 2000.
> *Describes MRI techniques, use, signs, and pitfalls for several common knee pathologic conditions.*

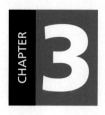

CHAPTER 3

Knee Arthroscopy

Indications

- Knee arthroscopy is an essential part of a variety of orthopaedic procedures.
- Arthroscopic partial meniscectomy is the most common procedure in orthopaedic surgery.
- In addition to meniscal surgery, arthroscopy is used for articular cartilage surgery, ligament reconstruction, synovectomy, loose body removal, and a variety of other procedures.

Arthroscopic Essentials (Figure 3–1)

- The arthroscope is an elongated lens that is attached to a camera.
  - A variety of lens angles are available.
  - For routine arthroscopy, a 30-degree angled arthroscope is used.
  - A 70-degree scope is helpful for viewing the posterior aspect of the knee.
- A variety of probes and instruments are used during arthroscopy (Figure 3–2).
  - These include hand-operated (probes, grabbers, baskets, etc.) and motorized instruments (shavers, burrs, etc.).
  - There are a variety of sizes, shapes, and designs for many of these instruments, and it is often a matter of experience in choosing appropriate instruments for any given task.
  - In general, baskets are chosen based on the ease of perpendicular access and shavers are chosen based on the task at hand—larger, more aggressive shavers are used for bigger tasks (synovectomy, debridement, etc.) and smaller shavers are used in tighter spaces (medial and lateral compartments).
- Specialized instruments continue to be developed for many common procedures.
  - These include guides, tools, and implants.
  - It is imperative that the surgeon stay educated on the proper use of these implants and devices to include their efficacy and complications.

- Irrigation systems allow control of arthroscopic fluid pressure during a case.
  - This has significant advantages in controlling hemostasis (Figure 3–3).
  - The use of fluid also aids in flushing debris and distending the joint capsule.
  - The judicious use of epinephrine to arthroscopic fluids can also be advantageous in maintaining hemostasis.
- Documentation of pathology and treatment can be accomplished with carefully planned arthroscopic still images and selected video segments.
  - Many systems create digital images that can be printed and saved on CDs and computer hard drives.
  - These images are helpful in documentation, clinical follow-up, and patient/surgeon education.

Positioning and Portal Placement

- Knee arthroscopy is typically accomplished with the patient in a supine position (Figure 3–4).
  - A post can be placed on the bed to stabilize the thigh when placing a valgus force on the knee to evaluate the medial compartment.
  - Alternatively, the surgical leg can be placed in an arthroscopic leg-holder, the foot of the bed can be dropped, and the leg can hang free.
  - Typically, the nonoperative leg is placed in a well-padded leg-holder.
- The two main portals are the (anterior) inferolateral (viewing) portal and the (anterior) inferomedial (instrument) portal (Figure 3–5).
- Superior portals can be used for inflow or outflow, but most modern pump systems are used without an outflow.
- Additional portals have been described and can be used for select indications.
- An accessory posteromedial portal is established with the scope in the back of the knee looking anterolaterally.
  - A spinal needle is used to localize this portal from outside-in prior to placing it.
  - Care is taken not to lacerate the saphenous vein or nerve, which is in this area.

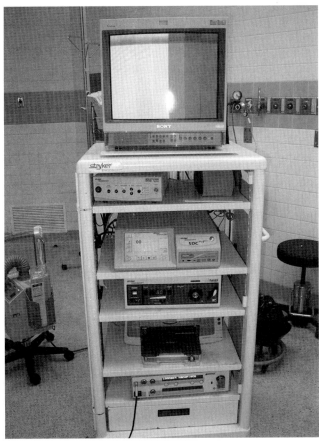

Figure 3–1:
Arthroscopy tower.

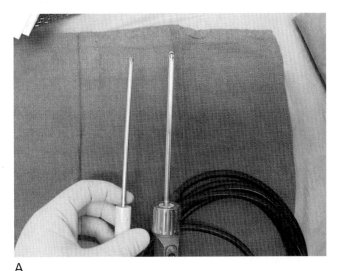

A

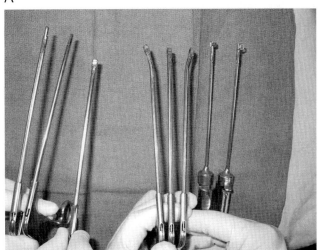

B

Figure 3–2:
A, Arthroscopic shavers. **B,** Arthroscopic baskets.

- The "nick and spread" method (a small skin incision is made and a hemostat is used to spread the tissues) can be applied to reduce the risk of neurovascular injury.
- An accessory posterolateral portal is used even less commonly but is helpful in cases that require a complete synovectomy or for removing posterolateral loose bodies.
  - The key to this portal is to make sure it is behind the lateral collateral ligament but in front of the biceps tendon (to protect the common peroneal nerve).
- A far-proximal portal (superomedial or superolateral) is used for evaluation of patellar tracking, and it is also established with the help of a spinal needle.

Diagnostic Arthroscopy

- A systematic, thorough evaluation of the knee joint includes completely visualizing the suprapatellar pouch; patellofemoral joint; medial and lateral gutters; intercondylar notch; medial and lateral compartments; and, when indicated, the posteromedial (and posterolateral) aspects of the knee (Figure 3–6).
- The knee is repositioned and stressed to allow the most beneficial access to each compartment.

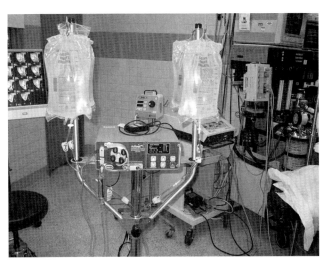

Figure 3–3:
Irrigation setup for knee arthroscopy.

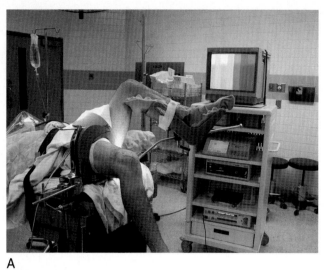

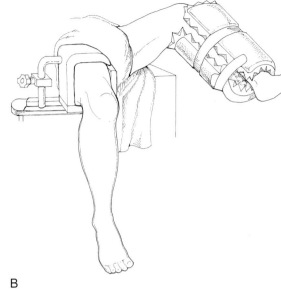

A   B

Figure 3–4:

A, General setup for knee arthroscopy. **B,** Patient setup for arthroscopy using standard leg-holder and padding the opposite leg in a second leg-holder. (**B** from Miller MD, Howard RF, Plancher KD: *Surgical atlas of sports medicine.* Philadelphia, 2003, WB Saunders.)

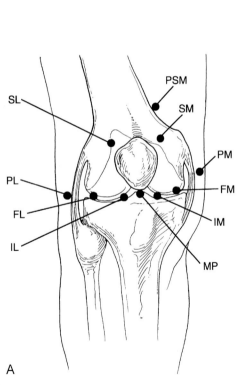

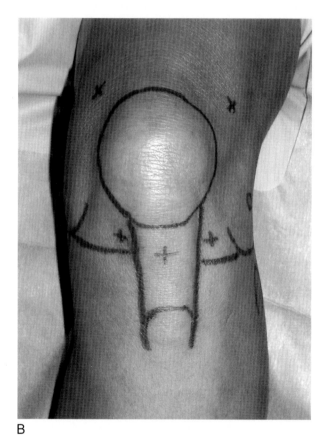

A   B

Figure 3–5:

A, Commonly used portals for knee arthroscopy. Arthroscopic portals. PSM, proximal superomedial (used to evaluate patellar tracking); SM, superomedial (optional inflow/outflow portal); PM, posteromedial (used to evaluate the posterior horn of the medial meniscus); FM, far medial (rarely used for perpendicular access to articular cartilage or menisci); IM, inferomedial (instrument portal); MP, midpatellar (used for instrumentation and traction during removal of large meniscal fragments); IL, inferolateral (primary viewing portal); FL, far lateral; PL, posterolateral (rarely used during complete synovectomy or loose body removal); SL, superolateral (alternative inflow/outflow portal). **B,** The approach to knee arthroscopy indicating sites of placement of the anteromedial, anterolateral, superomedial, superolateral, and transpatellar portals. (**A** from Miller MD, Osborne JR, Warner JJP, Fu FH, editors: *MRI-arthroscopy correlative atlas.* Philadelphia, 1997, WB Saunders; **B** from Ong BC, Shen FH, Musahl V, et al: Knee: patient positioning, portal placement, and normal arthroscopic anatomy. In Miller MD, Cole BC, editors: *Textbook of arthroscopy.* Philadelphia, 2004, WB Saunders.)

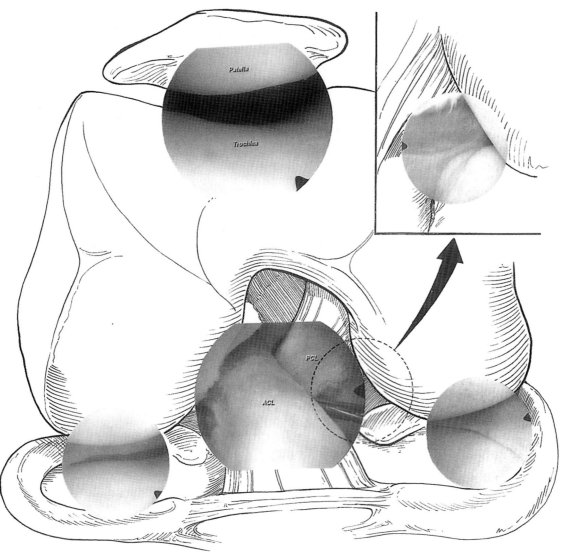

Figure 3–6:
Normal arthroscopic anatomy. Inset shows posteromedial aspect of the knee as seen through the intercondylar notch. (From Miller MD, Osborne JR, Warner JJP, Fu FH: *MRI-arthroscopy correlative atlas.* Philadelphia, 1997, WB Saunders.)

- The arthroscopic canula is introduced into the knee using a blunt obturator.
- It is often necessary to remove at least some synovium and fat pad in the front of the knee to access all areas. The suprapatellar pouch and gutters are examined with the knee in extension.
- The knee is then flexed to evaluate the intercondylar notch.
- Valgus stress is applied to the knee to access the medial compartment.
- Varus stress, or a "figure-4" position, is used to visualize the lateral compartment.
- When entering the lateral compartment, it is helpful to place the arthroscope in the intercondylar notch immediately adjacent to the lateral joint and then sweep the scope centrally and then into the lateral compartment (Figure 3–7).
- The probe allows the surgeon to "palpate" all surfaces.
- A complete examination of both menisci (posterior horn, body, and anterior horn; peripheral, middle, and central portions) and all articular surfaces is accomplished.
- Any abnormalities are quantified; documented; and, when appropriate, surgically addressed.

Complications

- Although the reported overall complication rate for knee arthroscopy is less than 2%, the incidence of "minor" complications (especially iatrogenic chondral injury) is probably much higher. This can be greatly reduced by

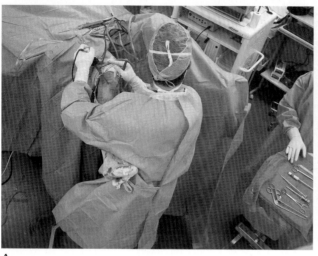
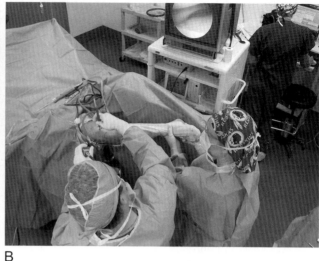

A

B

Figure 3–7:

Knee positioning for looking at medial and lateral compartments during arthroscopy. **A,** Valgus force is applied to allow easier visualization of the medial compartment. **B,** Figure-4 position is used to allow easier visualization of the lateral compartment.

Box 3–1	Complications Associated with Knee Arthroscopy

Postoperative hemarthrosis
Infection
Arthrofibrosis
Deep vein thrombosis
Anesthetic complications
Instrument failure
Complex regional pain syndrome
Iatrogenic injury (cartilage, ligaments, fracture)
Neurologic injury

From Ong BC, Shen FH, Musahl V, Fu F, Diduch DR: Knee: Patient positioning, portal placement, and normal arthroscopic anatomy. In Miller MD, Cole BC, editors: *Textbook of arthroscopy.* Philadelphia, 2004, WB Saunders.

gently introducing instruments into the joint and with experience.

• Complications include, but are not limited to, those presented in Box 3–1.

References

Bennett WF, Sisto D: Arthroscopic lateral portals revisited: a cadaveric study of the safe zones. *Am J Orthop* 24:546-551, 1995.

This is a cadaveric study in which the authors define five anatomic zones for lateral knee portal placement and discuss the anatomic structures at risk within these areas. Zone E is considered unsafe because it contains the long head of the biceps femoris and the peroneal nerve. Placement of the lateral portal at 90 degrees of flexion allows easier trocar insertion between the biceps femoris and the lateral collateral ligament.

Diduch DR, Shen FH, Ong BC, et al: Knee: diagnostic arthroscopy. In Miller MD, Cole BJ, editors: *Textbook of arthroscopy.* Philadelphia, 2004, WB Saunders.

This provides an overview of knee anatomy as seen during diagnostic arthroscopy. Descriptions in this text include patient positioning, portal placement, normal anatomy, and pathologic variants.

Kim TK, Savino RM, McFarland EG, Cosgarea AJ: Neurovascular complications of knee arthroscopy. *Am J Sports Med* 30:619-629, 2002.

This article provides an overview of neurovascular injury associated with knee arthroscopy. These injuries can be devastating after knee arthroscopy and can be prevented by understanding the anatomy and planning the procedure carefully. If a neurovascular injury does occur, it is important to recognize it early to initiate immediate treatment and/or referral for care.

Miller MD: Knee arthroscopy. In Miller MD, Osborne JR, Warner JJP, Fu FH, editors: *MRI-arthroscopy correlative atlas.* Philadelphia, 1997, WB Saunders.

This chapter provides a well-illustrated, diagrammatic approach to knee arthroscopy. Magnetic resonance imaging correlation of various knee disorders is a hallmark of this textbook.

Small NC: Complications of arthroscopic surgery performed by experienced arthroscopists. *Arthroscopy* 4:215-219, 1988.

This article reports a series of 8000 arthroscopic knee procedures done by experienced arthroscopists. Their overall complication rate was 1.68%. This number is probably lower than the actual incidence because of errors in self-reporting and higher rates expected with less-experienced arthroscopists.

Stetson WB, Templin K: Two-versus three-portal technique for routine knee arthroscopy. *Am J Sports Med* 30:108-111, 2002.

By studying 16 patients randomized into two- versus three-portal groups for routine knee arthroscopy, these authors find that patients who receive only two portals have a faster recovery time. The fact that this technique avoids injury to the vastus medialis muscle is the reason for this result.

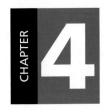

Meniscal Pathology

Introduction

- Menisci serve an important role in load sharing, shock absorption, stability, and lubrication of the knee joint.
- Incidents of meniscal tears have been reported at 60 to 70 per 100,000.
- Meniscal tears comprise approximately 50% of surgical knee injuries.
- Males are three times more likely to suffer from meniscal tears than females.
- Medial meniscal tears are three times more common than lateral meniscal tears.
- Anterior cruciate ligament (ACL) disruption is the most common associated injury with meniscal tears, occurring in up to one third of cases.
- The lateral meniscus is more likely to be injured during acute ACL tears, whereas medial meniscal tears are more frequently seen in chronic ACL-deficient knees.
- Peripheral tears, which are amenable to repair, are more frequently seen in traumatic injuries, especially when associated with ACL tears.
- Most tears affect the posterior half of the meniscus.

History, Physical Examination, and Imaging

- Diagnosis of meniscal tears can be derived from careful clinical evaluation (Box 4–1).
- Young patients require a traumatic event to tear a meniscus, whereas patients older than 40 years often develop degenerative tears without a history of significant trauma.
- History often consists of swelling, medial or lateral compartmental pain, locking, catching, decreased range of motion, and pain with squatting.
- Peripheral tears frequently present with acute swelling. In contrast, central and degenerative tears may demonstrate delayed or recurrent effusions, respectively.
- Physical examination findings consistent with a meniscal tear include mild swelling, pain with squatting, medial or lateral joint line tenderness, and a positive McMurray's sign and Apley's grind test.
- Concomitant ACL injury may reduce the accuracy of physical examination findings for meniscal tears.
- Occasionally, if there is a meniscal cyst associated with the meniscal tear, there is fullness of the corresponding medial or lateral joint line.
- Plain radiographs should be obtained and are usually normal; in cases of degenerative meniscal tears in older patients, there may be evidence of joint space narrowing, particularly on 45-degree flexion weight-bearing views, which can better visualize early changes.
- Magnetic resonance imaging (MRI) is highly sensitive and specific for meniscal tears if grade III changes are present and can complement clinical evaluation (Figure 4–1). The study can also assist with describing the location of the tear and identifying or confirming other injuries including chondral injuries, bone bruises, and associated ligament tears.
- MRI is less helpful in patients older than 60 years or with significant degenerative changes because they commonly demonstrate some meniscal abnormalities.
- Arthroscopy is the gold standard for definitive diagnosis and allows for immediate treatment of meniscal pathology (Figure 4–2).

Box 4–1	Symptoms and Clinical Findings Consistent with Meniscal Injury

Symptoms

Acute, delayed, or recurrent swelling
Medial or lateral compartment pain
Pain with squatting
Locking, limited range of motion (particularly extension)

Clinical Findings

Medial or lateral joint line tenderness
Positive McMurray's sign or Apley's grind test
Swelling

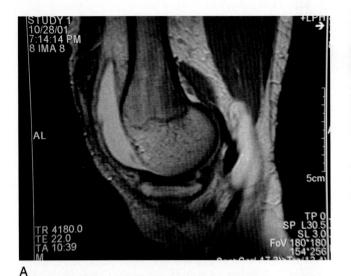

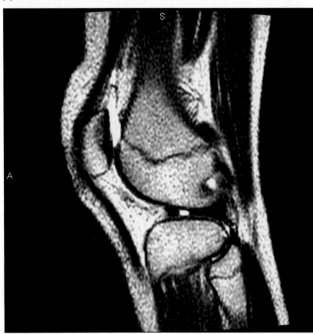

Figure 4–1:
Magnetic resonance imaging with a grade III (A) posterior horn and (B) radial meniscal tear.

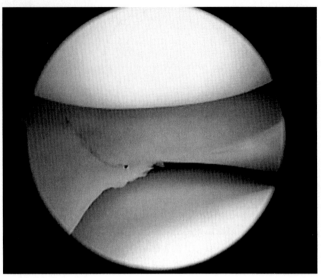

Figure 4–2:
Arthroscopy demonstrating a radial meniscal tear.

Types of Meniscal Tears

- Tears can be classified according to location and orientation/appearance (Figure 4–3A-E).
- Peripheral tears (red-red tears) have a superior blood supply and are therefore most amenable to surgical repair.
- Tears at the junction of the peripheral and middle thirds of the meniscus (red-white tears) have a moderate blood supply and, depending on the orientation and appearance, can also be repaired.

- Central tears occurring in the inner third of the meniscus (white-white tears) have the poorest blood supply and are usually not repairable.
- The orientation/appearance of tears can be described as longitudinal, horizontal, radial, oblique, degenerative, or any of the common haracteristically described tears.
- Bucket handle tears usually start at the posterior horn and can involve more than 50% of the meniscal length and often produce mechanical symptoms.
- Meniscal cysts are usually associated with lateral meniscus horizontal cleavage tears (Figure 4–4).
- Popliteal or Baker's cysts are more common forms of meniscal cysts, usually associated with degenerative medial meniscus tears. They are usually located in the popliteal fossa originating from the posteromedial joint line between the semimembranosus tendon and the medial head of the gastrocnemius. Resolution often occurs after partial meniscectomy of the tear with or without decompression of the cyst arthroscopically.
- Discoid menisci can be classified according to three types: type I—complete; type II—incomplete; type III—Wrisberg variant (deficiency of posterior horn meniscal tibial ligament) (Figure 4–5).
  - Type III discoid menisci have no attachment to the posterior tibia. Having an abnormal attachment to the medial femoral condyle by the Wrisberg ligament can make it unstable and vulnerable to displacement (into the intercondylar notch) with knee extension.
  - Diagnosis of discoid menisci can be made by MRI with three or more 5-mm sagittal images with meniscal continuity between anterior and posterior horns.

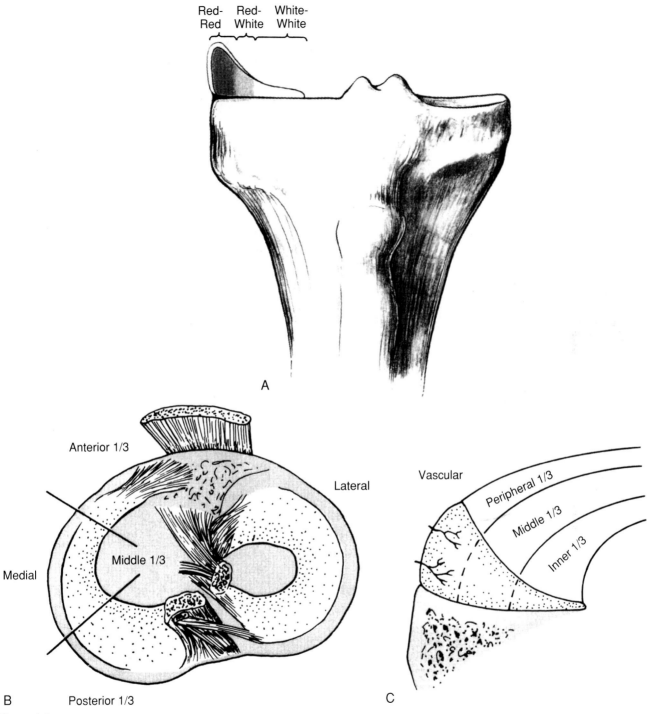

Figure 4–3:
Classification of meniscal tears according to location (**A–C**).

(*continued*)

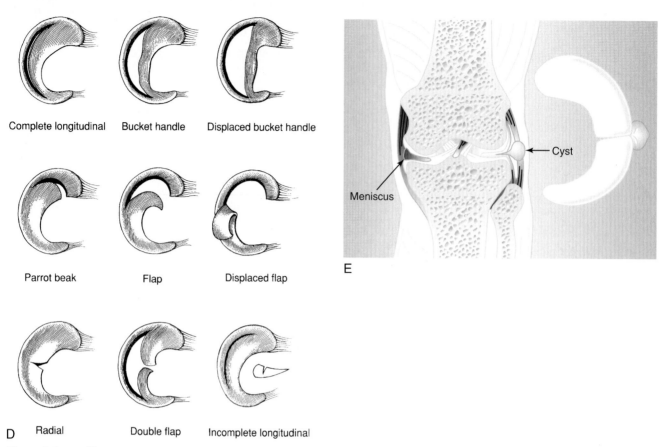

Complete longitudinal   Bucket handle   Displaced bucket handle

Parrot beak   Flap   Displaced flap

D   Radial   Double flap   Incomplete longitudinal

E   Cyst

Meniscus

Figure 4–3, cont'd:
Classification of meniscal tears according to orientation or characteristic appearance **(D-E).** (**A** from Miller MD, Warner JJP, Harner CD: Meniscal repair. In Fu FH, Harner CD, Vince KG, editors: *Knee surgery.* Baltimore, 1994, Williams & Wilkins; **B** and **C** from Siliski JM, Leffers D: Dislocations and soft tissue injuries of the knee. In Brown BD, Jupiter JB, Levine AM, Trafton PG, editors: *Skeletal trauma,* 2nd ed. Philadelphia, 1998, WB Saunders; **D** from Tria AJ Jr, Klein KS: *An illustrated guide to the knee.* New York, 1992, Churchill Livingstone; **E** from Safran M, Stone DA, Zachezewski J: *Instructions to sports medicine patients.* Philadelphia, 2002, WB Saunders.)

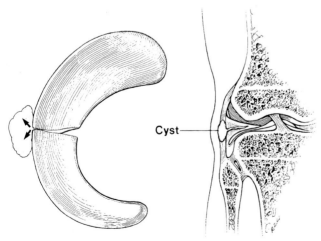

Cyst

Figure 4–4:
Meniscal cyst. (From Tria AJ Jr, Klein KS: *An illustrated guide to the knee.* New York, 1992, Churchill Livingstone.)

Treatment

- Options for treatment of meniscal tears include conservative therapy, arthroscopic partial meniscectomy, and meniscus repair.
- Age, occupation, activity level, and symptoms should all be considered during surgical evaluation. Young athletes and laborers who cannot afford loss of normal knee function may necessitate a more expedient course of treatment. However, meniscus preservation is usually the best course of treatment whenever feasible.
- Mechanically locked knees usually require prompt surgical treatment.
- Given the well-known progressive degenerative changes following complete or subtotal meniscectomy, meniscal tears are repaired whenever possible, and, if irreparable, only unstable and symptomatic portions of the meniscus tear are removed while preserving as much

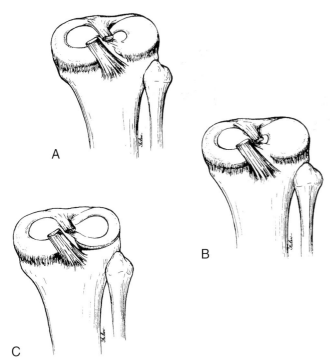

A

B

C

Figure 4–5:
Classification of discoid menisci. A, Type I (complete). B, Type II (incomplete). C, Type III (Wrisberg variant).
(From Neuschwander DC: Discoid lateral meniscus. In Fu FH, Harner CD, Vince KG, editors: *Knee surgery.* Baltimore, 1994, Williams & Wilkins.)

viable tissue as possible to limit loss of its mechanical properties.

- Bucket handle tears may be easier to resect by initially removing its posterior attachment, leaving the resection of the anterior horn until the end of the procedure to prevent displacement of the fragment into the posterior compartment (Figure 4–6).
- Short (<5 to 10 mm), stable (<3 mm displacement) tears can be managed by initial observation followed by surgery if symptoms persist.
- During arthroscopy, it is critical that the entire meniscus be probed for proper evaluation of all present tears to define their location and guide treatment.
- Incomplete longitudinal tears are usually stable and can be rasped to improve the chance for healing without the need for repair.
- Partial meniscectomy back to a stable, healthy rim can be performed with the use of basket forceps and shavers.
- Amount of meniscus removed should be well documented to assist with postoperative evaluation, complications, changes, and prognosis.
- Any tear's healing capacity can be improved by placing a fibrin clot into the repair site (Figure 4–7). A fibrin clot is sterile blood harvested and placed in a glass beaker with a

glass rod stirrer. This enhances the clotting ability of the blood. The clot has growth factors within its substance that have been shown in animal models to improve healing rates.

- Risk of progressive degenerative changes is proportional to the amount of meniscus removed.
- Meniscal cysts usually resolve with treatment of the meniscal pathology, occasionally requiring arthroscopic cyst decompression through the cyst (Figure 4–8).
- Treatment of discoid meniscus includes saucerization (if torn), repair of detachments (Wrisberg variant), or observation if asymptomatic (Figure 4–9).

Techniques for Repair

- Best performed in peripheral vertical tears in the red-red or red-white zone.
- Complete longitudinal, bucket handle, and displaced bucket handle tears of the meniscus can usually be repaired depending on the chronicity of the tear.
- Some patterns of meniscal tears are generally not repairable (Box 4–2).
- Improved healing has been observed with concomitant ACL reconstruction or the use of fibrin clots.
- Surgical repair can be performed inside-out, outside-in, open, all inside, and with the use of devices such as arrows or other peripheral fixation devices, determined by surgical preference and experience (Figures 4–10 to 4–14).
- All damaged menisci should be properly prepared ("freshened") with raspers and shavers prior to definitive repair.
- Open repairs are generally limited to tears involving the extreme periphery of the meniscus.
- Vertical mattress sutures are the strongest biomechanical configuration for meniscal repair.
- Arthroscopically placed inside-out vertical mattress sutures are still considered the gold standard for meniscus repair.

Meniscectomized Knee

- Knee realignment procedures including high tibial osteotomy and distal femoral osteotomy are considered in select, young patients with asymmetrical alignment and focal compartment degeneration.
- Meniscal allograft transplantation, a technically difficult procedure, is gaining popularity but is controversial as further investigation continues (with few long-term studies in the literature).
- Meniscal transplantation may be indicated in combined ACL and medial meniscus deficiency with significant anteromedial rotatory instability or in a young patient with symptomatic meniscus deficiency despite extensive

Text continued on p. 37

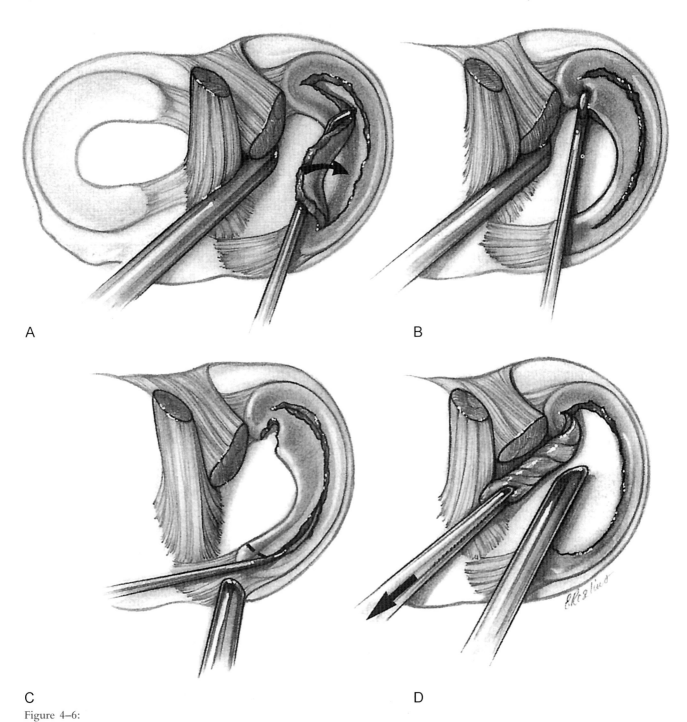

A

B

C

D

Figure 4–6:
Procedure for resection of bucket handle tears. **A,** The displaced fragment is repositioned back to its normal location. **B,** A biter is used to nearly transect its posterior attachment. **C,** Next, the anterior attachment is resected with a biter or knife. **D,** The fragment is then grasped, avulsed from its posterior attachment, and removed. (From Scott N: *The knee.* St Louis, 1994, Mosby-Year Book.)

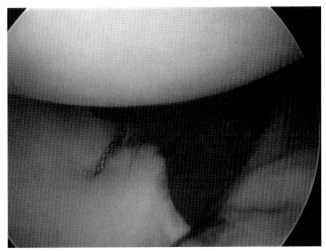

Figure 4–7:
Fibrin clot utilized in a meniscal repair.

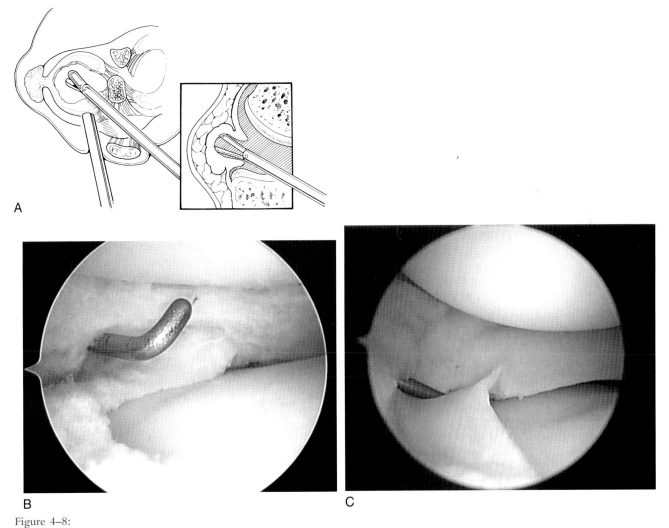

Figure 4–8:
A, Partial meniscectomy and cyst decompression through the tear. **B,** Decompression of cyst through a horizontal cleavage tear.
C, Decompression of a meniscal cyst through a radial tear. Note the spinal needle passed from outside in through the tear.
(A from Parisien JS: *Clin Orthop* 257:154-158, 1990.)

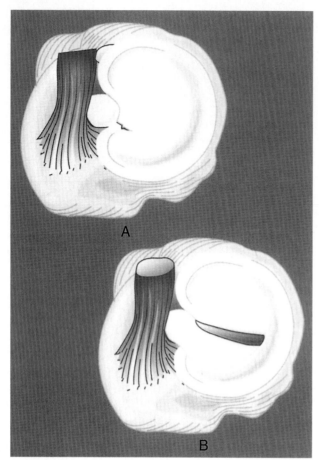

Figure 4–9:
Saucerization of a discoid menisci. **A,** The tear is extended to approximately 1 cm from the peripheral margin. **B,** The meniscus is then contoured anteriorly and posteriorly to approximate a normal-sized meniscus. (From Scott N: *The knee.* St Louis, 1994, Mosby-Year Book.)

Box 4–2	Patterns of Tears Generally Not Amenable to Repair

Parrot beak
Flap
Displaced flap
Radial
Double flap
Horizontal cleavage tear

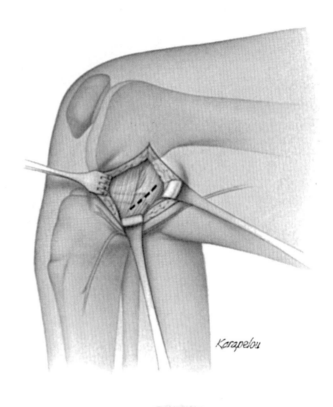

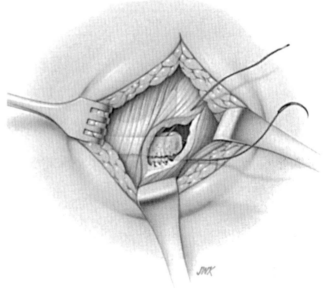

Figure 4–10:
Open meniscal repair. (From Miller MD: *Op Tech Orthop* 5(1):70-71, 1995.)

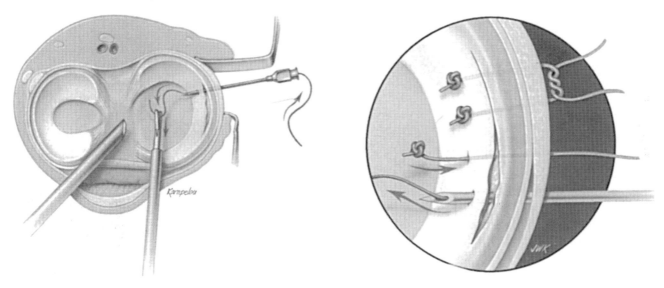

Figure 4–11:
Outside-in meniscal repair. (From Miller MD: *Op Tech Orthop* 5(1):70-71, 1995.)

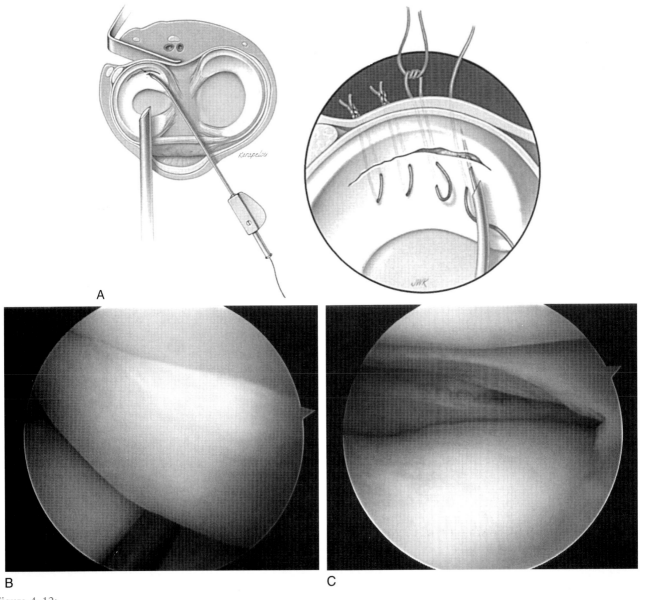

A

B

C

Figure 4–12:
A, Inside-out meniscal repair. **B,** Bucket-handle lateral meniscus tear displaced into the notch. **C,** Reduced bucket-handle tear.

(continued)

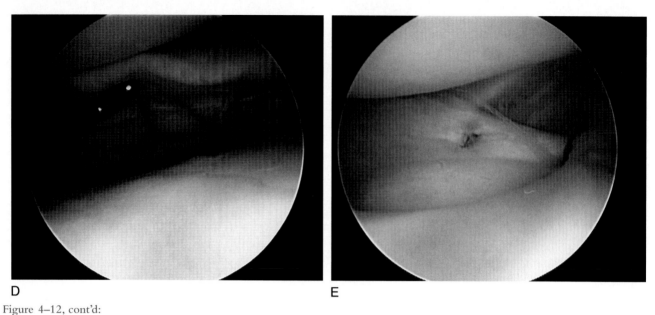

D   E

Figure 4–12, cont'd:
D, Arthroscopically placed inside-out vertical mattress sutures on the inferior surface of the tear. **E,** Corresponding superior inside-out vertical mattress sutures. (A from Miller MD: *Op Tech Orthop* 5(1):70-71, 1995.)

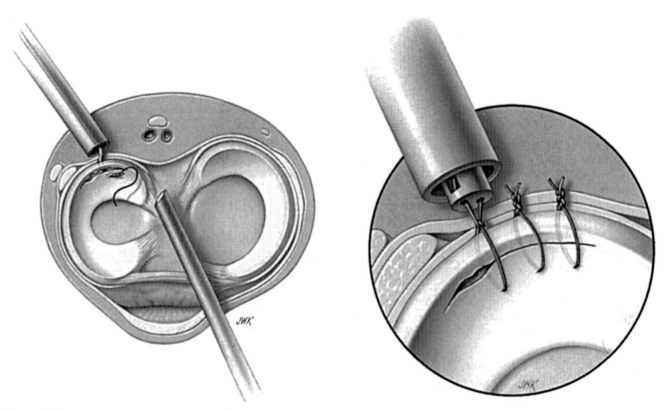

Figure 4–13:
All inside meniscal repair. (From Miller MD: *Op Tech Orthop* 5(1):70-71, 1995.)

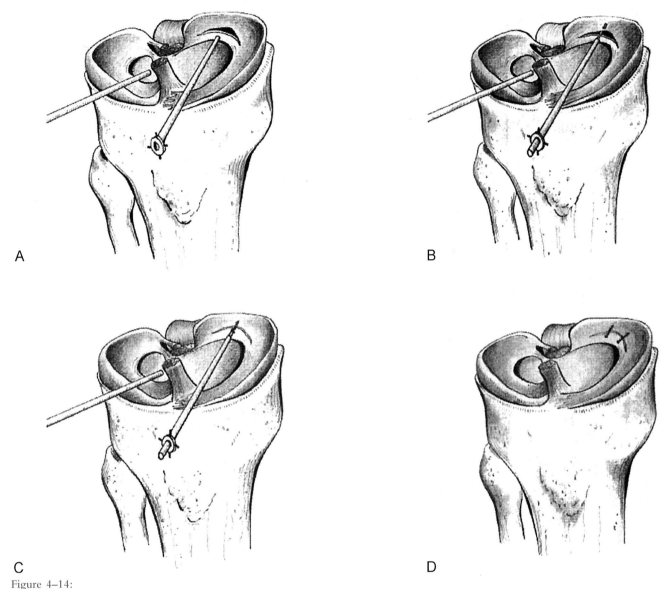

A

B

C

D

Figure 4–14:
Meniscal arrow repair. **A,** Cannula delivery. **B,** Perforator placed across tear. **C,** Arrow delivery across tear. **D,** Reduced tear. (From Miller MD, Cole BJ, editors: *Textbook of arthroscopy.* Philadelphia, 2004, Saunders.)

conservative measures and meniscectomy who have normal alignment and low-grade chondrosis.

- Several graft options are available including fresh-frozen, freeze-dried (lyophilized), and cryopreserved. Although future studies are still pending, deep-frozen allografts currently appear to be the best option.
- Standards for graft sizing have not been established but can be performed using plain radiographs, computed tomography (CT), or MRI.
- Generally, bone blocks are used for lateral meniscus allografts and bone plugs for medial meniscal allografts (Figures 4–15 and 4–16).
- Attachment of the allograft requires a good understanding of normal anatomic meniscal insertion sites (Figure 4–17).

Rehabilitation

- Variable from surgeon to surgeon.
- Most protect weight-bearing and/or range of motion to some degree in meniscal repairs until some degree of healing has occurred, usually by 4 to 6 weeks.
- Flexion of the knee past 90 degrees places increased loads across the posterior horns of the menisci.
- Full knee extension symmetrical to the contralateral knee is encouraged immediately.
- Allograft transplantation requires a period of protected weight-bearing between 4 to 8 weeks followed by extensive rehabilitation.
- Partial meniscectomies without concomitant procedures are allowed to immediately weight-bear as tolerated and

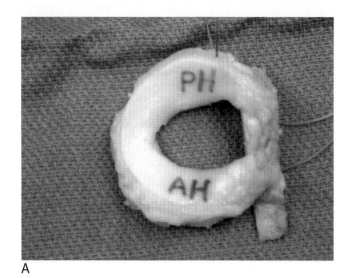

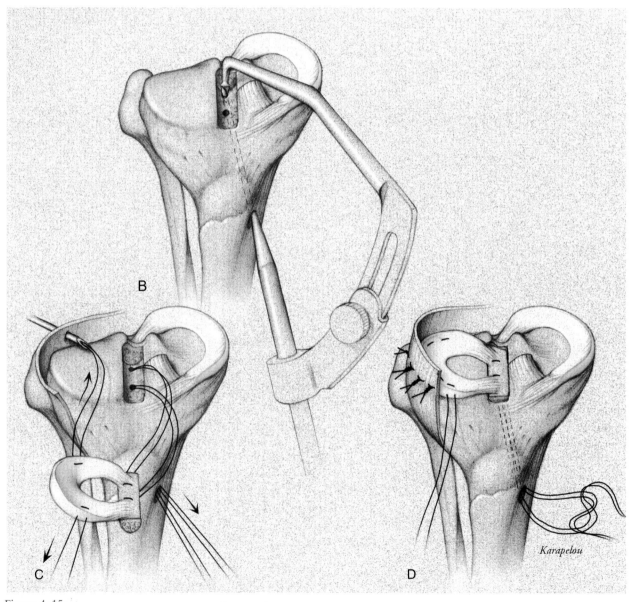

Figure 4–15:
A, Lateral meniscal allograft with bone bridge. **B-D,** Lateral bone block allograft insertion. (**B** to **D** from Goble M: *Op Tech Orthop* 10:220-226, 2000.)

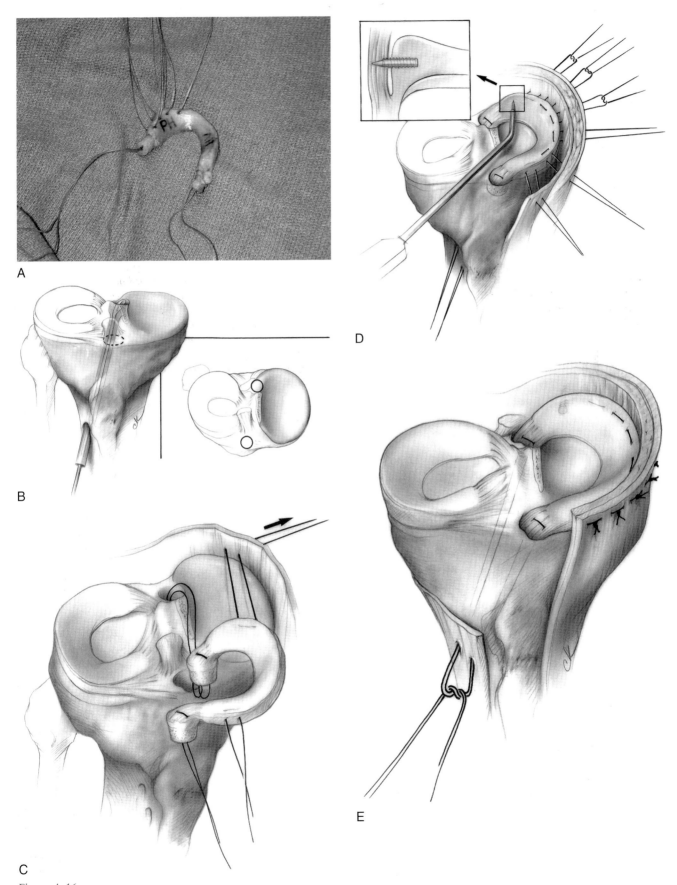

Figure 4–16:
A, Medial meniscal allograft with bone plugs. **B-E,** Medial bone plug allograft insertion. (**B** to **E** from Goble EM, Kane SM: Meniscal allograft transplantation. In Insall JN, Scott WN, editors: *Surgery of the knee,* 3rd ed. New York, 2001, Churchill Livingstone.)

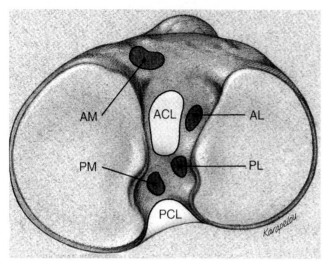

Figure 4–17:
Anatomy of the tibia plateau demonstrating the normal insertion sites of the lateral and medical menisci. (From Allen AA, Caldwell GL Jr, Fu FH: *Op Tech Orthop* 5:2-9, 1995.)

are progressed as strength and range of motion are obtained.

- Meniscal repairs performed in conjunction with ACL reconstruction usually follow postoperative ACL rehabilitation protocols with some limits to knee flexion and/or weight-bearing.

Complications

- Anatomic structures at risk during repair—medial: saphenous nerve/vein, popliteal vessels; lateral: peroneal nerve, popliteal vessels.
- Newer devices and techniques (arrows/peripheral fixation) have increased risks of breakage, migration, synovitis, chondral injury, and decreased strength.
- Entrapment of subcutaneous nerves is possible with meniscal repairs.
- Up to 50% of patients may demonstrate Fairbank changes after partial meniscectomies.

References

Bellabarba C, Bush-Josep CA, Back BR Jr: Patterns of meniscal injury in the anterior cruciate-deficient knee: a review of the literature. *Am J Orthop* 26:18-23, 1997.
Describes the greater incidence of lateral meniscal tears following acute ACL ruptures and medial meniscal tears in chronic ACL-deficient knees and the improved outcomes in medial meniscal repairs with ACL reconstruction using a review of the literature.

Boyd KT, Myers PT: Meniscus preservation; rationale, repair techniques and results. *Knee* 10:1-11, 2003.
Authors report that as meniscal criteria for repair continue to be defined, with the development of new techniques and adjuncts promot-

ing healing, surgeons have the opportunity to preserve as much normal tissue as possible and avoid alterations to the normal biomechanics of the knee. Several types of tears previously considered irreparable have seen successful results with surgical repair. Types of meniscal tears and surgical techniques for repair are discussed. The database of 288 meniscal repairs performed over 12 years by the senior author is reviewed. Most were performed in conjunction with ACL reconstruction (only 55 were isolated). Types of tears were longitudinal (243), radial (9), partial thickness (14), and complex (22). They report a 5.9% failure rate but with seven of these patients successfully treated after resuturing their tears. The authors conclude that repairs should be considered in good candidates with clinical indications, even in the face of unfavorable presentations.*

Farng E, Sherman O: Meniscal repair devices: a clinical and biomechanical literature review. *Arthroscopy* 20:273-286, 2004.
Literature review attempting to evaluate and compare different repair techniques and devices used in meniscal repairs. Biomechanical properties and clinical results are discussed. Vertical sutures were found to be superior to horizontal sutures biomechanically and under cyclic loading. The T-fix, Meniscus Arrow, and Mitek Meniscal Repair System were devices found to be comparable to suture techniques. However, some of these devices require further study to support their common use. Although healing rates have not improved, several of these new devices have been able to simplify surgical repairs and lower complication rates.

Greis PE, Holmstrom MC, Bardana DD, Burks RT: Meniscal injury: II. management. *J Am Acad Orthop Surg* 10(3):177-187, 2002.
Good review of operative management of meniscal tears. Includes descriptions, advantages, disadvantages, outcomes and complications of all current techniques including allograft transplantation.

Laprell H, Stein V, Petersen W: Arthroscopic all-inside meniscus repair using a new refixation device: a prospective study. *Arthroscopy* 18: 387-393, 2002.
Authors describe an all-inside meniscal repair technique using Mitek meniscus staples in 37 patients with unstable longitudinal meniscal tears in the middle or peripheral third with generally promising results. Seventeen patients with ACL ruptures underwent reconstruction 6 to 8 weeks after the meniscus repair at which time all of the repaired menisci were noted to be stable in their reduced position. Five patients experienced reruptures, all in the middle third of the menisci, with two of them reporting a history of significant trauma. The most common intraoperative complication was migration of the implant into the articular cavity. Long-term studies are still required to further evaluate the indications and outcomes of this technique.

Maitra RS, Miller MD, Johnson DL: Meniscal reconstruction. Part I: indications, techniques, and graft considerations. *Am J Orthop* 28:213-218, 1999.
Article discussing the anatomy and function of the meniscus and indications, techniques, and grafts available for meniscal transplantation. References several studies that have helped define and develop the relatively new technique of meniscal transplantation, which is still in its infancy.

Maitra RS, Miller MD, Johnson DL: Meniscal reconstruction. Part II: outcome, potential complications, and future directions. *Am J Orthop* 28:280-286, 1999.
Continuation of the previous article, outlining results from medical allograft transplantation studies and describing potential risks, complications, and fields of study that can help advance this relatively new procedure.

Noyes FR, Barber-Westin SD: Arthroscopic repair of meniscus tears extending into the avascular zone with or without anterior cruciate ligament reconstruction in patients 40 years of age and older. *Arthroscopy* 16:822–829, 2000.

Authors report relief of tibiofemoral joint symptoms in 26 (87%) of the 30 meniscal repairs (inside-out technique) performed in patients 40 years or older with meniscal tears involving the avascular zone. Although the 21 (72%) patients who required concomitant ACL reconstructions had better outcomes than the group with isolated meniscal tears, it was not found to be statistically significant. Observation of actual healing (by means of arthroscopy) was not performed or evaluated. Nevertheless, the authors recommend repairing meniscal tears that extend into the avascular zone in active patients regardless of age.

Rankin CC, Lintner DM, Noble PC, et al: A biomechanical analysis of meniscal repair techniques. *Am J Sports Med* 30:492–497, 2002.

Controlled laboratory study comparing the biomechanical strengths of Biofix meniscus arrows, anchor sutures (T-fix), and horizontal and vertical mattress sutures. Meniscal tears were created in bovine menisci and repaired with one of the four techniques above. Testing demonstrated the greatest displacement in the Biofix arrow group and the least displacement in the vertical mattress suture group, which provided the strongest repair.

Smith JP III, Barrett GR: Medial and lateral meniscal tear patterns in anterior cruciate ligament-deficient knees. *Am J Sports Med* 29:415 419, 2001.

Prospective study of 575 meniscal tears in acute and chronic ACL-deficient knees, evaluating the location of the tears. Incidence of medial and lateral meniscal tears in both acute and chronic ACL-deficient knees were not statistically different. Medial meniscal tears appeared to occur more often posterior (99.4% vs. 87.8%) and peripheral (75.4% vs. 44.1%) when compared with lateral meniscal tears.

Spindler KP, McCarty EC, Warren TA, et al: Prospective comparison of arthroscopic medial meniscal repair technique: inside-out suture versus entirely arthroscopic arrows. *Am J Sports Med* 31:929-934, 2003.

Prospective cohort study demonstrating similar success rates for suture and arrow repair (88% and 89%, respectively) of tears of the peripheral posterior horn of the medial meniscus during ACL reconstruction.

Van Arkel ER, de Boer HH: Survival analysis of human meniscal transplantations. *J Bone Joint Surg Br* 84:227-231, 2002.

Prospective study assessing the survival rate of meniscal allografts. Results demonstrated longer survival and fewer failures with lateral meniscal allografts compared with medial meniscal allografts. Furthermore, there was a significant negative correlation between the success of medial meniscal transplantation and ACL rupture. Authors report that survival may be improved with concomitant ACL reconstruction. They also believe that the success of meniscal transplantation is greatly dependent on alignment, stability, and fixation of the allograft.

Wirth CJ, Peters G, Milachowski KA, et al: Long term results after meniscal allograft transplantation. *Am J Sports Med* 30:174-181, 2002.

Allografts transplanted via soft tissue attachments— not a very good study.

Yoldas EA, Sekiya JK, Irrgang JJ, et al: Arthroscopically assisted meniscal allograft transplantation with and without combined anterior cruciate ligament reconstruction. *Knee Surg Sports Traumatol Arthrosc* 11:173-182, 2003.

Authors report on clinical and patient outcomes following meniscal transplantation in 31 patients (34 meniscal allografts) with or without ACL reconstruction. At a mean follow-up of 2.9 years, the Activities of Daily Living and Sports Activities Scale scores were 86 ±11 and 78 ±16, respectively, with no significant differences based on side of meniscus transplanted or whether concurrent ACL reconstruction was performed. Based on the Lysholm knee scale, results demonstrated 8 excellent, 13 good, 7 fair, and 3 poor results. Functional strength of the affected limb was determined to average 85% of the contralateral limb. The authors concluded that meniscal transplantation in carefully selected patients provides a good means of relieving symptoms and restoring function.

CHAPTER 5

Osteochondral Injuries to the Knee

Introduction

- Osteochondral lesions represent a wide variety of conditions ranging from partial thickness cartilage lesions to large defects involving the cartilage and underlying bone.
- Osteochondritis dissecans represents a subset of osteochondral lesions.
- Osteochondral defects should be discrete, focal areas of cartilage ± subchondral bone loss with normal adjacent articular cartilage. This should be distinguished from long-standing thinning of articular cartilage that represents osteoarthritis (Box 5–1, Figure 5–1).

Box 5–1	**Outerbridge Classification of Chondromalacia**

- Grade 0: normal cartilage
- Grade I: cartilage with softening and swelling
- Grade II: a partial-thickness defect with fissures on the surface that do not reach subchondral bone or exceed 1.5 cm in diameter
- Grade III: fissuring to the level of subchondral bone in an area with a diameter greater than 1.5 cm
- Grade IV: exposed subchondral bone

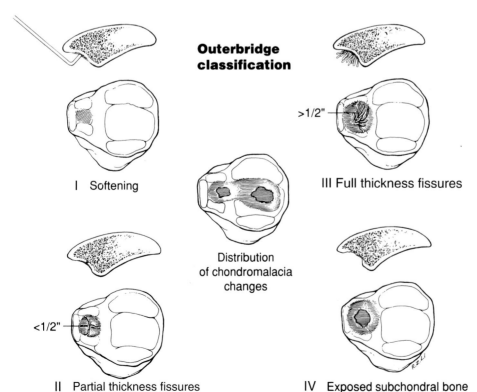

Outerbridge classification

I   Softening

III Full thickness fissures

Distribution of chondromalacia changes

<1/2"

II   Partial thickness fissures

>1/2"

IV   Exposed subchondral bone

Figure 5–1:
Outerbridge classification. (From Tria AJ Jr, Klein KS: *An illustrated guide to the knee.* New York, 1992, Churchill Livingstone.)

History, Physical Examination, and Imaging

- Patients typically present with recurrent knee effusions. Mechanical symptoms may or may not be present.
- Examination is often nonfocal. Patients may or may not have tenderness in the area where the defect is present.
- Radiographs (tunnel view or flexion weight-bearing posteroanterior [PA] view) may show defects, especially with osteochondritis dissecans, but will not be helpful in patients with chondral injury alone.
- Magnetic resonance imaging (MRI) is helpful to determine the size and extent of the lesion.
  - Bright signal on T2 images indicates an area of cartilage loss that is filled with synovial fluid.
  - Gradient echo (GRE) and fat-suppressed proton-density images help to identify associated abnormalities in the subchondral bone.
  - T1 and T2 images are useful in determining bony injury and increased marrow edema.

Osteochondritis Dissecans

- Osteochondritis dissecans is reserved for lesions of the articular cartilage and underlying bone that typically occur in adolescents and young adults.
- The etiology of osteochondritis dissecans is unknown, although trauma and possibly vascular injury have been implicated. Pathologic changes begin in the subchondral bone.
- The most common location of these lesions is the lateral aspect of the medial femoral condyle (Figure 5–2).
- Juvenile osteochondritis dissecans (JOCD) implies that the physis of the affected knee is still open.
- JOCD has a better prognosis than the adult osteochondritis dissecans (AOCD).
- Staging is based on the degree of detachment of the lesion (Box 5–2, Figure 5–3).
- Treatment of symptomatic patients who have failed rest and activity restriction includes primary repair of the lesion (which typically requires removing the piece, scraping fibrous tissue off the lesion and the bed where it was attached, bone grafting the defect, and fixing the

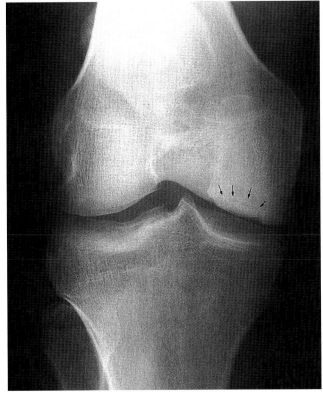

Figure 5–2:
Radiographic image of osteochondritis dissecans of the lateral aspect of the medial femoral condyle. (From Miller MD, Howard RF, Plancher KD: *Surgical atlas of sports medicine*. Philadelphia, 2003, WB Saunders.)

Box 5–2	Guhl Arthroscopic Classification of Osteochondritis Dissecans

A: Intact lesions
B: Lesions with early separation
C: Partially detached lesions
D: Crater with loose bodies

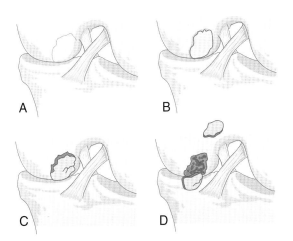

Figure 5–3:
Classification of osteochondritis dissecans.

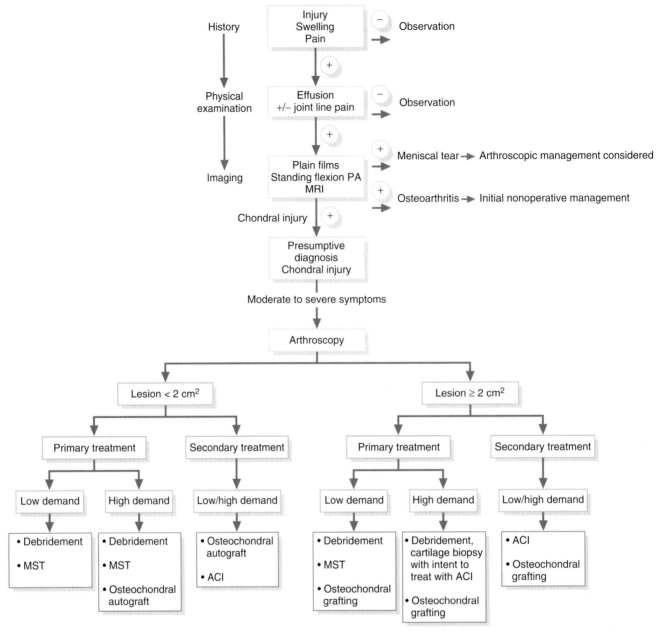

Figure 5–4:
Treatment algorithm for chondral injury. (From Miller MD, Cole B: *Op Tech Orthop* **11:145-150, 2001.)**

piece with absorbable or nonabsorbable fixation devices), removing of the lesion, drilling the lesion (antegrade or retrograde), and other techniques that are described in the section that follows (Figure 5–4).

Atraumatic Osteonecrosis

- Risk factors for developing this type of lesion include chronic use of steroids, deep-sea diving, and alcohol abuse.

- Usually a wedge-shaped lesion.
- Treated with core decompression/drilling techniques.

Spontaneous Osteonecrosis of the Knee (SONK)

- SONK involves a subchondral insufficiency fracture (Figure 5–5).

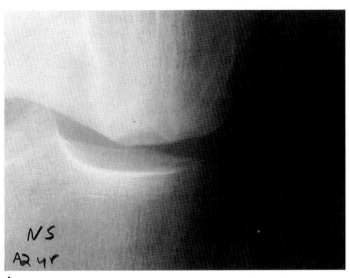
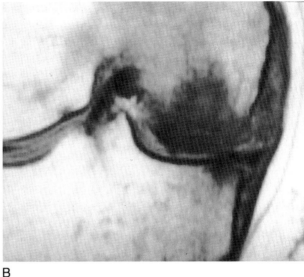

A   B

Figure 5–5:
Radiographic appearance of spontaneous osteonecrosis of the knee. **A,** x-ray. **B,** Magnetic resonance imaging. (From Lotke PA, Ecker ML, Lonner J: Spontaneous osteonecrosis. In Insall JN, Scott WN, editors: *Surgery of the knee,* 3rd ed. Philadelphia, 2001, Churchill Livingstone.)

- This usually occurs more commonly in the medial femoral condyle.
- Occurrence in females is three times greater than males and usually in patients older than 40 years (Table 5–1).
- Symptoms of a subacute onset of pain in the knee without provoking injury are suspect for this condition.
- SONK may occur after a surgical procedure such as an arthroscopy especially in older patients.

- Treatment is initially conservative with emphasis on pain control with medications.
- If conservative treatment fails, surgical options include unicompartmental or total knee replacement.

Focal Osteochondral Defects

- It is important to recognize that the treatment of focal defects is much different than diffuse thinning of the articular cartilage. The latter likely represents arthritis, which has been shown to not generally be amenable to arthroscopic treatment (Table 5–2).
- Treatment options include so-called marrow stimulating procedures (abrasion chondroplasty, drilling, and microfracture), which produce type I collagen; osteochondral transfer

Table 5–1:	Comparison of Spontaneous Osteonecrosis With Secondary Osteonecrosis	
CHARACTERISTIC	**SPONTANEOUS OSTEONECROSIS OF THE KNEE**	**SECONDARY OSTEONECROSIS OF THE KNEE**
Age	>55 to 60 years	<45 years
Pain onset	Acute	Gradual
Bilaterality	<5%	>80%
Lesion number	One	Multiple
Lesion size	Small	Large
Location	Usually medial femoral condyle	Multiple femoral and tibial condyles
Hip involvement	<1%	>90%
Associated factors	None	Corticosteroids, alcohol, tobacco
Associated diseases	None	Systemic lupus erythematosus and other immunocompromising disorders

From Mont MA, Rifia A, Baumgarten K, Hungerford DS: Osteonecrosis of the knee. In Insall JN, Scott WN, editor: *Surgery of the knee* 3rd ed., Philadelphia, 2001, Churchill Livingstone.

Table 5–2:	Factors in the Evaluation of Patients with Chondral Lesions
PATIENT-RELATED FACTORS	**DEFECT-RELATED FACTORS**
Age	Size
Activity level	Location
Alignment	Containment
Ligament instability	Cause
Expectations	Bone involvement
Time availability	Prior surgical treatment and response
	Associated degenerative changes

From Bonner KF, Bugbee WD: Osteochondral allografting in the knee. In Miller MD, Cole BJ, editors: *Textbook of arthroscopy.* Philadelphia, 2004, WB Saunders.

techniques (autografts and allografts); and chondrocyte implantation techniques (Box 5–3).

Abrasion Chondroplasty

- Abrasion chondroplasty involves using the arthroscopic shaver to remove loose flaps and "smooth" the margins of the chondral defect to stabilize the lesion and prevent propagation.
- Historically, this has been the only treatment used for full-thickness chondral lesions.
- Although there was some initial success with this treatment, it clearly deteriorates with time.

Drilling/Microfracture

- Although similar to abrasion chondroplasty, proponents of drilling/microfracture suggest that fibrocartilage formed by microfracture is superior to that formed following abrasion chondroplasty.
- Microfracture holes are drilled into the subchondral bone, which allows pluripotent cells to escape from the marrow cavity (Figure 5–6).

Box 5–3	Treatment Options for Focal Chondral Defects

Abrasion chondroplasty
Microfracture
Autogenous osteochondral transfer
Allograft osteochondral transfer
Autologous chondrocyte implantation

- A clot forms over the defect, and these cells become fibrochondrocytes that subsequently produce fibrocartilage.
- Emphasis has been placed on removing the calcified cartilage layer prior to microfracture.
- Although results appear to be better than abrasion chondroplasty, the fibrocartilage that forms is predominately type I collagen and is not as durable as articular cartilage (type II collagen).

Osteochondral "Plug" Transfer

- OsteoArticular Transfer System (commonly known as OATS) (Arthrex, Largo, FL), is one of three commercially available systems for articular cartilage and bone "plug" transfer.
- The other systems are COR (Mitek, Norwood, MA) and Mosaicplasty (Smith & Nephew Endoscopy, Andover, MA).
- Plugs of varying diameters (usually 4 to 10 mm) are harvested from a relatively low contact area of the knee (superolateral aspect of the lateral femoral condyle or notch) and are inserted into the defect that is prepared with matching cylindrical defects.
- The key to the operation is to harvest and deliver the plugs perpendicular to the articular surface.
- Defects up to 2.5 cm^2 can be addressed with this technique (Figure 5–7).

Chondrocyte Transplantation/Implantation

- Chondrocyte transplantation and implantation requires two steps.

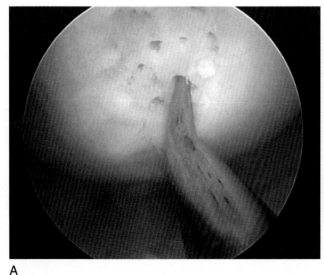
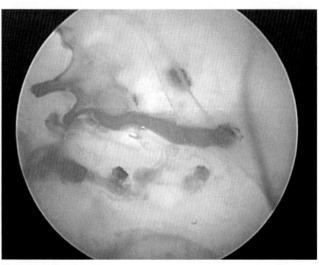

A

B

Figure 5–6:
Arthroscopic microfracture technique. A, Before. B, After. (From Freedman KB, Cole BJ: Microfracture technique in the knee. In Miller MD, Cole BJ, editors: *Textbook of arthroscopy.* **Philadelphia, 2004, WB Saunders.)**

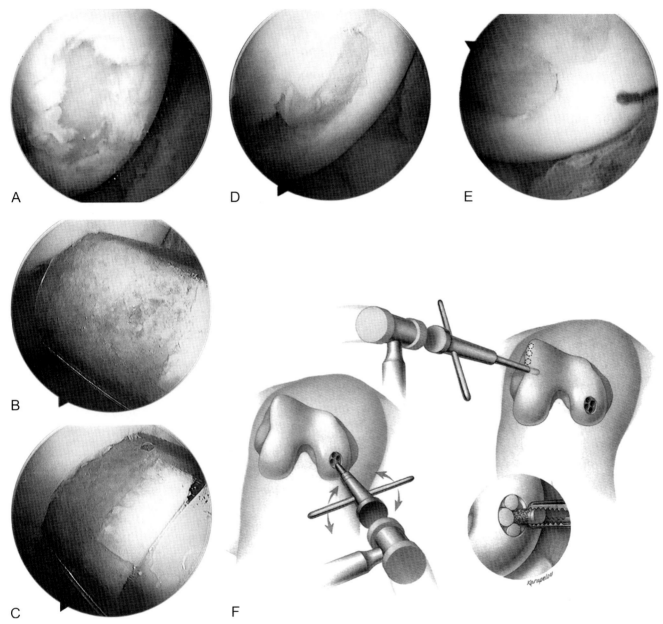

Figure 5–7:
OsteoArticular Transfer System (OATS) technique. **A,** Chondral defect is identified and debrided. **B,** Donor plug is drilled. **C,** Plug is delivered to area of chondral defect. **D,** First plug is placed flush with surface. **E,** Second plug is placed to finish the area. (From Miller MD, Howard RF, Plancher KD, editors: *Surgical atlas of sports medicine.* Philadelphia, 2003, WB Saunders.)

- The first step is to evaluate the defect and harvest a small amount of normal articular cartilage from a relatively low contact area of the knee.
- This cartilage is processed and chondrocytes are cultured in a laboratory.
- A second procedure is carried out in which the defect is prepared and a periosteal patch is carefully sewn over the defect.
- The cells are injected under the patch, which is sealed with fibrin glue (Figure 5–8).
- Results have been very encouraging, but the expense of cell culture (up to $16,000) and problems with patch

overgrowth have thwarted some of the enthusiasm for this technique.

Allograft

- Although there are different techniques, the most popular option is to transfer a giant osteochondral plug from a matched fresh allograft into the defect (Figure 5–9).
- This is reserved for large defects.
- Obtaining donor tissue has proven to be difficult in many centers.
- Other tissue processing options are being explored (Table 5–3, Figure 5–10).

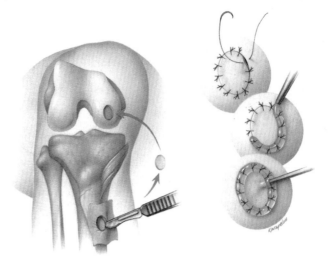

Figure 5–8:
Autologous chondrocyte implantation technique. (From Miller MD, Howard RF, Plancher KD, editors: *Surgical atlas of sports medicine*. Philadelphia, 2003, WB Saunders.)

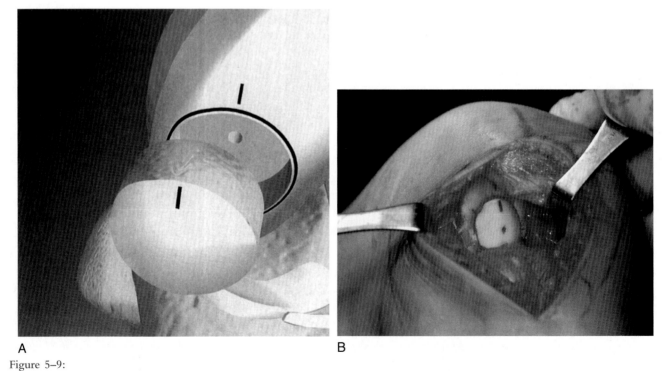

A

B

Figure 5–9:
A, Large osteochondral allograft plug being fitted into the prepared defect site. **B,** Intraoperative image of "fitted" allograft plug. (From Bonner KF, Bugbee WD: Osteochondral allografting in the knee. In Miller MD, Cole BJ, editors: *Textbook of arthroscopy*. Philadelphia, 2004, WB Saunders.)

Table 5–3: Summary of Decision Making in Articular Cartilage Injuries

Clinical Evaluation

History	Pain in ipsilateral compartment; recurrent effusions
Physical examination	Pain in ipsilateral compartment; rule out coexisting pathology
Imaging	Standing radiographs, including 45-degree posteroanterior, and mechanical axis views; magnetic resonance imaging commonly shows articular cartilage lesion
Classification	Outerbridge classification
Associated injuries	Evaluate for knee instability, meniscal deficiency, malalignment

Treatment Options

Nonoperative	Low-demand patients, small lesions (<1 cm²)
Operative	
Primary repair	Osteochondral lesions
Debridement and lavage	Low-demand patients
	Small to medium lesions (0.5-3 cm²)
Marrow stimulation (microfracture)	Moderate-sized lesions (1-3 cm²)
	Low- or high-demand patients
	Fibrocartilage repair tissue
Osteochondral autograft	Small to medium lesions (1-3 cm²)
	Autogenous tissue with normal hyaline architecture
	Consider donor site morbidity and availability
Autologous chondrocyte implantation	Medium to large lesions (2-10 cm²)
	Hyaline-like tissue
	Durable
Osteochondral allograft	Medium to large lesions (up to hemicondyle)
	Allograft tissue
	Good for lesions with bony defects
Postoperative rehabilitation	Protect repair tissue from weight-bearing for 6 wk
	Immediate range of motion
	Gradual return to weight-bearing and activities based on technique

From Freedman KB, Cole BJ: Microfracture technique in the knee. In Miller MD, Cole BJ, editors: *Textbook of arthroscopy.* Philadelphia, 2004, WB Saunders.

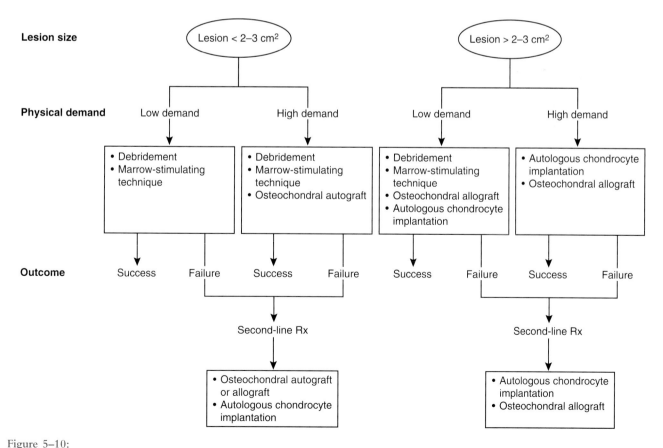

Figure 5–10:

Treatment algorithm for articular cartilage lesion. (From Freedman KB, Cole BJ: Microfracture technique in the knee. In Miller MD, Cole BJ, editors: *Textbook of arthroscopy.* Philadelphia, 2004, WB Saunders.)

References

Brittberg M, Lindhall A, Nilsson A, et al: Treatment of deep cartilage defects in the knee with autologous chondrocyte implantation. *N Engl J Med* 331:881-895, 1994.

This landmark article is the first report of successful autologous chondrocyte implantation. Although the authors reported excellent results in this series, other surgeons have been unable to replicate their results.

Chow JCY, Hantes ME, Houle JB, Zalavras CG: Arthroscopic autogenous osteochondral transplantation for treating knee cartilage defects: a 2- to 5-year follow-up study. *Arthroscopy* 20:681-690, 2004.

Following patients who were treated with autogenous osteochondral transplantation for approximately 4 years, these authors conclude that this procedure is a safe and effective treatment option but note that more long-term research is necessary to ensure that the transferred plug does not break down over time.

Freedman KB, Cole BJ: Microfracture technique in the knee. In Miller MD, Cole BJ, editors: *Textbook of arthroscopy.* Philadelphia, 2004, WB Saunders.

This is a well-illustrated review of different cartilage treatment options. This chapter includes several tables with useful information on each technique and an algorithm of treatment options.

Kuroki H, Nakagawa Y, Mori K, et al: Mechanical effects of autogenous osteochondral surgical grafting procedures and instrumentation on grafts of articular cartilage. *Am J Sports Med* 32:612-620, 2004.

In analyzing the mechanical properties of the bone plugs used for osteochondral transfer, there was no difference in the plug at the time of extraction or after implantation in terms of stiffness, surface irregularity, or thickness of the plug.

Lotke PA, Ecker ML, Lonner J: Spontaneous osteonecrosis. In Insall JN, Scott WN, editors: *Surgery of the knee,* 3rd ed. Philadelphia, 2001, Churchil Livingstone.

This is a chapter devoted entirely to spontaneous osteonecrosis. It provides a thorough review of this poorly understood diagnosis and includes a thorough discussion of the differential diagnoses and treatment options.

Mont MA, Rifia A, Baumgarten K, Hungerford DS: Osteonecrosis of the knee. In Insall JN, Scott WN, editors: *Surgery of the knee,* 3rd ed. Philadelphia, 2001, Churchill Livingstone.

This chapter begins with a very nice comparison of osteonecrosis and secondary osteonecrosis. It provides a thorough discussion of imaging and staging and describes treatment options for osteonecrosis of the knee.

CHAPTER

6

Synovial Lesions

Pigmented Villonodular Synovitis (PVNS)

- A proliferative disorder of the synovial membrane.
- Most commonly affects the knee joint but is an overall rare condition with an approximate annual incidence of 1.8 cases per million.
- Can be categorized into localized and diffuse forms, with the latter being more common.
- Diagnosis is difficult and often delayed.
- May present as an insidious onset of pain, swelling, and repeated hemarthrosis, potentially with a palpable mass.
- Plain radiographs may reveal bony erosions, but magnetic resonance imaging (MRI) usually can reveal the soft tissue lesions with great sensitivity (Figure 6–1).

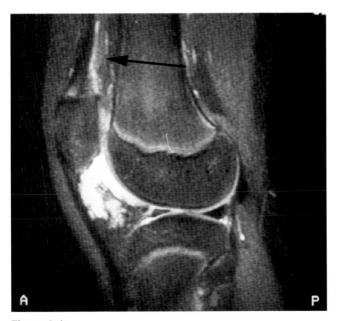

Figure 6–1:
Magnetic resonance imaging demonstrating diffuse pigmented villonodular synovitis. (From Sellards R, Stanley R, Bush-Joseph CA: Arthroscopic synovectomy in the knee. In Miller MD, Cole BJ, editors: *Textbook of arthroscopy*. Philadelphia, 2004, WB Saunders.)

- Histologic evaluation reveals foam cells (histiocytes), fibrous tissue, giant cells, and hemosiderin deposition (similar to giant cell tumor of the tendon sheath).
- Partial synovectomy of localized forms is usually successful.
- Treatment of diffuse forms requires complete synovectomy (arthroscopic or open).
- Recurrence is relatively common following resection and may necessitate more extensive surgical excision and/or chemotherapeutic agents.

Synovial Chondromatosis

- Proliferative synovial disease associated with cartilaginous or osteocartilaginous metaplasia resulting in loose bodies in the joint (Figure 6–2).
- The disease presents in three phases (Box 6–1).
- Treatment includes loose body removal along with synovectomy (which may be performed arthroscopically) to reduce the risk of recurrence.

Synovial Plicae

- Synovial folds are embryologic remnants of mesenchymal tissue that historically were thought to divide the knee into separate compartments.
- Not completely understood, with no definitive consensus on diagnostic and therapeutic criteria (making literature and studies difficult to interpret and compare).
- Four plicae have been described by their relationship to the patella: superior, inferior, lateral and medial, each with several subtypes defined in the literature (Box 6–2).
- Although the superior and inferior plicae are more common, they rarely are associated with symptoms.
- Medial plicae are the most clinically significant and studied (medial plica syndrome) (Figure 6–3).
- Lateral plicae are rare and generally not considered clinically relevant.
- There appears to be a greater prevalence of medial plicae in patients with lateral subluxation of the patella.

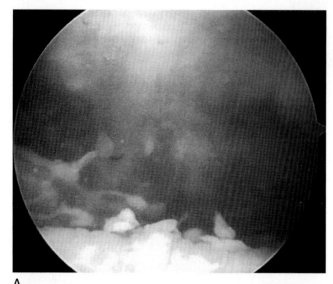

A

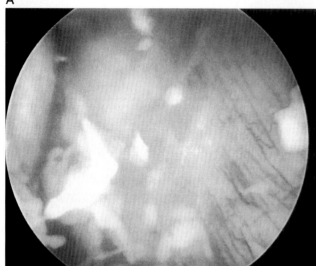

B

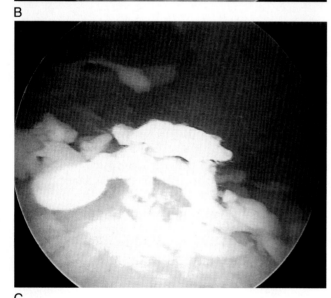

C

Figure 6–2:
Arthroscopic view of synovial chondromatosis. **A,** Suprapatellar pouch/trochlea. **B,** Medial gutter. **C,** Deep suprapatellar pouch.

Box 6–1 Phases of Synovial Chondromatosis

Early: Chondrometaplasia, no loose bodies
Transitional: Active synovial disease, loose bodies
Late: Loose bodies, no synovial disease

- Because of its clinical importance, several authors have attempted to define all the types of medial plicae and their association with symptoms and prognosis. However, the classification developed by Iino is most often referenced (Box 6–3).
- Symptoms classically present after blunt trauma, overuse, or twisting injuries but may also occur with no significant history.
- Young athletes, particularly those involved in activities requiring repetitive flexion and extension, are the most commonly affected.
- Often an incidental finding, symptomatic medial plicae present as a palpable click or catch anteromedially as the knee is brought into flexion and the plica passes over the medial femoral condyle.
- Pain is usually exacerbated with activity.
- On physical examination, a palpable cord that reproduces symptoms is almost pathognomonic.
- Tenderness of the medial plica is most often above the medial joint line.
- Other signs such as effusions, crepitus, catching, pseudolocking, and giving way (usually secondary to the pain) are not specific and are often confused with other pathologic conditions such as meniscal tears or patellar syndromes.
- Arthrography, computed tomography (CT) with arthrography, MRI, and ultrasound may all be used to further evaluate and diagnose plica.
- Arthroscopy allows visual and dynamic examinations and thorough assessment of the joint for other potential symptomatic pathology.
- Medial plica syndrome may demonstrate a thickened plica associated with medial impingement against the medial femoral condyle/trochlea and localized chondromalacia.

Box 6–2 Plicae of the Knee

- Superior: Originates anterior to the femoral metaphysis at the suprapatellar pouch and inserts above the patella, posterior to the quadriceps tendon
- Inferior: Runs from the anterior aspect of the intercondylar notch (above, anterior and parallel to the anterior cruciate ligament [ACL]) to the inferior aspect of the infrapatellar fat pad
- Medial: Originating from the medial wall of the synovial pouch or below the medial retinaculum, it runs parallel to the medial margin of the patella, approximately one fingerbreadth medially, to insert into the medial synovial lining of the infrapatellar fat pad
- Lateral: Runs a similar course as the medial plica, approximately 1 to 2 cm lateral to the patella from the lateral wall above the popliteus hiatus to the infrapatellar fat pad

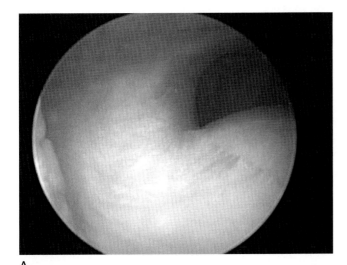

A

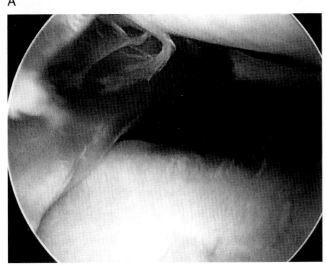

B

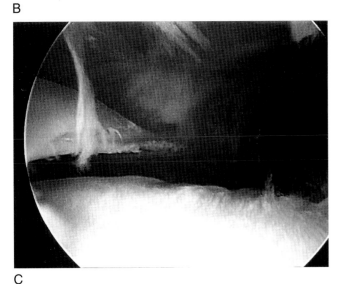

C

Figure 6–3:
Arthroscopic view of medial plica syndrome. **A,** Medial plica draping over the medial femoral condyle. **B,** Thickened medial plica abrading medial femoral condyle with evidence of chondrosis. **C,** Same thickened plica in full extension and lifted off the condyle.

Box 6–3 | **Iino Classification of the Medial Plica**

Type A: Thin elevation of synovium under the medial retinaculum
Type B: Narrow pleat without impingement on the medial condyle
Type C: Larger structure that partially covers the medial condyle
Type D: Fenestrated variant of type C, or bandlike structure
Types A and B are unlikely to result in symptoms
Types C and D are thought to be more likely to produce symptoms
  secondary to impingement on the medial condyle

From Dupont JY: *Clin Sports Med* 16:87-122, 1997.

- Initial treatment is generally conservative with rest, ice, avoidance of aggravating activities and use of nonsteroidal antiinflammatory drugs (NSAIDs).
- Arthroscopic resection, reserved for recalcitrant cases, is controversial and should not be performed if pathology is not observed during arthroscopic evaluation.
- If arthroscopic treatment is performed, resolution of symptoms should occur within 2 to 4 weeks. If symptoms persist, other possible conditions must be considered.
- Recurrence of plicae may occur after operative resection.

Arthroscopic Synovectomy

- Arthroscopic or open synovectomy can be performed for a variety of disorders including PVNS, synovial chondromatosis, hemophilia, and adult or juvenile rheumatoid arthritis.
- If an arthroscopic treatment is adopted, a thorough, systematic approach should be followed using as many as six portals depending on the pathology being treated: superomedial, superolateral, inferomedial, inferolateral, posteromedial, and posterolateral.
- Medial plicae are best addressed using anterolateral and superolateral portals.
- Whichever method is used, a thorough and complete synovectomy is essential to a successful treatment, using all necessary portals for full visualization and access (Box 6–4).

Box 6–4	Surgical Technique: Complete Synovectomy	
CAMERA PORTAL	**WORKING PORTAL**	**COMPARTMENTS**
Inferolateral	Superolateral	Suprapatellar pouch, lateral gutter
Inferolateral	Inferomedial	Suprapatellar pouch, medial gutter, intercondylar notch
Inferolateral	Superomedial	Suprapatellar pouch, medial gutter
Superolateral	Inferolateral	Retropatellar pouch, inferolateral gutter
Superolateral	Inferomedial	Retropatellar pouch, inferomedial gutter
Inferolateral	Posteromedial	Posteromedial
Inferomedial	Posterolateral	Posterolateral

From Sellards R, Stanley R, Bush-Joseph CA: Arthroscopic synovectomy in the knee. In Miller MD, Cole BJ, editors: Textbook of arthroscopy. Philadelphia, 2004, Saunders.

References

Akgun I, Ogut T, Kesmezacar H, Dervisoglu S: Localized pigmented villonodular synovitis of the knee. *Orthopedics* 26:1131-1135, 2003.

Authors review the controversy regarding the nomenclature of localized pigmented villonodular synovitis (LPVNS) and its relationship with the more common, and familiar, PVNS of the knee. Authors also report great success with local excision and partial synovectomy in eight patients with symptomatic LPVNS, with no recurrences at an average 24-month follow-up. LPVNS appears to occur most commonly in the anterior compartment and is best diagnosed with the use of MRI. Arthroscopy is considered the treatment of choice.

Al-Nakshabandi NA, Ryan AG, Choudur H, et al: Pigmented villonodular synovitis. *Clin Radiol* 59:414-420, 2004.

Article reviewing imaging findings associated with PVNS. Authors describe and provide figures of findings on plain radiographs, CT, and MRI.

Blanco CER, Leon HO, Guthrie TB: Combined partial arthroscopy synovectomy and radiation therapy for diffuse pigmented villonodular synovitis of the knee. *Arthroscopy* 17:527-531, 2001.

Prospective study evaluating the results of combined arthroscopic synovectomy and low-dose radiation therapy in 22 patients with diffuse PVNS of the knee. At an average of 33 months postoperatively, 19 patients (86%) had good to excellent results, similar to results seen with complete synovectomies. The authors propose that low-dose radiation therapy may serve as an adjunct to synovectomy procedures, possibly reducing rates of recurrence, particularly for lesions in locations where complete synovectomies are difficult to achieve.

Bojanic I, Ivkovic A, Dotlic S, et al: Localized pigmented villonodular synovitis of the knee: diagnostic challenge and arthroscopic treatment: a report of three cases. *Knee Surg Traumatol Arthrosc* 9:350-354, 2001.

Authors review the diagnostic challenges and typical presentation, findings, and treatment of LPVNS. Three patient cases are presented. These patients subsequently underwent arthroscopic resection of their lesions with postoperative resolution of symptoms.

De Ponti A, Sansone V, Gama Malcher M: Result of arthroscopic treatment of pigmented villonodular synovitis of the knee. *Arthroscopy* 19:602-607, 2003.

Retrospective analysis of 19 patients with localized (n = 4) and diffuse (n = 15) forms of PVNS of the knee who underwent arthroscopic treatment. Localized forms were treated with partial synovectomy and resulted in complete resolution of symptoms with no recurrence in all patients. Patients with the diffuse form were treated with either a partial or extended synovectomy. Extended synovectomy procedures provided significantly better results with 80% of patients reporting good results.

Dupont JY: Synovial plicae of the knee; controversies and review. *Clin Sports Med* 16:87-122, 1997.

Very complete discussion of plicae of the knee, reviewing the literature, embryology, anatomy, statistics, clinical significance, diagnosis, histology, treatment, and outcomes. Authors concentrate on the medial plica syndrome (noted to be the most clinically relevant) and offer suggestions deciding on arthroscopic treatment and technique.

Kim SJ, Choe WS: Arthroscopic findings of the synovial plicae of the knee. *Arthroscopy* 13:33-41, 1997.

Authors arthroscopically study and describe the anatomy of the plicae of the knee. The authors propose a classification system according to shape and size. Of 400 knees evaluated, incidence results demonstrated suprapatellar plica in 87%, infrapatellar plica in 86%, mediopatellar plica in 72%, and lateral patellar plica in 1.3% of cases.

Muscolo DL, Makino A, Costa-Paz M, Ayerza M: Magnetic resonance imaging evaluation and arthroscopic resection of localized pigmented villonodular synovitis of the knee. *Orthopedics* 23:367-369, 2000.

Authors review MRI findings and operative results of five patients with LPVNS. MRI demonstrated well-circumscribed lesions in all patients, although the authors warn that other conditions may have similar findings. Arthroscopy serves as an excellent diagnostic tool and effective therapy. All patients in the study were satisfied with their postoperative results except one who complained of intermittent pain and swelling.

CHAPTER 7

Anterior Cruciate Ligament Injuries

History

- Anterior cruciate ligament (ACL) injuries are typically the result of a noncontact pivoting injury (70%).
- A variety of mechanisms have been observed and described. Deceleration with internal rotation is the classically described mechanism with more recent literature supporting valgus and external rotation.
- Controversy exists regarding chronicity of ACL injuries with comparison between acute traumatic injuries versus chronic attritional subclinical injury with eventual low-energy event creating complete rupture.
- Predisposing factors for injury (particularly in female athletes) have been described and include a narrow intercondylar notch, genu valgum, higher Q angle, different neuromuscular control, and hormonal influences.
- The patient may feel or hear a "pop" and develop an acute hemarthrosis (>70% of acute hemarthroses are secondary to ACL injury).

Physical Examination and Imaging

- Patients may walk with a "quadriceps avoidance" gait. This is a reduced quadriceps contraction with the knee in 40 degrees or less of flexion to avoid anterior tibial translation.
- The most sensitive examination maneuver is the Lachman test (anterior translation of the tibia with the knee in 20 to 30 degrees of flexion) (Figure 7–1).
- A pivot shift test (best done as an examination under anesthesia) demonstrates reduction of a subluxated knee (due to internal rotation in extension) with valgus stress and flexion (Figure 7–2, Box 7–1).
- The classic O'Donoghue triad (ACL–medial collateral ligament [MCL]–medial meniscal tear) is less common than an acute ACL-MCL-lateral meniscal tear. Medial meniscal tears are more common in the chronically ACL-deficient knee secondary to the increased role of the medial meniscus as a secondary translational stabilizer.

- Arthrometry (KT-1000 or KT-2000) can be used for objectively measuring anterior translation in comparison with a contralaterally uninjured ligament.
- Plain radiographs are often normal, but a small fracture of the periphery of the proximal lateral tibia ("capsular sign" or Segond fracture) is highly associated with an ACL tear (Figure 7–3).
- Magnetic resonance imaging (MRI) is very sensitive and specific for ACL tears. An osteochondral contusion (bone bruise), which is located in the middle third of the lateral femoral condyle and the posterior third of the lateral tibial plateau, is seen in up to 50% of ACL-injured knees (Figures 7–4 and 7–5).

Treatment

- Factors in consideration of reconstruction include a patient's "functional age" (biologic age may not be indicative of activity level), activity level (noncutting sports may not require stabilization), degree of instability (functionally and on examination), and associated pathology (multiple ligament injuries).

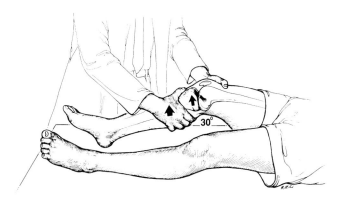

Figure 7–1:
The Lachman test.
(From Tria AJ Jr, Klein KS: *An illustrated guide to the knee.* **New York, 1992, Churchill Livingstone.)**

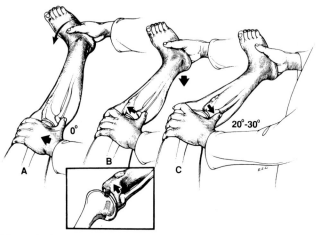

Figure 7–2:
The pivot shift test.
(From Tria AJ Jr, Klein KS: *An illustrated guide to the knee.* New York, 1992, Churchill Livingstone.)

Box 7–1	Grading the Pivot Shift Test

- Grade I: Slight subluxation—described as a "glide."
- Grade II: Subluxation with reduction—described as a "jump" or "clunk."
- Grade III: Subluxation with or without spontaneous reduction—marked "clunk" or transient lock.

- Although there is some controversy, ACL reconstruction is typically recommended for young, active patients who participate in cutting or pivoting activities. Nonoperative management is typically reserved for low-demand patients with less laxity.
- Patients experiencing instability during activities of daily life are also candidates for reconstruction and should be

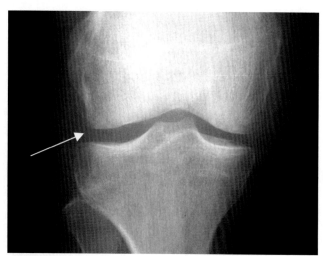

Figure 7–3:
Segond fracture.

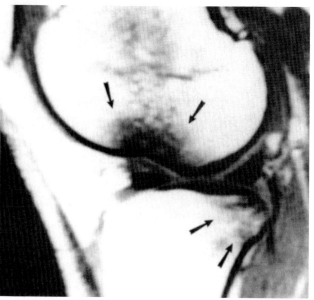

Figure 7–4:
Magnetic resonance imaging demonstrating bone bruises associated with acute anterior cruciate ligament tears.
(From Miller MD, Cooper DE, Warner JP: *Review of sports medicine and arthroscopy.* Philadelphia, 2002, WB Saunders.)

evaluated for other destabilizing-associated pathology (i.e., posterolateral corner injury).
- Nonoperative treatment includes hamstring strengthening (specifically the biceps femoris) and avoidance of unbalanced quadriceps strengthening to prevent anterior translation.
- Development of late arthrosis has not consistently been shown to be a result of chronic ACL deficiency. It appears to be more closely related to meniscal integrity.
- Recent literature has demonstrated an increase in late arthrosis in ACL-reconstructed knees thought to be due to overtensioning of the graft or continued subclinical rotational instability with single-bundle reconstruction.
- Development of meniscal tears and chondral injuries has been shown to be a result of chronic ACL deficiency.
- Timing of reconstruction is controversial with the common ground being that the patient must have full range of motion at the time of surgery to prevent stiffness postoperatively.
- ACL reconstruction consists of placing a tendinous graft through tunnels in the tibia and femur and fixing it on both ends with a variety of techniques.
- Primary repair of ACL tears is not effective for intrasubstance tears but has recently been advocated in conjunction with microfracture as an option for peel-off lesions from the femur.
- Treatment of "partial" ACL tears remains controversial. This diagnosis should be made arthroscopically under direct visualization in patients with a negative pivot shift.

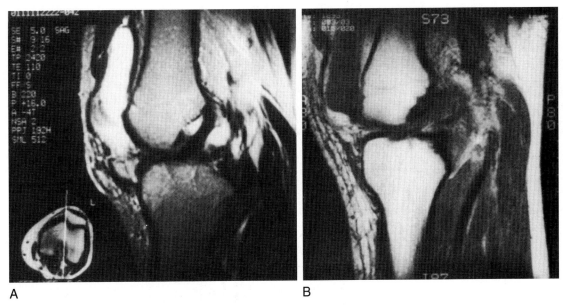

Figure 7–5:
Magnetic resonance imaging of normal and injured anterior cruciate ligament (ACL). A, Normal ACL. B, Injured ACL. (From Miller MD, Cooper DE, Warner JP: *Review of sports medicine and arthroscopy.* Philadelphia, 2002, WB Saunders.)

Some partial tears may be confused with a completely ruptured ligament that has scarred to the intercondylar roof and actually provides some translational stability. If the patient is clinically unstable, a partial tear should be reconstructed.

- Pediatric ACL injuries require more thorough evaluation including Tanner stage, estimate of remaining growth, radiographs to evaluate the open physis, and discussion with the parents about the possibility of physeal bar formation resulting in deformity.

- Although controversial, recent literature supports ACL reconstruction in the skeletally immature patient. Particular attention to crossing the physis as vertically as possible (smaller physeal defect), using hamstring grafts (although bone-patellar tendon-bone [BPTB] grafts without the bony ends crossing the physis have been shown to be effective), and fixation of the graft outside the physis (may consider an over-the-top technique in younger children) is required to reduce the risk of complications.

- Double-bundle ACL reconstruction has demonstrated biomechanical advantages over the standard single-bundle technique. The "anatomic" reconstruction is thought to provide improved rotational stability with clinical studies in process.

- Treatment of associated pathology at the time of ACL reconstruction is typically required to prevent early failure of the reconstruction. This includes excessive varus knee alignment with isolated medial compartment arthrosis, multiligament knee injuries (posterolateral corner, bicruciate, knee dislocation), meniscal pathology (particularly bucket-handle medial meniscus), and chondral injury.

Graft Choices

- The central one-third BPTB autograft has traditionally been thought of as the "gold standard" for ACL reconstruction. Its major advantage is good bony fixation with fast incorporation and is considered by some to be the graft of choice in athletes. There is an increased incidence of anterior knee pain with its use, however (Figure 7–6A).

- Quadrupled hamstring grafts (doubled semitendinosus and gracilis tendons) are becoming popular and are generally considered as a second gold standard for use in ACL reconstruction. These grafts are actually biomechanically stronger than BPTB grafts and not associated with as much harvest morbidity, but the inferior initial fixation and somewhat longer incorporation into bony tunnels may be an issue in athletes (Figure 7–6B).

- Many studies have compared BPTB with hamstring autografts finding similar short- and long-term results.

- Quadriceps tendon grafts are also a popular choice for some surgeons. There appears to be less morbidity with these grafts because some of the tendon can be left in place. These grafts are very strong biomechanically.

- Allografts are popular in some centers because they eliminate morbidity associated with harvesting autograft. However, cost, disease transmission (less than 1 in 1 million with optimal screening), and delayed incorporation must be considered. Allografts that are irradiated with greater than 2.5 mrad lose mechanical strength.

- Being prepared preoperatively with several graft options is necessary in the event that a harvested graft is suboptimal or is damaged during the reconstruction.

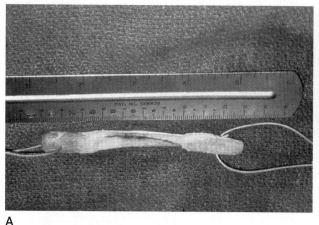

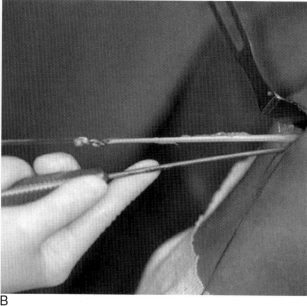

Figure 7–6:

Two common choices for anterior cruciate ligament autograft include (A) the middle one third of the patellar tendon and (B) the hamstring tendons (semitendinosus and gracilis).

- Preconditioning of grafts can reduce stress relaxation by up to 50%.

Tunnel Placement

- The tibial tunnel guide pin should be placed in reference to surrounding anatomic landmarks: posteromedial aspect of the ACL footprint, 7 to 10 mm in front of the PCL, adjacent to the medial eminence, and along a line in the coronal plane from the posterior aspect of the anterior horn of the lateral meniscus. The posterior cruciate ligament (PCL) appears to be the most reliable landmark (Figure 7–7A).
- When using the one-incision technique, the femoral tunnel placement should be planned so that a 1- to 2-mm posterior cortical rim will remain after drilling. It is important to identify the over-the-top position prior to drilling (Figure 7–7B).
- Anterior placement of either tunnel will result in strain in flexion. Posterior placement of either tunnel will result in strain in extension.

ACL Rehabilitation

- There has been no proven efficacy for braces in the postoperative ACL patient outside of those requiring concomitant meniscal repairs, chondral injury repair, or collateral ligament injury/reconstruction.

- Range of motion should be initiated early, and maintaining full extension emphasized in the early postoperative period. Some surgeons may use a brace locked in extension in the early postoperative period to protect against loss of extension.
- Isokinetic quadriceps strengthening (0 to 30 degrees) should be avoided in the early postoperative period (2 to 3 months) due to excessive strain on the graft.
- Return-to-play guidelines include return of the ipsilateral quadriceps peak torque force to 90% of the contralateral quadriceps, graft tunnel incorporation (approximately 5 months with BPTB grafts), and stability with progressive provocative drills including cutting and pivoting.
- Premature return to play may jeopardize graft tunnel incorporation, risk patellar fracture or patellar tendon rupture (BPTB autografts), or create further knee injury from lack of dynamic stabilization of the knee due to a deconditioned quadriceps.

ACL Complications

- Tunnel placement represents the most common technical error in ACL reconstruction with anterior tunnel placement the most common offender.
- An anterior tibial tunnel or suboptimal notchplasty (underresected roof or lateral femoral condyle) can cause impingement of the graft resulting in eventual failure.

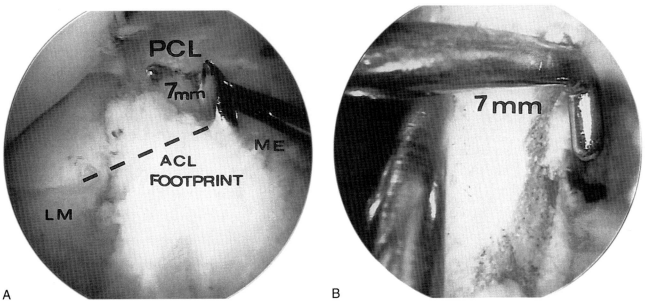

A   B

Figure 7–7:
Proper tibial and femoral tunnel placement in anterior cruciate ligament reconstruction. **A,** Tibial tunnel placement posteromedial to the anterior cruciate ligament footprint. **B,** Femoral tunnel placement. View confirms that the guide pin is 7 mm from the over-the-top position. (From Miller MD, Howard RF, Plancher KD: *Surgical atlas of sports medicine.* Philadelphia, 2003, WB Saunders.)

- Arthrofibrosis can be a result of performing surgery during the acute phase of injury or poor early postoperative rehabilitation. Lysis of adhesions and manipulation under anesthesia are indicated in patients who fail to regain reasonable motion 6 to 12 weeks postoperatively despite therapy.
- Hardware and graft fixation problems can occur in the early postoperative period. It is often a good practice to use two types of fixation, especially for the tibial side or both sides in the case of revision.
- Patellar fractures and patellar tendon ruptures can occur following patellar tendon harvesting.
- Saphenous nerve injuries can occur with hamstring harvesting.
- Tunnel osteolysis may occur late and may make revisions challenging.
- A "cyclops lesion" is fibroproliferative scar that can form in front of the notch and block full extension. When recognized, this can be arthroscopically debrided (Figure 7–8).
- Thermal devices should not be used to "shrink" ACLs or ACL grafts because of the risk of ACL rupture following this treatment.

ACL Prevention

- Plyometrics and neuromuscular training has been shown to reduce the incidence of ACL injuries in female athletes (which is significantly higher than that of males) (Figure 7–9).

- Prophylactic ACL functional bracing has only been shown to be beneficial in skiing and not other sports.
- Training reduced the incidence of ACL injuries in elite skiers in a Vermont study but did not affect the incidence in recreational skiers.

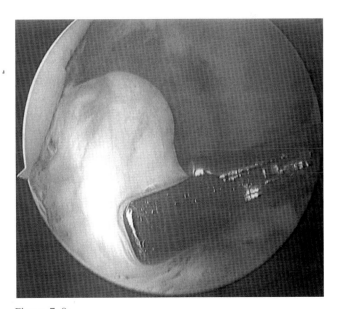

Figure 7–8:
The tibial stump of an injured anterior cruciate ligament graft can hypertrophy and become a cyclops lesion.
(From Diduch DR, Shen FH, Ong BC, et al: Knee: diagnostic arthroscopy. In Miller MD, Cole BJ, editors: *Textbook of arthroscopy.* Philadelphia, 2004, WB Saunders.)

Regular exercises to increase strength – and to keep muscles toned and flexible – are your best defense in preventing sports injuries. But even exercises, if done incorrectly, can cause damage. Before performing the jumping exercises listed here, be sure to warm up by stretching for 15–20 minutes, and cool down with a 2 minute walk and final stretch. Always do jumping exercises on a mat or other appropriate, non-skid, shock-absorbing surface. And take a 30 second rest between exercises to give the body time to recover. Your body will thank you for it!

The following exercise regimen is advocated by David Diduch, MD, Associate Professor of Orthopaedic Surgery and co-director of the Sports Medicine Division. This program is designed to be one in the "off season", six weeks before beginning participation in sports prone to ACL injuries. It has been shown by independent investigators to reduce the rate of ACL tears, especially in females. This regimen helps train the body in proper landing techniques in addition to building strength.

The jump training program and weight training programs are designed to be done on alternate days.

Weight Training Program
(complete 1 set of each exercise: 12 repetitions for upper body and 15 repetitions for the trunk and lower body)

Abdominal curl	Bench press
Back hyperextension	Latissimus doris pulldown
Leg press	Forearm curl
Calf raise	Warm-down/short stretch
Pullover	

Stretches
(perform 3 sets of 30 seconds each)

Calf stretch	Iliotibial band/lower back
Quadriceps	Posterior deltoids
Hamstring	Latissiumus dorsi
Hip flexors	Pectoral/biceps

Jump Training Program
Technique (Weeks 1 and 2)

	Week 1	Week 2
Wall jumps	20 sec	25 sec
Tuck jumps	20 sec	25 sec
Broad jumps stick (hold) landing	5 reps	10 reps
Squat jumps	10 sec	15 sec
Double-legged cone jumps	30 sec/ 30 sec	30 sec/30 sec (side to side and back to front)
180° jumps	20 sec	25 sec
Bounding in place	20 sec	25 sec

Fundamentals (Weeks 3 and 4)

	Week 3	Week4
Wall jumps	30 sec	30 sec
Tuck jumps	30 sec	30 sec
Jump, jump, jump vertical jump	5 reps	8 reps
Squat jumps	10 sec	15 sec
Bounding for distance	1 run	2 runs
Double-legged cone jumps	30 sec/ 30 sec	30sec/30 sec (side to side and back to front)
Scissors jump	30 sec	30 sec
Hop, hop, stick landing	5 reps/leg	5 reps/leg

Performance (Weeks 5 and 6)

	Week 5	Week 6
Wall jumps	30 sec	30 sec
Step, jump up, down, vertical	5 reps	10 reps
Mattress jumps	30 sec/ 30 sec	30 sec/30 sec (side to side and back to front)
Single-leg jumps distance*	5 reps/ leg	5 reps/leg
Squat jumps*	25 sec	25 sec
Bounding for distance	1 run	2 runs
Jump into bounding*	3 runs	4 runs
Hop, hop, stick landing	5 reps/	5 reps/leg

180° jumps: Rotate 180 degrees in mid-air. Hold landing for 2 seconds, then repeat in reverse direction.

Bounding for distance: Start bounding in place and slowly increase distance with each step, keeping knees high.

Bounding in place: Jump from one leg to the other straight up and down, increasing rhythm and height.

Broad jumps stick (hold) landing: Two-footed jump as far as possible. Hold landing for 5 seconds.

Double-legged cone jumps: With feet together, jump side to side over cones quickly, backward and forwards.

Hop, hop, stick landing: Single-leg hop. Stick second landing for 5 secs, increase distance as technique improves.

Jump into bounding: Land on single leg, then bound on two legs for distance.

Jump, jump, vertical: Three broad jumps with vertical jump immediately following last jump.

Mattress jumps: Two-footed jump on mattress, trampoline or similar device. Side to side, back to front.

Scissors jump: Start in stride position with one foot well in front. Jump up, alternating foot position in mid-air.

Single-leg jumps distance: Single-leg hop for distance, then hold landing with knees bent for 5 seconds.

Squat jumps: standing jump, raising both arms overhead, land in squatting position touching hands to floor.

Step, jump up, down, vertical: Two footed jump on 6–8 inch step. Jump off step with 2 feet, then jump up.

Tuck jumps: From Standing position, jump and bring both knees up to chest as high as possible. repeat quickly.

Wall jumps: With knees slightly bent and arms raised overhead, bounce up and down off toes.

Figure 7–9:
Plyometric training for anterior cruciate ligament prevention.

References

Cain EL Jr, Gillogly SD, Andrews JR: Management of intraoperative complications associated with autogenous patellar tendon graft anterior cruciate ligament reconstruction. *Instr Course Lect* 52:359-367, 2003.

Complications with graft harvest, tunnel placement, notch preparation, and graft fixation may be minimized with proper preoperative planning but are at times unavoidable. For this reason, it is important to have alternate graft options available.

Cascio BM, Culp L, Cosgarea AJ: Return to play after anterior cruciate ligament reconstruction. *Clin Sports Med* 23:395-408, 2004.

This is a review article that addresses the issue of return to play after ACL injury and reconstruction. It discusses principles of rehabilitation and specific criteria to return to athletic activity.

Costa-Paz M, Muscolo DL, Ayerza M, et al: Magnetic resonance imaging follow-up study of bone bruises associated with anterior cruciate ligament ruptures. *Arthroscopy* 17:445-449, 2001.

Twenty-one patients with rupture of the ACL and a documented bone bruise on initial MRI were followed with a second imaging study at 2 years after injury. Initial bone bruises were placed into three categories of severity with 100% resolution of grade I lesions but some persistent articular cartilage thinning and depression in all grade III lesions. Clinical scoring was not shown to be significantly different in these groups.

Griffin LY, Agel J, Albohm MJ, et al: Noncontact anterior cruciate ligament injuries: risk factors and prevention strategies. *J Am Acad Orthop Surg* 8:141-150, 2000.

ACL tears are most common in noncontact pivoting sports. It has been suggested that neuromuscular training programs may decrease the incidence of ACL injury in this population, especially in female athletes.

Harmon KG, Ireland ML: Gender differences in noncontact anterior cruciate ligament injuries. *Clin Sports Med* 19:287-302, 2000.

Much discussion has been given to the apparent gender differences associated with ACL injury. Risk factors are identified and prevention strategies suggested to minimize this difference.

Lopez MJ, Markel MD: Anterior cruciate ligament rupture after thermal treatment in a canine model. *Am J Sports Med* 31:164-167, 2003.

Thermal shrinkage was used on canine models with normal ACLs to evaluate the outcome over time. All ligaments ruptured by 55 days after the treatment.

Marcacci M, Molgora AP, Zaffagnini S, et al: Anatomic double-bundle anterior cruciate ligament reconstruction with hamstrings. *Arthroscopy* 19:540-546, 2003.

The technique of double-bundle hamstring ACL reconstruction involves harvesting the gracilis and semitendinosus tendon while leaving them attached on the tibial side and then passing the tendon through the femoral tunnel and into an over-the-top position. After looping and passing into the tibial tunnel, the graft is fixed with a transosseous suture knot. It is felt that this provides a more anatomic reconstruction while avoiding hardware fixation.

Wilson TC, Kantaras A, Atay A, Johnson DL: Tunnel enlargement after anterior cruciate ligament surgery. *Am J Sports Med* 32:543-549, 2004.

Tunnel lysis is a potential complication of ACL reconstruction and has implications during revision surgery. There are multiple causes of tunnel enlargement following ACL reconstruction including both mechanical and biologic factors. Identification of these causes is key to develop techniques to prevent this complication.

Medial Collateral Ligament Injuries

Introduction

- A good understanding of the anatomy of the medial collateral ligament (MCL) and surrounding structures is essential for proper diagnosis, treatment, and surgical correction.
- The medial structure of the knee has been described in three layers (Figures 8–1 and 8–2).
- The MCL complex is composed of the superficial (layer II) and deep (layer III) MCL, as well as the posterior oblique ligament.
- The MCL is a primary medial stabilizer of the knee against valgus stresses and a secondary stabilizer for anterior translation.
- Injury to the MCL places greater forces on the anterior cruciate ligament (ACL) to counteract valgus stresses, whereas ACL-deficient knees impose greater forces on the MCL when resisting anterior translation.

History, Physical Examination, and Imaging

- A history of trauma, in particular a valgus mechanism, is suggestive of injury to the MCL.
- External rotation is a less common mechanism of injury.
- Physical examination findings include tenderness over the medial aspect of the knee, soft tissue swelling in the presence of an acute injury, and medial joint space opening with valgus stressing at 30 degrees that is stable at 0 degrees.
- The evaluating surgeon should attempt to locate which portion of the MCL is likely injured (femoral vs. tibial).
- Injuries most commonly occur at the femoral insertion site of the ligament.
- Positive findings with valgus stress should be compared with the contralateral side.
- Medial joint line opening is classically graded according to American Medical Association guidelines (Box 8–1).
- If medial joint space opening is also present at 0 degrees, a combined ligamentous injury should be suspected in addition to severe injury to the MCL.

- Combined MCL and ACL injury produces significant anteromedial instability about the knee.
- Anterior drawer testing with the foot in external rotation may demonstrate anteromedial translation of the tibia that is accentuated with concurrent ACL tears. This test is often difficult to perform in the acute setting.
- Chronic injury may reveal a Pellegrini-Stieda lesion of the medial femoral epicondyle (a bony avulsion injury with calcification/heterotropic ossification of the femoral insertion of the MCL); otherwise, plain radiographs are often normal.
- In children with open physes, stress radiographs should be performed to rule out possible Salter-Harris fractures and validate potentially true ligamentous injury.
- Although physical examination is usually diagnostic, magnetic resonance imaging (MRI) can provide good visualization of the torn MCL, demonstrating the location of injury, which may assist in determining the prognosis of nonoperative treatment (Figure 8–3).
- A classification of MRI findings has been devised (Box 8–2).
- MRI can also be useful to diagnose other injured structures, most commonly the ACL.

Treatment

- Isolated MCL injuries usually respond to conservative therapy (Figure 8–4).
- Femoral-sided MCL injuries tend to respond better to conservative management than tibial-sided MCL injuries.
- Grade III tears that involve the entire length of the superficial layer may not respond to nonoperative management.
- Bracing may be helpful with protected, early range of motion.
- Prophylactic bracing in football players has been shown in some studies to be helpful in reducing the incidence of injuries in certain down lineman positions.
- MCL repair is considered with multiligamentous injuries.
- Treatment of combined ACL and MCL injuries is controversial—some studies have shown that early

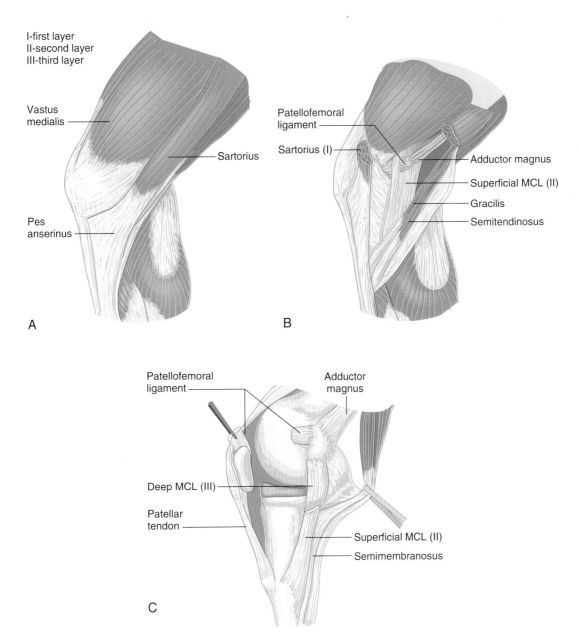

Figure 8–1:
Anatomy of the medial knee in layers. A, Layer I contains the tensor fascia lata and sartorius. B, Layer II contains the superficial medial collateral ligament (MCL), semimembranosus, and posterior oblique ligament. C, Layer III contains the deep MCL and capsule. (Redrawn from Warren RF, Arnockzy SP, Wickiewicz TL: Anatomy of the knee. In Nicholas JA, Hershman E, editors: *The lower extremity and spine in sports medicine,* 2nd ed. St Louis, 1995, Mosby-Year Book.)

surgical management of both injuries can lead to loss of motion.
- One therapeutic algorithm of combined MCL/ACL injury involves bracing with protected range of motion to allow the MCL to heal, followed by surgical reconstruction of the ACL when medial stability is restored and swelling and range of

motion has improved, minimizing the chance of developing an extension contracture and arthrofibrosis.
- Some authors recommend ACL reconstruction followed by a program of early weight-bearing, range of motion, and strengthening and allowing the MCL to heal without surgery.

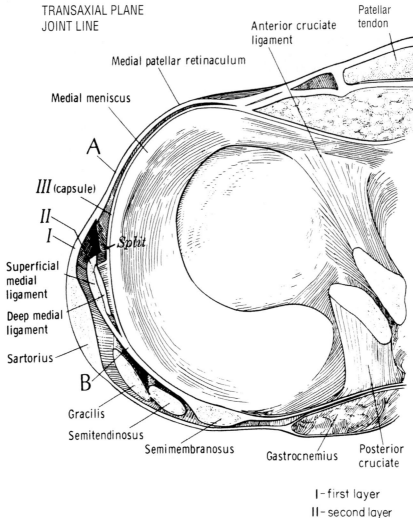

TRANSAXIAL PLANE
JOINT LINE

Patellar tendon

Anterior cruciate ligament

Medial patellar retinaculum

Medial meniscus

A

III (capsule)

II

I

Split

Superficial medial ligament

Deep medial ligament

Sartorius

B

Gracilis

Semitendinosus

Semimembranosus

Gastrocnemius

Posterior cruciate

I - first layer
II - second layer
III - third layer

Figure 8–2:
Cross sectional view of the medial knee.
(From Warren LF, Marshal JL: *J Bone Joint Surg Am* 61:56-62, 1979.)

- Other authors have reported success in surgical repair of acute MCL injuries with reconstruction of the ACL when conservative measures have failed.
- Conservatively treated MCL injuries (particularly grade III injuries) should be closely monitored and considered for surgical repair/reconstruction if instability continues to be present.

Box 8–1	Classification of Medial Joint Line Opening with Valgus Stress

Grade 0/Normal: 0 to 2 mm
Grade I: 3 to 5 mm
Grade II: 5 to 10 mm
Grade III: Greater than 10 mm

- Surgical repair techniques that have been described include proximal advancement of the MCL with repair and reinforcement of the posteromedial structures including the posterior oblique ligament (Figure 8–5).
- Reconstructions described have included patellar tendon or hamstring autografts and allograft tissue (Figure 8–6).

Rehabilitation

- The goal of rehabilitation is to regain full range of motion as soon as possible.
- Early, protected range of motion in a range of motion brace should be part of any rehabilitative program of conservatively or surgically managed MCLs.

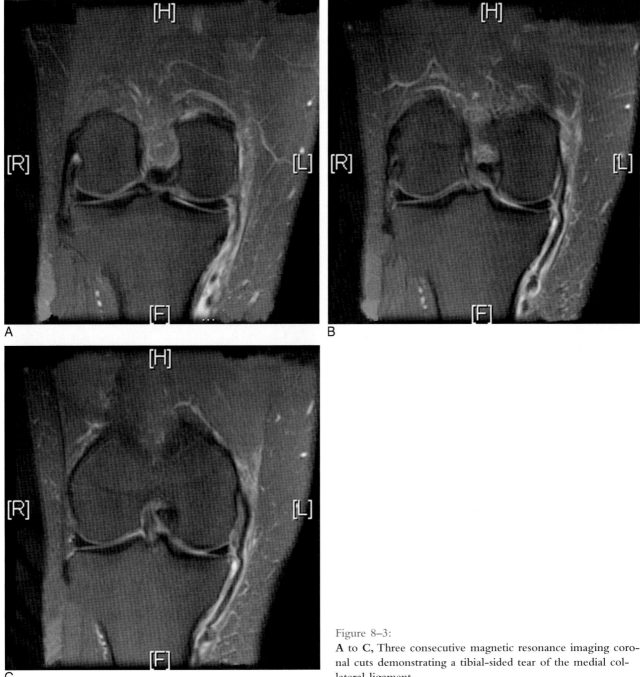

Figure 8–3:
A to **C,** Three consecutive magnetic resonance imaging coronal cuts demonstrating a tibial-sided tear of the medial collateral ligament.

- Full extension symmetrical to the contralateral, uninjured knee should be emphasized early.
- Patients may return to full activity when they have regained full strength and range of motion, with no signs of instability on examination.

Complications

- The most common complication of MCL injuries is loss of motion.

Box 8–2	**Magnetic Resonance Imaging Classification of Medial Collateral Ligament (MCL) injury**

Grade I: Minor tearing of MCL fibers
Grade II: Complete disruption of the superficial MCL
Grade III: Complete disruption of the superficial and deep MCL

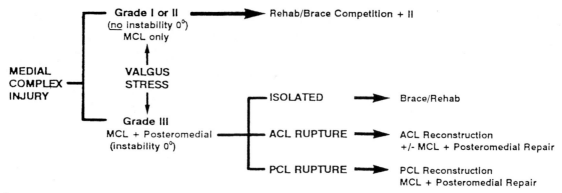

Figure 8–4:

Algorithm for the treatment of medial collateral ligament injuries.

(From Spindler KP, Walker RN: General approach to ligament surgery. In Fu FH, Harner CD, Vince KG, editors: *Knee surgery.* Baltimore, 1994, Williams & Wilkins.)

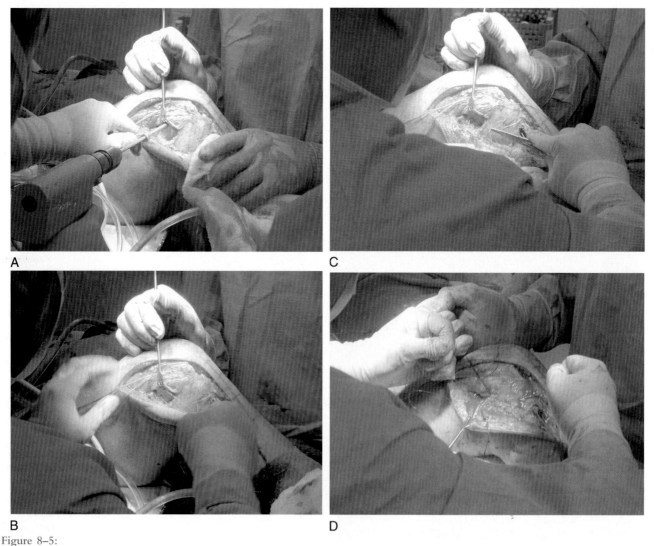

Figure 8–5:

Medial collateral ligament (MCL) repair. **A,** Suture anchor placement in the anatomic insertion of the proximal MCL (medial femoral epicondyle). **B,** Two suture anchors in place. The medial patellofemoral ligament and retinaculum were torn and are being retracted. **C,** The sutures from the suture anchors are being sutured through the proximal MCL and posterior oblique ligament. **D,** The sutures are being tied following repair of the MCL and posterior oblique ligament and medial patellofemoral ligament.

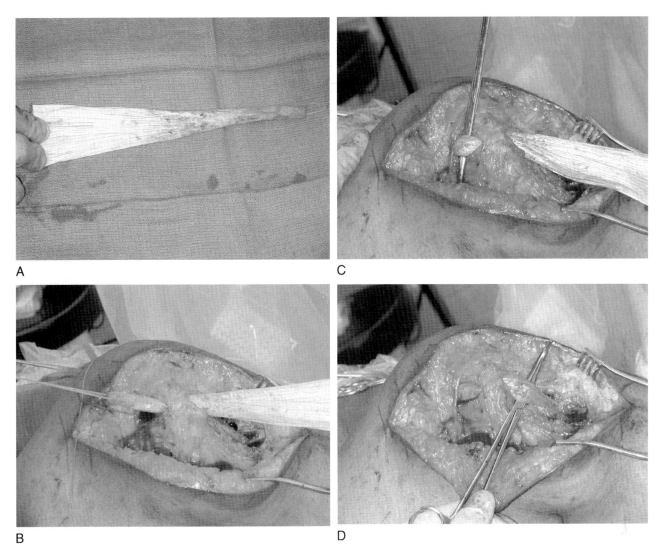

A

B

C

D

Figure 8–6:
Medial collateral ligament (MCL) reconstruction. **A,** Achilles tendon allograft used for the reconstruction. **B,** Achilles allograft is passed under the intact medial patellofemoral ligament. **C,** The bone plug on the Achilles allograft is fixed in a bone tunnel created in the anatomic insertion of the MCL at the medial femoral epicondyle. **D,** The tendinous portion of the Achilles allograft is then brought through a drill hole in the tibial insertion of the MCL. The hemostat is under the MCL graft. The sutures are brought out of the other side of the tibia and tensioned with the knee in 30 degrees of flexion and a varus force on the knee. The tibial MCL graft is then fixed using a bioscrew.

- Early, protected range of motion is essential to reduce the incidence of this complication.
- Loss of motion after surgery can be restored with physical therapy protocols and, when necessary, surgical management.

References

Borden PS, Kantaras AT, Caborn DN: Medial collateral ligament reconstruction with allograft using double-bundle technique. *Arthroscopy* 18(4):E19, 2002.
    Surgical technique using allograft tissue is described for isolated MCL and combined MCL/ACL ruptures. The authors use a double bundle allograft with two free ends to reconstruct and address the anterior and posterior components of the MCL, providing desired stability to valgus and rotational forces. The use of interference screws is reported to have the advantage of allowing immediate postoperative range of motion.

Frolke JP, Oskam J, Vierhout PA: Primary reconstruction of the medial collateral ligament in combined injury of the medial collateral and anterior cruciate ligaments. *Knee Surg Sports Traumatol Arthrosc* 6:103-106, 1998.
    Study in which 15 of 22 MCL- and ACL-injured knees demonstrated improvement after arthroscopic-guided repair of the MCL with nonoperative treatment of the ACL.

Hillard-Sembbell D, Daniel DM, Stone ML, et al: Combined injuries of the anterior cruciate ligament and medial collateral ligaments of the knee. *J Bone Joint Surg Am* 78:169-176, 1996.

Retrospective study evaluating valgus instability following different treatment modalities in 66 patients with combined injury of the anterior cruciate and medial collateral ligaments. Eleven patients underwent reconstruction of the ACL and MCL, 33 had only ACL reconstruction, and 22 were managed conservatively. Using clinical and radiographic evaluations, the authors were unable to demonstrate differences in late valgus instability between the treatment modalities used. Authors also compared the results of 22 of their 33 patients with combined injuries, treated with only ACL reconstruction, to 37 patients who had ACL reconstruction of isolated tears. Again, no differences in stability or function were demonstrated, leading the authors to conclude that patients with mild to moderate valgus instability and combined ligament tears do not require repair of the MCL.

Hughston, JC: The importance of the poterior oblique ligament in repairs of acute tears of the medial ligaments in knees with and without an associated rupture of the anterior cruciate ligament: results of long-term follow-up. *J Bone Joint surg Am* 76(9):1328-1344, 1994.

Forty-one patients who had acute medial knee injuries underwent surgical repair including repair of the posterior oblique ligament. The authors followed these patients for an average of 22 years and were able to conclude that this approach can lead to a low failure rate (7%) and a high level of return to sport.

Millet PJ, Wickiewicz TL, Warren RF: Motion loss after ligament injuries to the knee. Part II: prevention and treatment. *Am J Sport Med* 29:822-828, 2001.

Good review on the prevention and treatment of motion problems about the knee that may present after injury or surgery. Authors stress the importance of delaying reconstructive knee surgeries until full range of motion and swelling have resolved. Recommend delayed ACL reconstruction on patients with concomitant MCL injuries, supported by references.

Nakamura N, Horibe S, Toritsuka Y, et al: Acute grade III medial collateral ligament injury of the knee associated with anterior cruciate ligament tear. The usefulness of magnetic resonance imaging in determining a treatment regimen. *Am J Sport Med* 31:261-267, 2003.

Prospective cohort study assessing the ability of MRI to predict nonoperative outcome of MCL/ACL injured knees treated with only ACL reconstruction. Study demonstrated that 5 of the 6 patients (of 17 total patients) who required MCL repair (showing valgus laxity after a 6-week period of conservative treatment) demonstrated disruption over the entire length of the superficial MCL layer. All other patients had localized injury at the femoral attachment site.

Robins AJ, Newman AP, Burks RT: Postoperative return of motion in anterior cruciate ligament and medial collateral ligament injuries. *Am J Sports Med* 21:20-25, 1993.

Small retrospective study to determine a possible correlation between MCL tear location and postoperative outcomes. Twenty patients with combined anterior cruciate and medial collateral ligamentous injury underwent ACL reconstruction and MCL repair. Thirteen patients had tears at or proximal to the joint line, and seven patients had tears more distally. After analyzing their results, the authors concluded that patients with distal tears had an earlier return of and greater function. As a result, they recommended that patients with proximal tears be managed more aggressively from the start of treatment.

Sawant M, Murty AN, Ireland J: Valgus knee injuries: evaluation and documentation using a simple technique of stress radiography. *Knee* 11:25-28, 2004.

Describes using stress radiographs imaging both knees (on a single film) and taking the ratio of medial opening of the affected to the normal contralateral knee. The ratio of patients with an injured MCL ranged from 1.1 to 3.6. A ratio equal to or greater than 2 was indicative of concomitant ACL or posterior cruciate ligament injury (sensitivity 94%, specificity 86%).

Shelbourne KD, Porter DA: Anterior cruciate ligament-medial collateral ligament injury: nonoperative management of medial collateral ligament tears with anterior cruciate ligament reconstruction. A preliminary report. *Am J Sports Med* 20:283-286, 1992.

The authors follow 84 consecutive cases of combined ACL and MCL injury. Each patient had the ACL reconstructed, whereas the MCL was treated conservatively. Follow-up of up to 3 years, including subjective and objective measurements of pain, function, and instability, demonstrates that patients with combined ACL and MCL tears do very well without surgical treatment of the medial injury.

Shirakura K, Terauch, Katayama M, et al: The management of medial ligament tears in patients with combined anterior cruciate and medial ligament lesions. *Int Orthop* 24:108-111, 2000.

Retrospective study of 25 patients with combined ACL and MCL injury who were treated with either MCL repair with early immobilization (14) or conservative treatment with 2 weeks of immobilization (11). Results demonstrated no statistical differences when comparing clinical laxity, KT-1000 measurements, and Tegner activity score between the two groups. However, the operative group did demonstrate a statistically higher Lyshol function score (98.5 vs. 93.8). Site of MCL damage did not appear to influence outcomes.

Posterior Cruciate Ligament Injuries

Injury Mechanism and Diagnosis

- More common and associated with more morbidity than once believed.
- Intact posterior cruciate ligament (PCL) is a primary restraint to posterior tibial displacement and secondary restraint to varus, valgus, and rotatory instability.
- The two most common mechanisms of injury to the PCL are direct blow to the anterior tibia (motor vehicle crash dashboard injury), hyperflexion (noncontact), or hyperextension (bicruciate injury).
- The most obvious physical examination finding is the posterior sag sign (Figure 9–1). Patients will also commonly have anterior tibial contusions or popliteal ecchymosis if presenting acutely. Many patients present chronically and localize their complaints to a painful medial and/or patellofemoral compartment due to the degenerative process.
- The posterior drawer sign is the key examination finding for PCL deficiency and is performed at 90 degrees of knee flexion. It is graded I, II, or III on the basis of the amount of displacement of the tibial plateau in relation to the femoral condyle. Because the tibia typically is resting in a posteriorly subluxated position, the test should be initiated with the tibia reduced to prevent a misdiagnosis of anterior cruciate ligament (ACL) injury. The grade of injury has implications for treatment (Table 9–1).
- The quadriceps active test demonstrates that the posteriorly displaced tibia reduces with anterior force from contraction of the quadriceps.
- Tests to evaluate for commonly associated posterolateral corner instability include the Dial test at 30 and 90 degrees and the external rotation recurvatum test. These patients may also ambulate with a varus thrust. Failure to address and stabilize this associated pathology will likely result in failure of an isolated PCL reconstruction.
- Stress radiographs either manually or with the Telos device can provide an objective analysis of the amount of tibial displacement. Comparison with the contralateral stable knee corrects for differences due to ligamentous laxity (Figures 9–2 and 9–3).
- Magnetic resonance imaging (MRI) may be helpful to evaluate the integrity of the PCL and to evaluate for commonly associated pathology such as to the posterolateral corner. The PCL is much more dense and distinct than the ACL. The entire PCL is typically seen on coronal and sagittal scans as scanning is more commonly performed in the plane of the ligament. MRI can also demonstrate the meniscofemoral ligaments around the PCL (ligaments of Humphrey and Wrisberg). A "double PCL sign" is what appears to be two PCLs, but the

Figure 9–1:
Posterior sag sign in posterior cruciate ligament rupture.

Table 9–1:	Grades of Posterior Cruciate Ligament (PCL) Injury	
GRADE	AMOUNT OF DISPLACEMENT	TREATMENT
I	<5mm	Conservative
II	5-10 mm Flush with femoral condyle	Conservative
III	>10 mm Posterior to femoral condyle	Surgical (usually combined injury)

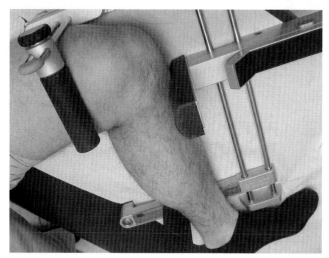

Figure 9–2:
Telos device for performing stress radiographs.

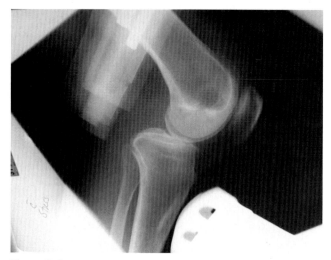

Figure 9–3:
Posterior displacement demonstrated on stress radiographs with Telos device.

anterior structure is actually a flipped bucket-handle medial meniscal tear retained in the notch (Figure 9–4).

Treatment Options

- Selection of appropriate treatment is dependent on the type of injury sustained (Figures 9–5 and 9–6).
- A bony avulsion of the ligamentous insertion may be treated by open reduction and internal fixation if the bony fragment is large enough to accommodate the hardware. Transtibial suture fixation over a button on the anteromedial aspect of the tibia can be used when comminution of the bony fragment is encountered. These must be fixed acutely.

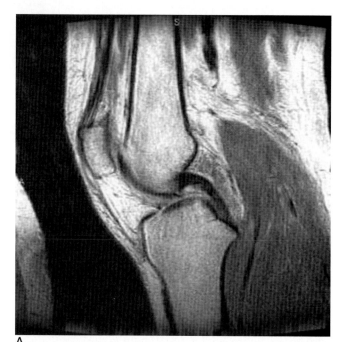

A

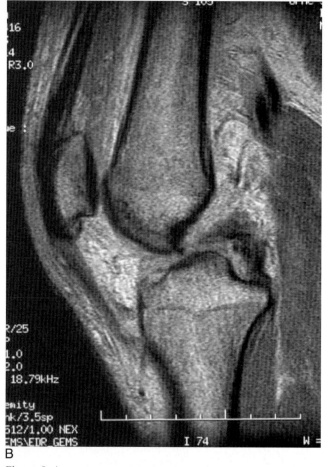

B

Figure 9–4:
A, Sagittal magnetic resonance imaging (MRI) view demonstrating a normal posterior cruciate ligament (PCL). **B,** Sagittal MRI demonstrating a torn PCL. (From Miller MD, Cole BJ: *Textbook of arthroscopy.* Philadelphia, 2004, WB Saunders.)

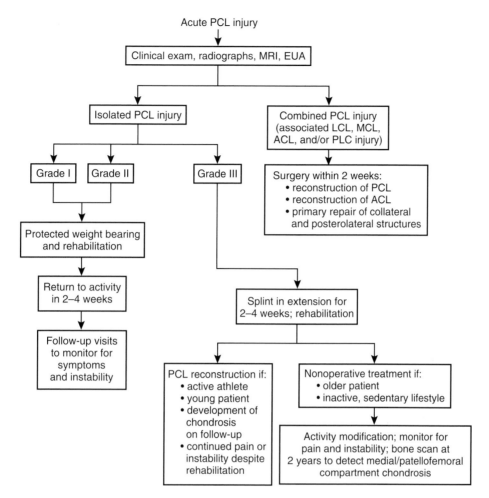

Figure 9–5:
Treatment algorithm for acute posterior cruciate ligament (PCL) injury.
(From Miller MD, Cole BJ: *Textbook of arthroscopy.* Philadelphia, 2004, WB Saunders.)

- Isolated PCL injuries may be treated nonoperatively, especially if determined to be grade I or II.
  - In these cases, an extension brace should be used for 2 to 4 weeks and physical therapy should concentrate on quadriceps strengthening to compensate for posterior translation.
  - The risk of treating grade III PCL deficient knees nonoperatively is the late development of chondrosis of the medial femoral condyle and patellofemoral articulation.
  - The use of bone scan to evaluate these compartments if the patient becomes symptomatic is useful in making operative decisions (Figure 9–7).
  - Operative thresholds for reconstruction continue to be controversial with a trend toward more aggressive management, particularly in younger patients.
- Partial PCL tears are treated conservatively and monitored for development of symptoms.

Surgical Reconstruction

- Transtibial technique (Figure 9–8*A*).
  - Involves a traditional ACL-type approach with a transtibial anterior to posterior tunnel.
  - Risk is to the posterior neurovascular structures with passage of the tibial tunnel guidewire or reamer, or both. The neurovascular bundle is anatomically 4 mm posterior to the posterior horn of the lateral meniscus. Recommendations to prevent injury include visualization both fluoroscopically and through a posteromedial portal, protecting the tissues with a curette or similar device, and hand reaming through the posterior cortex for greater control.
  - There is a potential for graft abrasion at anterior edge of the tibial tunnel ("killer curve" phenomenon). A maximally vertically placed tibial tunnel and placement of the tunnel intraarticular aperture in the more distal

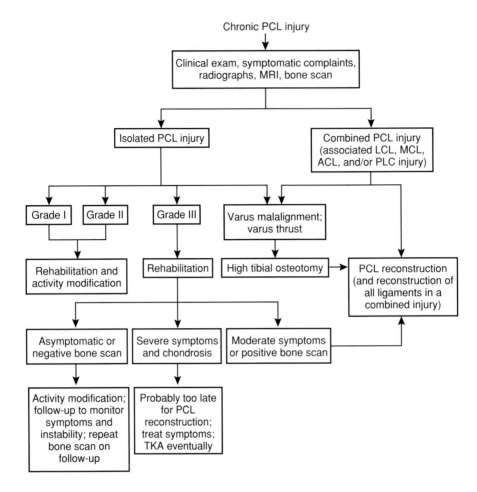

Figure 9–6:
Treatment algorithm for chronic posterior cruciate ligament (PCL) injury.
(From Miller MD, Cole BJ: *Textbook of arthroscopy.* Philadelphia, 2004, WB Saunders.)

portion of the tibial upslope (true insertion of anterolateral bundle) reduces this angle and theoretical stress on the graft.

- Tibial inlay technique (Figure 9–8*B*).
  - Considered to be a more "anatomic" reconstruction.
  - Quicker incorporation of tibial bone block compared with soft tissue graft used with transtibial technique.
  - Literature supports less graft attrition and failure.
  - Popliteal fossa dissection theoretically places neurovascular structures at greater risk and may not be an option with extensive soft tissue injury.
  - Transverse skin incision in the popliteal fossa prevents wound complications associated with an S-type or L-type incision (ischemic corner in already traumatized tissue due to initial injury).
  - Natural anatomic interval between the semimembranosus and medial head of the gastrocnemius allows for blunt dissection over the posterior capsule to PCL insertion. Retraction of entire

posterior soft tissue envelope laterally with the use of K-wires placed in the posterior tibia protects the neurovascular bundle during the reconstruction.

- Newer techniques are currently in development to perform a transtibial arthroscopic inlay technique. This technique uses a reverse reamer through the tibia to create a trough for the graft bone block, and transtibial suture fixation is tied over a button on the anteromedial tibia to fix the graft.
- Double-bundle technique (Figure 9–8*C*).
  - Transtibial tunnel or tibial inlay technique with two transfemoral tunnels to re-create the posteromedial and anterolateral bundles.
  - Hypothetically results in better rotational and translational stability throughout both flexion and extension.
  - Theorized possibility of medial femoral condylar fracture, collapse, or avascular necrosis due to the amount of bone removed for tunnel preparation

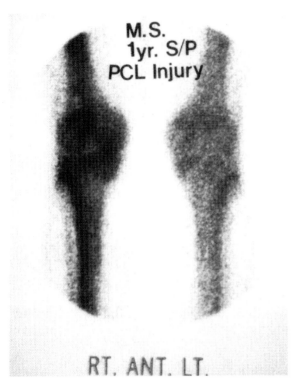

Figure 9–7:
Technetium bone scan of a patient with a chronic posterior cruciate ligament (PCL) injury. Note the diffuse uptake in the affected right knee. The association of chondral injury with chronic PCL injuries is well documented with bone scan images. (From Miller MD, Cooper DE, Warner JP: *Review of sports medicine and arthroscopy.* Philadelphia, 2002, WB Saunders.)

creating a larger stress riser and greater disruption of the blood supply. This can be avoided by not placing the femoral tunnel extraarticular aperture too close to the articular surface (Figure 9–9).

Postoperative Rehabilitation

- Postoperative rehabilitation is somewhat dependent on the technique used to reconstruct the PCL and the fixation involved.
- Generally, the patient is left at 50% weight-bearing for the first 4 weeks of the postoperative period.
- Initial bracing in extension relaxes the anterolateral component of the PCL and minimizes gravitational forces.
- Emphasis on early progression of motion. Initially, flexion exercises should be done in the prone position only to prevent an increased gravitational stress on the graft. These patients tend to lose full extension unless this is

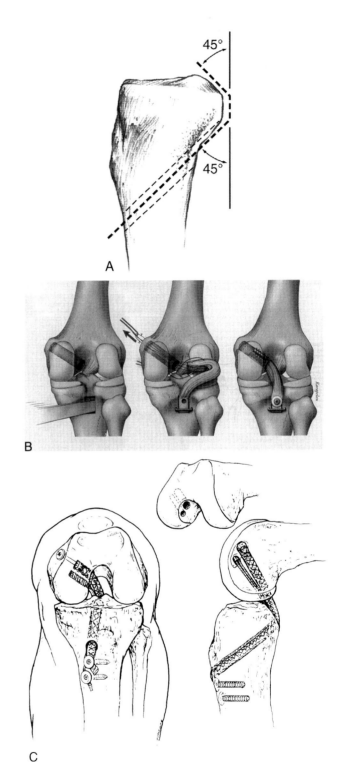

Figure 9–8:
A, Desired turning angles of the posterior cruciate ligament (PCL) graft using the transtibial tunnel technique. **B,** Tibial inlay technique. (**A** from Miller MD, Cole BJ: *Textbook of arthroscopy.* Philadelphia, 2004, WB Saunders; **B** from Gill SS, Cohen SB, Miller MD: PCL inlay and posterolateral corner reconstruction. In Miller MD, Cole BJ, editors: *Textbook of arthroscopy.* Philadelphia, 2004, WB Saunders.) **C,** Double-bundle technique. (**C** from Miller MD, Howard RF, Plancher KD: *Surgical atlas of sports medicine.* Philadelphia, 2003, WB Saunders.)

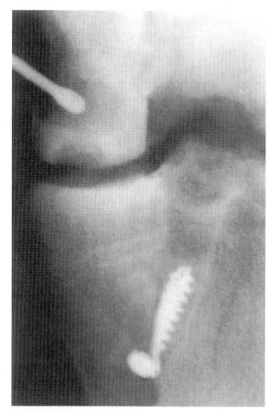

Figure 9–9:
Intraoperative fluoroscopic view of medial femoral condyle avascular necrosis. The area of necrosis is distal to the femoral tunnel used for posterior cruciate ligament (PCL) reconstruction. This area was drilled and bone grafted 9 months following the PCL reconstruction. (From Veltri DM, Warren RF, Silver G: *Op Tech Sports Med* 1:157, 1993.)

emphasized from the beginning of their rehabilitative course.

- Quadriceps strengthening may begin immediately with straight leg raises and quad sets.
- Hamstring isometrics should be avoided for the first 6 weeks postoperatively.

References

Andrews JR, Edwards JC, Satterwhite YE: Isolated posterior cruciate ligament injuries. History, mechanism of injury, physical findings, and ancillary tests. *Clin Sports Med* 13:519-530, 1994.
This paper provides a comprehensive review of the basics in understanding and identifying PCL injuries. It discusses the importance of plain and stress radiographs in making the diagnosis of a PCL tear, as well as the importance of MRI as the most sensitive objective evaluation of PCL integrity.

Borden PS, Nyland JA, Caborn DN: Posterior cruciate ligament reconstruction (double bundle) using anterior tibialis tendon allograft. *Arthroscopy* 17(4):E14, 2001.
In this paper, the author introduces the concept of using a cryopreserved anterior tibialis tendon allograft with bioabsorbable fixation. Other graft choices such as autograft quadriceps tendons and hamstring tendons have also been described (see Richards RS et al. and Stahelin AC et al.).

Cooper DE, Stewart D: Posterior cruciate ligament reconstruction using single-bundle patella tendon graft with tibial inlay fixation. *Am J Sports Med* 32:346-360, 2004.
This study looks at 2-year outcomes of patients with PCL reconstructions with the tibial inlay technique. They demonstrate a mean improvement of two grades of translation from the PCL-injured state. They show an improved average side to side displacement distance measured with Telos of 4.11 mm postoperatively (compared with a minimum displacement of 12 mm preoperatively) and marked improvements in patient satisfaction.

Fanelli GC, Edson CJ: Combined posterior cruciate ligament-posterolateral reconstructions with Achilles tendon allograft and biceps femoris tenodesis: 2 to 10 year follow-up. *Arthroscopy* 20:339-345, 2004.
This is a case series of 41 patients with combined reconstruction of the PCL with Achilles tendon allograft and posterolateral corner reconstruction with biceps femoris tenodesis and capsular shift. Follow-up evaluation at 2 to 10 years using objective data from arthrometry, stress radiography, and physical examination shows significant improvement in patient function with this technique.

Johnson DH, Fanelli GC, Miller MD: PCL 2002: indications, double-bundle versus inlay technique and revision surgery. *Arthroscopy* 18(9 suppl 2):40-52, 2002.
This article gives an overview of PCL injury and surgical indications, as well as technique guides to two of the most commonly performed reconstructive techniques. Both techniques are evaluated and found to have significant improvements in patient symptoms and stability.

Miller MD, Kline AJ, Gonzales J, Beach WR: Vascular risk associated with a posterior approach for posterior cruciate ligament reconstruction using the tibial inlay technique. *J Knee Surg* 15:137-140, 2002.
Because the approach to a tibial inlay type of PCL reconstruction is directly posterior, the authors of this paper look at the relative risk to the popliteal artery. They used cadavers and injected the femoral arteries with barium. The standard inlay approach was performed and a bicortical screw was placed posterior to anterior. Radiographs were used to measure the distance from the screw to the popliteal artery with the closest distance being 18.1 mm. From this, the authors concluded that there is a low relative risk to the popliteal artery from this posterior approach.

Richards RS, Moorman CT: Use of autograft quadriceps tendon for double-bundle posterior cruciate ligament reconstruction. *Arthroscopy* 19:906-915, 2003.
These authors are proponents of the use of quadriceps tendon autografts if the aforementioned tendon is adequate. Reasons for this include having a bone plug configuration for fixation, and the paper serves as a technique guide for harvest and fixation of the graft.

Seitz H, Schlenz I, Pajenda G, Vecsei A: Tibial avulsion fracture of the posterior cruciate ligament: k-wire or screw fixation? A retrospective study of 26 patients. *Arch Orthop Trauma Surg* 116:275-278, 1997.
Bony avulsions encompass only a small portion of total PCL injuries, but they are significant because treatment may often be by open reduc-

tion, internal fixation rather than reconstruction. These authors look at two common methods of fixation of the distal bony fragment and are unable to identify a difference in terms of stability or symptomatic outcome.

Stahelin AC, Sudkamp NP, Weiler A: Anatomic double-bundle posterior cruciate ligament reconstruction using hamstring tendons. *Arthroscopy* 17:88-97, 2001.

These authors give another graft choice for PCL reconstruction. They emphasize that the double-bundle technique is biomechanically superior to that of a single-bundle. They feel that their technique is more anatomically and functionally related to the normal PCL because the semitendinosus portion of the graft is fixed in flexion and the gracilis tendon part is fixed in extension.

CHAPTER 10

Lateral Collateral Ligament and Posterolateral Corner Injuries

Introduction

- Lateral collateral ligament (LCL) and posterolateral corner (PLC) injuries are more common than previously thought due to an increased awareness of these injuries.
- LCL injuries are much less common than medial collateral ligament (MCL) injuries and rarely occur in isolation.
- PLC injuries most often present with other ligamentous injury.

- Similar to the medial side of the knee, the lateral anatomy can also be divided into three layers (Figure 10–1, Box 10–1).
- The PLC complex includes several structures (Box 10–2).
- The LCL is a primary stabilizer of the knee for varus loads.
- The PLC (most notably the popliteofibular ligament and popliteus) is critical in providing the knee with stability against external rotation and posterior translation.

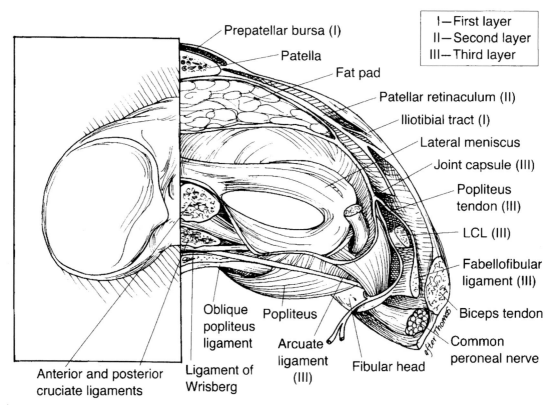

Figure 10–1:
Anatomy of the lateral side of the knee.
(From Seebacher JR, Inglis AE, Marshall FL, Warren RF: *J Bone Joint Surg Am* 64:536-541, 1982.)

Box 10–1	Structures of the Three Layers of the Lateral Knee

Layer I: Lateral fascia, Iliotibial tract, biceps tendon
Layer II: Patellar retinaculum, patellofemoral ligament
Layer III: Lateral collateral ligament, popliteofibular ligament, fabellofibular ligament, popliteus tendon, arcuate ligament, capsule

Box 10–2	Structures of the Posterolateral Corner

Popliteus tendon
Popliteofibular ligament
Arcuate ligament
Fabellofibular ligament
Biceps femoris tendon
Iliotibial band
Lateral gastrocnemius tendon

History, Physical Examination, and Imaging

- Mechanism of injury is variable and can include a varus load to the knee, an external rotational torque, or a combined force resulting in a knee dislocation and subsequent multiple ligament knee injury.
- Severe injuries may be associated with peroneal nerve injury and produce symptoms of paresthesias on the dorsum of the foot, foot drop, or weak dorsiflexion.

Box 10–3	Clinical Findings and Tests Associated with Lateral Collateral Ligament (LCL) or Posterolateral Corner (PLC) Injury

LCL injury

Lateral compartment tenderness
Lateral knee swelling
Varus laxity at 30 degrees (isolated injury)
Varus laxity at 0 degrees with combined ligamentous injury

PLC injury

External rotation test ("Dial test") positive at 30 degrees
External rotation test positive at 90 degrees with concomitant PCL injury
External rotation recurvatum test
Increased posterolateral translation with posterolateral drawer test
Reverse pivot-shift test
Posterolateral Lachman
Varus thrust gait
Genu varus

- Physical examination is the key to diagnosis (Box 10–3).
- In the acute setting, an examination under anesthesia may be required for proper ligamentous assessment/evaluation.
- Acute injuries of the LCL present with pain and soft tissue swelling along the lateral aspect of the knee, with varus laxity at 30 degrees and at 0 degrees if a combined cruciate injury is present. Increasing varus laxity is appreciated with concomitant PLC injury.
- Patients with PLC injuries may complain of instability and demonstrate a varus thrust gait that can be compensated by internally rotating the foot and flexing the knee and enhanced with the foot in external rotation.
- Grading of lateral joint line opening and posterolateral translation is performed similar to MCL injuries.
- Injury to the PLC results in increased external rotation of the tibia on the femur at 30 degrees ("Dial test") that improves at 90 degrees when compared with the contralateral knee (Figure 10–2).
- Further asymmetry with external rotation at 90 degrees suggests a combined PLC and posterior cruciate ligament (PCL) injury.
- A reverse pivot shift is performed with the knee in flexion and a valgus and external rotational force applied to the knee. In PLC injuries, this subluxes the tibia posterolaterally, and, as the knee is brought to full extension, the knee suddenly reduces by the pulling action of the iliotibial band, creating a "reverse pivo." (Figure 10–2).
- The external rotation recurvatum test for PLC injury is performed by lifting the extended leg by the great toe and comparing the amount of recurvatum to the contralateral knee. This test is commonly positive in patients with combined PLC and anterior cruciate ligament (ACL) or PCL injuries (Figure 10–2).
- A posterolateral Lachman may be performed to assess the amount of posterolateral translation of the tibia.
- The posterolateral rotation drawer test is performed similar to the posterior drawer but with the foot externally rotated (approximately 15 degrees) and force directed to the PLC (Figure 10–2).
- Because PLC injuries rarely occur in isolation, a comprehensive examination is essential to evaluate the integrity of all other ligaments about the knee.
- Plain radiographs are very useful to rule out bony avulsions such as those of the fibular head—these represent significant LCL and PLC injuries with injury to the LCL, popliteofibular ligament, and the biceps femoris tendon (Figure 10–3).
- Stress radiography and arthroscopic findings may also be useful to demonstrate lateral joint line opening (Figure 10–4).
- In chronic PLC injuries, a fixed varus malalignment or dynamic varus thrust may be present and necessitates evaluation with long leg alignment films.

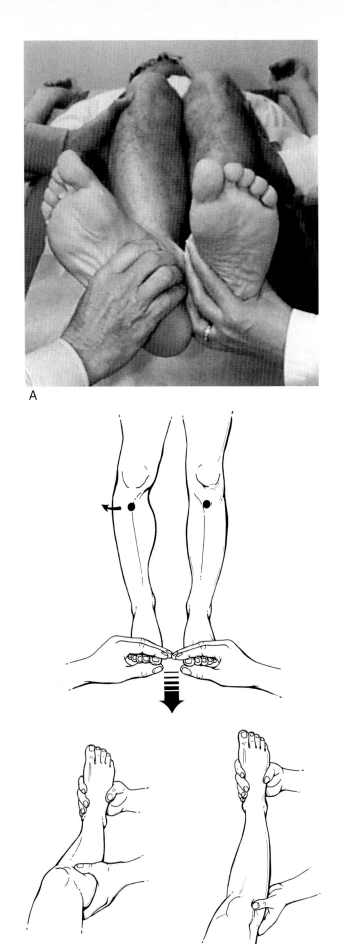

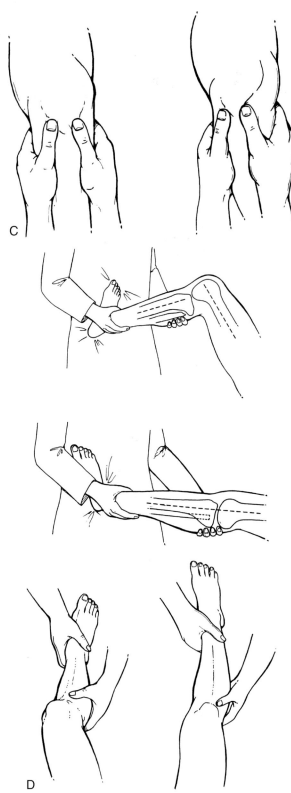

Figure 10–2:

Physical examination maneuvers testing for posterolateral corner (PLC) injury. **A,** Dial test. **B,** External rotation recurvatum test. **C,** Posterolateral drawer test. **D,** Reverse pivot-shift test. (**A** from DeLee JC, Drez D Jr, Miller MD, editors: *DeLee and Drez's orthopaedic sports medicine: principles and practice,* 2nd ed. Philadelphia, 2003, WB Saunders; **B** from Jakob RP, Hassler H, Staubli HU: *Acta Orthop Scand* 191[suppl]:1-32, 1981; Hughston JC, Norwood LA Jr: *Clin Orthop* 147:82-87, 1980; **C** from Hughston JC, Norwood LA Jr: *Clin Orthop* 147:82-87, 1980; **D** from Jakob RP, Hassler H, Staubli HU: *Acta Orthop Scand* 191[Suppl]:1-32, 1981.)

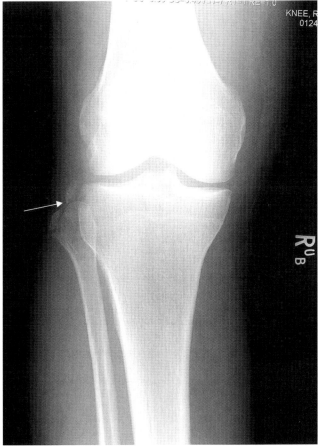

Figure 10–3:
Anteroposterior radiograph demonstrates bony avulsions of the fibular head and proximal lateral tibia (Segund sign) representing disruption of the lateral meniscotibial ligament and posterolateral corner attachments on the fibula.

- Long-leg standing radiographs can further evaluate varus malalignment and are particularly helpful in chronic injuries.
- Magnetic resonance imaging (MRI) can be very accurate in acute injuries showing the location of the tears (femoral/fibular/midsubstance) and can assist the surgeon in making surgical decisions but is less helpful in the chronic setting (Figure 10–5).
- MRI should include coronal oblique views of the entire fibular head and styloid.

Treatment

- Grades I and II LCL and PLC injuries usually do not require surgery unless in conjunction with other ligament injuries (Figure 10–6).
- Treatment of grade I and II PLC injuries includes knee immobilization in extension for approximately 3 weeks followed by progressive rehabilitation.
- Grade III LCL and PLC injuries usually require surgical treatment, particularly if they are in combination with other ligament injuries.
- Acute injuries (less than 3 weeks) are best treated with surgical repair, producing the best outcome in most clinical scenarios.
- Avulsions of the popliteus tendon or fibular collateral ligament can be anatomically repaired directly to bone with suture anchors, recess procedures, or use of cancellous screws (Figure 10–7).
- Careful neurolysis of the peroneal nerve may be required to access, evaluate, and repair structures that lie close to the proximal fibula (Figure 10–8).
- Severe acute injuries may require graft augmentation or reconstruction.

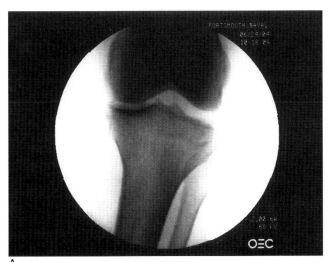

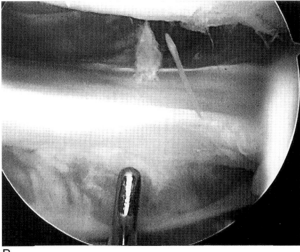

A   B

Figure 10–4:
Lateral joint line opening. A, Lateral joint line opening on a fluoroscopic image during examination under anesthesia. B, Arthroscopic lateral drive through sign revealing greater than 15 mm of lateral compartment opening.

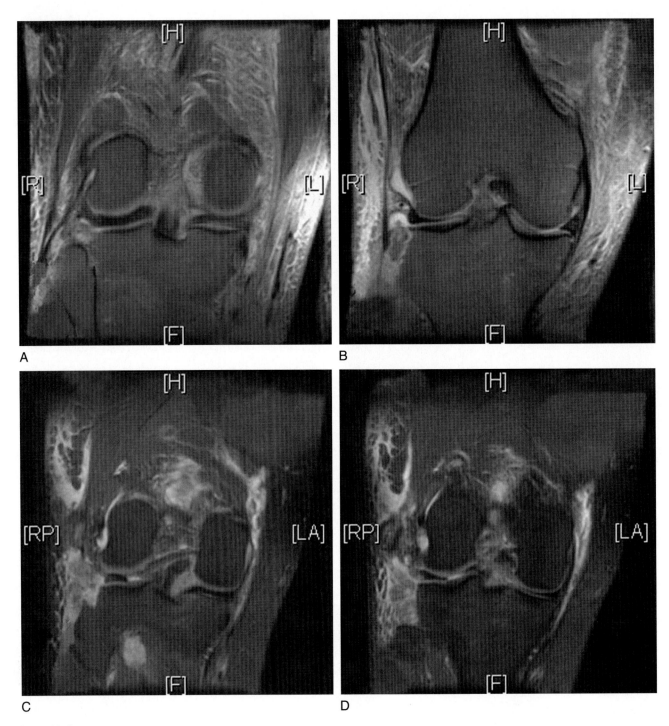

Figure 10–5:
Magnetic resonance imaging (MRI) depicting several different types of lateral collateral ligament (LCL)/posterior lateral corner (PLC) injuries. **A** and **B,** Serial MRI images depicting an acute iliotibial band avulsion from Gerdy's tubercle and biceps femoris avulsion from the fibular head. **C-E,** Serial images demonstrating a complete disruption of the biceps femoris, iliotibial band, LCL, meniscotibial ligaments, and popliteofibular ligament with proximal retraction off the fibular head and proximal lateral tibial.

(continued)

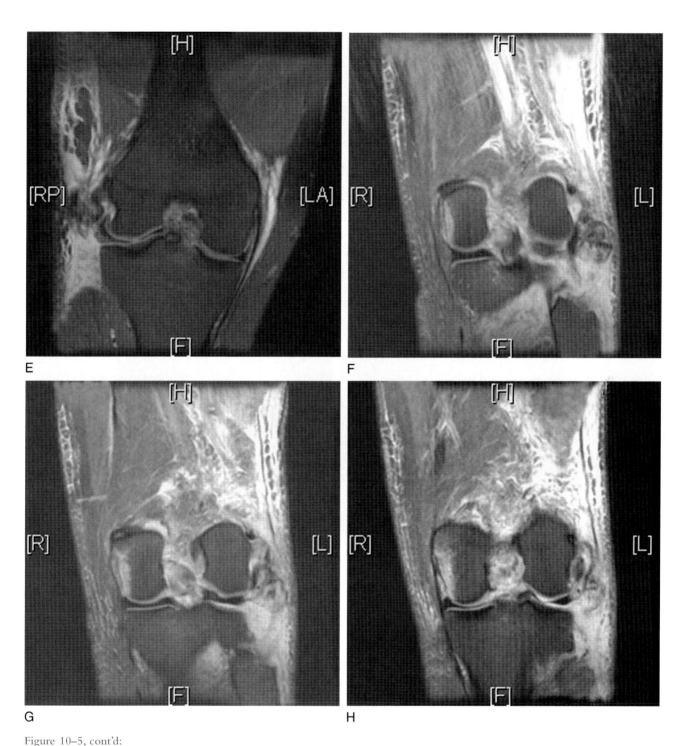

E

F

G

H

Figure 10–5, cont'd:
C-E, Serial images demonstrating a complete disruption of the biceps femoris, iliotibial band, LCL, meniscotibial ligaments, and popliteofibular ligament with proximal retraction off the fibular head and proximal lateral tibial. **F-H,** Similar injury pattern to C-E with a bony avulsion of the fibular head.

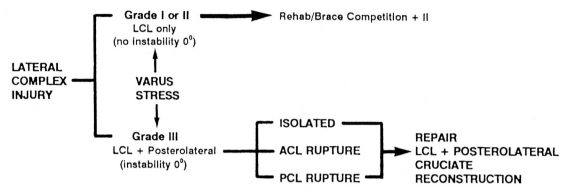

Figure 10–6:

Algorithm for management of lateral collateral ligament (LCL) injuries.

(From Spindler KP, Walker RN: General approach to ligament surgery. In Fu FH, Harner CD, Vince KG, editors: *Knee surgery.* Baltimore, 1994, Williams & Wilkins.)

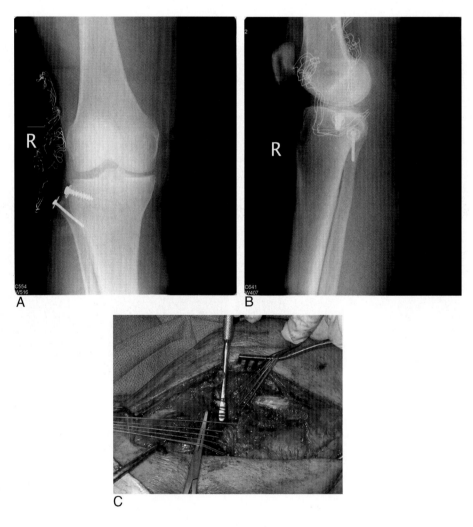

Figure 10–7:

A and **B,** Internal fixation of posterolateral corner injury with screws and washers. **C,** Acute repair of injured posterolateral corner structures.

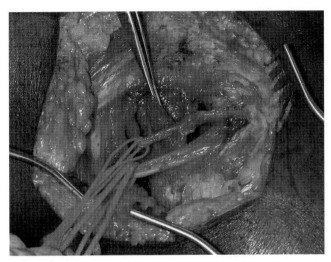

Figure 10–8:
Deep and superficial peroneal nerves dissected, marked, and protected throughout the procedure.

- Subacute and chronic injuries (greater than 2 to 3 weeks) are complicated to repair because of the significant scarring and difficulty in identifying individual structures to be repaired and often necessitate surgical reconstruction.
- Osteotomy of the femoral attachment of the lateral structures with proximal advancement to restore proper tension of the complex has also been described.
- Ensuring proper repair or reconstruction of the posterolateral complex is extremely difficult, with a large learning curve for surgeons new to the procedure.
- In the chronic setting, fixed or dynamic malalignment such as a varus thrust must be addressed with corrective osteotomy before any soft tissue reconstruction is attempted to restore the normal mechanical axis. Failure to correct genu varus may stretch repaired/reconstructed structures, predisposing them to fail over time (Figure 10–9).

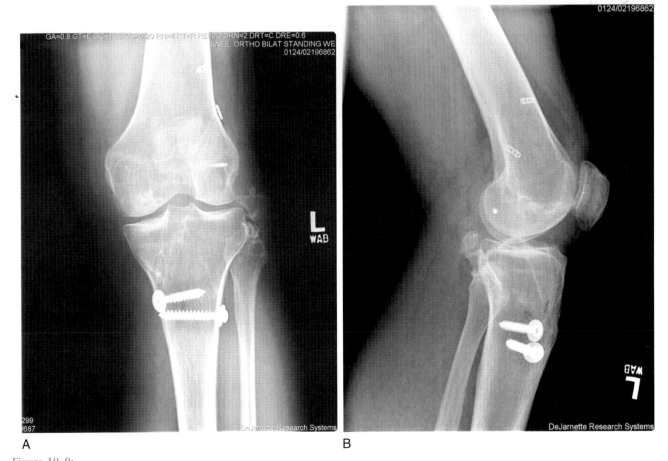

A   B

Figure 10–9:
Realignment of chronic posterolateral corner knee injury. **A** and **B**, Preoperative anteroposterior and lateral x-rays of patient with anterior cruciate ligament (ACL), posterior cruciate ligament (PCL), and lateral collateral ligament (LCL)/posterolateral corner (PLC) following two surgeries with persistent chronic PLC insufficiency and varus thrust.

(continued)

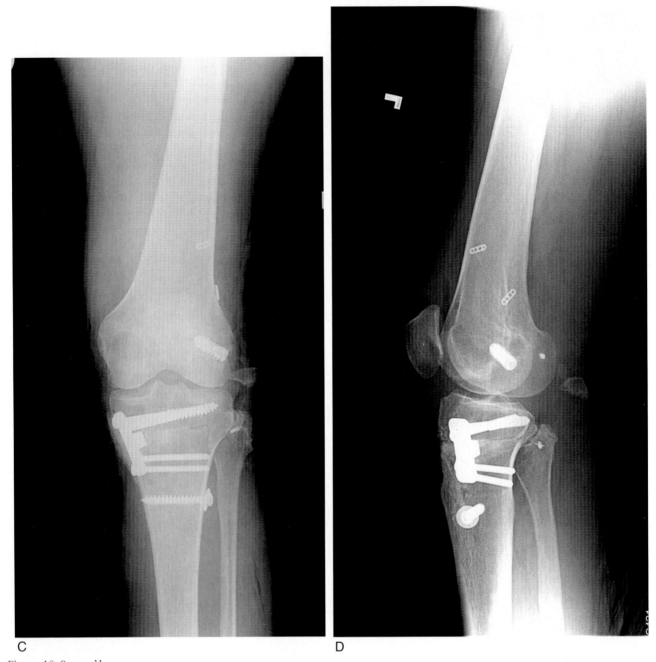

C

D

Figure 10–9, cont'd:
C and **D,** High tibial osteotomy with concomitant PLC reconstruction was performed and resolved the chronic instability.

- Opening medial tibial wedge osteotomies are preferred over lateral tibial closing osteotomies when the PLC is to be repaired.
- Reconstructions primarily concentrate on re-creating the popliteofibular ligament, LCL, and/or popliteus.
- Several techniques for reconstruction are available and include the following (Figure 10–10):
  - Biceps tenodesis
  - Popliteal bypass and popliteofibular ligament reconstruction
  - Figure eight
  - Patellar tendon or Achilles tendon autograft or allograft
- Several other grafts have been described for the purpose of reconstructing the LCL and PLC (Box 10–4): semitendinosus, gracilis, double-loop hamstrings, iliotibial band, biceps femoris tendon, bone-patellar tendon-bone, and quadriceps tendon-patellar bone grafts.
- Anatomic reconstructions appear to be the most favorable according to biomechanical studies (see LaPrade et al., 2004).

Rehabilitation

- The knee is usually kept in a range of motion brace locked in extension to reduce the tibia and prevent posterolateral stress on the repair/reconstruction.
- Operative assessment of range of motion that limits undue tension can assist with postoperative rehabilitation recommendations.
- The knee is initially held in full extension postoperatively with passive flexion begun between 1 and 4 weeks.
- Passive flexion only is performed for a period of 4 to 6 weeks to decrease firing of the hamstrings and any subsequent posterolateral moment force on the repair/reconstruction.
- Hamstring exercises are usually restricted for 2 months because of the stresses they place on the PLC.
- Patients may perform quadriceps exercises and straight leg raises early on.
- Reconstructions usually allow earlier range of motion than repairs.

- Combined ligamentous repairs normally must remain nonweight-bearing for a period of 6 to 8 weeks to allow proper healing and should then follow the customary protocols followed for the specific structures repaired or reconstructed.
- Early range of motion regimens should be instituted as soon as possible to decrease the chance of developing arthrofibrosis.
- When weight-bearing is begun, a medial unloader brace can be used to again decrease the forces on the repaired or reconstructed tissue until it has completely healed.

Complications

- Because of the close proximity to the LCL and PLC, peroneal nerve injuries can be a consequence of the injury itself or of the surgical repair or reconstruction technique.
- Careful attention to anatomy is critical to avoid injury, particularly when some of the normal anatomy is disrupted.
- When peroneal nerve dysfunction occurs in association with the knee trauma, exploration of the nerve both proximally and distally is indicated to identify the nature of the injury (laceration—uncommon, stretch—common) and to free any potential areas of constriction.
  - If a laceration is present, surgical repair is appropriate by a surgeon trained in microvascular repair; however, prognosis is guarded.
  - If a stretch injury is present, observation is performed for a minimum of 6 months to see what function will return, with late tendon transfers as an option to restore ankle dorsiflexion if the patient desires.
- Intraarticular and bone damage, particularly with tunnel placement, is a potential complication during repair/reconstruction procedures.
- Arthrofibrosis can be prevented with proper physical therapy and frequent follow-up.
- Failure to recognize and repair PLC injuries when reconstructing the cruciate ligaments may place them at an increased risk of failure.
- Autograft procedures may result in pain over the donor site or weakness of the donor muscle.
- Instability may persist.

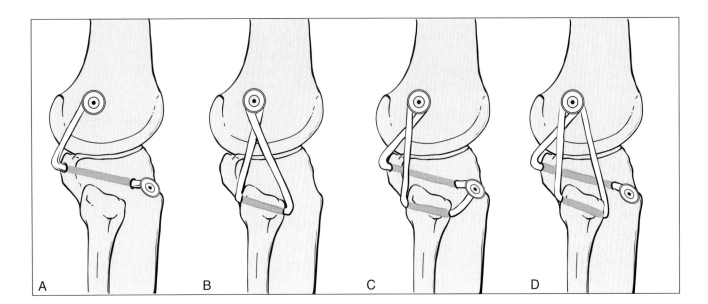

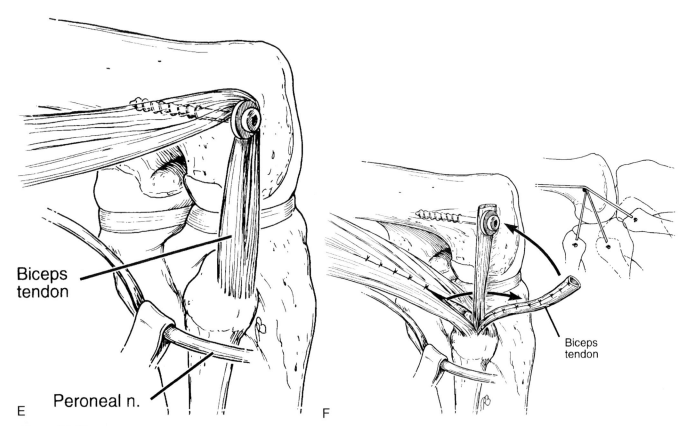

Figure 10–10:
Techniques for posterolateral reconstruction. **A,** Popliteal bypass (Muller). **B,** Figure eight (Larsen). **C,** Two tail (Warren).
D, Three tail (Warren/Miller). **E,** Biceps tenodesis for posterolateral corner (PLC) reconstruction. **F,** Biceps tendon lateral
collateral ligament (LCL) reconstruction. **G,** Popliteus and popliteofibular reconstruction with patellar tendon graft.   *(continued)*

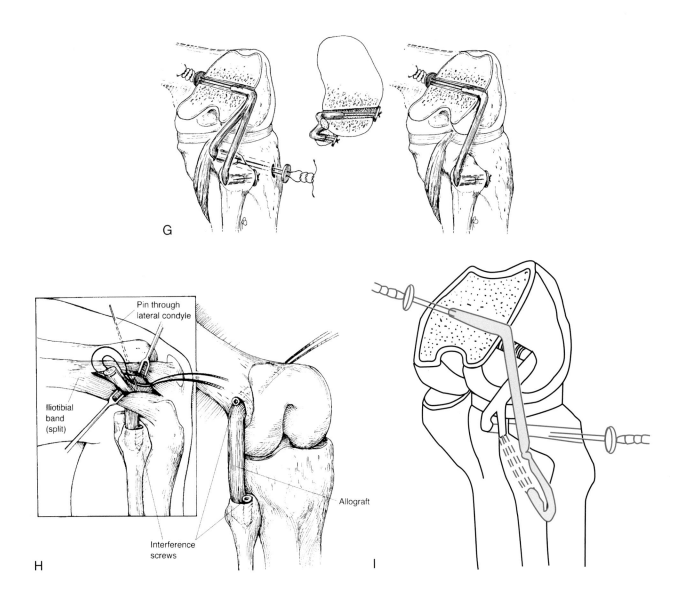

Figure 10–10, cont'd:
H, Bone-patella-bone LCL reconstruction using interference screws. **I,** Sekiya technique.
(**A** to **D** from Miller MD, Cooper DE, Warner JP: *Review of sports medicine and arthroscopy,* 2nd ed. Philadelphia, 2002, WB Saunders; **E** to **G** from Veltri DM, Warren RF: *Op Tech Sports Med* 4:174-181, 1996; **H** from Latimer HA et al: *Am J Sports Med* 26:656-662, 1998; **I** from Arthroscopy [accepted].)

Box 10–4	Grafts Available for Lateral Collateral Ligament (LCL) and Posterolateral Corner (PLC) Reconstruction

Achilles tendon
Patellar tendon
Semitendinosus
Gracilis
Biceps femoris
Double-loop hamstrings
Iliotibial band
Bone-patellar tendon-bone
Quadriceps tendon-patellar bone
Allografts

References

Chen CH, Chen WJ, Shih CH: Lateral collateral ligament reconstruction using quadriceps tendon-patellar bone autograft with bioscrew fixation. *Arthroscopy* 17:551-554, 2001.

Technical article describing the use of quadriceps tendon-patellar bone autograft as a good alternative in reconstructing the LCL in knees requiring multiple ligament and/or PLC reconstruction. Referenced anatomic and biomechanical studies reveal that the quadriceps tendon has a greater tensile failure load and cross-sectional area than patellar tendon grafts. The authors conclude that the quadriceps tendon-patellar bone autograft is a reasonable option for surgeons with limited allograft resources and patients not suitable for bone-patellar tendon-bone autografts.

Covey DC: Injuries of the posterolateral corner of the knee. *J Bone Joint Surg Am* 83:106-118, 2001.

Review article with more than 100 references detailing the anatomy and biomechanics of the PLC and diagnosis and treatment of PLC injury. Acute repair of PLC injuries is recommended when combined with cruciate ligament injury. Reconstruction techniques for severe chronic injuries are reviewed. Author points out that anatomic reconstruction potentially offers the best outcomes. Furthermore, if the PLC is not repaired, cruciate ligament reconstruction is more likely to fail.

LaPrade RF, Johansen S, Wentorf FA, et al: An analysis of an anatomical posterolateral knee reconstruction: an in vitro biomechanical study and development of a surgical technique. *Am J Sports Med* 32:1405-1414, 2004.

A novel, near-anatomic reconstruction of the popliteus tendon, LCL, and popliteofibular ligament is developed and tested biomechanically with excellent stability to external rotatory and varus loads.

Latimer HA, Tibone JE, ElAttrache NS, McMahon PJ: Reconstruction of the lateral collateral ligament of the knee with patellar tendon allograft. Report of a new technique in combined ligament injuries. *Am J Sports Med* 26:656-662, 1998.

Retrospective study on 10 patients with combined cruciate ligament and posterolateral instability who underwent reconstruction. The technique of LCL reconstruction using a bone-patellar tendon-bone allograft and interference screws is described. Nine of the 10 patients had reductions in varus laxity at 30 degrees of knee flexion and all

demonstrated improvement in external rotation at 30 degrees of knee flexion. The authors conclude that their method for LCL reconstruction can correct the varus and external rotatory instability associated with the above injuries. These authors also mention that their allograft, which was much larger than the native LCL, may have served as a functional substitute for the arcuate and popliteofibular ligaments that lie in close proximity to the LCL.

Lee J, Papakonstantinou O, Brookenthal KR, et al: Arcuate sign of the posterolateral knee injuries: anatomic, radiographic, and MR imaging data related to patterns of injury. *Skeletal Radiol* 32:619-627, 2003.

Radiographic and MRI images of 12 patients with isolated PLC injuries were reviewed, all demonstrating some radiographic finding. Injury to the arcuate or popliteofibular ligament was associated with small avulsion fractures of the styloid process of the fibula on plain radiographs or localized bone marrow edema in the medial aspect of the fibular head. Disruption of the fibular collateral ligament or conjoint tendon was associated with larger fibular avulsion fractures and more generalized edema about the proximal fibula.

Lee MC, Park YK, Lee SH, et al: Posterolateral reconstruction using split Achilles tendon allograft. *Arthroscopy* 19:1043-1049, 2003.

New surgical technique using a split Achilles tendon allograft for posterolateral reconstruction in patients with concomitant PCL injury is described. One of the limbs is used to re-create the popliteofibular ligament and LCL and the other to re-create the popliteus. The authors comment on this procedure's ability to reconstruct the important posterolateral structures and regain the isometry of the LCL with good fixation, which they believe addresses the pitfalls of previous techniques.

Maynard MJ, Deng X, Wickiewicz TL, Warren RF: The popliteofibular ligament: rediscovery of a key element in posterolateral stability. *Am J Sport Med* 24:311-316, 1996.

A biomechanical study highlighting the importance of the popliteofibular ligament in addition to the LCL and popliteus tendon with regard to knee posterolateral stability.

McGuire DA, Wolchok JC: Posterolateral corner reconstruction. *Arthroscopy* 19:790-793, 2003.

Authors describe posterolateral reconstruction using a semitendinosus allograft and bioabsorbable interference screws. This technique approximates the anatomy of the popliteofibular ligament, which has been shown to be an important stabilizer against external rotation forces about the knee. Authors suggest that autograft is a viable alternative, although it potentially exposes the patient to greater morbidity.

Noyes FR, Barber-Westin SD: Surgical reconstruction of severe chronic posterolateral complex injuries of the knee using allograft tissues. *Am J Sports Med* 23:2-12, 1995.

Clinical results following allograft reconstruction of the PLC in severe, chronic injuries in which insufficient soft tissues are present for repair and suitable autogenous tissue was not available. Success rate following surgery was 76% by examination and stress radiographs.

Noyes FR, Barber-Westin SD: Surgical restoration to treat chronic deficiency of the posterolateral complex and cruciate ligaments of the knee joint. *Am J Sports Med* 24:415-426, 1996.

Clinical results of combined cruciate ligament reconstruction and PLC complex advancement when lax but sufficient tissue is present for repair. The proximal advancement represents a simplified method to restore tension to the posterolateral complex.

Sekiya JK, Jacobson JA, Wojtys EM: Sonographic imaging of the posterolateral structures of the knee: findings in human cadavers. *Arthroscopy* 18:872-881, 2002.

> *Review of relevant PLC knee structures in cadavers and unique methods of evaluation using ultrasonography. Anatomic dissection of key PLC knee elements depicted.*

Sekiya JK, Kurtz CA: Posterolateral corner reconstruction of the knee: surgical technique utilizing a bifid Achilles tendon allograft and a double femoral tunnel. *Arthroscopy* (in press).

> *A novel technique of the PLC using a double femoral tunnel to reconstruct the LCL, popliteus tendon, and popliteofibular ligament.*

Veltri DM, Deng XH, Torzilli PA, et al: The role of the popliteofibular ligament in stability of the human knee: a biomechanical study. *Am J Sports Med* 24:19-27, 1996.

> *A biomechanical study of the popliteus tendon and its fibular attachment, the popliteofibular ligament. This study describes the biomechanical importance of both of these structures to knee stability in posterior translation and varus and external rotation.*

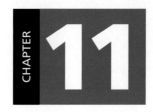

Multiple Ligament Injuries

Introduction

- Multiple ligament injuries of the knee can result from either low- or high-energy mechanism.
- "Ultra-low velocity" knee dislocations can occur in obese patients with minor energy mechanisms.
- Knee dislocations are named by the direction of the dislocation: anterior, posterior, lateral, medial, or rotational (Figure 11–1).
  - Anterior dislocations are the most common, although they are only slightly more common than posterior dislocations.
  - Lateral dislocations are more frequent than medial dislocations.
- Grading systems (Table 11–1).
- You must maintain a high level of suspicion for neurovascular trauma with these injuries as incidence has been reported to be anywhere from 30% to 50%.
  - Popliteal artery or peroneal nerve, or both, are the most commonly injured structures.
  - Popliteal artery injury can occur due to direct transection of the artery (posterior dislocations) or from intimal tearing due to traction of the vessel (anterior dislocations).

- A thorough neurovascular examination is vital.
- Vascular surgery consult/arteriogram should be considered.
- Initial treatment includes reduction of the knee, which is most easily performed with traction. Definitive treatment centers on reconstruction of the injured soft tissue structures.

Table 11–1:	Schenck Classification of Multiple Ligament Injuries
CLASS	INVOLVED LIGAMENTS
KDI	ACL + MCL or LCL
KDII	ACL + PCL
KDIII	
KDIIIM	ACL + PCL + MCL
KDIIIL	ACL + PCL + LCL
KDIV	ACL + PCL + MCL + LCL

ACL, anterior cruciate ligament; LCL, lateral collateral ligament; MCL, medial collateral ligament; PCL, posterior cruciate ligament.

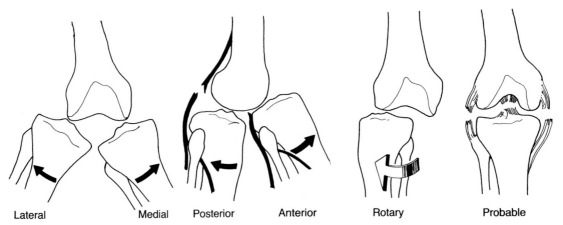

Lateral Medial Posterior Anterior Rotary Probable

Figure 11–1:

Classification of knee dislocations by direction of dislocation—anterior, posterior, medial, lateral, rotational. (From Miller MD, Cooper DE, Warner JJP: *Review of sports medicine and arthroscopy.* **Philadelphia, 2002, WB Saunders.)**

Cruciate and Collateral Ligament Injury

- The anterior and posterior cruciate ligaments are the most commonly involved ligaments in knee dislocation because of the anterior or posterior translation that must occur as the tibiofemoral joint is disrupted.
- Lachman and anterior/posterior drawer tests may be difficult to grade if both the anterior and posterior cruciate ligaments are injured because the neutral position is difficult to determine.
- Medial collateral ligament (MCL) injury may also occur if valgus force is applied during the injury. Although isolated MCL injuries are often treated nonoperatively, combined injury is more likely to require surgical repair or reconstruction, especially if the knee opens to valgus stress in full extension (implies injury to the posterior oblique ligament [POL]).
- Although an isolated injury to the lateral collateral ligament (LCL) is relatively rare, this ligament can be disrupted during a knee dislocation because of varus or rotational force. In the majority of cases, this results in both lateral and rotational instability, which will require surgical reconstruction for definitive treatment.
- If an LCL injury is suspected, the posterolateral corner structures should also be critically evaluated (as follows).

Posterolateral Corner Injury

- The posterolateral corner (PLC) is composed of the LCL, popliteus, popliteofibular ligament, posterolateral capsule, biceps femoris tendon, and iliotibial band/tract (Box 11–1).
- The most common method of injury to these structures is a rotational force.
- PLC injuries are commonly found in association with posterior cruciate ligament (PCL) injuries and less often with anterior cruciate ligament (ACL) injuries.
- The PLC injury is rarely an isolated injury.
- The best diagnostic physical examination finding is that of asymmetry on external rotation testing (Figures 11–2 and 11–3).

- This test is performed after reduction of the tibia with the patient in a prone position.
- This test should be done at 30 degrees of knee flexion and may also be repeated at 90 degrees of knee flexion.
- A positive test is described as increased external rotation when compared with the normal side.
- Asymmetry only at 30 degrees suggests an isolated PLC injury, whereas asymmetry at both 30 and 90 degrees of knee flexion suggests a combined PLC and PCL injury.
- Other pertinent physical examination findings may include positive external rotation recurvatum and posterolateral drawer.

Proximal Tib-Fib Dislocation

- The mechanism of injury usually involves falling on the flexed and adducted knee.
- These are commonly anterolateral in direction.
- These injuries may be treated initially with closed reduction techniques. Manually, the fibula is reduced with posterior pressure while the knee is in flexion.
- Operative treatment involves stabilization of the joint.
- Postoperatively or postreduction, the patient should have the knee immobilized in extension for 2 to 4 weeks.
- If this condition becomes a recurrent problem symptomatically for the patient, fibular head resection may become necessary.

Box 11–1	Structures That Compose the Posterolateral Corner

Lateral collateral ligament (LCL)
Popliteus
Popliteofibular ligament
Posterolateral capsule
Biceps femoris tendon
Iliotibial band/tract

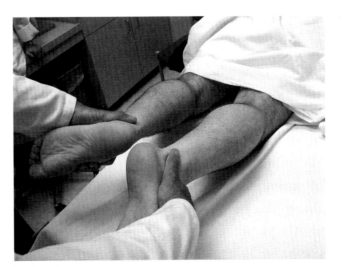

Figure 11–2:
External rotation examination at 30 degrees of knee flexion to diagnose posterolateral corner injury.

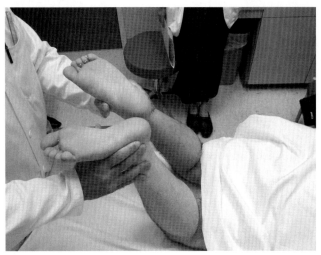

Figure 11–3:
External rotation examination at 90 degrees of knee flexion to diagnose posterolateral corner injury.

Imaging and Diagnostic Studies in Knee Dislocations

- Plain radiographs are helpful in determining the direction of the dislocation, adequacy of the reduction, and presence of associated fracture (Figure 11–4).
- Arteriography may be necessary to diagnose possible popliteal artery injury and should be considered along with a vascular consultation for all knee dislocation patients (Figure 11–5).
- Electromyographic studies may be beneficial in determining the degree of peroneal nerve injury.
- Magnetic resonance imaging (MRI) is very useful in preoperative planning (Figure 11–6).
  - Visualization of both cruciate and collateral ligaments.
  - Visualization of the meniscus.
  - Determination of chondral injury.

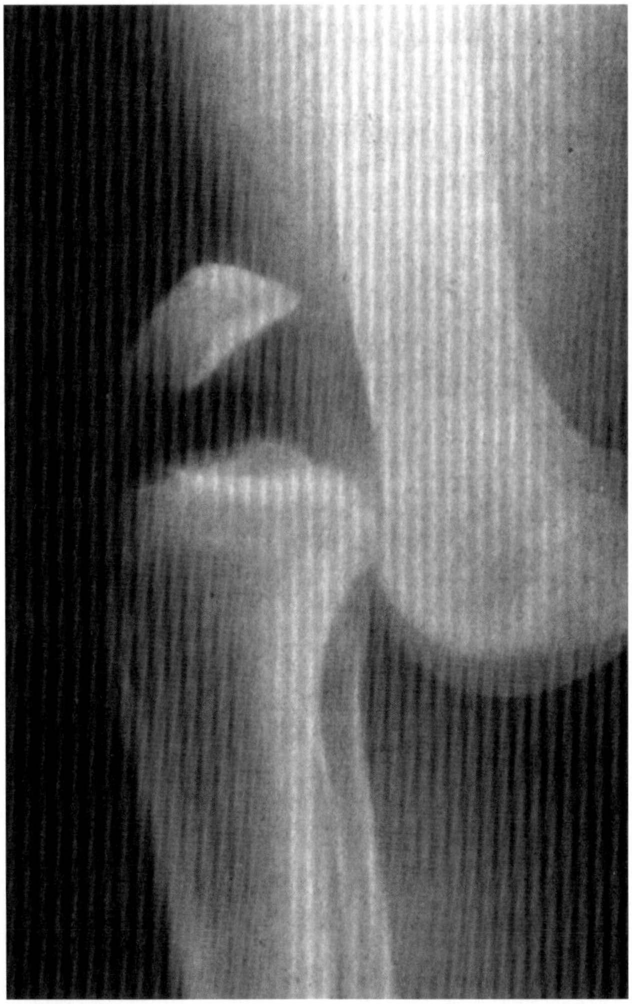

Figure 11–4:
Dislocated knee.

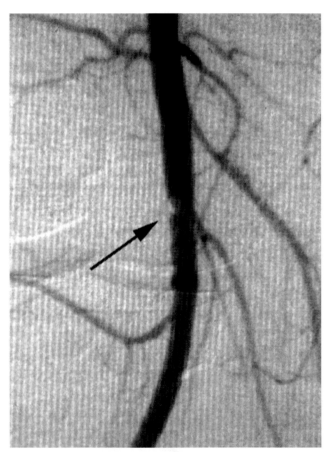

Figure 11–5:
Intimal popliteal artery injury after knee dislocation.

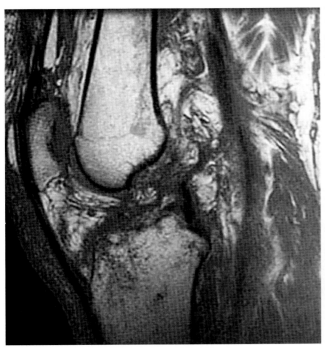
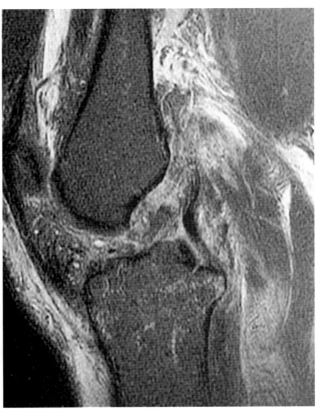

A   B

Figure 11–6:
Magnetic resonance imaging appearance of anterior cruciate ligament (ACL) and posterior cruciate ligament (PCL) injury in knee dislocation. **A,** T$_1$-weighted image of an ACL and PCL tear. **B,** T$_2$-weighted image of an ACL and PCL tear. (From Miller MD, Howard RF, Plancher KD: *Surgical atlas of sports medicine.* Philadelphia, 2003, WB Saunders.)

Surgical Reconstruction of the Dislocated Knee

- Immediate surgery is indicated for repairable vascular injuries and open knee dislocations.
  - Extraarticular procedures (posterolateral or posteromedial, or both) can be done concurrently with vascular procedures after the knee is stabilized with an external fixator.
  - Open injuries require irrigation and debridement with delayed surgical intervention. External fixation is usually indicated.
- Current recommendations for surgical intervention include primary repair of posterolateral/posteromedial injuries within 2 weeks of injury. Some studies have suggested that augmentation will result in improved outcomes. Timing of cruciate ligament reconstruction is somewhat more controversial, but most authors recommend reconstruction of either one (posterior) or both of the cruciates at the time of surgery. Primary repair is usually not possible unless there is a bony avulsion or a "peel off" lesion of the PCL off the femur with minimal intraligamentous injury.

Complications Associated with Multiple Ligament Injuries

- Delayed diagnosis may in turn delay surgical reconstruction. This is especially true in cases with a low-velocity injury because these often are associated with a lower index of suspicion for knee dislocation.
- Vascular injuries are unfortunately a relatively common complication of knee dislocation.
  - The most commonly injured vessel is the popliteal artery.
  - To minimize this risk, the examiner needs to recognize the injury as being a knee dislocation and keep a high index of suspicion for arterial compromise.
  - It is a good rule of thumb to get a vascular consultation or arteriogram, or both, on all knee dislocation patients early in the management.
  - Ideally, the artery should be repaired within 6 to 8 hours of injury to prevent ischemia to the soft tissues of the leg.
  - If the popliteal artery injury is not promptly recognized and treated, the ischemia could progress to the point that amputation is necessary.

- Neurologic injury may be a complication of the dislocation itself or may even occur as a result of the surgery to reconstruct the knee.
  - The most commonly injured nerve is the peroneal nerve.
  - This injury often results from traction on the nerve as it wraps around the fibular neck and is most frequently associated with posterior, posterolateral, or medial dislocations.
  - Treatment involves exploration of the peroneal nerve with possible repair or decompression.
  - The tibial nerve may also be injured, although this is much more rare and tends to be associated with high-velocity injuries.
- Infection or delayed wound healing is a serious complication that may be more prevalent in knee dislocation patients because of the extensive soft tissue damage associated with the initial injury.
- Compartment syndrome is a complication of concern in any trauma to an extremity.
  - The high velocities and vascular injury associated with many cases of knee dislocation predispose the patient to the development of compartment syndrome.
  - Observation and serial neurovascular checks help to diagnosis a developing compartment syndrome.
  - If any signs or symptoms of compartment syndrome develop, compartment pressure testing is indicated.
  - Treatment involves complete four-compartment fasciotomy.
- Anterior knee pain can arise in these patients for several reasons:
  - Patellar tendon harvesting.
  - Prominent hardware.
  - Persistent posterior sag.
  - Chondral damage at the time of the injury.
- Chondral damage can range from initial bone bruising to more involved defects that may require additional surgical treatment such as microfracture, autologous chondrocyte implantation (ACI), or osteochondral autogenous transfer (OATS). These procedures were discussed in more detail in Chapter 5.
- Persistent instability may be a result of graft failure or improper tensioning during the reconstruction.
- Heterotopic ossification (HO) is a frustrating complication that can severely limit the range of motion of the knee postoperatively. This is discussed more fully in Chapter 13.

References

Fanelli GC: The multiple ligament injured knee (part I). *Op Tech Sports Med* 11(3), 2003.
This is a collection of articles discussing the anatomy and pathology associated with multiple ligament injuries of the knee, classification systems, and treatment of complications.

Fanelli GC: The multiple ligament injured knee (part II). *Op Tech Sports Med* 11(3), 2003.
This is a collection of articles discussing the surgical management of the multiple ligament injured knee. It includes discussion of the treatment of the various classifications of ligament injuries.

Hagino R, DeCrapio J, Valentine R: Spontaneous popliteal vascular injury in the morbidly obese. *J Vasc Surg* 28:458-462, 1998.
This is an article that discusses arterial injury in morbidly obese patients. In these patients (body mass index >35kg/m² or 100 lb overweight), these authors find that the obesity is itself a risk factor for spontaneous knee dislocation and is associated with an extremely high rate of popliteal artery injury. Obesity also contributes to a poor postoperative course due to delayed healing and tissue hypoperfusion.

Hegyes MS, Richardson, MW, Miller MD: Knee dislocations: complications of nonoperative and operative management. *Clin Sports Med* 19:519-543, 2003.
This is a review article discussing the various complications associated with knee dislocation. However, great care should be taken in every case to match treatment to that particular injury. In addition, experience of the surgeon and familiarity of operative technique will help to minimize potential complications of this injury.

Liow RY, McNicholas MJ, Keating JF, Nutton RW: Ligament repair and reconstruction in traumatic dislocation of the knee. *J Bone Joint Surg Br* 85:845-851, 2003.
This article discusses the appropriate decision making for the timing of surgery after knee dislocation. Clinical outcomes of ACL reconstruction after knee dislocation are better if performed during the first 2 weeks following injury. No such difference is shown in the PCL if reconstructed early or late. General outcome in terms of patient activity and knee function are better if surgery is performed during the acute phase of the injury.

Mills WJ, Tejwani N: Heterotopic ossification after knee dislocation: the predictive value of the injury severity score. *J Orthop Trauma* 17:338-345, 2003.
This article discusses HO after knee dislocation. Injury Severity Score (ISS) above 26 seems to correlate with the development of HO. Closed head injury at the time of the injury also may be a factor that predisposes the patient to the development of HO. There is no connection shown between number of ligaments reconstructed or time until surgery and the development of HO.

Perron AD, Brady WJ, Sing RF: Orthopedic pitfalls in the ED: vascular injury associated with knee dislocation. *Am J Emerg Med* 19:583-588, 2001.
Recognition of vascular injury after knee dislocation is crucial. Clinical presentation, diagnostic tests, and appropriate treatment are discussed in detail.

Potter HG, Weinstein M, Allen AA, et al: Magnetic resonance imaging of the multiple-ligament injured knee. *J Orthop Trauma* 16:330-339, 2002.
MRI has been shown to have excellent correlation with surgical findings in patients after knee dislocation. In addition, magnetic resonance angiogram and angiograms demonstrate excellent correlation with vascular injury found as a result of the injury.

Schenck R: The dislocated knee. *Instruct Course Lect* 43:127-136, 1994.
This lecture provides an overview of the initial diagnosis and management of knee dislocations including a method of classification of these injuries in terms of anatomic structures involved.

Schenck R: Classification of knee dislocations. *Op Tech Sports Med* 11:193-198, 2003.

The author argues that proper classification of knee dislocations leads to better communication between referring and accepting physicians and leads to better operative management of these patients. Classification should be based on direction of dislocation, force involved in the injury, and ligamentous structures injured.

Tom JA, Miller MD: Complications in the multiple-ligament injured knee. *Op Tech Sports Med* 11:302-311, 2003.

This is a review of the most common complications associated with multiple ligament injuries of the knee. Among the topics discussed are neurovascular injuries, compartment syndrome, fractures and dislocations, delayed wound healing, HO, and osteonecrosis.

12

Patellofemoral Disorders

Introduction

- Patellofemoral disorders are a broad group of problems surrounding the patellofemoral joint often characterized by anterior knee pain exacerbated by activities that produce extra loads across the knee.
- They can be roughly divided into traumatic and atraumatic conditions, each with subcategories. Idiopathic chondromalacia patella, osteochondritis dissecans, and synovial plicae are given separate categories to complete the differential (Box 12–1).
- Chondromalacia describes a pathology that is often a result of an underlying condition that must be evaluated and diagnosed.
- Several conditions about the knee have no underlying articular damage.
- Undetected trauma to the knee may result in future patellofemoral disorders.

Box 12–1   **Classification of Patellofemoral Disorders**

I. Trauma (conditions caused by trauma in the otherwise normal knee)
   A. Acute trauma
      1. Contusion (924.11)
      2. Fracture
         a. Patella (822)
         b. Femoral trochlea (821.2)
         c. Proximal tibial epiphysis (tubercle) (823.0)
      3. Dislocation (rare in the normal knee) (836.3)
      4. Rupture
         a. Quadriceps tendon (843.8)
         b. Patellar tendon (844.8)
   B. Repetitive trauma (overuse syndromes)
      1. Patellar tendinitis ("jumper's knee") (726.64)
      2. Quadriceps tendinitis (726.69)
      3. Peripatellar tendinitis (e.g., anterior knee pain of the adolescent due to hamstring contracture) (726.699)
      4. Prepatellar bursitis ("housemaid's knee") (726.65)
      5. Apophysitis
         a. Osgood-Schlatter disease (732.43)
         b. Sinding-Larsen-Johansson disease (732.42)
   C. Late effects of trauma (905)
      1. Posttraumatic chondromalacia patellae
      2. Posttraumatic patellofemoral arthritis
      3. Anterior fat pad syndrome (posttraumatic fibrosis)
      4. Reflex sympathetic dystrophy of the patella
      5. Patellar osseous dystrophy

      6. Acquired patella infera (719.366)
      7. Acquired quadriceps fibrosis
II. Patellofemoral dysplasia
   A. Lateral patellar compression syndrome (LPCS) (718.365)
      1. Secondary chondromalacia patellae (717.7)
      2. Secondary patellofemoral arthritis (715.289)
   B. Chronic subluxation of the patella (CSP) (718.364)
      1. Secondary chondromalacia patellae (717.7)
      2. Secondary patellofemoral arthritis (715.289)
   C. Recurrent dislocation of the patella (RDP) (718.361)
      1. Associated fractures (822)
         a. Osteochondral (intraarticular)
         b. Avulsion (extraarticular)
      2. Secondary chondromalacia patellae (717.7)
      3. Secondary patellofemoral arthritis (715.289)
   D. Chronic dislocation of the patella (718.362)
      1. Congenital
      2. Acquired
III. Idiopathic chondromalacia patellae (717.7)
IV. Osteochondritis dissecans
   A. Patella (732.704)
   B. Femoral trochlea (732.703)
V. Synovial plicae (727.8916) (anatomic variant made symptomatic by acute or repetitive trauma)
   A. Medial patellar ("shelf") (727.89161)
   B. Suprapatellar (727.89163)
   C. Lateral patellar (727.89165)

Orthopaedic ICD-9-CM Expanded Diagnostic Codes in parentheses.
From Merchant AC: *Arthroscopy* 4:235, 1988.

- Physical examination should include a careful evaluation of the patellofemoral joint (see Chapter 2) and an assessment of lower extremity alignment, Q angle, and detection for pes planus.

Types

Patellar Fracture

- Fractures of the patella can be described according to their pattern, which in turn can assist in deciding the most optimal technique for repair (Figure 12–1).
- They usually result from a direct blow or fall but may also be the consequence of indirect trauma.
- Patients often present with swelling and inability to ambulate.
- Physical examination should document any skin abrasions or lacerations, palpable defects of the patella or extensor mechanism tendons, and ability to perform a straight leg raise.
- Inability to perform a straight leg raise in the face of a patellar fracture may indicate disruption of the medial and lateral retinaculum.
- Significant hematomas often require aspiration.

- Standard radiographs can confirm the diagnosis and assist with classification.
- Nondisplaced fractures may be treated by immobilization in extension for 6 weeks followed by rehabilitation to regain range of motion.
- Several techniques exist for patellar fracture repair (Figure 12–2).
- Arthroscopic reduction and repair, primarily using percutaneous screws, is an option for some fracture patterns and offers several advantages (Figure 12–3 and Boxes 12–2 and 12–3).
- Surgical repair allows early range-of-motion exercises, reducing the risk of arthrofibrosis.

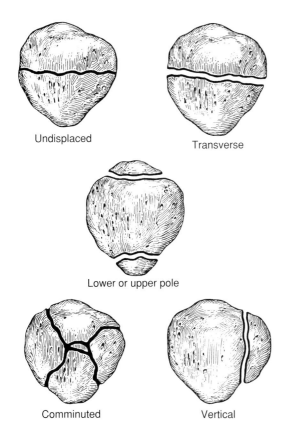

Figure 12–1:
Fractures of the patella. (From Tria AJ Jr, Klein KS: *An illustrated guide to the knee*. New York, 1992, Churchill Livingstone.)

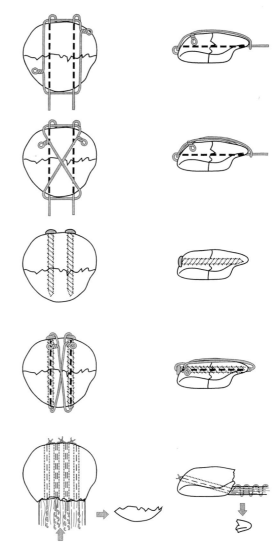

Figure 12–2:
Techniques for patella fracture open reduction internal fixation (ORIF). (From Ross PW, Miller MD: Extensor mechanism injuries of the knee. In Brinder MR, editor: *Review of orthopaedic trauma*. Philadelphia, 2001, WB Saunders.)

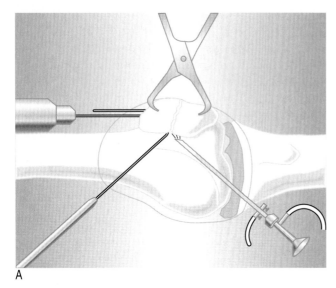

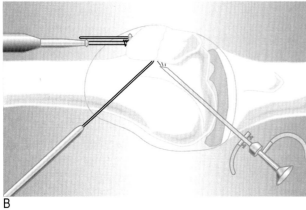

Figure 12–3:
Arthroscopic-assisted reduction and cannulated screw fixation of a transverse patellar fracture. **A,** The fracture is reduced and held in place with forceps while guidepins for the cannulated screws are passed across the fracture. The arthroscope is used to verify anatomic reduction of the articular fracture. **B,** The partially threaded, cannulated leg screws are then passed across the fracture site and the fracture is compressed. This is all done under direct arthroscopic visualization. (From Tandogan RN, Demirors H, Tuncay CL, et al: *Arthroscopy* 18:156-162, 2002.)

Anterior Fat Pad Syndrome

- Trauma to the anterior fat pad of the knee can cause pain and limited extension of the knee when it undergoes fibrous change and squeezes itself within the patellofemoral joint.
- It is more common in patients with genu recurvatum.
- This condition is distinct from fat pad fibrosis, a complication seen after knee ligament surgery.
- Initially, it is managed with ice, padding, and activity modifications; symptoms normally resolve with time.
- Occasionally, excision is performed to alleviate pain and recover motion about the knee.

Box 12–2	Indications for Arthroscopic Treatment of Patellar Fractures

Displacement > 3 mm, stepoff > 2 mm (displacement < 8 mm)
Transverse fractures (rarely sagittal split fractures)
Noncomminuted
Good-quality bone
Intact extensor mechanism (ability to perform straight leg raise)

From Berkowitz MJ, Bottoni CR: Arthroscopically assisted fracture repair for intra-articular knee fracture. In Miller MD, Cole BJ, editors: *Textbook of arthroscopy.* Philadelphia, 2004, Saunders.

Box 12–3	Advantages of Arthroscopic Fixation of Patellar Fractures

Avoids long incision, soft tissue disruption
Avoids traumatized anterior skin
Improved cosmesis
Preserves blood supply to patella
Shortens anesthesia and operative time
Improves postoperative pain control
Allows perfect articular reduction without arthrotomy
Facilitates early range of motion
Prevents intraarticular adhesions

From Berkowitz MJ, Bottoni CR: Arthroscopically assisted fracture repair for intra-articular knee fracture. In Miller MD, Cole BJ, editors: *Textbook of arthroscopy.* Philadelphia, 2004, Saunders.

- This condition is classically described in three phases (Box 12–4).
- In the knee, classic symptoms and findings may be varied and not conform to this classical description and up to 50% of patients may demonstrate normal motion.
- Some patients may have a "flamingo gait," in which they walk on one leg with crutches and the affected leg flexed at the knee.
- Radiologic evaluation may reveal osteopenia.
- Complex regional pain syndrome does best when recognized and treated early.
- Initial treatment should include counseling, nonsteroidal antiinflammatory drugs (NSAIDs), low-dose antidepressants, range-of-motion exercises, hot-cold soaks, and transcutaneous electrical nerve stimulation.
- Some patients benefit from lumbar sympathetic or epidural blocks.

Box 12–4	Classic Stages of Complex Regional Pain Syndrome

I (3 months): Swelling, edema, warmth, hyperhidrosis, allodynia
II (6 months): Brawny edema, loss of motion, trophic changes
III (indefinite): Pale, cool, dry, glossy skin, stiffness

From Miller MD, Cooper DE, Warner JJP: *Review of sports medicine and arthroscopy.* Philadelphia, 2002, WB Saunders.

- Surgery is initially contraindicated because it may exacerbate symptoms and preclude resolution. However, patients with persistent symptoms that respond to a series of blocks can be considered for surgical elimination of the triggering pathology.

Tendon Ruptures

- Quadricep tendon ruptures occur three times more frequently than patellar tendon ruptures.
- Quadricep tendon ruptures usually result from indirect trauma, such as falling on a partially flexed knee, and occur in patients older than 40 years, whereas patellar tendon ruptures are most often seen in younger patients from direct trauma.
- Underlying conditions such as infection, arthritis, metabolic disease, fatty degeneration, and calcific tendinitis may predispose patients to tendon injury.
- On physical examination, effusions are commonly present, a palpable defect may be appreciated, and displacement of the patella may also occur.
- Active extension of the knee should be performed with the knee and hip flexed at 90 degrees in the starting position. Limited extension suggests injury to the extensor mechanism.
- Most patients are also unable to perform a straight leg raise.
- Radiographs may demonstrate an inferiorly displaced patella with quadriceps ruptures and superiorly displaced with patellar tendon ruptures.
- Effusions may be aspirated to provide relief of tension and enhance range of motion.
- Anatomic repair of acute tendon ruptures provides the best results and may avoid severe tendon retraction and development of adhesions.
- Delayed repair of the quadriceps tendon can be performed by either the Scuderi or Marti techniques (Figure 12–4). If necessary, hamstring tendons or other exogenous tissue can supplement the repair.
- Temporary stabilization of the patella tendon rupture can be performed by the McLaughlin technique using wire or nonabsorbable suture (Figure 12–5).
- Generally, results of quadriceps tendon repairs are superior to patellar tendon repairs.

Tendinitis

- Patellar and quadriceps tendinitis are both caused by overuse.
- Patellar tendinitis, also known as jumper's knee, is commonly diagnosed in jumping athletes such as basketball and volleyball players. A history of forced contraction of the quadriceps may precede the onset of tendinitis symptoms.
- Patellar tendinitis is more common than quadriceps tendinitis.
- Patients present with anterior knee pain and tenderness near their patella attachment sites, best appreciated with the knee extended, which improves with the knee flexed.
- Pain can be elicited by stressing the extensor mechanism with hyperflexion of the knee or by testing resisted extension.
- Magnetic resonance imaging (MRI) can be useful to rule out a partial tear if weakness and a lack of a palpable defect are present.
- Semimembranous tendinitis is most frequently diagnosed in young male athletes who complain of pain at its insertion site at the posterior tubercle of the tibia.
- Peripatellar tendinitis has been attributed to hamstring tightness in adolescents.
- Tendinitis is primarily managed conservatively with NSAIDs and rehabilitation, including therapeutic modalities.
- Isokinetic and plyometric exercises should initially be avoided because they may exacerbate the condition.
- A patellar tendon strap may provide some relief for patellar tendinitis.
- Rarely is operative debridement and removal of damaged tendon necessary. (Ultrasound may assist in locating areas of damaged tendon.)
- Extracorporeal shock wave therapy has also been described for the treatment of recalcitrant patellar tendinitis with good success.
- Peripatellar tendinitis responds best to hamstring stretching exercises.

Bursitis

- Bursae about the knee can be subjected to aggravation (acutely or from overuse), producing symptoms of pain and swelling (Figure 12–6).
- Prepatellar bursitis (housemaid's knee), the most common bursitis of the knee, is associated with prolonged kneeling.
- Direct trauma is less of a causal factor.
- The bursa is located between the skin and patella.
- Thickening of the skin and swelling over the bursa may be appreciated on physical examination.
- Pain can be exacerbated with flexion of the knee, which imposes stress over the bursa.
- If abrasions or punctures are noticed over the area, one must first rule out the possibility of infection.

Iliotibial Band

- Iliotibial band syndrome is caused by excessive friction between the iliotibial band and the lateral femoral condyle.
- It is commonly seen in runners and cyclists.
- Patients often present with complaints of pain and tenderness along the lateral aspect of the knee.

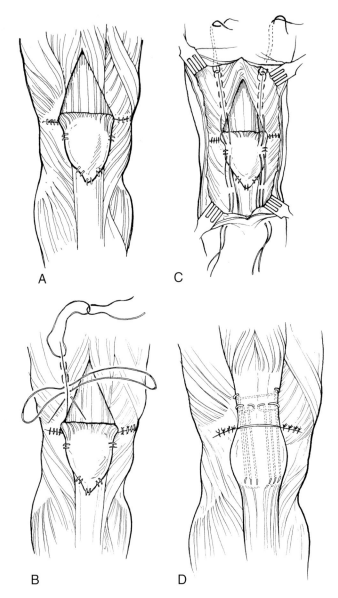

A

C

B

D

Figure 12–4:
(A-C) Scuderi and **(D)** Marti techniques for quadriceps tendon repair. (From Miller MD, Cooper DE, Warner JJP: *Review of sports medicine and arthroscopy*. Philadelphia, 2002, WB Saunders.)

- The Ober test may demonstrate tightness of the iliotibial band and reproduce pain. It is performed by instructing the patient to lie on the contralateral side and flexing the hip and knee. The hip is then abducted and extended and the leg is released. Failure of the leg to fall into adduction suggests a contracture of the fascia lata or iliotibial band (Figure 12–7).
- Conservative treatment, including activity modifications, stretching, and use of NSAIDs, usually provides adequate treatment.
- Rarely is partial excision of its posterior aspect recommended, except in refractory cases that have failed extended conservative therapy (Figure 12–8).

Lateral Patellar Compression Syndrome

- Lateral patellar compression syndrome is a condition characterized by malalignment of the patella without instability secondary to a tight lateral retinaculum (Box 12–5).
- This may cause the patient pain, which is accentuated when the retinaculum is strained during knee flexion (Figure 12–9).
- On physical examination, findings include a tight lateral retinaculum (negative patellar tilt) with normal mobility (decreased medial glides) and a normal Q angle.

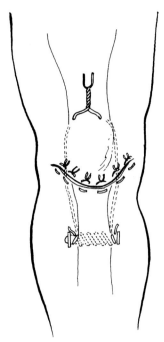

Figure 12–5:
McLaughlin technique for temporary wire augmentation of patellar tendon repairs. (From Miller MD, Cooper DE, Warner JJP: *Review of sports medicine and arthroscopy,* 2nd ed. Philadelphia, 2002, WB Saunders.)

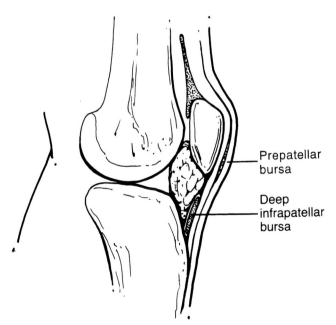

Prepatellar bursa

Deep infrapatellar bursa

Figure 12–6:
Bursae about the knee. (From Walsh WM: Patellofemoral joint. In DeLee JC, Drez D Jr, editors: *Orthopaedic sports medicine: principles and practice.* Philadelphia, 1994, WB Saunders.)

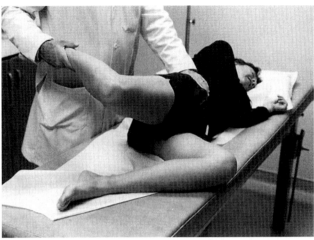

Figure 12–7:
The Ober test. (From Safaran MR, Fu FH: *Orthop Clin North Am* 26:547-559, 1995.)

- Merchant views will demonstrate an abnormal patellar tilt without subluxation (Figure 12–10*A* and *B*). This is revealed when lines drawn through the lateral facet of the patella and across the femoral condyle are parallel or form an angle that opens medially.
- If arthroscopy is performed, classical findings include lack of medial patellar articulation by 40 degrees of flexion and no subluxation with full range of motion (Figure 12–11).
- A tight lateral retinaculum initially is treated with activity modifications, NSAIDs, and rehabilitation.
- Bracing, with a medial buttress, can assist during initial rehabilitation and subsequently be used with aggravating activities.
- The use of taping and electrical stimulation may also be considered.
- An open or arthroscopic lateral release extending from the lateral joint line to the superior pole of the patella should only be performed on patients who have exhausted their conservative options. The surgeon should ensure that the retinaculum is completely released and the patella can be passively tilted at least 30 to 40 degrees but preferably up more.

Patellar Instability

- Patellar instability results from an excessively mobile patella that frequently subluxates or dislocates (Box 12–6).
- The most severe chronic form prevents the patella from returning to the trochlea throughout the knee range of motion.
- Increased symptoms are found in patients with genu valgum, pronated feet, and femoral anteversion.
- The apprehension and J signs (abnormal tracking) are often present on examination. Radiographic evaluation commonly demonstrates a lateral tilt.

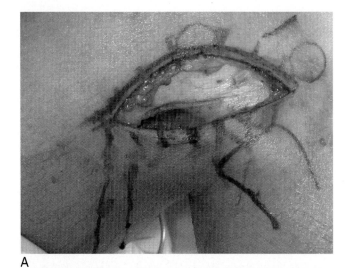

A

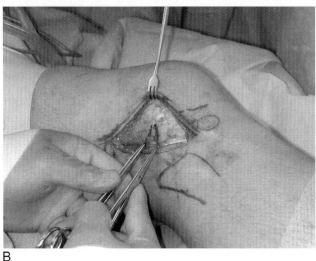

B

Figure 12–8:
Iliotibial band release in a 28-year-old Navy SEAL with a 2-year history of iliotibial band syndrome refractory to extensive conservative therapy. **A,** Iliotibial band before release. **B,** Iliotibial band following release at the lateral femoral epicondyle. The patient's symptoms completely resolved following surgery.

Box 12–5	History and Clinical Findings Associated with Lateral Patellar Compression Syndrome

Lateral patellar pain, particularly with knee flexion
Negative patellar tilt
Focal lateral retinaculum tenderness
Decreased medial patellar glide
Normal Q angle/alignment
Lack of instability and subluxation
Abnormal patellar tilt on merchant views
Lack of medial patellar articulation by 40 degrees of flexion under arthroscopy

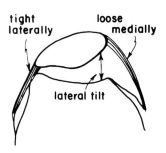

Figure 12–9:
Tight lateral retinaculum and excessive patellar tilt that is exacerbated during knee flexion. (From Fu FH, Maday MG: *Orthop Clin North Am* 23:601, 1992.)

- Merchant views at 20, 40, and 60 degrees are recommended when a maltracking patella is suspected.
- Axial computed tomography (CT) can further assess the relationship of the patella and trochlea in different degrees of motion (Figure 12–12).
- Repeated subluxation or dislocation of the patella may stretch or tear the restraining medial ligaments and cause hemarthrosis and further loss of motion.
- A malaligned, subluxating, or dislocating patella could exacerbate symptoms and lead to more severe damage in a knee already affected by arthritis or articular damage.
- Various techniques for restoring patellar stability are available.
- The medial patellofemoral ligament has been described as the most important restraining structure to lateral patellar mobility and, if disrupted, must be repaired anatomically (Figure 12–13). Other supporting structures include the patellotibial and patellomeniscal ligaments.
- Several other procedures are recommended in a knee with severe cartilage damage (chondromalacia) and patellar malalignment or increased Q angles including tibial tubercle osteotomy (anterior transfer of tibial tubercle [Maquet]), anteromedial transfer of tibial tubercle (Fulkerson), and straight medial transfer (Figure 12–14).
- Generally, bony realignment procedures are contraindicated in the skeletally immature patient. Procedures with soft tissue augmentation have been described for these patients.

Patella Alta/Infera

- Abnormal patellar height, best measured using lateral radiographs, can be congenital or acquired (Figure 12–15).
- Evaluation may be misinterpreted secondary to various patellofemoral bony deformities, spurring, and knee position.
- The Insall-Salvati and Blackburne-Peel ratios are the most reliable—with the latter recommended in knees with patellar or tubercle deformity.

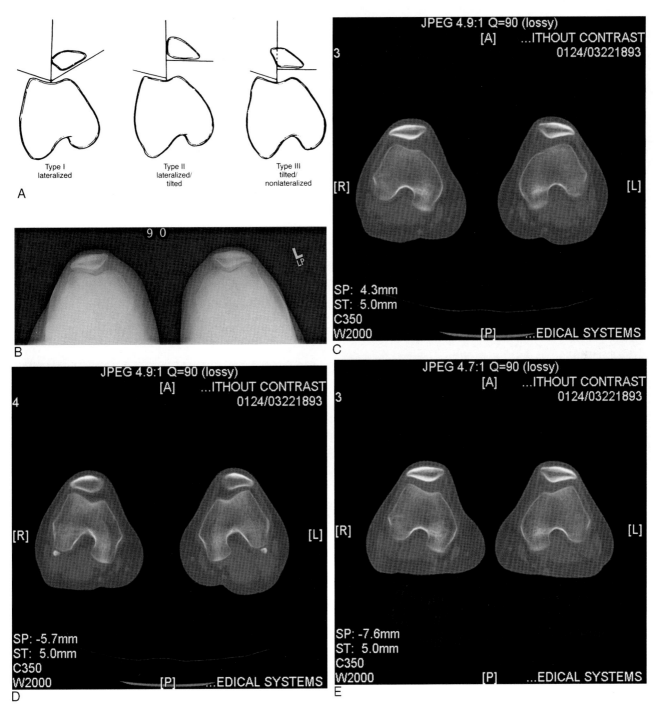

Figure 12–10:
Evaluation of patellar tilt and alignment using radiographs or computed tomography (CT). **A,** Schematic drawing evaluating patellar tilt. **B,** Sunrise views. C-E, CT scan axial images in various degrees of flexion. (**A** From Scott WN: *Arthroscopy of the knee.* Philadelphia, 1990, WB Saunders.)

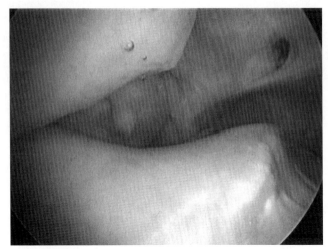

Figure 12–11:

View from the superolateral portal and a 70-degree arthroscope of a severe lateral patellar tilt.

- Patella alta, a high-riding patella, is associated with instability, whereas patella baja, a low-riding patella, usually develops with fibrosis and contracture of the fat pad, patellar tendon, or retinaculum.

Chondromalacia

- The pathology of chondromalacia can be classified according to the scheme developed by Outerbridge or modified by Insall (Box 12–7, Figure 12–16).
- Arthroscopic debridement and drilling (or curettage) of chondromalacia lesions are advocated by some after patients report no significant relief from nonoperative management.
- Patellofemoral arthroplasty is not indicated for isolated arthritis.

Treatment

- Except for fractures of the patella and tendon ruptures, most patellofemoral disorders are initially treated conservatively with activity modifications, NSAIDs, and rehabilitation including modalities.

Box 12–6	History and Findings Associated with Patellar Instability

Recurrent patellar subluxations or dislocations or both
Medial patellar pain and tenderness
Effusions or hemarthrosis or both
Increased lateral glide
Apprehension sign
J sign (abnormal patellar tracking)
Lateral malalignment with or without patellar tilt on radiographs

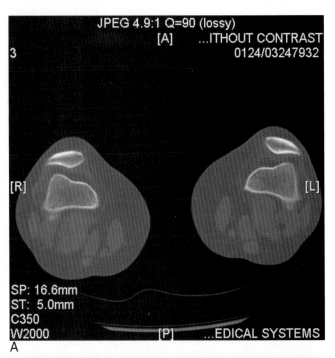

A

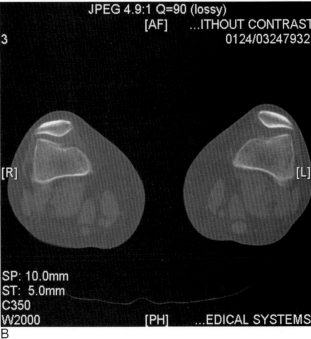

B

Figure 12–12:

A-B, Axial computed tomography scans of the patellofemoral joint showing lateral patellar subluxation.

(continued)

Rehabilitation

- Modalities such as ultrasound, phonophoresis, and hot/cold baths can aid in initial treatment of several conditions and can be continued through the rehabilitation program if necessary.
- Only after the symptoms have been well controlled can the patient begin range of motion exercises.

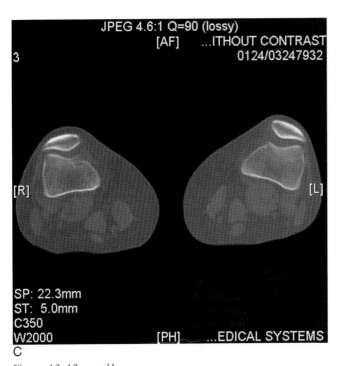

Figure 12–12, cont'd:
C, Axial computed tomography scans of the patellofemoral joint showing lateral patellar subluxation.

- When full, pain-free range of motion is restored, strengthening of the quadriceps and hamstrings can be initiated with the goal of returning the patient to the previous activity level.
- Patients with a tight lateral retinaculum should concentrate on strengthening the vastus medialis to counteract the lateral stress placed on the patella.
- Heat prior to exercise and ice after is often beneficial.

Complications

- Uncontrolled pain can lead to secondary weakness.
- Prolonged patellar instability and malalignment can cause and accelerate patellofemoral arthrosis.

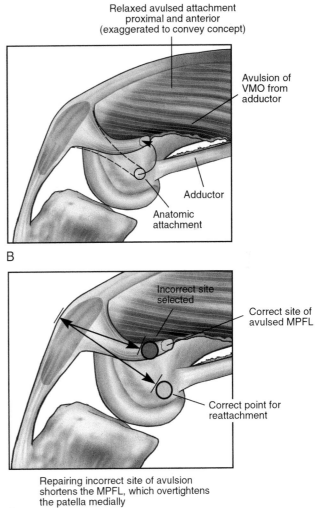

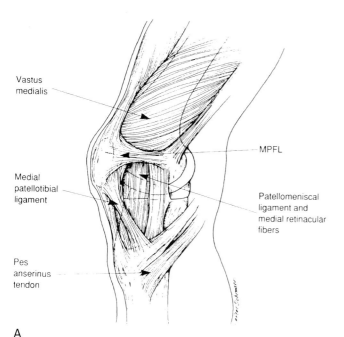

Figure 12–13:
A, Anatomy of medial patellofemoral ligament. **B** and **C,** Medial patellofemoral ligament injury pattern and correct anatomic site for repair. (**A** from Boden BP, Pearsall AW, Garrett WE Jr, Feagin JA Jr: *J Am Acad Orthop Surg* 5:47, 1997. **B** and **C** from Farr J: Lateral release and medial repair for patellofemoral instability. In Miller MD, Cole BJ, editors: *Textbook of arthroscopy.* Philadelphia, 2004, WB Saunders.)

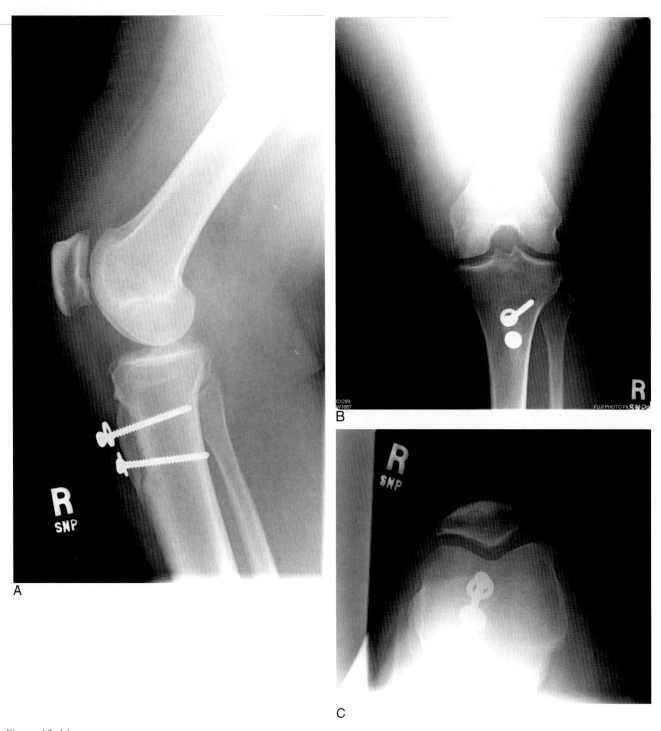

Figure 12–14:
Healed Fulkerson osteotomy for patellar subluxation. **A** and **B,** Healed anteroposterior and lateral radiographs of a tibial tubercle anteromedialization. **C,** Sunrise view showing the patella centered in the trochlear groove.

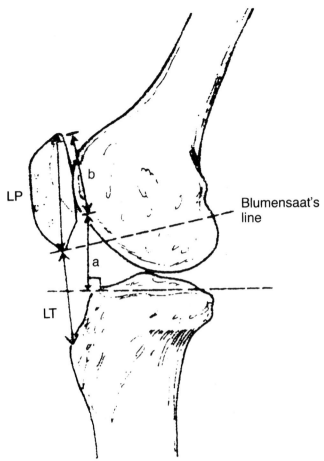

Figure 12–15:
Radiographic measurements for the evaluation of patella height. (From Harner CD, Miller MD. Irrgang JJ: Management of the stiff knee after trauma and ligament reconstruction. In Siliski JM, editor: *Traumatic disorders of the knee.* New York, 1994, Springer-Verlag.)

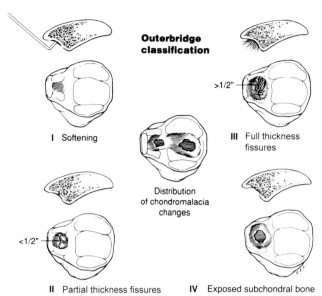

Figure 12–16:
Outerbridge classification of chondromalacia. (From Tria AJ Jr, Klein KS: *An illustrated guide to the knee.* New York, 1992, Churchill Livingstone.)

- Overtightening of the patella tendon during repair may result in patella infera and can be avoided with intraoperative lateral radiographs that can be compared with the uninjured knee.
- Delayed repair of tendon ruptures makes surgical repair more difficult and can result in a poor outcome.
- Failure to ensure adequate hemostasis during surgery may result in a subsequent hemarthrosis.
- Undetected and untreated septic bursitis can spread to the knee joint.
- The superior lateral geniculate artery, a branch off the popliteal artery, is at risk for injury during lateral release procedures.
- In lateral release procedures, surgeons are cautioned not to perform overzealous release of the lateral retinaculum or overtighten the medial structures, which can result in persistent instability and pain symptoms.

References

Biedert RM, Sanchis-Alfonso V: Sources of anterior knee pain. *Clin Sports Med* 21:335-347, 2002.
Authors provide a good pathophysiologic review of the structures around the knee including the cartilage, subchondral bone, synovium, fat pad, retinacula, capsule, and tendons as potential causes of anterior knee pain.

Fu FH, Maday MG: Arthroscopic lateral release and the lateral patellar compression syndrome. *Orthop Clin North Am* 23:601-612, 1992.
Review of lateral patellar compression syndrome, the diagnostic criteria for this condition, and the treatment of this disorder with an arthroscopic lateral release.

Box 12–7	Classification of Articular Injury

Grade	Description
Outerbridge System	
I	Softening and swelling of cartilage
II	Fragmentation and fissuring, <0.5 inch in diameter
III	Fragmentation and fissuring, >0.5 inch in diameter
IV	Erosion of cartilage down to exposed subchondral bone
Insall Modification	
I	Softening and swelling of cartilage
II	Fissuring to subchondral bone
III	Fibrillation of articular surface
IV	Erosion of cartilage down to exposed subchondral bone

From Diduch DR et al: Knee: diagnostic arthroscopy. In Miller MD, Cole BJ, editors: *Textbook of arthroscopy.* Philadelphia, 2004, WB Saunders.

Fulkerson JP: Diagnosis and treatment of patients with patellofemoral pain. *Am J Sports Med* 30:447-456, 2002.

Excellent review of the diagnosis and management of patients with patellofemoral pain. The author comments on several current concepts of nonoperative treatment that successfully manage most patellofemoral conditions. Surgery, when considered, must be supported by specific indications.

Fulkerson JP, Becker GJ, Meaney JA, et al: Anteromedial tibial tubercle transfer without bone graft. *Am J Sports Med* 18:490-496, 1990.

Clinical results following anteromedial tibial tubercle transfer in 30 patients with patellofemoral pain associated with patellar chondrosis. Good or excellent results were achieved in 93% of patients subjectively assessed with a minimum follow-up of 2 years.

Holmes JC, Pruitt AL, Whalen NJ: Iliotibial band syndrome in cyclists. *Am J Sports Med* 21:419-424, 1993.

Authors report on the incidence of iliotibial band syndrome among cyclists seen at their institution and the results of nonoperative and surgical management. The etiology was found to be similar to that seen in runners. Nonoperative treatment, which included bicycle and training modifications in addition to general conservative measures, successfully treated 57.4% of the cyclists. Percutaneous release of the iliotibial band was successful in only one case. However, the open elliptical excision release technique described in the article, which was used on 21 cyclists, returned 81% of patients (17 patients) to preinjury levels. As a result, the author recommends this surgical method as an effective method of treatment in cases refractory to nonoperative management.

Kelly MA: Algorithm for anterior knee pain. *AAOS Instruct Course Lect* 4:339-343, 1998.

Author provides and describes an algorithm that can be used for the evaluation, diagnosis, and treatment of anterior knee pain, a common orthopaedic complaint with a wide differential.

Merchant AC: Classification of patellofemoral disorders. *Arthroscopy* 4:235-240, 1988.

Author offers a classification table of patellofemoral disorders to guide the physician in the difficult task of anterior knee pain evaluation. He stresses that chondromalacia should be thought of as a secondary process and not be used as a primary diagnostic term. He divides the differential into traumatic, atraumatic, osteochondritis dissecans, and synovial plicae categories, reserving the category of idiopathic chondromalacia patella for conditions in which no causative factor is found.

Rasul AT, Fischer DA: Primary repair of quadriceps tendon ruptures. *Clin Orthop Related Res* 289:205-207, 1993.

Authors report on the results of primary surgical repair of quadriceps tendon ruptures in 19 patients. Seventy-five percent of patients older than 40 (9 of 12) were found to have tears at the tendon bone junction, whereas 71% of patients younger than 40 (5 of 7) had midtendinous tears. Surgical treatment consisted of nonabsorbable suture repair followed by immobilization for 6 weeks and physical therapy. All patients treated acutely (range 0 to 5 days) demonstrated excellent results compared with only good results in the two patients with delayed repairs (30 and 70 days postinjury).

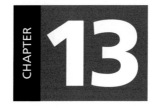

Arthrofibrosis of the Knee

Introduction

- Arthrofibrosis refers to the development of postsurgical or posttraumatic scar tissue leading to a loss of motion of the affected joint (Figure 13–1).
- Impairment of function may follow if the situation cannot be resolved by either conservative or surgical methods.
- Researchers have discovered a possible genetic predisposition to the development of arthrofibrosis.
- Incidence of arthrofibrosis has decreased with improved surgical techniques for anterior cruciate ligament (ACL) reconstruction and postoperative rehabilitation emphasizing early range of motion.
- Infrapatellar contraction syndrome is a related condition that involves the development of vigorous scar formation in the anterior soft tissue structures of the knee.
  - This fibrous tissue acts as a tether on the patella that draws it into a position of patella baja.
  - Knee flexion is sometimes limited by this condition, and it can be recognized on examination or radiograph.
- A classification system for arthrofibrosis was described by Shelbourne in 1999:
  - Type 1: ≤10 degrees of extension loss with normal flexion.
  - Type 2: >10 degrees of extension loss with normal flexion.
  - Type 3: >10 degrees of extension loss with >25 degrees of flexion loss and decreased patellar mobility.
  - Type 4: >10 degrees of extension loss with ≥30 degrees of flexion loss and decreased patellar mobility with evidence of patella baja.

Prevention

- Prevention is the first step to minimizing complications associated with the development of arthrofibrosis.
- Understanding and recognizing the factors that may predispose a patient to the development of this problem is an important first step (Box 13–1, Table 13–1).

- In conditions such as ACL tear, which do not require immediate surgical attention, effusion and motion loss associated with the initial injury should be allowed to resolve prior to considering operative intervention.
- In patients who exhibit a loss of motion at initial presentation, a formal physical therapy program should be considered prior to the surgery.
- Combined ligament injuries such as the medial collateral ligament (MCL) and medial patellofemoral ligament (MPFL) can predispose the patient to the development of arthrofibrosis.
- Intraoperatively, concern should be taken to properly place tunnels and tension grafts to help avoid motion difficulties in the postoperative period.

Postoperative Considerations

- Postoperatively, hemarthrosis should be minimized with good intraoperative hemostasis, judicious use of drains, and cryotherapy. If the hemarthrosis is persistent and affecting motion, aspiration may become necessary.
- Range of motion exercises should begin immediately in the postoperative period with emphasis on extension.
  - Loss of only 5 to 10 degrees of extension can result in quadriceps weakness, patellofemoral pain, and a "bent knee" gait.
  - Loss of up to 20 degrees of flexion is usually well tolerated, except in sprinting athletes.
- Even immediately postoperatively, patients should not be allowed to keep their knee in a flexed position. Beginning in the recovery room, the pillow should be placed under the heel and not the knee!
- Continuous passive motion (CPM) machines may be beneficial in the early postoperative period.
  - This is especially true if other surgical or patient-related factors will impede an early passive motion rehabilitation program.
  - The use of CPM machines may be restricted by cost and insurance authorization and should therefore be reserved for cases when obtaining early motion might otherwise be difficult.

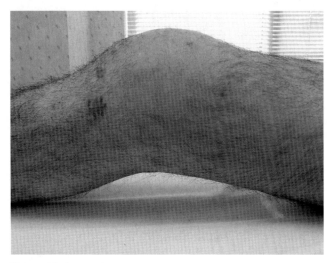

Figure 13–1:
Postsurgical arthrofibrosis.

- If restricted weight-bearing is not an essential part of the postoperative course, patients should be encouraged to return to normal ambulation as early as possible. This allows for a faster return of quadriceps function, which may assist the return of motion as well.
- Reflex sympathetic dystrophy (RSD), also known as complex regional pain syndrome (CRPS), may contribute to postoperative motion restriction, so symptoms of this should be remembered and recognized as early as possible (Box 13–2).

Box 13–1	Risk Factors for the Development of Arthrofibrosis

Prior surgery
Presence of an effusion
Decreased quadriceps muscle tone
Associated head injury
Associated fracture
Gait disturbances
Graft impingement

Table 13–1:	Anterior Cruciate Ligament Graft Placement Problems	
PROBLEM	POSSIBLE CAUSE	TREATMENT
Limited flexion	Shallow femoral tunnel	Revision reconstruction
Extension block	Anterior tibial tunnel	Notchplasty/possible revision
	Or inadequate notchplasty	Revision notchplasty
	Cyclops lesion	Debridement of Cyclops
Loss of motion	Overtensioning of graft	Revision reconstruction

Box 13–2	Signs and Symptoms of Complex Regional Pain Syndrome

Pain out of proportion to injury
Hyperesthesia
Changes in skin color
Changes in skin temperature
Changes in skin texture
Changes in local hair distribution

Treatment

- Physical therapy is the first-line treatment for arthrofibrosis.
- The use of an extension brace (Figure 13–2) or an extension drop-out cast (Figure 13–3) can be helpful in gaining extension in the early postoperative period.
- Surgical lysis of adhesions (Figure 13–4) and manipulation under anesthesia (Figure 13–5) may be necessary if other measures fail after 6 weeks.
  - Loss of extension should be addressed with aggressive release of adhesions including the anterior surface of the tibia.
  - Revision notchplasty should be considered in cases of graft/roof impingement.
- Patients should be instructed that aggressive physical therapy will need to be started as soon as possible after surgical intervention for arthrofibrosis to maintain the motion that was obtained.
- Patients also need to be instructed on such techniques as prone hangs, heel slides, wall slides, and manual pressure so that these may be done at home in addition to the formal supervised physical therapy.

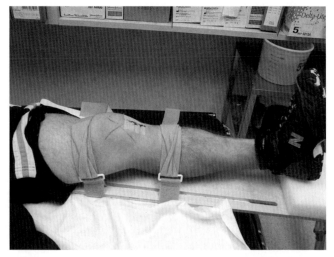

Figure 13–2:
Commercially available extension brace. Note that heel is placed on elevated surface and straps are used to achieve extension. This brace is typically worn three times a day for 10- to 15-minute intervals.

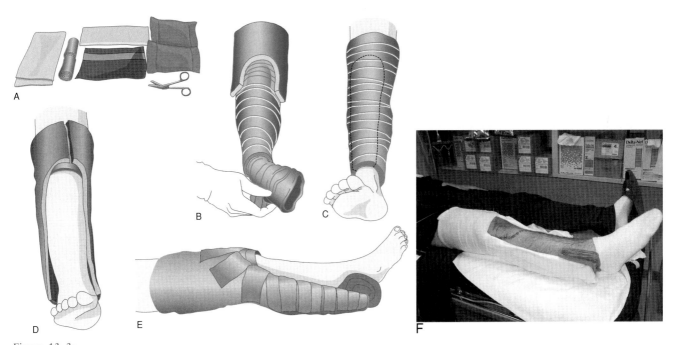

Figure 13–3:
Extension drop-out cast. **A,** Lay necessary supplies out before beginning cast. **B,** Cast is applied. **C,** Area to be cut out is marked as shown. **D,** Anterior portion is cut out as marked. **E,** Edges are padded to prevent skin irritation. **F,** Final cast appearance.

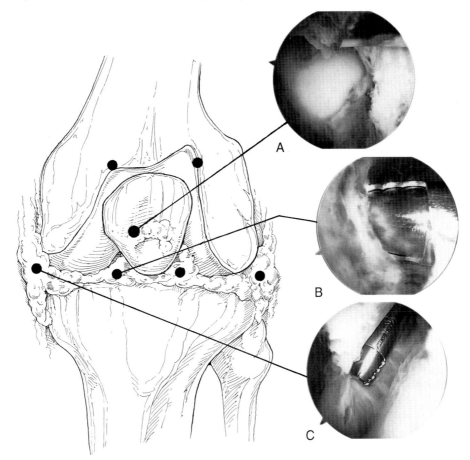

Figure 13–4:
Arthroscopic lysis of adhesions. **A,** Area in front of lateral femoral condyle. **B,** Notch. **C,** Medial gutter. (From Miller MD, Howard RF, Plancher KD: *Surgical atlas of sports medicine.* Philadelphia, 2003, WB Saunders.)

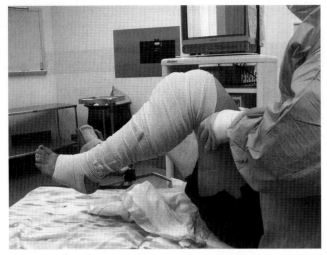

Figure 13–5:
Range of motion following lysis of adhesions and manipulation under anesthesia.

References

DeHaven KE, Cosgarea AJ, Sebastianelli WJ: Arthrofibrosis of the knee following ligament surgery. *Instruct Course Lect* 52:369-81, 2003.

This instructional course lecture discusses the development of arthrofibrosis as a potentially disabling complication of anterior ligament reconstructive surgeries. Aggressive physical therapy has been shown to decrease the rates of incidence. Another factor that has shown to be beneficial is waiting to perform surgery until after the acute inflammation from the injury has resolved.

Lindenfeld TN, Wojtys EM, Husain A: Operative treatment of arthrofibrosis of the knee. *J Bone Joint Surg Am* 81:1772-1783, 1999.

This is another instructional course lecture providing an overview of operative management of knee arthrofibrosis.

Mills WJ, Tejwani N: Heterotopic ossification after knee dislocation: the predictive value of the injury severity score. *J Orthop Trauma* 17:338-345, 2003.

This study looks at factors that affect the development of heterotopic ossification (HO) and shows that a higher injury severity score (ISS) and concurrent head injury are significant predictable risk factors in the development of heterotopic ossification. Increased length of time from injury to surgery and higher number of ligaments reconstructed are not risk factors for the development of HO.

Mohtadi NG, Webster-Bogaert S, Fowler PJ: Limitation of motion following anterior cruciate ligament reconstruction. A case-control study. *Am J Sports Med* 19:620-624, 1991.

Postsurgical loss of motion is a difficult complication of ACL reconstruction. Surgeries performed less than 2 weeks after injury are more likely to develop stiffness, whereas other factors such as age, sex, and associated

ligament or meniscal injury do not tend to contribute to the development of knee stiffness postoperatively.

Noyes FR, Barber-Westin SD: Reconstruction of the anterior and posterior cruciate ligaments after knee dislocation. Use of early protected postoperative motion to decrease arthrofibrosis. *Am J Sports Med* 25:769-78, 1997.

These authors demonstrate that when a combined knee cruciate ligament and medial or lateral collateral ligament are reconstructed, there is a very high rate of developing decreased motion in that knee. However, treatment with manipulation or lysis of adhesions or both, is helpful in the prevention of permanent arthrofibrosis.

Noyes FR, Berrios-Torres S, Barber-Westin SD, Heckmann TP: Prevention of permanent arthrofibrosis after anterior cruciate ligament reconstruction alone or combined with associated procedures: a prospective study in 443 knees. *Knee Surg Sports Traumatol Arthrosc* 8:196-206, 2000.

These authors conclude that early range-of-motion exercises following ACL surgery effectively prevent the development of arthrofibrosis. In the 5% of patients who do go on to develop arthrofibrosis, intervention from extension casting to arthroscopic lysis of adhesions can restore normal motion and function.

Recht MP, Piraino DW, Cohen MA, et al: Localized anterior arthrofibrosis (cyclops lesion) after reconstruction of the anterior cruciate ligament: MR imaging findings. *Am J Roentgenol* 165:383-385, 1995.

Magnetic resonance imaging (MRI) is a useful tool in diagnosing a patient with having focal arthrofibrosis (Cyclops lesion) after an ACL reconstruction. The MRI appearance is that of soft tissue within the notch just anterior to the ACL graft.

Shelbourne KD, Patel DV: Treatment of limited motion after anterior cruciate ligament reconstruction. *Knee Surg Sports Traumatol Arthrosc* 7:85-92, 1999.

These authors define arthrofibrosis and establish a treatment algorithm for their patients who develop this condition following anterior cruciate ligament reconstruction.

Skutek M, Elsner H, Slateva K, Mayer H, et al: Screening for arthrofibrosis after anterior cruciate ligament reconstruction: analysis of association with human leukocyte antigen. *Arthroscopy* 20:469-473, 2004.

Because of the serious nature of arthrofibrosis as a postsurgical complication, it is concerning that some patients develop this problem regardless of an otherwise appropriate rehabilitative course. The authors suggest that there is a genetic predisposition to the condition as they find a link between certain loci in DNA samples and arthrofibrosis.

Stannard JP, Wilson TC, Sheils TM, et al: Heterotopic ossification associated with knee dislocation. *Arthroscopy* 18:835-839, 2002.

These authors demonstrate that the incidence of arthrofibrosis after knee dislocation is 26% with 12% of cases exhibiting severe arthrofibrosis (>50% of joint involved). The also demonstrate no increased risk of developing arthrofibrosis in patients who also sustained a head injury or fracture at the time of their injury.

Pediatric Knee Injuries

CHAPTER 14

Physeal Injuries

- Injury to the distal femoral physis is more frequent than to the proximal tibial physis. This may be explained by the greater amount of activity found in the distal femoral physis, which is responsible for approximately 70% of total femoral growth.
- Salter-Harris type II fractures, in which the fracture line runs from the epiphysis and into the metaphysis, is the most common type (Figure 14–1).
- Patients are often unable to ambulate and complain of swelling and pain.
- Deformity may be present on examination with displaced injuries.
- Neurovascular examination must be carefully performed to rule out any damage to the popliteal vessels or peroneal nerve, which is more commonly found with proximal tibial physeal injury.
- Standard radiographs may be normal in nondisplaced fractures. In such cases, oblique or stress views may aid in the diagnosis.
- Magnetic resonance imaging (MRI) may also be helpful in more occult fractures that occur in the coronal or sagittal plane.
- Salter-Harris types I and II respond well to closed reduction and immobilization for 4 to 6 weeks in a long leg or hip spica cast.
- Salter-Harris III or IV fractures that are stable and nondisplaced may also be managed by cast immobilization and frequent follow-up to ensure there is no displacement.
- Stabilization of fractures with pins or screws is recommended by some authorities.
- Salter-Harris types III and IV with displacement, as well as types I and II with poor closed reduction, should undergo open reduction and internal fixation.

Ligament Injuries

- Medial collateral ligament (MCL) injuries are common in children and are successfully treated with bracing and early motion, similar to adults.

- Anterior cruciate ligament (ACL) injuries have been diagnosed with greater frequency in children.
  - Treatment is problematic given that optimal reconstruction of this ligament requires drilling through the femur and tibia, which in children disturbs the growth plates.
  - Many recommend an initial trial of conservative management with activity modification and bracing.
  - Patients with persistent symptoms or unstable meniscal tears often require surgery.
  - Several techniques have been described to avoid the disturbance of the growth plates but have not achieved the success of the standard method used in adult ACL reconstruction.
  - Physeal sparing reconstruction techniques unfortunately do not reproduce the normal isometry and kinematics of the knee but can provide a temporary or permanent solution in some patients. Hybrid reconstructions, such as those using hamstring or other soft tissue grafts secured to a central tibial tunnel and over the top of the femur, may provide successful results (Figure 14–2).
  - Transphyseal reconstructions closely resemble the normal ACL anatomy and are similar to adult procedures. However, this procedure requires producing tunnels across both the proximal tibia and distal femoral physes (Figure 14–3).
  - Some surgeons advocate delaying surgery until less than 1 cm of growth remains in the femoral physis.
- ACL avulsion fracture of the intercondylar eminence has been most commonly described in children between 8 and 15 years of age involved in bicycle accidents.
- Classification of tibial eminence fractures (Box 14–1, Figure 14–4).
  - Initial management is closed reduction and long leg cast immobilization for 4 to 6 weeks.
  - Unsatisfactory reduction (>2 mm) (and type III) or persistent symptoms require arthroscopic reduction and fixation of the fractured fragment followed by immobilization in the position that results in the best anatomic reduction, usually between 20 and 30 degrees of flexion.

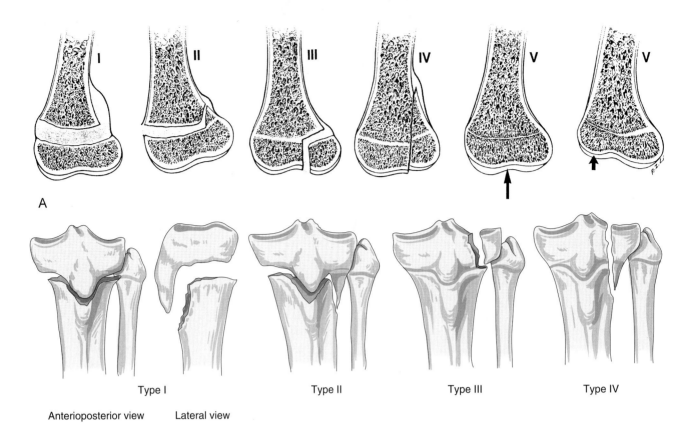

Figure 14–1:
A, Salter-Harris classification of distal femoral epiphyseal fractures. **B,** Same classification is used for proximal tibia epiphyseal fractures. (**A** from Tria AJ Jr, Klein KS: *An illustrated guide to the knee.* New York, 1992, Churchill Livingstone; **B** redrawn from Zionts LE: *J Am Acad Orthop Surg* 10:348, 2002 and from Hensinger RN, editor: *Operative management of lower extremity fractures in children.* Rosemont, IL, 1992, American Academy of Orthopaedic Surgeons.)

- Care should be taken not to disrupt or entrap the surrounding menisci during operative treatment.

Extensor Mechanism Disorders

Acute

- Patellar dislocation is more common in adolescents than adults but responds well to immobilization for 3 weeks and quadriceps strengthening.
- Patients involved in high-energy trauma or those with suspected chondral or osteochondral injuries can be considered for arthroscopic evaluation.
- Patients with minimally displaced tibial tuberosity fractures (type I) and retained full range of motion can be treated with closed reduction and immobilization in extension in a cylinder or long leg cast for 4 to 6 weeks (Box 14–2).
- Open reduction and internal fixation ensures the best results in type II and III fractures and is recommended in type I fractures when range of motion is affected (Figure 14–5).

- Patellar fractures, rare in children (because the patella is predominantly composed of cartilage), are classified according to the location, pattern, and degree of displacement.
- Patellar sleeve fractures, identified as an avulsion fracture of the patella with a large cartilaginous segment, are unique to the pediatric population (particularly in children 8 to 12 years of age) (Figure 14–6).
  - Most frequently occur along the medial border (47%—often associated with patellar dislocations) followed by the inferior pole (38%).
  - The small bony fragment can be missed on radiographic evaluation.
- Most commonly result from a sudden contraction of the extensor mechanism or direct blow.
- Hemarthrosis, swelling, tenderness, extensor lag, and patella alta are common physical examination findings.
- Minimally displaced (≤ 2 mm) fractures with an intact extensor mechanism can be treated by immobilization in extension.

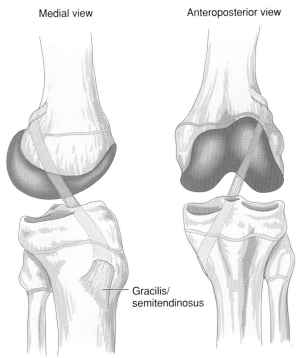

Medial view   Anteroposterior view

Gracilis/
semitendinosus

Figure 14–2:
Partial (over the top) transphyseal anterior cruciate ligament (ACL) reconstruction. (Redrawn from Stanitski CL: *J Am Acad Orthop Surg* **3:146-158, 1995.)**

- Displaced fractures or a disrupted extensor mechanism, or both, require open reduction and internal fixation using tension band wiring or screw fixation.

Overuse Injuries

- Bipartite patellae is usually discovered incidentally on radiographic evaluation.

Box 14–1	Meyers and McKeever Classification of Tibial Eminence Fractures

Type I: Fracture with no displacement
Type II: Fracture with elevation of the anterior portion of the tibial eminence and intact posteriorly
Type III: Completely displaced fracture

- It is most commonly located at the superolateral pole of the patella and is the result of an accessory ossification center that failed to fuse (Box 14–3, Figure 14–7).
- The fragment is usually attached to the remainder of the patella by thick fibrous tissue.
- Although primarily asymptomatic, in selected patients it may be the cause of anterior knee pain, especially with activities demanding jumping or squatting or after direct trauma.
- It is believed that stretching or tearing of the fibrous union is the principle source of pain.
- Conservative management with activity modifications and nonsteroidal antiinflammatory drugs (NSAIDs) is the standard.
- Protected weight-bearing with crutches and an immobilizer can initially be recommended with range-of-motion exercises out of the brace several times a day for up to 3 to 4 weeks.
- Large displaced fragments associated with direct trauma may require open reduction and internal fixation.
- Rarely is excision of the fragment recommended.
- Osgood-Schlatter disease is a traction apophysis thought to be the result of repetitive stress placed on the immature patellar tendon insertion site into the secondary ossification center of the tibial tuberosity.

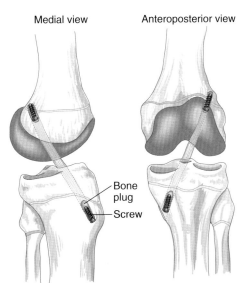
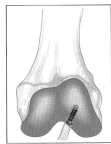

Medial view   Anteroposterior view

Bone
plug
Screw

Figure 14–3:
Transphyseal anterior cruciate ligament (ACL) reconstruction. (Redrawn from Stanitski CL: *J Am Acad Orthop Surg* **3:146-158, 1995.)**

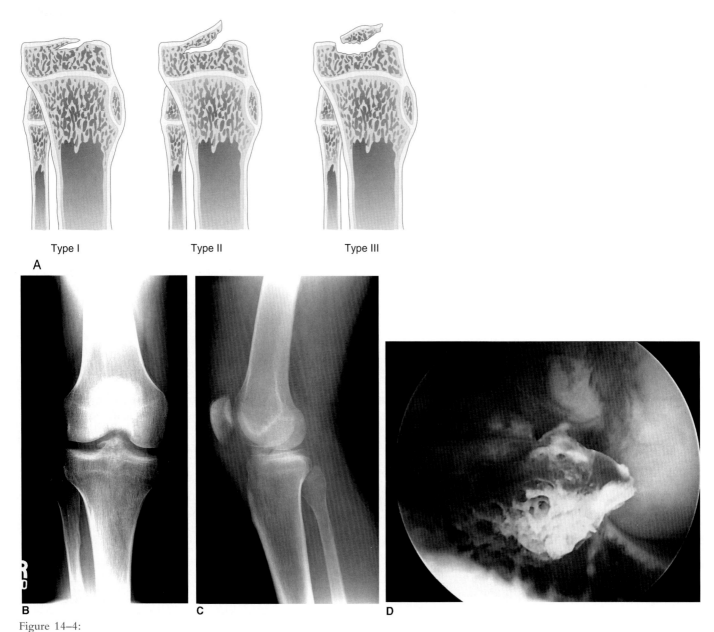

Type I   Type II   Type III

A

B   C   D

Figure 14–4:
Anterior cruciate ligament (ACL) avulsion/tibial eminence fractures. **A,** Schematic of Meyers and McKeever classification of tibial eminence fractures. Type I: fracture with no displacement, Type II: fracture with elevation of the anterior portion of the tibial eminence and intact posteriorly, Type III: completely displaced fracture. **B** and **C,** Anteroposterior (AP) and lateral radiographs of a type II ACL avulsion injury. **D,** Arthroscopic view of the displaced tibial eminence. (**A** redrawn from Zionts LE:. *J Am Acad Orthop Surg* 10:345-355, 2002.)

(continued)

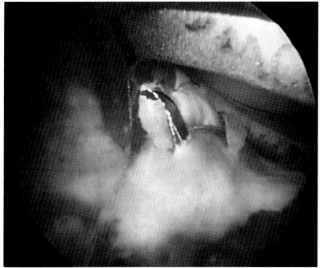

E

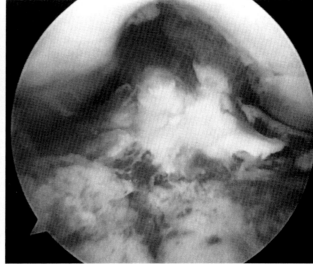

G

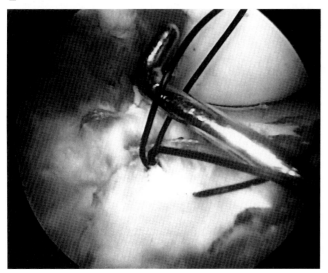

F

Figure 14–4, cont'd:
E, An ACL guide is used to drill a guide pin through the bony fragment. **F,** A suture passer is used to shuttle suture through the tibial eminence arthroscopically. **G,** The tibial eminence is secured anatomically using several No. 2 sutures.

- It is most common in adolescent male athletes 13 to 14 years old and is reported to be bilateral in 20% to 30% of patients. Girls affected are most commonly 10 to 11 years old.
- Pain, particularly with kneeling, and a prominent tibial tubercle may persist into adulthood.
- Swelling and tenderness may be appreciated at the tendon insertion site.
- Standard radiographs may reveal heterotropic ossification at the site of the tubercle (Figure 14–8A).
- Activity modification, NSAIDs, and occasionally immobilization with daily range of motion exercises (for 4 to 8 weeks) often are adequate for treatment.

- In some instances, surgical removal of symptomatic ossicles may produce resolution of persistent symptoms.
- Sinding-Larsen-Johansson disease, which closely resembles the adult form of jumper's knee, results from repetitive

Box 14–2	Watson-Jones Classification of Tibial Tuberosity Fractures

Type I: Occurs before fusion of the epiphyseal and secondary ossification center of the tuberosity with the fracture line running between both centers
Type II: Occurs after the ossification centers have fused with the fracture line dividing the tuberosity and proximal tibial plateau
Type III: Fracture line extends through the proximal tibial plateau

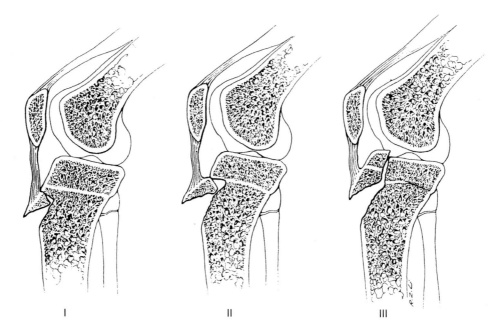

Figure 14–5:

Watson-Jones classification of tibial tuberosity fractures. Type I: Occurs before fusion of the epiphyseal and secondary ossification center of the tuberosity with the fracture line running between both centers, Type II: Occurs after the ossification centers have fused with the fracture line dividing the tuberosity and proximal tibial plateau, Type III: Fracture line extends through the proximal tibial plateau. (From Tria AJ Jr, Klein KS: *An illustrated guide to the knee.* **New York, 1992, Churchill Livingstone.)**

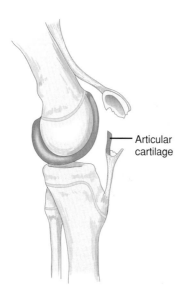

Figure 14–6:

Sleeve fracture of the patella. Small portion of the inferior pole of the patella is avulsed with a large segment of the articular cartilage. (Redrawn from Zionts LE: *J Am Acad Orthop Surg* 10:352, 2002 and from Tolo VT: Fractures and dislocations around the knee. In Green NE, Swiontkowski MF, editors: *Skeletal trauma in children.* Philadelphia, 1994, WB Saunders.)

traction on the immature inferior pole of the patella where the patellar tendon originates.

- It is most frequently seen in patients 11 to 13 years old, slightly younger than those with Osgood-Schlatter disease.
- Pain likely results from microtears within the patella.
- Heterotropic ossification may be demonstrated on plain films at the symptomatic site (Figure 14–8*B*).
- Nonoperative management is the standard treatment.
- As the patella continues to grow and ossify, the bone-tendon bond is usually healed and strengthened.
- Only in older children should surgery be considered because further patellar growth is limited and recovery may be more predictable.

Box 14–3	**Saupe's Classification of Accessory Ossification Centers of the Patella (and Approximate Prevalence)**

Type I: Inferior pole (5%)
Type II: Lateral margin (20%)
Type III: Superolateral pole (75%)

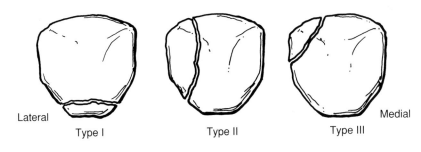

Lateral   Medial

Type I   Type II   Type III

Figure 14–7:
Saupe's classification of accessory ossification centers of the patella. (From Miller MD, Cooper DE, Warner JJP: *Review of sports medicine and arthroscopy,* 2nd ed. Philadelphia, 2002, WB Saunders and from Bottoni CR, Taylor DC, Arciero RA: Patella fractures in the adult. In DeLee JC, Drez D Jr, editors: *Orthopaedic sports medicine: principles and practice.* Philadelphia, 1994, WB Saunders.)

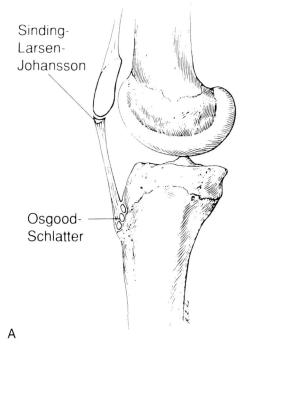

Sinding-
Larsen-
Johansson

Osgood-
Schlatter

A

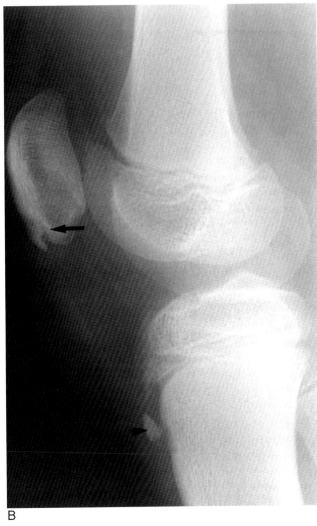

B

Figure 14–8:
A, Schematic drawing demonstrating sites of Osgood-Schlatter and Sinding-Larsen-Johansson disease. **B,** Radiograph of patient with concomitant Osgood-Schlatter and Sinding-Larsen-Johansson disease. (**A** from Miller MD, Cooper DE, Warner JJP: *Review of sports medicine and arthroscopy,* 2nd ed. Philadelphia, 2002, WB Saunders; **B** from DeLee JC, Drez Jr D, Miller MD, editors: *DeLee and Drez's orthopaedic sports medicine: principles and practice,* 2nd ed. Philadelphia, 2003, WB Saunders.)

Rehabilitation

- Initial isometric quadriceps exercises should be performed with the immobilizer after patellar dislocations.
- Reevaluation should occur approximately every 2 weeks.
- On resolution of medial tenderness, the patient can begin more aggressive range-of-motion and strengthening exercises.

Complications

- Angular deformity and shortening may occur with physeal injury.
- Leg-length discrepancy and thigh atrophy is commonly seen after fractures of the distal femoral physis.
- ACL laxity (translation) may persist after tibial spine fractures despite healing anatomically.
- Residual prominence of the tibial tubercle may occur in patients with a history of Osgood-Schlatter disease.

References

Beasley LS, Chudik SC: Anterior cruciate ligament injury in children: update of current treatment options. *Curr Opin Pediatr* 15:45-52, 2003.

Author reports on the current treatment trends in ACL injury in the skeletally immature, which has become more prevalent. As a result of poor outcomes with conservative treatment, several techniques have been developed to reconstruct the ACL without significantly disturbing the growth plates. Although initial reports appear promising, long-term studies and general consensus on surgical reconstruction are still under much debate.

Dorizas JA, Stanitski CL: Anterior cruciate ligament injury in the skeletally immature. *Orthop Clin North Am* 34:355-363, 2003.

Another article addressing the difficulty in managing ACL injury in the skeletally immature. The authors provide a three-phase nonoperative plan and review several of the technical points, advantages, and concerns of several surgical techniques currently being studied for pediatric ACL reconstruction.

Eid AM, Hafez MA: Traumatic injuries of the distal femoral physis. Retrospective study on 151 cases. *Injury* 33:251-255, 2002.

Authors review results of 151 cases of distal femoral physis fractures, divided into Salter-Harris classifications, treated conservatively and surgically. They noted that Salter-Harris type II fractures were most common and after Salter-Harris type V fractures (only 6 total) had the poorest outcomes (46% with poor results) with the surgical group (fixation by Kirschner wires or cancellous screws) performing only slightly better than the conservative group, which was insignificant. Type II fractures were also noted to have a high incidence of angular and shorten-

ing deformities. The authors concluded that further studies are still necessary to determine when nonoperative management is adequate and surgery is indicated.

Kocher MS, DiCanzio J, Zurakowski D, Micheli LJ: Diagnostic performance of clinical examination and selective magnetic resonance imaging in the evaluation of intraarticular knee disorders in children and adolescents. *Am J Sports Med* 29:292-296, 2001.

Authors compared the diagnostic performance of clinical examination and MRI in the evaluation of pediatric intraarticular knee disorders. Results demonstrated no significant difference between clinical examination and MRI for overall sensitivity and specificity (71.2% and 91.5% vs. 72.0% and 93.5%, respectively) and agreement with arthroscopic findings (70.3% vs. 73.7%). However, clinical examination had a significantly greater sensitivity for lateral discoid meniscus (88.9% compared with 38.9% with MRI) and MRI demonstrated greater specificity of medial meniscal tears (92.0% compared with 80.7% with clinical examination). MRI was less sensitive and specific in children younger than 12 years. As a result, the authors stress that MRI should be used judiciously in cases in which clinical diagnosis is difficult to determine or when it may alter treatment. The authors do comment that clinical examinations were performed by pediatric sports medicine specialists, whereas MRIs were evaluated by radiologists with varying experiences.

Strouse PJ, Koujok K: Magnetic resonance imaging of the pediatric knee. *Top Magn Reson Imaging* 13:277-294, 2002.

A comprehensive review, with several example images, discussing the indications, techniques, and findings of MRI in the pediatric knee. A wide range of disorders, with an emphasis on traumatic conditions, are evaluated. Authors provide a systemic approach to image interpretation and note differences between the adult and pediatric knee on MRI.

Wessel LM, Scholz S, Rusch M: Characteristic patterns and management of intra-articular knee lesions in different pediatric age groups. *J Ped Orthop* 21:14-19, 2001.

Retrospective study evaluating 1273 patients up to 16 years of age with knee trauma to define specific injury patterns and effective diagnostic techniques according to age. Soft tissue injuries prevailed in all age groups (10 years or younger, 11-12, 13-16) but significantly decreased with age. Metaphyseal fractures of the femur and tibia were more common in patients 10 or younger. Conversely, the incidence of hemarthrosis, cruciate ligament ruptures, intraligamentous injury, and meniscal lesions increased with age. Physical examination, radiographs, and judicious use of MRI were often sufficient to define knee injuries in patients younger than 13 years. Arthroscopy is generally reserved for patients older than 13 years requiring further evaluation when it can lead to therapeutic options.

Zionts LE: Fractures around the knee in children. *J Am Acad Orthop Surg* 10:345-355, 2002.

Author reviews the diagnosis, classification, treatment, and outcome of fractures around the pediatric knee.

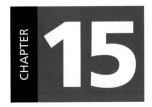

Hip Anatomy and Biomechanics

Anatomy

Joint

- The hip joint is composed of the acetabulum, which is formed from portions of the ilium, ischium, and pubis, and the femoral head.
- The hip is perhaps the best example of a "ball and socket" joint. The lunate articular surface surrounds the majority of the joint in an inverted horseshoe shape.
- The labrum is a fibrocartilaginous structure adding stability to the hip and deepens the articular socket of the acetabulum. It is contiguous with the transverse acetabular ligament (Figure 15–1).
- The ligamentum teres attaches the acetabulum to the femoral head and offers a limited blood supply to the head. It attaches at the fovea capitis.
- The femoral head forms two thirds of a sphere.
- The neck-shaft angle of the proximal femur is approximately 130 degrees.
- The femoral head/neck is anteverted approximately 15 degrees relative to the bicondylar axis of the knee (Figure 15–2).
- The anterior hip capsule (composed primarily of the iliofemoral ligament [of Bigelow]) (Figure 15–3A) is much stronger and inserts farther distal than the posterior hip capsule (ischiofemoral ligament) (Figure 15–3B).

Muscles

- Superficial muscles (Figure 15–4A).
  - Tensor fascia lata.
    - Bridges over greater trochanter (implicated in "external snapping hip").
    - Becomes iliotibial band distally to attach to Gerdy's tubercle.
  - Sartorius.
    - Insertion onto tibia is one of three muscles making up pes anserinus.
    - Insertion forms facial covering over semitendinosus and gracilis.
    - Longest muscle in the body.
  - Gluteus maximus.
    - Major hip external rotator and abductor.
    - "Pelvic deltoid."
    - Largest muscle in the body.
- Gluteus medius.
  - Transition layer.
  - Internal rotator of hip and pelvic girdle stabilizer.
  - Weakness secondary to pain and neurologic dysfunction results in Trendelenburg sign/gait.
- Deep muscles.
  - Posterior group (Figure 15–4B).
    - Piriformis, obturator internus and externus, superior and inferior gemmulae, and quadratus femoris.
    - Short external rotators.
    - Sciatic nerve exits hip between piriformis and remaining short external rotators.
  - Lateral group (gluteus minimus).
  - Anterior group (Figure 15–4C).
    - Rectus femoris, iliopsoas.
    - Implicated on "internal snapping hip."
  - Medial group (adductors [longus, magnus, brevis], pectineus, gracilis).

Neurovascular Structures

- Anterior structures (Figure 15–5A).
  - The femoral nerve, artery, vein (and lymph vessels) (Lateral to medial: NAVL) lie on the surface of the iliopsoas muscle under the inguinal ligament.
- Posterior structures (Figure 15–5B).
  - Key structures that enter the lower extremity below the piriformis muscle (the so-called key to the sciatic foramen) include the sciatic nerve, inferior gluteal nerve and artery, pudendal nerve, posterior femoral cutaneous nerve, and the medial circumflex femoral artery (more distal).
  - The medial and lateral circumflex femoral arteries supply the main blood supply to the femoral head.

Biomechanics

- Hip range of motion (average).
  - Flexion 115 degrees.
  - Extension 30 degrees.

Text continued on p. 126

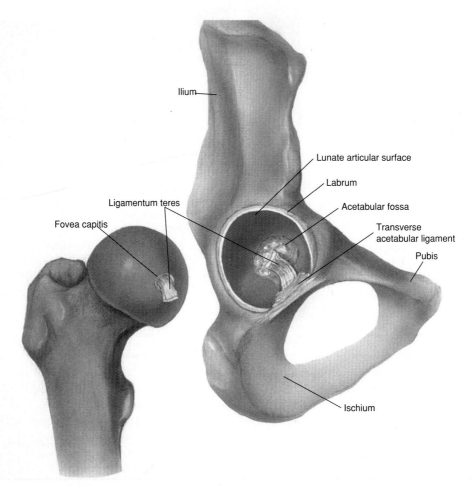

Figure 15–1:
Hip joint anatomy. (From Byrd JWT: Gross anatomy. In Byrd JWT, editor: *Operative hip arthroscopy.* New York, 1998, Thieme.)

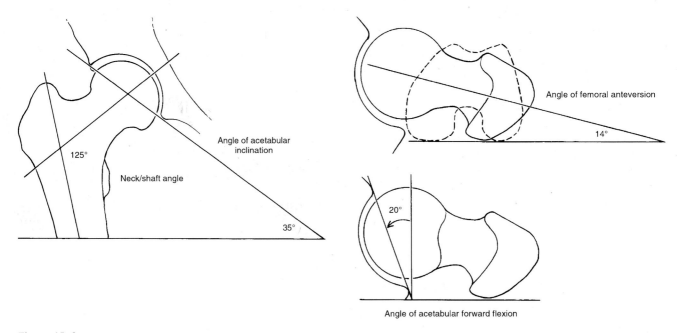

Figure 15–2:
Acetabular orientation. (From Byrd JWT: Gross anatomy. In Byrd JWT, editor: *Operative hip arthroscopy.* New York, 1998, Thieme.)

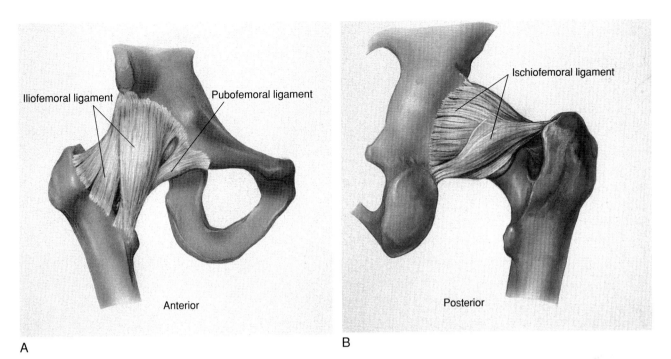

Figure 15–3:
A, Anterior hip capsule. **B,** Posterior hip capsule. (From Byrd JWT: Gross anatomy. In Byrd JWT, editor: *Operative hip arthroscopy.* New York, 1998, Thieme.)

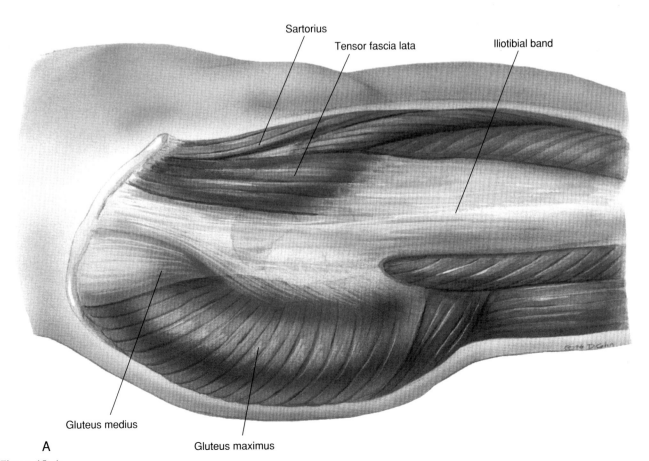

Figure 15–4:
Hip muscle anatomy. A, Superficial muscle layer.

(continued)

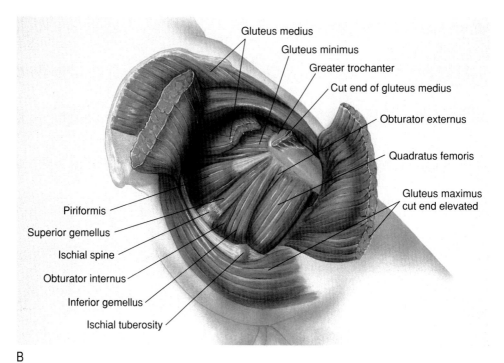

Gluteus medius
Gluteus minimus
Greater trochanter
Cut end of gluteus medius
Obturator externus
Quadratus femoris
Gluteus maximus cut end elevated
Piriformis
Superior gemellus
Ischial spine
Obturator internus
Inferior gemellus
Ischial tuberosity

B

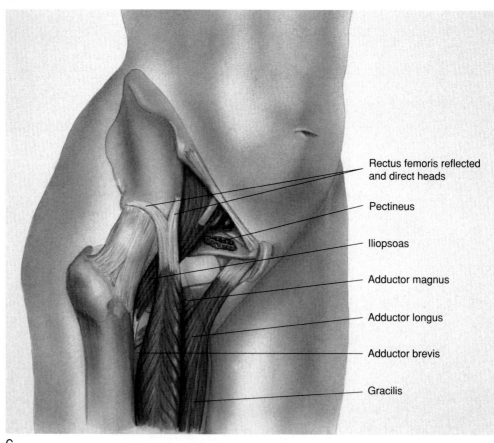

Rectus femoris reflected and direct heads
Pectineus
Iliopsoas
Adductor magnus
Adductor longus
Adductor brevis
Gracilis

C

Figure 15–4, cont'd:
B, Deep structures (posterior view). **C,** Deep structures (anterior view). (From Byrd JWT: Gross anatomy. In Byrd JWT, editor: *Operative hip arthroscopy.* New York, 1998, Thieme.)

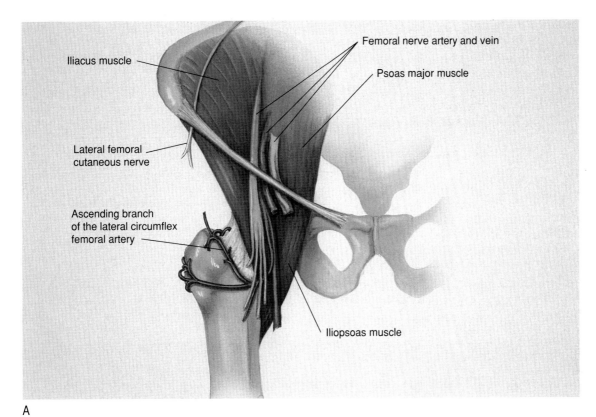

Femoral nerve artery and vein

Psoas major muscle

Iliacus muscle

Lateral femoral
cutaneous nerve

Ascending branch
of the lateral circumflex
femoral artery

Iliopsoas muscle

A

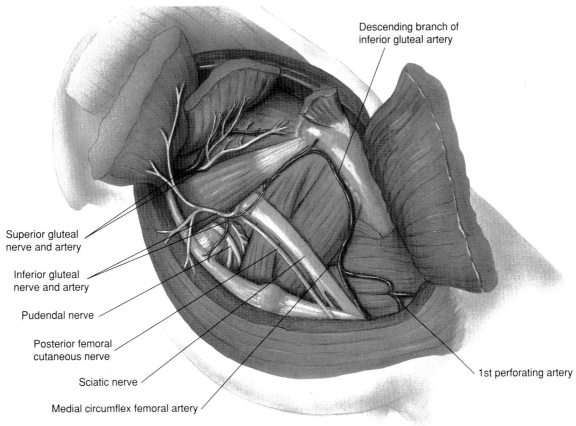

Descending branch of
inferior gluteal artery

Superior gluteal
nerve and artery

Inferior gluteal
nerve and artery

Pudendal nerve

Posterior femoral
cutaneous nerve

Sciatic nerve

Medial circumflex femoral artery

1st perforating artery

B

Figure 15–5:
A, Hip neurovascular anatomy (anterior view). **B,** Hip neurovascular anatomy (posterior view). (From Byrd JWT: Gross anatomy. In Byrd JWT, editor: *Operative hip arthroscopy.* New York, 1998, Thieme.)

- Abduction 50 degrees.
- Adduction 30 degrees.
- Internal rotation 45 degrees.
- External rotation 45 degrees.
- Joint reaction force.
  - Up to three to six times body weight.
  - Greatest with standing from seated position.
  - 1.5 times body weight with "non–weight-bearing."
  - Concentrated at sourcil (superomedial acetabulum).

References

Byrd JWT: Gross anatomy. In Byrd JWT, editor: *Operative hip arthroscopy.* New York, 1998, Thieme.

   This is an excellent reference with clear illustrations. Several of these figures have been reproduced, with permission, in this chapter.

Dienst M, Godde S, Seil R, et al: Hip arthroscopy without traction: in vivo anatomy of the peripheral hip joint cavity. *Arthroscopy* 17:924-931, 2001.

   By performing 35 hip arthroscopies without distraction, these authors clearly identify anatomic structures and suggest a systematic approach to ensure that all intraarticular areas are explored during the procedure.

Henry AK: *Extensile exposure,* 2nd ed. New York, 1973, Churchill Livingstone.

   This is a classic reference for orthopaedic surgical approaches and has an excellent section on hip anatomy.

Hoppenfeld S, DeBoer P, editors: *Surgical exposures in orthopaedics: the anatomic approach,* 2nd ed. Philadelphia, 1994, JB Lippincott.

   Another well-illustrated classic for all orthopaedic surgeons.

Krebs DE, Robbins CE, Lavine L, Mann RW: Hip biomechanics during gait. *J Orthop Sports Phys Ther* 28:51-59, 1998.

   Using gait analysis in an elderly patient with a femoral head prosthesis, these authors are able to define changes in hip gait and biomechanics with and without the use of a cane by the patient. They demonstrate that the use of a cane in the contralateral hand can be beneficial in decreasing the amount of pressure on the acetabulum as well as in decreasing the amount of activity exerted by the gluteus medius during normal gait.

Sweeney HJ: Arthroscopy of the hip. Anatomy and portals. *Clin Sports Med* 20:697-702, 2001.

   Again the authors describe the normal anatomy of the hip as viewed through the arthroscope, emphasizing both a supine patient positioning and lateral decubitus positioning.

Hip Arthroscopy

Introduction

- Since its establishment, hip arthroscopy has allowed the identification and treatment of several intraarticular conditions that were previously difficult to detect.
- Technically difficult procedure because of the deep location of the hip joint within dense soft tissues and a thick capsule (Figure 16–1).
- Neurovascular structures are at minimal risk.
- Lower morbidity than formal arthrotomy, with an easier postoperative course.
- Indications (Box 16–1).
- Contraindications (Box 16–2).

Surgical Technique

- Supine or lateral decubitus position.
- Traction setup required. Traction vector should be in line with the femoral neck, which can be produced from lateral distraction using the perineal post and distal distraction (Figure 16–3).

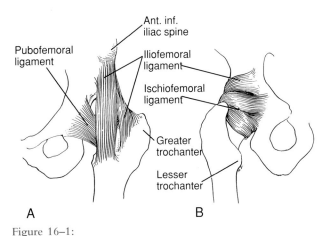

Figure 16–1:
Ligamentous constraints of the hip. Anterior (A) and posterior (B) views of the hip joint. (From Jenkins DB, Hollinshead WH: *Hollinshead's functional anatomy of the limbs and back.* Philadelphia, 2002 Saunders.)

Box 16–1	Surgical Indications

Diagnostic (undiagnosed hip pain failing conservative management)
Labral tear (Figure 16–2)
Loose bodies (ossified or nonossified)
Synovial disease such as synovitis, pigmented villonodular synovitis, or synovial chondromatosis
Degenerative joint disease
Chondral injuries
Osteonecrosis
Joint infection/septic arthritis
Ligamentum teres injuries
Instability
Snapping hip syndrome/iliopsoas bursitis
Staging for femoral head avascular necrosis

Box 16–2	Surgical Contraindications

Generally any condition that limits capsular mobility, proper distraction, and/or introduction of arthroscopic instruments
Hip ankylosis
Advanced osteoarthritis
Significant joint contracture
Inability to undergo traction to involved lower extremity
Severe osteoporotic bone
Significant wound condition or abnormal anatomy
Grade III or grade IV heterotropic ossification
Significant protrusio acetabuli

- A well-padded perineal post placed against the proximal medial thigh improves lateral distraction and reduces the risk of pudendal nerve palsy.
- Time is monitored as soon as traction is applied to the operative lower extremity.
- Image intensification (e.g., C-arm) is recommended for spinal needle placement (to be used for insufflation of the hip joint with saline), evaluation/confirmation of adequate distraction, and guidewire and initial portal placement (Figure 16–4).
- Hip arthroscopy instrumentation is specially made to be longer and stouter, with cannulated trocars so guidewires can be used, and to provide adequate reach to the surgical site.

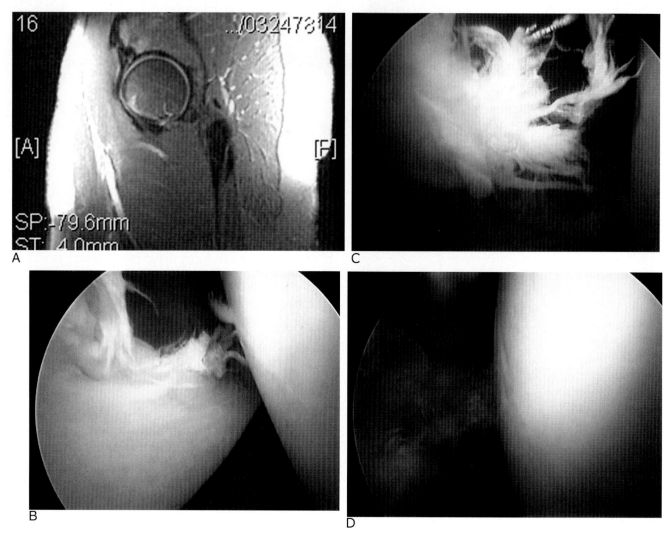

Figure 16–2:
Labral debridement. **A,** Magnetic resonance imaging of a labral tear. **B,** Arthroscopic view of an acetabular labral tear. **C,** Close-up view. **D,** After arthroscopic debridement.

- Usually both a 30- and 70-degree arthroscope are necessary for complete visualization of the hip joint.
- Prior to establishing any portals, distention of the joint should be performed, using saline fluid through a spinal needle placed under fluoroscopy, releasing the negative pressure vacuum created by joint distraction, and assisting placement of trocars and cannulas and allowing greater maneuverability of instruments.
- During portal placement, the trocar and cannula should be directed toward the femoral head.
- The first portal is usually a paratrochanteric portal: anterior, proximal, or posterior. Generally, the anterior paratrochanteric (anterolateral) portal is recommended as the initial portal because it runs the least risk of injury to neurovascular structures (Figure 16–5).
- The anterior paratrochanteric portal is placed under fluoroscopic guidance approximately 1 to 2 cm superior

and 1 to 2 cm anterior to the anterosuperior border of the greater trochanter.
- The anterior portal is then made with a starting point in line with the tip of the greater trochanter intersecting a line distally from the anterior superior iliac spine and inserted into the joint under arthroscopic visualization. Placement is directed 45 degrees cephalad and 30 degrees medially into the joint (Figure 16–6).
- Flexing and internally rotating the hip relaxes the anterior capsule and can assist anterior arthroscope placement.
- The second portal can be used as a working portal with various shavers, graspers, and specially made radiofrequency ablation devices that can bend 90 degrees at the tip for increased maneuverability.
- The arthroscopic visualization and working portals are then switched to have a complete view of the hip joint.

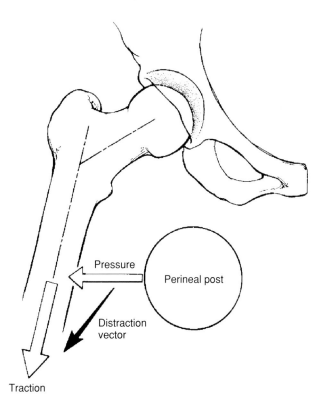

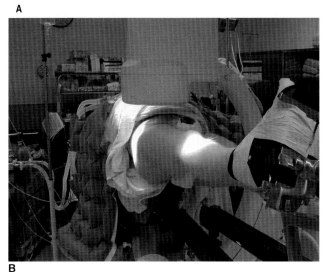

B

Figure 16–3:
Positioning for hip arthroscopy. **A,** The perineal post is placed as far lateral as possible against the medial thigh to provide a lateral force vector. The addition of distal traction produces the desired distraction vector force. **B,** Actual traction setup with foot internally rotated. (**A** from Byrd JWT: *Hip arthroscopy: principles and application.* Andover, MA, 1996 Smith & Nephew Endoscopy.)

- The posterolateral (posterior paratrochanteric) portal is entered 2 to 3 cm posterior to the tip of the greater trochanter (Figure 16–7).

- If needed, additional portals can be placed (usually under arthroscopic visualization) to improve visualization and access all areas of the hip joint.

Mini-Open Technique

- Because of the significant technical difficulties with gaining arthroscopic access to the hip joint, an alternative technique has been developed (Figure 16–8).
- A small, cosmetic, 3- to 4-cm skin incision is made in the groin skin crease centered over the anterior inferior iliac spine.
- The interval between the sartorius and tensor fascia lata is developed while protecting the lateral femoral cutaneous nerve.
- The rectus femoris muscle is identified and retracted, followed by the iliopsoas tendon.
- This exposes the anterior hip capsule for arthroscopic access.
- Manual traction is usually adequate, and range of motion of the hip is allowed during the arthroscopic examination, which may improve visualization of difficult areas to access.

Rehabilitation

- Considerably shorter rehabilitation than with open procedures, providing quicker return to full activity.
- Depending on the procedure performed, protected weight-bearing with crutches is usually begun immediately postoperatively and weight-bearing is advanced to full over a period of a week.
- Passive, active-assisted, and then active range-of-motion exercises are begun and advanced along with hip isometric strengthening exercises.
- Once range of motion is full, strengthening can be advanced with progressive resistance exercises, strengthening all muscles of the hip girdle.
- Full activities are usually allowed by 3 months post-operatively as long as strength and range of motion are full.

Complications

- Neuropraxia or direct injury of nerves can be reduced with careful orientation and attention to landmarks. (Table 16–1, Figure 16–9).
  - Anterior portal placement risks injury to the femoral artery and nerve, branches of the lateral circumflex femoral artery, and femoral cutaneous nerve.
  - Anterolateral portal may place the superior gluteal nerve at risk.
  - Excessive posterior placement of the posterolateral portal may injure the underlying sciatic nerve and nearby superior gluteal nerve.

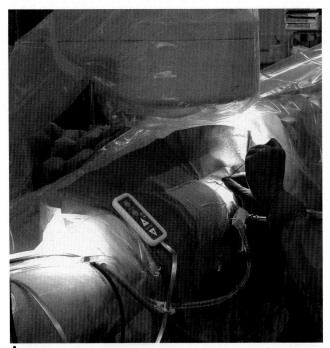

A

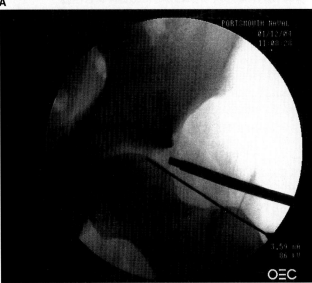

B

Figure 16–4:
A, Setup of the patient intraoperatively for image intensification. **B,** Fluoroscopic view of the hip for the anterior portal placement using a spinal needle.

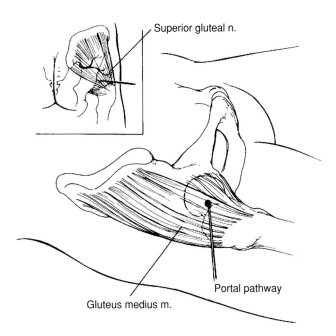

Figure 16–5:
Anterolateral portal. (From Byrd JWT: *Hip arthroscopy: principles and application.* Andover, MA, 1996, Smith & Nephew Endoscopy.)

- Traction and compression injuries (to the peroneal, femoral, sciatic, lateral femoral cutaneous, and pudendal nerves) can be decreased with proper positioning, use of a well-padded perineal post, minimized traction force, and limiting traction time to less than 2 hours.
  - Intermittent release of traction is recommended for longer procedures.
  - Adequate anesthesia (providing muscle relaxation) and fluid distention reduces the forces required for adequate distraction.

- Use of a tensiometer can assist with monitoring traction forces during the procedure.
- Pressure necrosis of the scrotum, perineum, and foot have been described.
- Fluid extravasation into the intraabdominal or intrapelvic cavity.
- Iatrogenic intraarticular damage or trauma to the articular surfaces may occur from portal placement or instrumentation during the procedure.
- Instrument breakage.

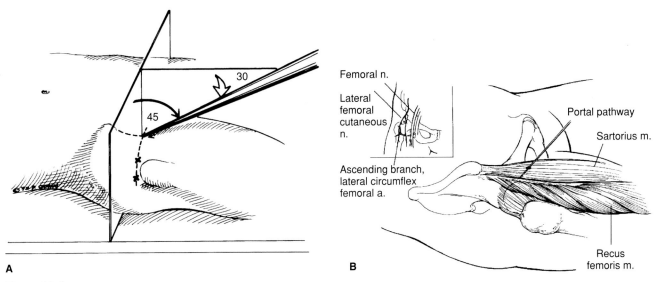

A   B

Figure 16–6:
A, Anterior portal landmarks and direction. Placement coincides with the intersection of a line drawn distally from the anterior superior iliac spine and transverse line drawn from the superior margin of the greater trochanter. The portal is directed approximately 45 degrees cephalad and 30 degrees toward the midline. **B,** Anterior portal placement and relationship to the neurovascular structures. (**A** from Byrd JWT: *Arthroscopy* 10:275-280, 1994; **B** from Byrd JWT: *Hip arthroscopy: principles and application.* Andover, MA, 1996, Smith & Nephew Endoscopy.)

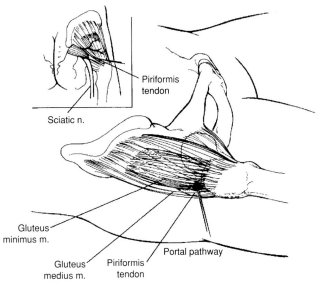

Figure 16–7:
Posterolateral portal placement and relationship to neurologic structures. (From Byrd JWT: *Hip arthroscopy: principles and application.* Andover, MA, 1996 Smith & Nephew Endoscopy.)

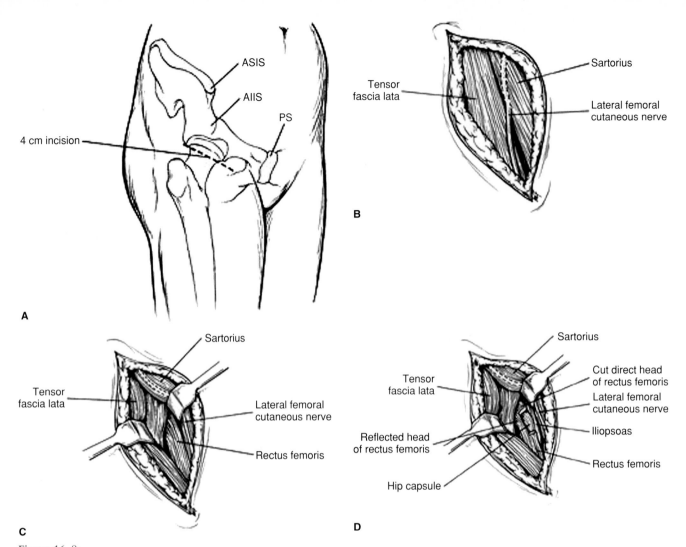

Figure 16-8:

A, Mini-open approach for hip arthroscopy. AIIS, Anterior superior iliac spine; ASIS, anterior inferior iliac spine; PS, pubic symphysis. **B,** Interval between the tensor fascia lata and sartorius muscle. **C,** Rectus femoris muscle is identified and retracted. **D,** Iliopsoas muscle is identified and retracted, exposing the anterior hip capsule. (From Sekiya JK, Wojtys EM, Loder RT, Hensinger RN: *Arthroscopy* 16:16-20, 2000.)

PORTALS	ANATOMIC STRUCTURE	AVERAGE (CM)	RANGE (CM)
	Anterior superior iliac spine	6.3	6-7
	Lateral femoral cutaneous nerve[†]	0.3	0.2-1.0
Anterior	Femoral nerve[‡]		
	Level of sartorius	4.3	3.8-5
	Level of rectus femoris	3.8	2.7-5
	Level of capsule	3.7	2.9-5
	Lateral circumflex femoral artery		
	Ascending branch	3.7	1-6
	Terminal branch[§]	0.3	0.2-0.4
Anterolateral	Superior gluteal nerve	4.4	3.2-5.5
Posterolateral	Sciatic nerve	2.9	2-4.3

Table 16-1: Distance from Portal to Anatomic Structures*

*Based on an anatomic dissection of portal placements in 8 fresh cadaver specimens.
[†]Nerve had divided into three or more branches and measurement was made to the closest branch.
[‡]Measurement made at superficial surface of sartorius, rectus femoris, and capsule.
[§]Small terminal branch of ascending branch of lateral circumflex femoral artery identified in three specimens.
From Byrd JWT, Pappas JN, Pedley MJ: *Arthroscopy* 11:418-123, 1995.

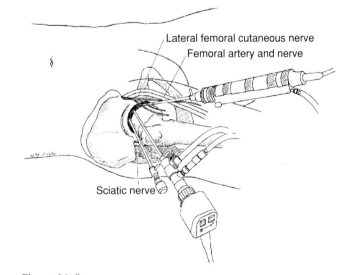

Figure 16-9:

Relationship of major neurovascular structures to the three standard portals. (From Miller MD, Cooper DE, Warner JJP: *Review of sports medicine and arthroscopy,* 2nd ed. Philadelphia, 2002, WB Saunders.)

References

Byrd JW, Chen KY: Traction versus distension for distraction of the joint during hip arthroscopy. *Arthroscopy* 13:346-349, 1997.

> *Study assessing the additive effects of traction and distension on attaining distraction of the hip during arthroscopy. Results demonstrated distention significantly changed the amount of distraction (from 0% to 81% with an average of 22%) when compared with traction alone, although the degree was greatly variable.*

Byrd JW, Jones KS: Hip arthroscopy in the presence of dysplasia. *Arthroscopy* 19:1055-1060, 2003.

> *Prospective clinical study evaluating the results of hip arthroscopy for various conditions in 48 patients with acetabular dysplasia. Given the favorable postoperative outcomes, the authors concluded that hip dysplasia is not a contraindication to arthroscopy. Prognosis appears to be more associated with the underlying condition for which operative treatment is considered.*

Byrd JWT, Pappas JN, Pedley MJ: Hip arthroscopy: an anatomic study of portal placement and relationship to the extra-articular structures. *Arthroscopy* 11:418-423, 1995.

> *Authors define the relationship of significant neurovascular structures to common portals used in hip arthroscopy using cadaver specimens. Average distances of the structures from the portal sites are provided. Although the hips were not distracted, this study reinforces the importance of accurate anatomic orientation and portal placement during hip arthroscopy.*

Clarke MT, Arora A, Villar RN: Hip arthroscopy: complications in 1054 cases. *Clin Orthop Related Res* 406:84-88, 2003.

> *Prospective study of 1054 (between 1989 and 2001) consecutive hip arthroscopies demonstrating a 1.4% overall complication rate. This rate increased to 4.2% if the 30 hips that could not be accessed (primarily because of severe dysplasia or osteoarthritis) were included.*
> *Neuropraxias, primarily resulting from traction injury, comprised the greatest number of complications in agreement with several previous studies. Other complications included trochanteric bursitis, portal site bleeding and hematoma, instrument breakage, and infection.*

Kelly BT, Williams RJ, Philippon MJ: Hip arthroscopy: current indications, treatment options, and management issues. *Am J Sports Med* 31:1020-1037, 2003.

> *A comprehensive review of current clinical and radiographic evaluation methods of sports-related hip conditions and the indications and techniques of hip arthroscopy. Authors report that patients with reproducible symptoms and limited function recalcitrant to conservative measures are likely to have the best outcomes after surgical management.*

Krebs VE. The role of hip arthroscopy in the treatment of synovial disorders and loose bodies. *Clin Orthop Related Res* 406:48-59, 2003.

> *Author reviews the pathology, symptoms, and clinical and radiographic evaluation of synovial disorders about the hip. The role of arthroscopic management is highlighted, with references of initial favorable results as this technique undergoes further advancements and future studies.*

Mason JB, McCarthy JC, O'Donnell J, et al: Hip arthroscopy: surgical approach, positioning, and distraction. *Clin Orthop Related Res* 406:29-37, 2003.

> *Detailed description of positioning, portal placement, and approaches of hip arthroscopy.*

McCarthy JC, Day B, Busconi B: Hip arthroscopy: application and technique. *J Am Acad Orthop Surg* 3:115-122, 1995.

> *Review of hip arthroscopy including indications, contraindications, surgical technique, and complications.*

Sampson TG: Complications of hip arthroscopy. *Clin Sports Med* 20:831-835, 2001.

> *Review of 530 hip arthroscopy cases (since 1977) revealed complications in 34 cases. Authors reported 20 neuropraxias, 9 cases with fluid extravasation, 2 incidents of instrument breakage, 2 iatrogenic articular injuries, and 1 case of avascular necrosis of the femoral head. Authors note that most complications can be avoided with careful attention to traction and fluid management.*

Sekiya JK, Ruch DS, Hunter DM, et al: Hip arthroscopy in staging avascular necrosis of the femoral head. *J South Orthop Assoc* 9:254-261, 2000.

> *Authors propose an arthroscopic staging system for avascular necrosis of the femoral head with specific attention to the status of the articular cartilage in terms of prognosis and implications of further management options.*

Sekiya JK, Wojtys EM, Loder RT, Hensinger RN: Hip arthroscopy using a limited anterior exposure: an alternative approach for arthroscopic access. *Arthroscopy* 16:16-20, 2000.

> *Authors describe a hip arthroscopy technique using a limited anterior exposure and manual traction that they propose may reduce the risk of neurovascular and articular damage. Five cases are reported without any postoperative complications.*

Groin Pain

Introduction

- Understanding of groin pathology has lagged behind that of the knee and shoulder.
- Often goes undiagnosed unless specifically recognized as a potential problem.
- Differential diagnoses should include such things as adductor strain, inguinal hernia, osteitis pubis, femoral neck stress fracture, intraarticular hip problems, and "snapping hip," to name a few (Box 17–1).
- Differential diagnoses must also include nonmusculoskeletal etiologies such as endometriosis, inflammatory bowel disease, urologic problems, and ovarian cysts.

Athletic Pubalgia

- The term *athletic pubalgia* refers to chronic inguinal or pubic-area pain in athletes that is exertional only and not explained by a palpable hernia or other diagnosis.
- Thought to involve a tear in the attachment of the adductor longus or the rectus abdominis muscles, or both (Figure 17–1).
- Sometimes called "chronic symphysis syndrome" when a combination of abdominal, groin, and adductor pain is present.
- Adductor component is most likely a secondary phenomenon subsequent to rectus abdominus tear with resulting anterior pelvic tilt.
- Similarly described in Europe as "Gilmore's groin."
- Found more frequently in males than females.

History

- Initial hyperextension injury with the pivot point being the anterior pelvis or pubic symphysis is commonly reported.
- Disabling, lower-abdominal/inguinal pain at extremes of exertion.
- Pain resolves with cessation of activity over a period of minutes to hours.
- Progression of pain over months or years.

- Specific sports participation such as soccer or ice hockey, which requires frequent change of direction.

Physical Examination

- Tenderness to palpation of the peripubic area, pubic symphysis, or adductor tendon.
- No palpable hernia.
- Pain with restricted adduction or resisted sit-ups.
- Painful Valsalva maneuver may be seen, but this is more frequently associated with frank hernia.
- Hamstring tightness or limitation of hip motion may be seen.
- Neurologic examination will help to differentiate athletic pubalgia from spinal pathology such as herniated disc, which can produce radiating pain into the pelvis and groin.

Imaging

- Imaging may be helpful in ruling out other possible causes of pelvic and groin pain, but findings are generally not specific for athletic pubalgia.
- Radiography can help to narrow the differential diagnosis.
- Magnetic resonance imaging (MRI) may reveal rectus tear, avulsion fracture, pubic symphyseal edema, or musculotendinous asymmetry or may be completely normal.
- Bone scan can be useful in demonstrating the presence of osteitis pubis.
- Herniography is becoming less favorable but may be helpful in diagnosing occult hernia.

Treatment

- Initially conservative with rest, ice, nonsteroidal antiinflammatory drugs (NSAIDs), physical therapy, and fluoroscopically guided injection.
- Once an adequate trial of conservative treatment fails, surgery may be indicated.
- "Pelvic floor repair."
  - Reattachment of inferolateral edge of the rectus abdominus muscle to the pubis and adjacent anterior ligaments.

Inguinal hernia
Sports hernia
Iliopsoas bursitis
Stress fracture of the femoral neck
Apophyseal avulsion fractures
Nerve compression
Osteitis pubis
Piriformis syndrome
Athletic pubalgia

- Some authors describe imbrication techniques using the transversalis fascia.
- Adductor release.
  - Division of anterior epimysial fibers of the adductor longus muscle about 2 to 3 cm from pubic insertion.

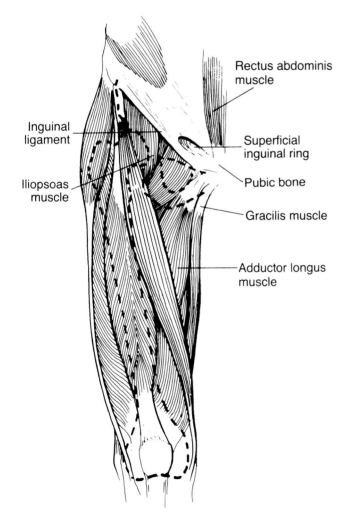

Figure 17–1:
Groin muscular anatomy demonstrating the relationship of the adductor longus and rectus abdominis. (From DeLee JC, Drez DD, Miller MD: *DeLee & Drez's orthopaedic sports medicine principles and practice,* **2nd ed. Philadelphia, 2003, Saunders.)**

Labels in figure:
Rectus abdominis muscle
Inguinal ligament
Superficial inguinal ring
Iliopsoas muscle
Pubic bone
Gracilis muscle
Adductor longus muscle

- Muscle belly left intact.
- Performed independently or concomitantly with pelvic floor repair.
- Rarely successful independently.
- Surgeons experienced with these techniques report success rates as high as 95%.

Hernias

- Inguinal hernias may be seen in all populations, and athletes are no exception.
  - Athletes with an inguinal hernia typically present with groin pain that may radiate to the upper thigh.
  - Pain is typically worse with Valsalva maneuvers, which help to differentiate this diagnosis from others discussed in this chapter.
  - Differential diagnosis should include other scrotal abnormalities such as epididymitis, scrotal abscess, testicular torsion, varicocele, spermatocele, and hydrocele.
  - Physical examination is the mainstay of diagnosis for this condition, with hernia being palpable in the inguinal ring with Valsalva maneuver.
  - Surgical repair of the defect is necessary, which is typically done through laparoscopic techniques.
- Sports hernia (Figure 17–2).
  - This is still a controversial diagnosis.
  - Generally, the term *sports hernia* refers to refractory pain in the abdominal wall or groin during exertion that is thought to be caused by injury to the muscle wall, specifically the rectus muscle and transversalis fascia.
  - Pain may be severe and typically limits or completely impedes athletic activity.
  - Typically the area is tender, but no palpable hernia is present in most cases.
  - Conservative treatment does not typically reduce pain.
  - Operative treatment may include an open repair of the defect, but more often laparoscopic techniques are being described.

Osteitis Pubis

- Osteitis pubis simply refers to a painful inflammatory process of the pubic symphysis.
- The mechanism is thought to be microtrauma from athletic activity involving repetitive motion at the pubic symphysis including kicking and running (Figure 17–3).
- Also implicated as a possible etiology of this process is an imbalance between the muscles of the abdominal wall and the hip adductors.
- The onset of this condition may be after an acute event but more often is insidious and may progress to a degree significant enough to impede athletic performance.
- This condition may or may not be associated with instability of the pubic symphysis.

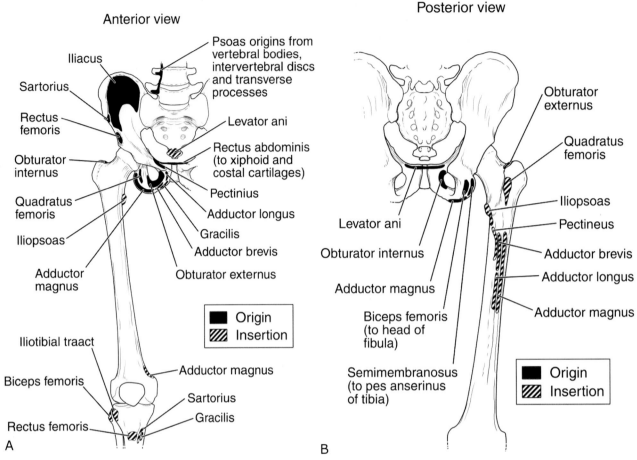

Figure 17–2:
A, Anterior pelvic muscles. **B,** Posterior pelvic muscles. (From Meyers WC, Greenleaf R, Saad A: *Op Tech Sports Med* 13:55-61, 2005.)

- Physical examination findings include localized tenderness in the area of the pubic symphysis but may also include more generalized tenderness in the surrounding soft tissue structures.
- Plain radiographs are typically normal but may include some irregularity and sclerosis at the pubic symphysis in later stages of the process (Figure 17–4).
- MRI findings are nonspecific but may include local bone marrow edema.
- Ultrasound and computed tomography (CT) scan may be helpful to exclude other conditions that may cause groin pain including infectious, gynecologic, and urologic sources.
- Treatment of this condition is generally conservative and may include rest, activity modification, physical therapy with emphasis on core strengthening and muscle balance, NSAIDs, and/or fluoroscopically guided injections of the pubic symphysis.
- Surgical options for this process are limited and should be reserved for patients who have failed extensive conservative treatment and are experiencing debilitating pain.

- Wedge resections of the pubic symphysis have been reported in the literature with care to preserve the ligamentous attachment at the inferior aspect of the symphysis to prevent instability.
- Pubic symphysis arthrodesis has also been reported, but both of these procedures have limited follow-up and low study numbers to report.

Piriformis Syndrome

- Piriformis syndrome describes a condition of sciatic nerve irritation caused by its compression by the piriformis muscle as both structures exit the sciatic notch (Figure 17–5).
- The cause for this compression is variable but may be influenced by several factors, which include the following:
  - Variation of normal anatomy of the sciatic nerve or piriformis muscle, or both.
  - History of repetitive sports activity that may allow for hypertrophy of the muscle belly.
  - Acute trauma to the gluteal area.

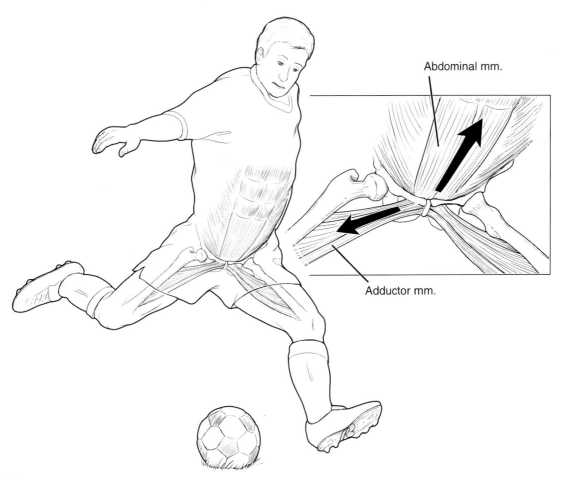

Figure 17–3:
Core muscle imbalance and repetitive trauma in sports involving kicking and running are thought to be the major contributing factors in the development of osteitis pubis. (From Mandelbaum B, Mora SA: *Op Tech Sports Med* 13:62-67, 2005.)

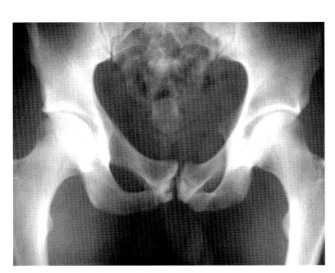

Figure 17–4:
Radiographic findings of osteitis pubis. (From Mandelbaum B, Mora SA: *Op Tech Sports Med* 13:62-67, 2005.)

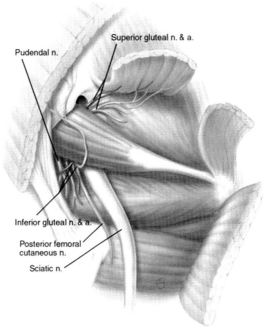

Figure 17–5:
Sciatic notch anatomy. (From Byrd JWT: *Op Tech Sports Med* 13:71-79, 2005.)

- Postural problems associated with sitting on an overly firm surface, the so-called wallet neuritis.
- Leg-length discrepancy or lower extremity mechanical malalignment, or both.
- Physical examination findings are often nonspecific.
  - Posterior tenderness near the sciatic notch.
  - Straight-leg raise testing may be positive, but the absence of this common sign does not exclude the diagnosis of piriformis syndrome.
  - Provocative maneuvers such as performing resisted abduction of the flexed hip may reproduce the pain. Another described maneuver involves flexing the hip to 90 degrees and passively adducting and internally rotating the hip.
- Plain radiographs and MRI studies are generally the most helpful in determining the presence of other lesions that may produce sciatic-type pain but are rarely helpful in the specific diagnosis of piriformis syndrome.
- Nerve conduction studies may be helpful to rule out other sites of nerve entrapment.
- Treatment of piriformis syndrome is generally conservative and includes activity modification, NSAIDs, and physical therapy with emphasis on piriformis stretching.

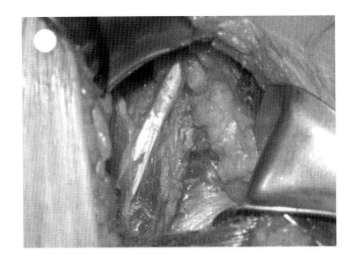

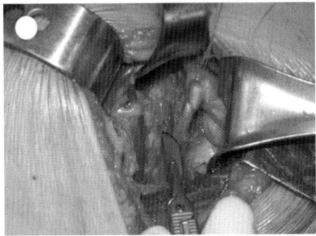

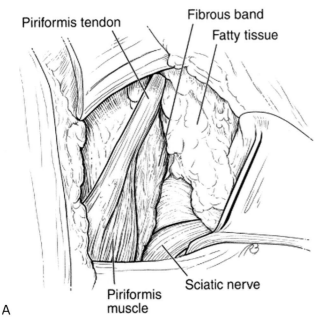

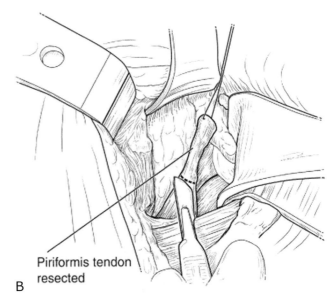

Figure 17–6:
Piriformis release. A, The gluteus maximus muscle is split and retracted. The piriformis tendon is isolated and the sciatic nerve is seen passing beneath its muscle belly. **B,** The piriformis tendon is released off of its insertion and a portion is resected. (From Byrd JWT: *Op Tech Sports Med* 13:71-79, 2005.)

- Corticosteroid injections at the point of maximal tenderness near the sciatic notch have also been advocated.
- Surgical treatment is reserved for refractory cases and involves release of the piriformis muscle and sciatic nerve decompression (Figure 17–6).

Stress Fracture of the Hip

- A stress fracture of the hip should be considered in any athlete, especially those involved in endurance running.
- Not recognizing this clinical entity could result in a catastrophic displaced femoral neck fracture.
- Stress fractures of the hip are discussed in more detail in Chapter 27.

References

Akermark C, Johansson C: Tenotomy of the adductor longus tendon in the treatment of chronic groin pain in athletes. *Am J Sports Med* 20:640-643, 1992.

With a 35-month follow-up after adductor longus tenotomy, all subjects demonstrated symptom improvement and all but one returned to sports activity. This demonstrates good long-term results of this procedure with pain localized to the area of the adductor longus without any significant clinical compromise in strength.

Biedert RM, Warnke K, Meyer S: Symphysis syndrome in athletes: surgical treatment for chronic lower abdominal, groin, and adductor pain in athletes. *Clin J Sports Med* 13:278-284, 2003.

These authors propose treatment of what they term "symphysis syndrome" with spreading of the lateral border of the rectus sheath and adductor release. They have good results with this technique, demonstrating 23 of 24 subjects returning to full sports activity.

Byrd JW: Piriformis syndrome. *Op Tech Sports Med* 13:71-79, 2005.

This is a review of the etiology, diagnosis, and treatment of piriformis syndrome, especially in the athletic population. Surgical indications are discussed, as well as a description of operative techniques used by the author.

Diaco JF, Diaco DS, Lockhart L: Sports hernia. *Op Tech Sports Med* 13:68-70, 2005.

This article reviews the experience of the authors in treating athletes with refractory abdominal/groin pain both conservatively and surgically.

Harner CD, Rihn JA, Vogrin TM: Specialty update: what's new in sports medicine. *J Bone Joint Surg Am* 85:1173-1181, 2003.

Short review of current approaches to hip and groin injuries.

Larson CM, Lohnes JH: Surgical management of athletic pubalgia. *Op Tech Sports Med* 10:228-232, 2002.

This article reviews the mechanism, history, and physical examination findings most commonly associated with athletic pubalgia and then describes a surgical techniques used by the authors to address the inguinal/rectus pathology, as well as that of the adductor tendon.

Mandelbaum B, Mora SA: Osteitis pubis. *Op Tech Sports Med* 13:62-67, 2005.

This article serves as a review of the diagnosis and treatment of osteitis pubis. The discussion includes both conservative and surgical treatment techniques including pubic symphysis compression plate arthrodesis.

Meyers WC, Foley DP, Garrett WE: Management of severe lower abdominal or inguinal pain in high-performance athletes. *Am J Sports Med* 28(1):2-8, 2000.

These authors look at a large number of cases of athletes with both abdominal and groin pain. Many of these athletes had undergone procedures to reinforce the pelvic floor or adductor releases, or both. By looking at patient history and surgical outcome, they conclude that the cause of combination abdominal and groin pain in athletes is abdominal hyperextension and thigh hyperabduction.

Meyers WC, Greenleaf R, Saad A: Anatomic basis for evaluation of abdominal and groin pain in athletes. *Op Tech Sports Med* 13(1):55-61, 2005.

This article provides an overview of the anatomy of the pelvis and proximal femur with specific consideration of the origins and insertions of the muscles in the area. Correlation is given between these anatomic areas and the pathology that is most commonly seen here in the athletic population.

Meyers WC, Ricciardi R, Busconi BD: Athletic pubalgia and groin pain. In Garrett WE, Speer KP, Kirkendall DT, editors: *Orthopaedic sports medicine.* Philadelphia, 2000, Lippincott Williams & Wilkins.

This chapter discusses groin pain in athletes and summarizes the authors' belief that athletic pubalgia results from repetitive trunk hyperextension during athletic activities, which leads to periostitis or frank injury at the site of the rectus abdominis insertion.

Srinivasan A, Schuricht A: Long-term follow-up of laparoscopic preperitoneal hernia repair in professional athletes. *J Laparosc Adv Surg Tech* 12:101-106, 2002.

These authors show that laparoscopic preperitoneal hernia repair is a very effective method for treating sports hernias in professional athletes. Long-term follow-up at an average of 46 months shows no evidence of recurrence or adverse event. Eighty-seven percent of athletes may return to full sports participation in as little as 4-weeks postoperatively.

CHAPTER 18

Hip Overuse Syndromes

History, Physical Examination, and Imaging

- Increased or repetitive activity can cause several conditions about the hip involving bone and muscle, ranging from mild tendinitis to stress fractures.
- Thorough history and physical examination can direct one to a proper diagnosis.
- Leg-length discrepancies, foot abnormalities, and abnormal joint angles can be the cause of pain.
- One must also consider referred pain from the lumbar spine, hernias, visceral disorders, or tumors.
- Initial radiographic evaluation should include standard anteroposterior (AP) and lateral views of either the pelvis or affected hip to assess bony alignment and condition.
- Suspicion of stress fractures must be ruled out first with plain radiographs with supplementation if needed from either bone scans or magnetic resonance imaging (MRI), with the latter being more specific.
- MRI can assist in confirming certain diagnoses and ruling out any intraarticular pathology.

Types

- Bursitis often results from repetitive friction with a nearby muscle and may result in symptoms of severe pain, especially with continued activity.
  - It can be difficult to differentiate it from tendinitis or other soft tissue inflammatory processes, and they can often coexist.
  - There are several bursae about the hip, but we primarily concern ourselves with the four major bursae (Figure 18–1).
  - Trochanteric bursitis is often associated with friction of the iliotibial band and is typically seen in runners. Patients complain of pain over the trochanter and inability to lie on the affected side. A wider pelvis and more prominent trochanter may explain why it is more common in females.
  - Iliopsoas bursitis may be associated with a snapping iliopsoas tendon and usually presents with anterior hip pain.
  - Ischial bursitis can develop after trauma or prolonged sitting.
  - Iliopectineal bursitis is also associated with the iliopsoas tendon and causes anterior hip pain.
- Stress fractures have the ability to become complete if not recognized and treated appropriately.
  - Seen in athletes that participate in sports or activities that require repetitive motion, such as running.
  - Commonly, patients complain of pain with activity that subsides with a period of rest.
  - Radiographs are frequently normal until bone remodeling occurs.
  - Bone scan and MRI are both sensitive in evaluating stress fractures, but MRI is more specific and can assist in ruling out neoplasms.
  - Localization of femoral neck stress fractures will guide treatment recommendations on the basis of the different forces involved. Medial femoral neck stress fractures occur along the compressive cortex of bone and are considered more stable. The lateral neck represents the tensile surface, which is more prone to fracture completely (Figure 18–2).
  - Stress fractures of the pelvis (including the sacrum and pubis) do occur but are inherently more stable than stress fractures of the femur.
- Apophysitis can occur anywhere within the hip girdle of a skeletally immature athlete.
  - Commonly thought to result from overuse, although acute trauma or increased intense activity may produce similar pathology.
  - Characterized by tenderness overlying the affected area.
  - Radiographs may reveal mild asymmetric physeal widening on the affected side.
- Osteitis pubis, an inflammatory disorder, can develop from repetitive intense activity, usually in sports such as soccer, hockey, and running.
  - Localized tenderness around the symphysis occasionally is associated with spasms and tenderness of the adductor muscles.

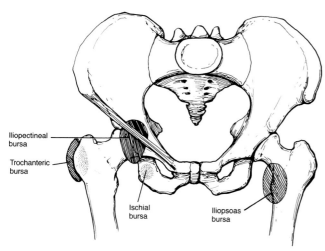

Figure 18–1:
Major bursae about the pelvis. (From Gross ML, Nasser S, Finerman GAM: Hip and pelvis. In DeLee JC, Drez D Jr, editors: *Orthopaedic sports medicine.* Philadelphia, 1994, Saunders.)

- Sclerosis or cystic changes may be appreciated on radiographic evaluation.
- Bone scan and MRI will also show positive findings.
- Degenerative disease can be associated with or exacerbated by a very intense athletic lifestyle and can lead to labral tears, chondral injuries, loss of hip motion, and intractable pain.

Treatment

- As with most overuse syndromes, control of symptoms is attempted with activity modifications, nonsteroidal antiinflammatory drugs (NSAIDs), and physical therapy when appropriate.
- A cane may be provided for ambulatory assistance if pain is severe.
- Steroid injections should be used judiciously and reserved for symptomatic pain unresponsive to conservative management. Bursography is recommended when injecting into deep bursae.

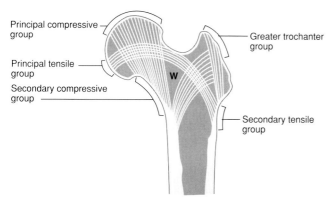

Figure 18–2:
Compressive and tensile surfaces about the proximal femur.

- Bursectomy is rarely recommended. Surgical procedures for iliopsoas or iliopectineal bursitis concentrate on relaxing the iliopsoas tendon overlying the symptomatic bursa.
- All stress fractures can initially be treated conservatively with protected weight-bearing except for stress fractures along the lateral femoral neck. Pain control and protected weight-bearing with crutches for a period of 3 to 6 months is generally recommended, with frequent radiographic evaluation to monitor the healing process. Surgical correction is recommended to poor responders. Surgical fixation of lateral neck stress fractures is recommended as initial treatment to prevent progression of the fracture.
- Patients with recalcitrant osteitis pubis and instability of the pubic symphysis may benefit from arthrodesis.
- Patients should be advised that degenerative changes are irreversible and lifestyle modifications are important to slow its progression. They must be told to avoid high-impact activities such as running, jumping, and heavy lifting and be offered alternative low-impact exercises such as swimming, biking, golf, and elliptical machines.
- Arthroscopic debridement of labral tears can provide great results.
- Chondral injuries may benefit from excision or microfracture procedures.

Rehabilitation

- Generally, patients with overuse syndromes initially should refrain from any aggravating activity but may participate in other activities that are not associated with symptoms.
- Patients may advance their activities as tolerated once symptoms have resolved.
- It is recommended that patients with stress fractures implement nonimpact exercises into their routine to maintain conditioning as recovery may take up to 6 months.

Complications

- Chronic pain and a limp are possible.
- Return to intense activity too soon risks ongoing symptoms and morbidity.
- Improper management of stress fractures may lead to complete fractures.
- Evaluating physicians must rule out other possible etiologies that would require different treatment.

References

Holt MA, Keene JS, Graf BK, Helwig DC: Treatment of osteitis pubis in athletes. *Am J Sport Med* 23:601-606, 1995.
Report on the use of corticosteroid injections acutely (within 2 weeks) or delayed (after 16 weeks) in patients with osteitis pubis unresponsive

to conservative measures. All three acutely treated patients were able to return to full athletic participation within 2 weeks. Among the patients with chronic osteitis pubis (>16 weeks), three athletes only required one injection and returned to full activity within 3 weeks, three necessitated two injections with resolution of symptoms within 11 to 16 weeks, one athlete required three injections and 24 weeks to become symptom free, and one remained symptomatic. The authors concluded that corticosteroid injections should be used within 2 weeks for optimal results.

Miller C, Major N, Toth A: Pelvis stress injuries in the athlete. *Sports Med* 33:1003-1012, 2003.

Review of the etiology, diagnosis, treatment and prevention of pelvis stress fractures. Authors prefer the use of MRI (rather than bone scan) for diagnosis in high-suspect cases with normal radiographs because of its great specificity and sensitivity. Authors recommend the use of a three-phase protocol for treatment with a cyclical training program. Prevention of these injuries is advocated by guiding athletes on proper training, shoeware, and nutrition. Additionally, normal hormonal balances should be ensured among female athletes.

Slawski DP, Howard RF: Surgical management of refractory trochanteric bursitis. *Am J Sport Med* 26:86-89, 1997.

Review of five patients (seven hips) with refractory trochanteric bursitis treated surgically with longitudinal release of the iliotibial band over the greater trochanter and subgluteal bursectomy. All patients experienced a great improvement and were satisfied with their results. Authors comment that although most cases can be successfully managed nonoperatively, the surgical technique described is an effective option for intractable cases.

Williams PR, Thomas DP, Downes EM: Osteitis pubis and instability of the pubic symphysis. *Am J Sport Med* 28:350-355, 2000.

Authors report on the use of arthrodesis in patients with recalcitrant cases of osteitis pubis and vertical instability of the pubic symphysis. Arthrodesis is performed by bone grafting and use of a compression plate. All seven rugby players treated were freed of symptoms with radiographic evidence of successful arthrodesis and no residual instability.

CHAPTER 19

Snapping Hip

Introduction

- Coxa saltans, or snapping hip, is so named because of the characteristic "snap" sound made with active hip flexion and extension.
- Three types: internal, external, and intraarticular (Figures 19–1 and 19–2).
  - Internal coxa saltans is caused as the iliopsoas snaps over the iliopectineal eminence.
  - External is the most common and is characterized by snapping as the iliotibial (IT) band or gluteus maximus tendon passes over the greater trochanter of the femur. This may also result in inflammation of the greater trochanteric bursa.

- Intraarticular involves more of a clicking, and causes are multiple including labral tears, loose bodies, and osteochondral injury.

Diagnosis

- History and physical examination are key in making the diagnosis of snapping hip.
- Patients typically describe a painful snapping.
- Snapping is usually reproducible by the patient.
- A history of trauma may be reported, but more frequently coxa saltans is a more chronic condition with an insidious onset.
- Physical examination.

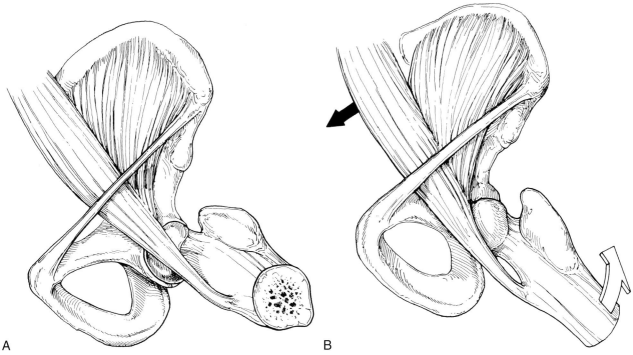

A B

Figure 19–1:
Internal snapping hip. **A,** With flexion of the hip, the iliopsoas tendon is lateral, in its groove. **B,** With hip extension, the tendon shifts medially. (From Miller MD, Howard RF, Plancher KD: *Surgical atlas of sports medicine.* Philadelphia, 2003, WB Saunders.)

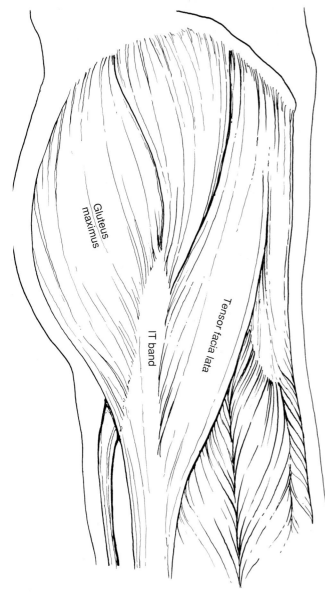

Gluteus maximus

IT band

Tensor facia lata

Figure 19–2:
External snapping hip. (From Miller MD, Howard RF, Plancher KD: *Surgical atlas of sports medicine.* **Philadelphia, 2003, WB Saunders.)**

○ Internal—the examiner passively flexes and extends the hip with the patient in a supine position to reproduce the snapping.
  ■ This may be more obvious if the patient moves the hip from an abducted/flexed position to an adducted/extended position.
  ■ Applying gentle pressure over the iliopsoas tendon where it passes over the femoral head will usually stop the snapping and help to confirm the diagnosis.
○ External—the examiner palpates the area where the tendon crosses the greater trochanter of the femur as the patient actively flexes the hip.

  ■ This may be best reproduced when the patient is standing. The Ober test may also be useful (Figure 19–3).
  ■ With this maneuver the patient lies on his or her side with the affected hip up and in a flexed and abducted position.
  ■ A positive test is when the hip is unable to be fully adducted from this position.
  ○ Intraarticular—this is more difficult to diagnose by physical examination because there are multiple causes.
    ■ Sometimes a click is able to be noted with active or passive flexion, abduction, and external rotation (Figure 19–4).
    ■ Radiologic studies are more useful in cases of intraarticular coxa saltans.
• Radiographs are usually normal.
• Bursography can be a useful procedure in the diagnosis of coxa saltans. With this technique contrast material is injected into the iliopsoas bursa under fluoroscopy. The tendon is then easily visualized as the hip is moved through its full range of motion. A sudden jerking of the tendon is diagnostic of internal coxa saltans (Figure 19–5).
• Dynamic ultrasound has been used in some cases to demonstrate the tendon "snapping" over the bony prominence. The difficulty with this diagnostic test is that a good result is dependent on the experience of the examiner.
• Magnetic resonance imaging (MRI) is useful in cases of intraarticular coxa saltans. MRI arthrogram is best for detecting pathology of the labrum.

Conservative Treatment

• Coxa saltans should be treated conservatively before any surgical intervention is considered. The exception to this is the case of intraarticular coxa saltans with a definable lesion amenable to arthroscopic treatment.
• The mainstay of conservative treatment of snapping hip is rest and avoidance of symptom-provoking activities.
• Stretching the involved muscle may help to reduce symptoms.
• Nonsteroidal antiinflammatory medications may be used.
• Local injection of corticosteroids may reduce pain and inflammation associated with this condition.
• It should be emphasized to the patient early that, even with full compliance, resolution of symptoms may take 6 to 12 months.

Surgical Treatment

• Internal.
  • Iliopsoas fractional lengthening is the gold standard of surgical treatment of internal coxa saltans (Figure 19–6).

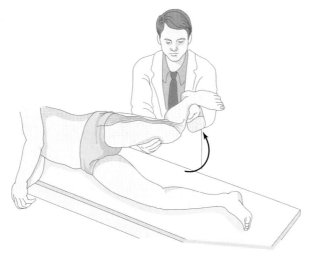

A   To test for contraction of the fascia lata.

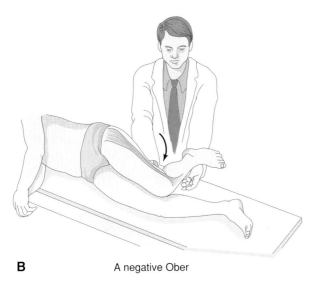

B   A negative Ober

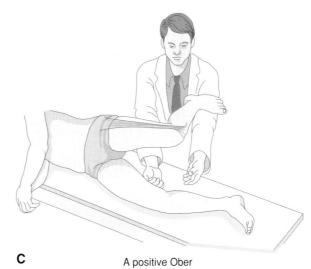

C   A positive Ober

Figure 19–3:
Examination of external snapping hip. The Ober test.

- In this technique an open groin incision is made and the iliopsoas tendon is identified and four partial tenotomies of the posterolateral tendon are made at 2-cm intervals beginning 1 cm proximal to the lesser trochanter and moving proximally, ending at the superior femoral head.
- Fractional lengthening has also been described with a more proximal approach. In this case, the initial incision is made just inferior to the iliac crest and requires dissection through the tensor fascia latae and external oblique muscles at the attachment to the iliac apophysis. This approach is felt by some to involve less risk to the lateral femoral cutaneous nerve.
- Postoperative rehabilitation is specific to each individual as tolerated. No specific weight-bearing or range of motion restrictions are necessary during the postoperative period.
- Iliopsoas fractional lengthening has shown reasonable improvement in patient symptoms with estimated return to play at 3 to 6 months.
- Complications include recurrence of symptoms, motor and sensory changes, bursal swelling, hematomas, and infection.
- External.
  - Z-plasty of the IT band is the most commonly described treatment of external coxa saltans (Figure 19–7).
- In this technique the incision is made over the greater trochanter with the patient in a lateral decubitus position. A longitudinal incision is made through the

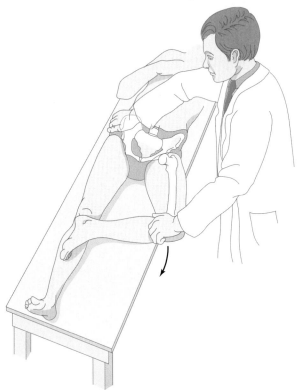

The Patrick or Faber test.

Figure 19–4:
Examination of intraarticular snapping hip (flexion, abduction, external rotation).

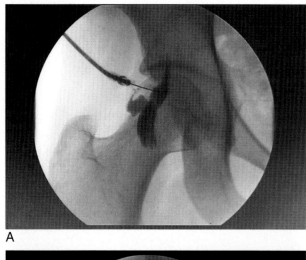

A

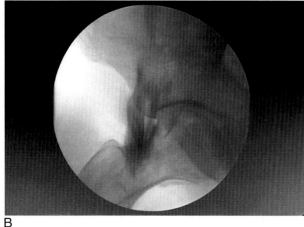

B

Figure 19–5:
Iliopsoas bursography. A, Normal location of the tendon with hip in neutral position. **B,** Snapping of the tendon over the bone with external rotation. (From Miller MD, Howard RF, Plancher KD: *Surgical atlas of sports medicine.* Philadelphia, 2003, WB Saunders.)

tensor fascia latae and proximal and distal incisions of the IT band complete the z-plasty.
- Another surgical technique has been described that involves excising an elliptical area of the IT band as well as excision of the bursa. Mixed results have been reported.
- Intraarticular.
  - Surgical treatment is variable, depending on the exact pathology identified. Often hip arthroscopy is a useful tool in this setting.

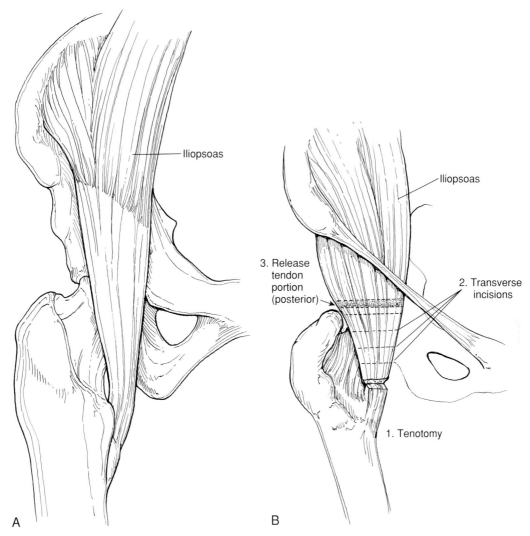

A

B

Figure 19–6:
Iliopsoas fractional lengthening. A, Iliopsoas is isolated. B, Tenostomy is performed. (From Miller MD, Howard RF, Plancher KD: *Surgical atlas of sports medicine.* Philadelphia, 2003, WB Saunders.)

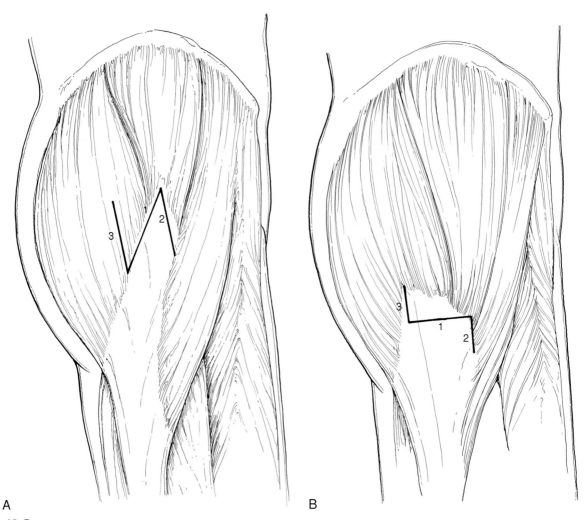

A   B

Figure 19–7:
Z-plasty of the iliotibial band. **A,** Z-plasty before transposition. **B,** Z-plasty after transposition. (From Miller MD, Howard RF, Plancher KD: *Surgical atlas of sports medicine.* Philadelphia, 2003, WB Saunders.)

References

Allen WC, Cope R: Coxa saltans: the snapping hip revisited. *J Am Acad Orthop Surg* 3:303-308, 1995.

This article provides a description of the three types of coxa saltans. Physical examination is the key to diagnosis of this process with radiography being less helpful. Bursography, computed tomography, MRI, and arthrography may be helpful especially in ruling out other potential causes. Conservative treatment options should be exhausted prior to consideration for surgical intervention.

Choi YS, Lee SM, Song BY, et al: Dynamic sonography of external snapping hip syndrome. *J Ultrasound Med* 21:753-758, 2002.

This article discusses the use of dynamic ultrasound as a diagnostic tool in cases of external snapping hip. In seven cases of symptomatic patients, dynamic ultrasound showed the cause to be the IT band snapping over the greater trochanter of the femur in five cases. The other two cases demonstrated abnormality involving the gluteus maximus.

Dobbs MB, Gordon JE, Luhmann SJ, et al: Surgical correction of the snapping iliopsoas tendon in adolescents. *J Bone Joint Surg Am* 84:420-424, 2002.

Using a modified iliofemoral approach to perform iliopsoas fractional lengthening in adolescent patients, these authors show good results in terms of symptom relief. Patients return to normal activity with no notable loss of strength as a result of the procedure.

Gruen GS, Scioscia TN, Lowenstein JE: The surgical treatment of internal snapping hip. *Am J Sports Med* 30:607-613, 2002.

The authors demonstrate by reviewing 30 patients with snapping hip at 3-years' follow-up that 63% improved with conservative treatment. Those who did not improve underwent iliopsoas-lengthening procedures. The surgical group had resolution of the symptoms in all cases.

Hoskins JS, Burd TA, Allen WC: Surgical correction of internal coax saltans: a 20-year consecutive study. *Am J Sports Med* 32:998-1001, 2004.

This is a review of 92 cases of snapping hip treated with primary surgical repair by iliopsoas tendon fractional lengthening shows a complication or recurrence rate of 43%. Complications include recurring symptoms, persistent pain, sensory deficit, motor weakness, bursal swelling, hematoma formation, and superficial infection.

Provencher MT, Hofmeister EP, Muldoon MP: The surgical treatment of external coxa saltans (the snapping hip) by z-plasty of the iliotibial band. *Am J Sports Med* 32:470-476, 2004.

Although conservative treatment is the mainstay for managing external coxa saltans, surgery may be indicated if symptoms are persistent. In cases of refractory snapping hip, these authors show good results with z-plasty of the IT band with all subjects being relieved of the snapping and only one having some persisting groin pain.

Zoltan DJ, Clancy WG, Keene JS: A new operative approach to snapping hip and refractory trochanteric bursitis in athletes. *Am J Sports Med* 14:201, 1986.

A newly described technique for treatment of snapping hip involves excising an elliptical section of the IT band and removal of the bursa. Four of five subjects show significant improvement.

Hip and Thigh Muscle Strains and Contusions

History, Physical Examination, and Imaging

- Contusions and strains are one of the most common injuries seen in sports participation and can debilitate an athlete.
- These injuries vary in severity.
- Patients may present with pain, swelling, ecchymosis, and spasms over the affected area.
- Contusions are the result of direct injury from either a collision or fall.
- Strains are usually the result of a forceful contraction while the muscle is on stretch and typically occur at the myotendinous junction.
- Occasionally, strains develop from repetitive microtrauma.
- A contused muscle that has not healed properly is susceptible to strain or tear at the injured site.
- Determining the type of activity during the injury and location of pain can help to isolate the affected muscle, tendon, or bone.
- Muscles that span two joints, such as the hamstrings, are usually composed of more fast-twitch muscle fibers and are more susceptible to injury than single-joint muscles that have greater strength and slow contracting fibers, as seen in the gluteal muscles.
- Muscle that cross two joints are also more likely to be less flexible, which predisposes them to greater stress with certain activities.
- Patients present with pain over the injured area and can often describe exacerbating activities or movements.
- Knowledge of the muscles and their insertion sites about the hip is essential when performing a clinical examination (Figures 20–1 and 20–2, Boxes 20–1 to 20–4).
- Physical examination often demonstrates tenderness over the injured site.
- Precise localization of an injured muscle is not always possible during the examination given the deep location of the hip muscle groups.
- Diagnosis can be confirmed by reproducing the pain on examination by placing the affected muscle on stretch or

testing the muscle group strength against resistance. Muscles that cross two joints (e.g., the hamstring and rectus femoris) must be stretched at both joints for proper evaluation.
- Imaging is typically not necessary, especially with an adequate history and physical.
- Standard radiographs can be used to rule out any bony abnormality or fracture.
- Magnetic resonance imaging (MRI) can confirm the diagnosis and aid in defining the location and severity of the injury but is rarely performed except, perhaps, in elite athletes.

Types

- Iliac crest contusion is also known as the "hip pointer" in football and usually results from a direct blow or fall.
  - Hematomas are common and can sometimes present as a fluctuant mass although they may not be visible.
  - Occasionally, this will lead to periostitis or exostosis at the site of injury.
  - In growing children, it is critical to rule out an avulsion of the iliac apophysis.
- Quadriceps contusions are very common in contact sports. Occasionally, they may progress to myositis ossificans and restrict knee motion. Initially, quadriceps contusions should be immobilized in flexion.
- Groin contusions are seen less frequently. During evaluation, traumatic phlebitis, thrombosis, and femoral neuropathy must be considered.
- Hamstring strain is perhaps the most common injured muscle in the lower extremity.
  - The hamstring, a hip extensor and knee flexor, spans two joints and is under stretch with hip flexion and knee extension.
  - With its varied myotendinous junction sites, pain can present practically anywhere along the posterior thigh.
  - Complete avulsions from its origin on the ischium can occur and cause considerable pain and weakness.
- The adductor longus is the most commonly strained muscle of the adductors about the hip.

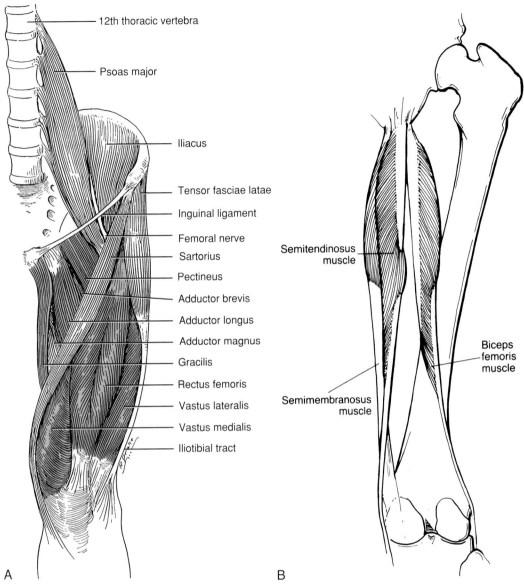

Figure 20–1:
Anterior **(A)** and **(B)** posterior views of thigh and hip musculature. **(A** from Jenkins DB, Hollinshead WH: *Hollinshead's functional anatomy of the limbs and back.* Philadelphia, Saunders, 2002; **B** from Brunet ME, Hontas RB: The thigh. In DeLee JC, Drez D Jr, editors: *Orthopaedic sports medicine.* Philadelphia, Saunders, 1994.)

- The rectus femoris, the only two-joint muscle within the quadriceps, is the most commonly injured of the group. This muscle can be placed under stretch with the prone rectus femoris test where the knee is flexed as the patient lies prone on the examining table.
- Iliopsoas strains are not common and can be distinguished from rectus femoris strains if pain is absent with resisted knee extension.

Treatment

- Treatment of contusions is directed at reducing swelling with rest, ice, elevation, and compression and alleviating pain with antiinflammatories.

- Crutches are suggested for ambulatory assistance if necessary.
- If appropriate, rehabilitation that concentrates on returning the affected extremity to full range of motion and strength can be offered to the patient. For most patients, a home exercise program is sufficient for rehabilitation. Elite athletes usually are provided with more aggressive and personal regimens.
- Return to sports is only recommended after the patient is pain free and has full function and strength of the extremity.
- Steroid injections for iliac crest contusions have been advocated by some surgeons. Padding over the affected area during activity may also prevent recurrence or further injury.

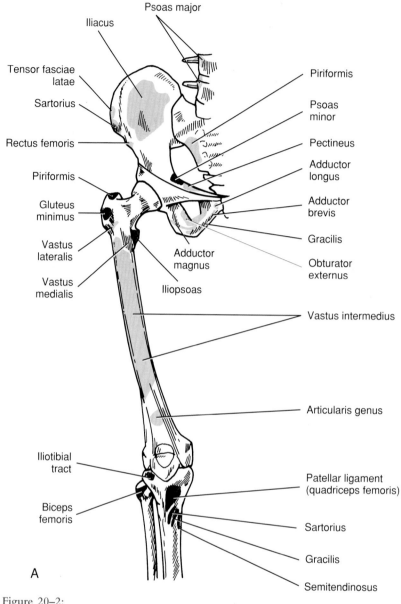

Figure 20–2:
(A) Anterior and

(continued)

- It is recommended that patients with quadriceps contusions rest the extremity with the knee flexed to provide tension on the muscle and thus inhibit blood pooling and muscle contracture.
- Myositis ossificans often requires more aggressive physical therapy but rarely requires operative excision.
- Complete avulsed muscles may require anatomical surgical correction.

Rehabilitation

- Rehabilitation for muscle injuries in athletes has been described in five phases with an average of 6 weeks to complete (Box 20–5).

- It is essential that the patient follows the regimen sequentially and avoids simultaneous efforts that could stress an injured muscle.
- The sequence of most rehabilitation programs begins with reducing pain and inflammation; advances to regaining pain free range of motion; and finally concentrates on rebuilding muscle strength, flexibility, and endurance to preinjury levels.
- Strengthening is initiated with isometric exercises and, when appropriate, advanced to isotonic and isokinetic regimens.
- Isokinetic testing can be used to assess muscle strength and imbalances after rehabilitation and to assist in determining if an athlete is ready to return to play.

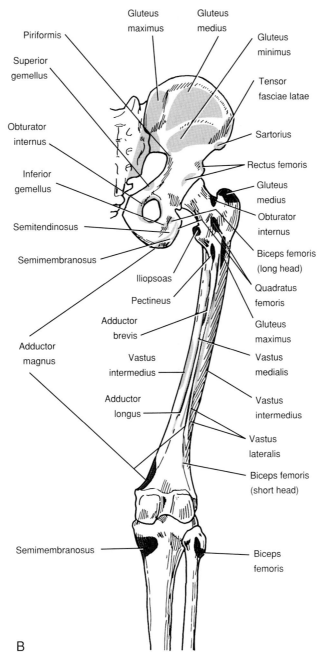

Figure 20–2, cont'd:
(B) posterior views of bones of the pelvis and thigh illustrating muscle origins and insertions. (From Jenkins DB, Hollinshead WH: *Hollinshead's functional anatomy of the limbs and
back.* Philadelphia, 2002, Saunders.)

Complications

- Chronic injuries can debilitate an athlete and occasionally affect the gait.
- Returning athletes to activities too early may predispose them to reinjury, which tends to be more severe and require an even longer recovery period.

- Contusions of the quadriceps can occasionally progress to myositis ossificans and restrict knee motion.
- Recurrence of myositis ossificans most often occurs after the lesion is excised, before it is fully matures. Delayed surgery is recommended.

Box 20–1	Anterior Muscles of the Thigh

Muscle	Origin (proximal attachment)	Insertion (distal attachment)	Action	Innervation
Sartorius	Anterior superior iliac spine	Medial surface—proximal end of tibia just distal to tibial tuberosity	Flexion, abduction, and lateral rotation of thigh; flexion of leg	Femoral nerve
Tensor fasciae latae	Iliac crest posterior to anterior superior iliac spine	Iliotibial tract	Flexion, medial rotation, and abduction of thigh	Superior gluteal nerve
Quadriceps femoris				
1. Rectus femoris	Anterior inferior iliac spine; ilium above acetabulum	Patella and through patellar ligament to tibial tuberosity	Extension of leg; flexion of thigh	Femoral nerve
2. Vastus medialis	Medial lip of linea aspera; lower part of intertrochanteric line	Patella and through patellar ligament to tibial tuberosity	Extension of leg	Femoral nerve
3. Vastus lateralis	Lateral lip of linea aspera of femur; limited origin from intertrochanteric line	Patella and through patellar ligament to tibial tuberosity	Extension of leg	Femoral nerve
4. Vastus intermedius	Anterior and lateral surfaces of femur	Patella and through patellar ligament to tibial tuberosity	Extension of leg	Femoral nerve
Articularis genus	Distal part of anterior surface of femur	Synovial membrane of knee joint	Pulls synovial membrane of knee proximally during extension of leg	Femoral nerve (nerve to vastus intermedius)
Iliopsoas				
1. Psoas major	Bodies and transverse processes of lumbar vertebrae (and possibly last thoracic vertebra)	Lesser trochanter of femur	Flexion of thigh; slight adduction of thigh of free limb	Second to fourth lumbar nerves
2. Iliacus	Iliac fossa	Lesser trochanter (with psoas major) of femur	Flexion of thigh; slight adduction of thigh of free limb	Femoral nerve
Psoas minor	Twelfth thoracic and first lumbar vertebrae	Superior ramus of pubis	Upward rotation of pelvis	First or second lumbar nerve (or both)
Pectineus	Superior ramus of pubis	Femur just distal to lesser trochanter	Flexion and adduction of thigh	Femoral nerve; possibly obturator or accessory obturator nerve, or both

From Jenkins DB, Hollinshead WH: *Hollinshead's functional anatomy of the limbs and back.* Philadelphia, 2002, Saunders.

Box 20–2	Adductor Group of Muscles

Muscle	Origin (Proximal attachment)	Insertion (Distal attachment)	Action	Innervation
Adductor longus	Pubic tubercle	Medial lip of linea aspera of femur	Adduction and flexion of thigh	Obturator nerve
Gracilis	Inferior ramus of pubis; ramus of ischium	Medial surface—proximal end of tibia just distal to medial condyle	Adduction of thigh; flexion of leg; medial rotation of flexed leg	Obturator nerve
Adductor brevis	Body and inferior ramus of pubis	Pectineal line; proximal part of linea aspera of femur	Adduction and flexion of thigh	Obturator nerve
Adductor magnus	Inferior ramus of pubis; ramus of ischium; ischial tuberosity	Linea aspera (anterior fibers); adductor tubercle of femur (posterior fibers)	Adduction of thigh; flexion of thigh (anterior fibers); extension of thigh (posterior fibers)	Obturator nerve (anterior fibers); sciatic nerve (posterior fibers)
Obturator externus	Obturator membrane; bone around obturator foramen on external surface of pelvis	Trochanteric fossa of femur	Lateral rotation of thigh	Obturator nerve

From Jenkins DB, Hollinshead WH: *Hollinshead's functional anatomy of the limbs and back.* Philadelphia, 2002, Saunders.

Box 20–3	Muscles of the Gluteal Region			
Muscle	**Origin (proximal attachment)**	**Insertion (distal attachment)**	**Action**	**Innervation**
Gluteus maximus	Lateral surface of ilium behind posterior gluteal line; dorsal sacroiliac and sacrotuberous ligaments; dorsal surface of sacrum	Iliotibial tract; gluteal tuberosity of femur	Extension, lateral rotation, abduction (upper fibers), and adduction (lower fibers) of thigh	Inferior gluteal nerve
Gluteus medius	Lateral surface of ilium between anterior and posterior gluteal lines	Greater trochanter of femur	Abduction of thigh; medial rotation and flexion (anterior fibers) and lateral rotation and extension (posterior fibers) of thigh	Superior gluteal nerve
Gluteus minimus	Lateral surface of ilium between anterior and inferior gluteal lines	Greater trochanter of femur	Abduction of thigh; medial rotation and flexion of thigh	Superior gluteal nerve
Piriformis	Sacrum (pelvic surface)	Greater trochanter of femur	Lateral rotation of thigh; abduction of thigh when thigh is flexed	S1 and S2
Obturator internus	Obturator membrane; bone around obturator foramen on internal surface of pelvis	Medial surface of greater trochanter above trochanteric fossa of femur	Lateral rotation of thigh; abduction of thigh when thigh is flexed	Nerve to obturator internus
Superior gemellus	Ischial spine	Superior border of obturator internus tendon	Lateral rotation of thigh; abduction of thigh when thigh is flexed	Nerve to obturator internus
Inferior gemellus	Ischial tuberosity	Inferior border of obturator internus tendon	Lateral rotation of thigh; abduction of thigh when thigh is flexed	Nerve to quadratus femoris
Quadratus femoris	Ischial tuberosity	Posterior surface of femur between greater and lesser trochanters	Lateral rotation and adduction of thigh	Nerve to quadratus femoris

From Jenkins DB, Hollinshead WH: *Hollinshead's functional anatomy of the limbs and back.* Philadelphia, 2002, Saunders.

Box 20–4	Posterior Muscles of the Thigh			
Muscle	**Origin (proximal attachment)**	**Insertion (distal attachment)**	**Action**	**Innervation**
Semitendinosus	Ischial tuberosity	Medial surface of proximal end of tibia	Extension of thigh; flexion of leg; medial rotation of flexed leg	Sciatic nerve—tibial part
Semimembranosus	Ischial tuberosity	Medial condyle of tibia	Extension of thigh; flexion of leg; medial rotation of flexed leg	Sciatic nerve—tibial part
Biceps femoris	Long head—ischial tuberosity	Head of fibula	Extension of thigh (long head); flexion of leg; lateral rotation of flexed leg	Sciatic nerve—tibial part to long head; common fibular part to short head
	Short head—linea aspera of femur and lateral interm uscular septum			

From Jenkins DB, Hollinshead WH: *Hollinshead's functional anatomy of the limbs and back.* Philadelphia, 2002, Saunders.

Box 20–5	Rehabilitation Guidelines for Muscle Injuries in Elite Athletes		
	Goals	**Treatment**	**Time frame**
Phase I	Reduce pain, inflammation, and bleeding	Rest, ice, and compression; crutches if needed	48 to 72 hours
Phase II	Regain range of motion	Passive range of motion, heat, ultrasound, electrical muscle stimulation	72 hours to week 1
Phase III	Increase strength, flexibility, and endurance	Isometrics, well-leg cycling	Weeks 1 to 3
Phase IV	Increase strength and coordination	Isotonic and isokinetic exercises	Weeks 3 to 4
Phase V	Return to competition	Sport-specific training	Weeks 4 to 6

From Delee JC, Drez D J, editors: *Orthopaedic sports medicine: principles and practice.* vol 2. Philadelphia, 1994, WB Saunders.

References

Clanton TO, Coupe KJ: Hamstring strains in athletes: diagnosis and treatment. *J Am Acad Orthop Surg* 6:237-248, 1998.

Detailed review of hamstring strain injury including anatomy, physiology, mechanism of injury, clinical evaluation and diagnosis, and treatment. Authors offer a five-phase treatment protocol that can be followed to return players back to competition after a hamstring injury.

Croisier JL, Forthomme B, Namurois MH, et al: Hamstring muscle strain recurrence and strength performance disorders. *Am J Sports Med* 30:199-203, 2002.

Authors evaluate the relationship between muscle/strength imbalance and hamstring injury. Twenty-six athletes with recurrent histories of hamstring strain/pain are assessed by isokinetic testing, revealing 18 patients with strength deficits. These patients underwent individual rehabilitation programs, resulting in isokinetic normalization in all but one of the subjects. Authors conclude that muscle weakness or imbalance may predispose athletes to recurrent hamstring injury that may be prevented with proper rehabilitation, particularly using eccentric exercises.

Hughes C, Hasselman CT, Best TM, et al: Incomplete, intrasubstance strain injuries of the rectus femoris muscle. *Am J Sports Med* 23:500-506, 1995.

Authors report on 10 cases with intrasubstance rectus femoris strains, located proximal to the more common (classical) site of injury at the distal muscle-tendon junction. Authors review the patients' presentations and clinical findings and differentiate intrasubstance rectus femoris strains from distal strains and soft tissue neoplasms in an effort to increase awareness of this less common injury.

Klingele KE, Sallay PI: Surgical repair of complete proximal hamstring tendon rupture. *Am J Sport Med* 30:742-747, 2002.

Retrospective cohort study of 11 patients who underwent acute (<4 weeks) or delayed repair of proximal hamstring tendon ruptures with suture anchors. Ten (91%) of the patients were satisfied with their

results. Muscle testing revealed an average return of 83% in the acute group (n = 7) and 89% in the chronic group (n = 4) when compared with the uninjured extremity. Authors conclude that good results can be produced from early or late repairs of hamstring ruptures.

Nicholas AJ, Tyler TF: Adductor muscle strains in sport. *Sports Med* 32:339-344, 2002.

Comprehensive review of adductor strains including anatomy, diagnosis, epidemiology, risk factors, prevention, and conservative and surgical management options. The authors stress that such injuries may be prevented if risk factors are identified early and addressed appropriately. Prevention primarily concentrates on strengthening the adductor group of muscles. Recommended prevention and postinjury programs are outlined.

Ryan JB, Wheeler JH, Hopkinson WJ, et al: Quadriceps contusions: West Point update. *Am J Sports Med* 19:299-304, 1991.

Three-year study of 117 quadriceps contusions in West Point cadets using their three-phase therapy program that documented excellent results in returning these young athletes back to full duty. Salient point of their rehabilitation protocol involved resting the injured leg in flexion and emphasizing early flexion exercises.

Verrall GM, Slavotinek JP, Barnes PG, Fon GT: Diagnostic and prognostic value of clinical findings in 83 athletes with posterior thigh injury. *Am J Sports Med* 31:969-973, 2003.

Prospective study following posterior thigh injuries in Australian football player for two seasons. MRI confirmed hamstring injury in 82% of the 83 players with posterior thigh injuries. Typical history and examination findings included sudden onset of symptoms, usually associated with a history of running or acceleration activity, pain, posterior thigh tenderness, and pain with resisted hamstring testing. Patients with positive MRI findings had a poorer prognosis (greater pain and longer absence from play) than those with negative findings. The authors propose fatigue as a possible causative risk factor for hamstring injury.

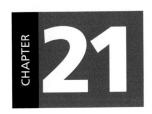

Nerve Entrapment Syndromes of the Hip and Knee

Introduction

- Symptoms are varied based on nerve involved (Box 21–1).
- Involvement may be sensory or motor, or both.
- Other etiologies of neurologic symptoms must be considered (Figure 21–1).
- Treatment is often controversial but includes removing external restrictive clothing or equipment and may ultimately require surgical release of offending internal structures.

Pudendal Nerve

- Numbness of the shaft of the penis and impotence have been cause by prolonged bicycle riding.
  - Compression of pudendal nerve between bicycle seat and pubic symphysis.
- Symptomatic treatment (seat modifications, etc.) is often effective.

Ilioinguinal Nerve

- Entrapment of the nerve occurs as a result of hypertrophied abdominal muscles in athletes, especially in bodybuilding.
- Pain or paresthesias, or both, may be reproduced with active hip extension.
- Surgical release may be beneficial.

Sciatic Nerve

- Entrapment occurs in gluteal region.
- Hip injury is commonly implicated.
- Transient neuropathy can be seen in cyclists.
- Complete injury can cause paralysis of hamstrings and all muscles below knee.
- Electromyography (EMG)/nerve conduction studies (NCS) are often helpful.
- Piriformis syndrome (entrapment in this muscle) is a controversial cause of this and is discussed more fully in Chapter 17 (Figure 21–2).
- Surgical decompression may be helpful in some cases.

Obturator Nerve

- Entrapment occurs as the obturator nerve enters the thigh.
- Classic presentation is pain or paresthesias, or both, in the medial thigh that is worsened with exercise.
- Adductor weakness may be evident on physical examination but is not always present.
- EMG may be helpful as it shows decreased latency of the obturator nerve and decreased innervation to the adductor muscle group.
- Surgical release of the tight fascia is successful and is associated with a high rate of return to sport within as little as a month.

Femoral Nerve

- Femoral nerve entrapment is seen in gymnasts, dancers, judoists, and parachuters.
- Weakness and atrophy of quadriceps, loss of knee jerk reflex, and sensory loss over anteromedial thigh and leg may occur.
- Treatment includes nonsteroidal antiinflammatory drugs (NSAIDs), physical therapy, bracing, and rarely surgical decompression.

Box 21–1	Etiologies of Lower Extremity Neurologic Signs and Symptoms

Local compression
   Tight clothing
   Compression against equipment
   Soft tissue swelling or mass
Lumbar disc disease
Lumbar plexopathy
Systemic disease
   Thyroid disease (hyporeflexia or hyperreflexia)
   Diabetes mellitus (sensory loss)
Rapid weight loss
Compartment syndrome
Contusion/traction

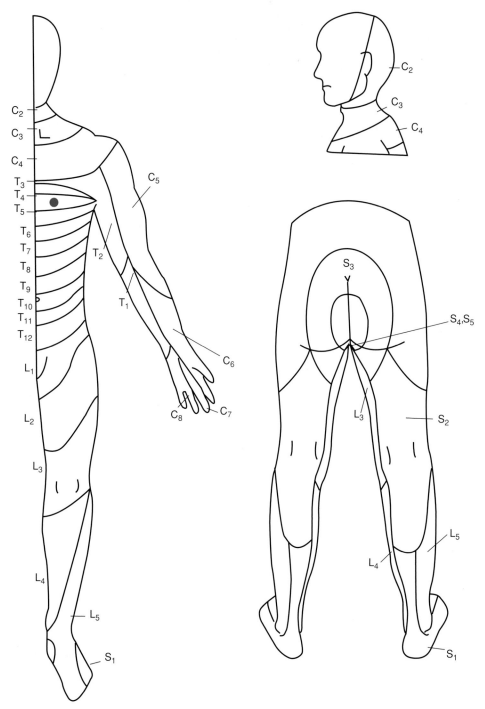

Figure 21-1:
Dermatomes of the lower extremity. (Redrawn from Masear VR: *Primary care orthopaedics.* Philadelphia, 1996, WB Saunders.)

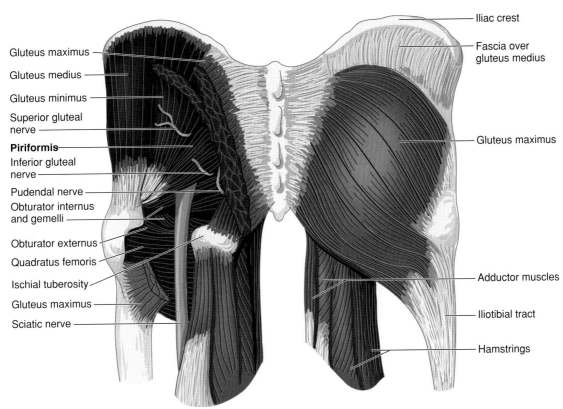

Gluteus maximus
Gluteus medius
Gluteus minimus
Superior gluteal nerve
Piriformis
Inferior gluteal nerve
Pudendal nerve
Obturator internus and gemelli
Obturator externus
Quadratus femoris
Ischial tuberosity
Gluteus maximus
Sciatic nerve

Iliac crest
Fascia over gluteus medius
Gluteus maximus
Adductor muscles
Iliotibial tract
Hamstrings

Figure 21-2:
Piriformis syndrome. (Redrawn from Jenkins DB: *Hollinshead's functional anatomy of the limbs and back.* **Philadelphia, 1991, WB Saunders.)**

Lateral Femoral Cutaneous Nerve (Meralgia Paresthetica)

- This is often reported in runners but may also be a result of restrictive belts or other equipment that produces focal pressure on the nerve (Figure 21–3).
- Symptoms include anterolateral thigh numbness/paresthesias.
  - Burning, aching pain common.
  - No motor symptoms.
- Etiologies include constricting clothing/belts, rapid weight change, systemic diseases affecting nerves (e.g., thyroid disease and diabetes).
- Differential diagnosis includes focal muscular injury, lumbosacral plexus injury, and systemic disease.
- Treatment should first involve removal of offending constrictive clothing or equipment but may also include local injections and occasionally surgical release.

Common Peroneal Nerve

- The common peroneal nerve can be compressed at fibular head.

- Signs and symptoms include dorsiflexion weakness, foot drop, steppage gait, and ankle sprains.
- Differential diagnosis includes disc disease, compartment syndrome, and lumbosacral plexopathy.
- Electrodiagnostic testing is helpful.
- Magnetic resonance imaging (MRI) may be helpful if nerve impingement by cysts or other soft tissue mass is expected.
- Treatment includes use of transcutaneous electrical nerve stimulation (TENS), biomechanical interventions, and change in running style.

Saphenous Nerve

- The branch of the femoral nerve most commonly entrapped at the medial knee (Figure 21–4).
- Etiologies include entrapment at the adductor canal, pes anserine bursitis, and contusion.
  - External pressure can cause neuropathy in certain sports such as surfing (surfer's neuropathy).
- Signs/symptoms include neuropathic pain and numbness in medial knee/calf.
  - No motor defects.

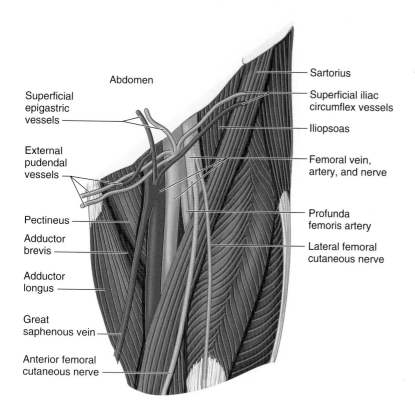

Abdomen

Superficial
epigastric
vessels

External
pudendal
vessels

Pectineus

Adductor
brevis

Adductor
longus

Great
saphenous vein

Anterior femoral
cutaneous nerve

Sartorius

Superficial iliac
circumflex vessels

Iliopsoas

Femoral vein,
artery, and nerve

Profunda
femoris artery

Lateral femoral
cutaneous nerve

Figure 21-3:
Lateral femoral cutaneous nerve (meralgia paresthetica). (Redrawn from Jenkins DB: *Hollinshead's functional anatomy of the limbs and back*. Philadelphia, 1991, WB Saunders.)

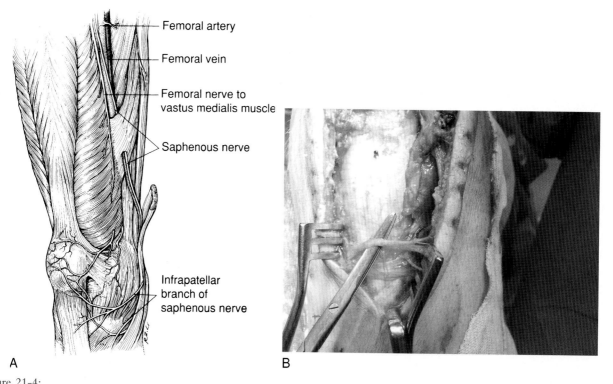

Femoral artery

Femoral vein

Femoral nerve to
vastus medialis muscle

Saphenous nerve

Infrapatellar
branch of
saphenous nerve

A   B

Figure 21-4:
Saphenous nerve entrapment at the medial aspect of the knee. **A,** Entrapment of the infrapatellar branch of the saphenous nerve can occur. **B,** Intraoperative view of the infrapatellar branch of the saphenous nerve. (A from Tria AJ, Klein KS: *An illustrated guide to the knee.* New York, 1992, Churchill Livingstone.)

- Percussion may localize area of entrapment.
- Differential diagnosis.
  - Proximal femoral nerve entrapment.
  - Intraarticular knee injuries.
- Treatment.
  - Reduction of offending constriction.
  - Surgical release.

References

Bradshaw C, McCrory P, Bell S, Brukner P: Obturator nerve entrapment—a cause of groin pain in athletes. *Am J Sports Med* 25:402-408, 1997.

This reviews the authors' experiences with 32 athletes diagnosed with obturator neuropathy. Discussion includes a review of the most pertinent history and physical examination findings, as well as the reported success of surgical nerve decompression.

Harvey G, Bell S: Obturator neuropathy—an anatomic perspective. *Clin Orthop Related Res* 363:203-211, 1999.

This is a cadaveric study that reviews the relationship between the obturator nerve, its associated vascular structures, and the fascia that is commonly thought to cause entrapment as the nerve exits the pelvis.

House JH, Ahmed K: Entrapment neuropathy of the infrapatellar branch of the saphenous nerve. *Am J Sports Med* 5:217-224, 1977.

This is a review of the anatomy of the saphenous nerve, its branches, and its path into the thigh. Discussion includes possible causes of entrapment and treatment.

Leach RE, Purnell MB, Saito A: Peroneal nerve entrapment in runners. *Am J Sports Med* 17:287-291, 1989.

Runners are one athletic group that have been identified to have an increased incidence of peroneal nerve compression. This article discusses the most common history and physical examination findings in this group and also outlines appropriate treatment for these athletes.

McCrory P, Bell S: Nerve entrapment syndromes as a cause of pain in the hip, groin, and buttock. *Sports Med* 27:261-274, 1999.

This is a helpful article that summarizes proximal nerve entrapment syndromes in the lower extremity.

Mitra A, Stern JD, Perrotta VJ, Moyer RA: Peroneal nerve entrapment in athletes. *Ann Plast Surg* 35:366-368, 1995.

These authors discuss 12 of their patients with peroneal nerve entrapment syndrome in terms of the diagnostic workup performed, treatment strategies used, and outcome.

Romanoff ME, Cory PC, Kalenak A, et al: Saphenous nerve entrapment at the adductor canal. *Am J Sports Med* 17:478-481, 1989.

This study is a retrospective review of cases of saphenous nerve entrapment and discusses the diagnosis of the problem, as well as results of treatment in this group.

Schon L: Nerve entrapment neuropathy and nerve dysfunction in the athlete. *Orthop Clin North Am* 25:47-59, 1994.

This article discusses nerve entrapment and dysfunction as these conditions affect the athletic population. Discussion includes etiology, diagnosis, and proper management of these conditions.

Worth RM, Kettelkamp DB, Defalgue RJ, Duane KU: Saphenous nerve entrapment. A cause of medial knee pain. *Am J Sports Med* 12:80-81, 1984.

This article reviews cases of patients with medial-sided knee pain caused by entrapment of the saphenous nerve including clinical course and outcomes.

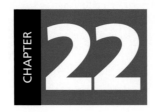

CHAPTER **22**

Leg, Ankle, and Foot Anatomy and Biomechanics (Including Gait)

Introduction

- The leg, composed of the tibia and fibula, connects the knee and ankle joints.
- Muscles that originate in the leg all attach distally on the foot and are arranged into anterior, lateral, and posterior compartments with the posterior compartment further characterized by superficial and deep subdivisions.
- The ankle joint is a uniaxial hinge joint whose primary movements are dorsiflexion and plantarflexion.
- The foot, with a total of 26 bones, contains the tarsus, metatarsus, and phalanges.
- Because the lower extremity is responsible for supporting a person's weight during ambulation, pathologic conditions may manifest in gait. Therefore a firm understanding of normal and abnormal gait is required by the evaluating surgeon.
- Certain injuries are more common in specific sports (Box 22–1).

Tibia

- As the second longest bone in the body, the tibia ("shin bone") bears most of the weight of the leg and articulates superiorly with the femoral condyles and inferiorly with the talus (Figure 22–1).
- It is derived from three ossification centers.
- Its proximal surface consists of medial and lateral plateaus divided by the intercondylar eminence, which also separates the anterior and posterior cruciate ligaments.
- Its prominent anterior tubercle serves as an attachment site for the patellar tendon.
- Gerdy's tubercle is found along the proximal, lateral aspect of the tibia into which the iliotibial band inserts.
- The shaft is triangular in transverse section and can be said to have medial, lateral, and posterior surfaces.
- Distally, the tibia forms the medial malleolus and has a quadrilateral surface that articulates with the talus.
- Laterally, the tibia gives rise to an interosseous membrane that unites the leg bones and both proximal and distal facets that articulate with the fibula.

Fibula

- The fibula ("calf bone") primarily serves as an attachment site for muscles and its lateral malleolus provides some ankle stability (Figure 22–1).
- Derived from three ossification centers.
- May help brace the tibia, affording it to withstand some bending and twisting.
- The lateral malleolus lies more inferior and posterior than the medial malleolus.

Muscles of the Leg

- The muscles of the leg can be grouped according to compartments (Boxes 22–2 to 22–5, Figures 22–2 to 22–5).
- In general, each major compartment shares the same function and nerve supply and receives its blood supply from branches off the anterior and posterior tibial

Box 22–1	Common Sport-Associated Injuries of the Leg, Foot, and Ankle
Sport	**Common Injuries**
Aerobic dance	Sesamoid fractures, tendinitis, stress fractures
Ballet	Sesamoid fractures, tendinitis, stress fractures
Baseball	Talonavicular joint injury, ankle sprains, osteophytes
Basketball	Fifth metatarsal base fractures, stress fractures, tendinitis
Bicycling	Lacerations, strains, sprains
Football	Sesamoid fractures, ankle fractures, sprains, turf toe, tarsometatarsal fractures and dislocations
Hockey	Puck injuries and fractures, contusions, ankle and hindfoot injuries, exostoses, bursitis
Racket sports	Ankle sprains, Achilles tendon injuries, tendinitis
Running	Ankle sprains, overuse injuries, stress fractures
Skiing	Ankle fractures, peroneal tendon dislocation
Soccer	Forefoot injuries, tendinitis, ankle sprains
Wrestling	Fifth metatarsal base fractures, Achilles tendinitis, ankle sprains

From Miller MD, Cooper DE, Warner JJP: *Review of sports medicine and arthroscopy.* Philadelphia, 2002, Saunders.

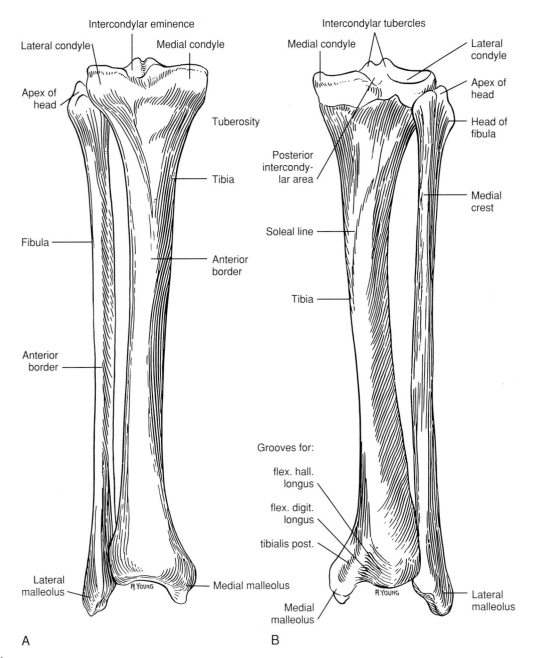

Figure 22–1:
(**A**) Anterior and (**B**) Posterior views of the tibia and fibula. (From Jenkins DB, Hollinshead WH: *Hollinshead's functional anatomy of the limbs and back,* 8th ed. Philadelphia, 2002, Saunders.)

arteries, which are divisions of the popliteal artery (Box 22–6, Figure 22–6).

- The anterior compartment is bounded by the lateral surface of the tibia and the anterior crural intermuscular septum.
  - Its muscles primarily serve to dorsiflex the foot and extend the toes.
  - Supplied by the deep peroneal nerve.
- The lateral compartment is formed by the lateral surface of the fibula, anterior and posterior intermuscular septa, and the crural fascia.

- Its two peroneal muscles help plantarflex and evert the foot.
- Receives nerve supply from the superficial peroneal nerve.
- The deep posterior compartment is located posterior to the interosseous membrane, fibula, and posterior crural intermuscular septum.
  - Although the popliteus muscle acts to flex the knee, all the other muscles are responsible for plantar flexion of the foot and toes.
  - This compartment receives its innervation from the tibial nerve.

Box 22–2	Muscles in the Anterior Compartment of the Leg			
Muscle	**Proximal Attachments**	**Distal Attachments**	**Innervation**	**Main Actions**
Tibialis anterior	Lateral condyle and superior half of lateral surface of tibia	Medial and inferior surfaces of medial cuneiform bone and base of first metatarsal bone	Deep fibular (peroneal) nerve (L4 and L5)	Dorsiflexes and inverts foot
Extensor hallucis longus	Middle part of anterior surface of fibula and interosseous membrane	Dorsal aspect of base of distal phalanx of great toe (hallux)		Extends great toe and dorisiflexes foot
Extensor digitorum longus	Lateral condyle of tibia, superior three-fourths of anterior surface of fibula, and interosseous membrane	Middle and distal phalanges of lateral four digits	Deep fibular (peroneal) nerve (L5 and S1)	Extends lateral four digits and dorsiflexes foot
Fibularis (peroneus) tertius	Inferior third of anterior surface of fibula and interosseous membrane	Dorsum of base of fifth metatarsal bone		Dorsiflexes foot and aids in eversion of it

From Jenkins DB, Hollinshead WH: *Hollinshead's functional anatomy of the limbs and back*, 8th ed. Philadelphia, 2002, Saunders.

Box 22–3	Muscles in the Lateral Compartment of the Leg[1]			
Muscle	**Proximal**	**Distal**	**Innervation**	**Main Actions**
Fibularis (peroneus) longus	Head and superior two thirds of lateral surface of fibula	Base of first metatarsal bone and medial cuneiform bone	Superficial fibular (peroneal) nerve (L5, S1, and S2)	Evert foot and weakly plantarflex it
Fibularis (peroneus) brevis	Inferior two thirds of lateral surface of fibula	Dorsal surface of tuberosity on lateral side of base of fifth metatarsal bone		

From Jenkins DB, Hollinshead WH: *Hollinshead's functional anatomy of the limbs and back*, 8th ed. Philadelphia, 2002, Saunders.
[1]The fibularis (peroneus) longus and brevis were named because their proximal attachment is to the fibula. *Peroneus* is the Greek word for the Latin term *fibula* and was formerly used to describe these muscles.

Box 22–4	Muscles in the Superficial Posterior Compartment of the Leg			
Muscle	**Proximal Attachment**	**Distal Attachment**	**Innervation**	**Main Actions**
Gastrocnemius	*Lateral head:* Lateral aspect of lateral condyle of femur *Medial head:* Popliteal surface of femur, superior to medial condyle	Posterior surface of calcaneus via tendo calcaneus	Tibial nerve (S1 and S2)	Plantarflexes foot, raises heel during walking, and flexes knee joint
Soleus	Posterior aspect of head of fibula, superior fourth of posterior surface of fibula, soleal line, and medial border of tibia			Plantarflexes foot and steadies leg on foot
Plantaris	Inferior end of lateral supracondylar line of femur and oblique popliteal ligament			Weakly assists gastrocnemius in plantarflexing foot and flexing knee joint

From Jenkins DB, Hollinshead WH: *Hollinshead's functional anatomy of the limbs and back*, 8th ed. Philadelphia, 2002, Saunders.

Box 22–5	Muscles in the Deep Posterior Compartment of the Leg			
Muscle	**Proximal Attachment**	**Distal Attachment**	**Innervation**	**Main Actions**
Popliteus	Lateral surface of lateral condyle of femur and lateral meniscus	Posterior surface of tibia, superior to soleal line	Tibial nerve (L4, L5, and S1)	Weakly flexes knee and unlocks it
Flexor hallucis longus	Inferior two-thirds of posterior surface of fibula and inferior part of interosseous membrane	Bases of distal phalanx of great toe (hallux)	Tibial nerve (S2 and S3)	Flexes great toe at all joints and plantarflexes foot; supports longitudinal arch of foot
Flexor digitorum longus	Medial part of posterior surface of tibia, inferior to soleal line, and by a broad aponeurosis to fibula	Bases of distal phalanges of lateral four digits		Flexes lateral four digits and plantarflexes foot; supports longitudinal arch of foot
Tibialis posterior	Interosseous membrane, posterior surface of tibia inferior to soleal line, and posterior surface of fibula	Tuberosity of navicular, cuneiform, and cuboid bones, and bases of second, third, and fourth metatarsal bones	Tibial nerve (L4 and L5)	Plantarflexes and inverts foot

From Jenkins DB, Hollinshead WH: *Hollinshead's functional anatomy of the limbs and back,* 8th ed. Philadelphia, 2002, Saunders.

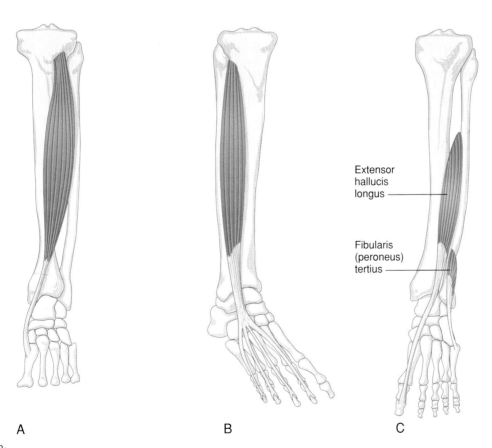

Extensor hallucis longus

Fibularis (peroneus) tertius

A   B   C

Figure 22–2:
Muscles in the anterior compartment of the leg. **A,** Tibialis anterior. **B,** Extensor digitorum longus **C,** Extensor hallucis longus and peroneus tertius. (Redrawn from Jenkins DB, Hollinshead WH: *Hollinshead's functional anatomy of the limbs and back.* Philadelphia, 2002, Saunders.)

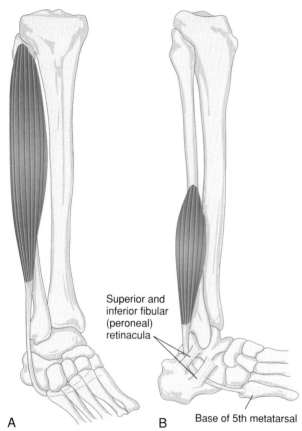

A B

Figure 22–3:

Muscles in the lateral compartment of the leg. A, Peroneus longus. **B,** Peroneus brevis. (Redrawn from Jenkins DB, Hollinshead WH: *Hollinshead's functional anatomy of the limbs and back.* Philadelphia, 2002, Saunders.)

- The superficial posterior compartment encloses muscles that assist in foot plantar flexion and lie posterior to the transverse crural intermuscular septum.
  - The posterior tibial tendon is a major supporter of the medial ankle and arch of the foot and maintains the hindfoot in 7 to 10 degrees of valgus in the neutral position.
  - Supplied by the tibial nerve.

Nerves

- All nerves to the inferior lower limb derive from divisions of the sciatic nerve (Figure 22–7).
- The tibial nerve is the larger terminal branch of the sciatic nerve.
  - Runs through the popliteal fossa over the popliteus muscle and down the median plane of the calf muscles, deep to the soleus, eventually terminating along the posteroinferior aspect of the medial malleolus, under the flexor retinaculum, where it branches into the medial and plantar nerves that run along the second layer of the foot (Figure 22–9*A*).

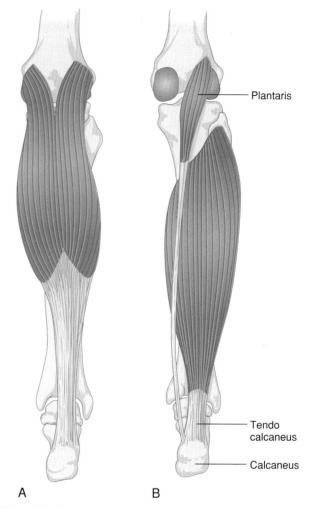

A B

Figure 22–4:

Muscles in the superficial posterior compartment of the leg. A, Gastrocnemius. **B,** Soleus and plantaris. (Redrawn from Jenkins DB, Hollinshead WH: *Hollinshead's functional anatomy of the limbs and back.* Philadelphia, 2002, Saunders.)

- The medial plantar nerve acts much like the median nerve of the hand, supplying the medial 3½ digits with sensation and motor function to a few plantar muscles. This nerve usually travels deep to the abductor hallucis.
- The lateral plantar nerve is similar to the ulnar nerve in the hand, providing sensation to the lateral 1½ digits and motor function to the remaining intrinsic muscles of the foot.
- The common peroneal nerve is the smaller of the terminal branches off the sciatic nerve (Figure 22–8).
- It runs along the lateral aspect of the popliteal fossa between the medial border of the biceps femoris and lateral head of the gastrocnemius, winds around the neck of the fibula, and dives deep to the peroneus longus where it further divides into the superficial and deep peroneal nerves that will supply the lateral and anterior compartments of the leg, respectively.

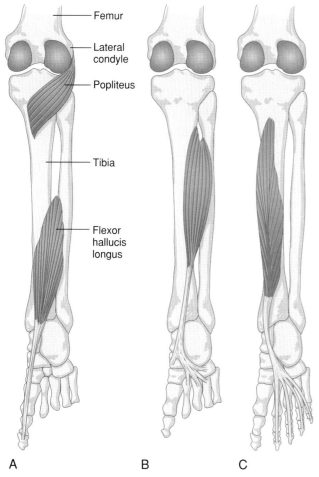

Femur

Lateral condyle

Popliteus

Tibia

Flexor hallucis longus

A   B   C

Figure 22–5:
**Muscles in the deep posterior compartment of the leg.
A, Popliteus and flexor hallucis longus. B, Tibialis posterior.
C, Flexor digitorum longus. (Redrawn from Jenkins DB, Hollinshead WH:** *Hollinshead's functional anatomy of the limbs and back.* **Philadelphia, 2002, Saunders.)**

- The deep peroneal nerve runs inferomedially on the fibula, deep to the extensor digitorum longus until it pierces through the anterior crural intermuscular septum and continues down the anterior surface of the interosseous membrane where it will be accompanied by the anterior tibial artery (Figure 22–9B).

- At the end of its course, after it passes deep to the extensor retinaculum, it will divide into medial and lateral branches.
- The medial terminal branch will supply sensation to the first web space, and the lateral terminal branch will innervate the extensor digitorum brevis muscle.
- The superficial peroneal nerve runs posterolateral to the anterior crural intermuscular septum and courses between the peroneal muscles and extensor digitorum longus prior to becoming more superficial in the distal third of the leg, eventually also innervating the skin of the anterior, distal leg and the dorsal foot and toes.
- The saphenous nerve is the largest cutaneous branch of the femoral nerve and is subcutaneous between the sartorius and gracilis along the medial knee.
  - Supplies the skin of the medial leg and foot.
- The sural nerve is usually formed by cutaneous branches of the tibial and common peroneal nerves at the popliteal fossa and then runs down between the heads of the gastrocnemius muscle.
  - Supplies sensation to the posterolateral aspect of the distal leg and lateral foot.
  - Is frequently a source for nerve grafting.

Vessels

- The leg receives its blood supply from branches of the popliteal artery (Figure 22–9).
- The popliteal artery, a continuation of the femoral artery, crosses the popliteal fossa inferolaterally between the biceps and semimembranosus, passing under the tibial nerve. It then divides at the distal border of the popliteus muscle between the medial and lateral heads of the gastrocnemius muscle into the anterior and posterior tibial arteries.
- The anterior tibial artery is the smaller terminal branch of the popliteal artery and is the primary source of blood supply to the anterior compartment. It runs along the anterior surface of the interosseous membrane alongside the deep peroneal nerve, between the tibialis anterior and extensor hallucis longus, and ends at the ankle joint midway between the malleoli and turns into the dorsalis pedis artery.

Box 22–6	Tests for Assessment of Peripheral Nerves and Compartments of the Leg*		
Nerve	**Compartment**	**Motor Function**	**Sensory Function**
Deep peroneal	Anterior	Toe dorsiflexion	Dorsal I–II web space
Superficial peroneal	Lateral	Foot eversion	Lateral dorsum of foot
Tibial	Deep posterior	Toe plantar flexion	Sole of foot
Sural	Superficial posterior	Gastrocsoleus	Lateral heel

*By testing each nerve and associated muscle group, it is possible to assess the status of myoneural tissue within each compartment.
From Canale ST, editor: *Campbell's operative orthopaedics*, 10th ed. Philadelphia, 2003, Saunders.

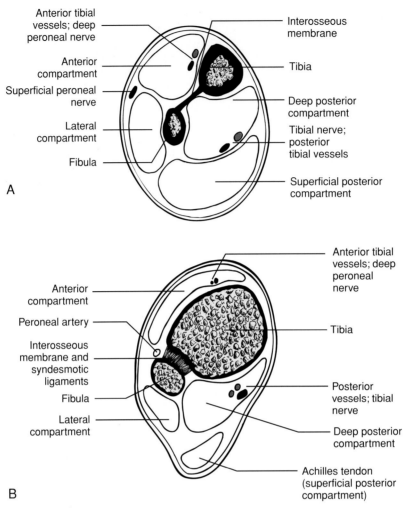

Figure 22–6:
Transverse section through the leg showing its compartments. A, Mid-shaft. **B,** At ankle. (From Browner BD et al., editors: *Skeletal trauma: basic science, management and reconstruction,* 3rd ed. Philadelphia, 2003, Saunders.)

- The dorsalis pedis artery continues to supply the dorsum of the foot via several branched arteries. The deep plantar artery, its largest branch, travels between the first two metatarsals and forms part of the plantar arch.
- The posterior tibial artery, the larger terminal branch of the popliteal artery, continues down the posterior compartment and, after giving off the peroneal artery approximately 2.5 cm distal to the popliteal fossa, travels inferomedially on the posterior surface of the tibialis posterior muscle. It terminates under the abductor hallucis longus after passing the medial malleolus inferiorly by dividing into the medial and lateral plantar arteries. The larger lateral plantar artery, together with the deep plantar artery, forms the plantar arch, which is located in the fourth layer of the plantar foot.
- The fibular artery, which runs between the tibialis posterior and flexor hallucis longus, ends by giving off calcaneal branches.

Ankle Joint

- This hinge joint is composed of a three-sided mortise defined by the medial and lateral malleoli and the talus. The joint can often be palpated between the tendons along the anterior surface of the ankle.
- The talus has three articular facets that articulate with the malleoli and the inferior surface of the tibia.
- Primary movements of the ankle involve dorsiflexion and plantarflexion, with a greater range of plantarflexion.
- Some rotation, including abduction and adduction, is possible when the foot is planted.
- The talus is wider anteriorly than superiorly and thus attempts to spread the malleoli apart with extreme ankle dorsiflexion. However, this is counteracted by the interosseous and anterior and posterior tibiofibular ligaments that unite the tibia and fibula.

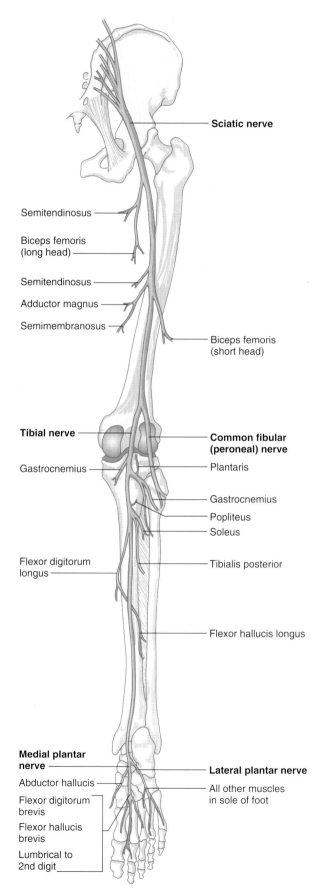

Sciatic nerve

Semitendinosus

Biceps femoris
(long head)

Semitendinosus

Adductor magnus

Semimembranosus

Biceps femoris
(short head)

Tibial nerve

**Common fibular
(peroneal) nerve**

Gastrocnemius

Plantaris

Gastrocnemius

Popliteus

Soleus

Flexor digitorum
longus

Tibialis posterior

Flexor hallucis longus

**Medial plantar
nerve**

Abductor hallucis

Lateral plantar nerve

All other muscles
in sole of foot

Flexor digitorum
brevis

Flexor hallucis
brevis

Lumbrical to
2nd digit

Figure 22–7:
Nerves of the lower extremity.

- There is greater stability with dorsiflexion given the arrangement and types of ligaments, retinacula, and tendons and the fact that there is a greater filling of the mortise with the talus in this position.
- Blood supply to the joint is provided by articular arteries that derive from malleolar branches of the peroneal and anterior and posterior tibial arteries.
- Innervation of the joint is received from the tibial and peroneal nerves.
- There are 13 tendons that cross the ankle joint.

Ankle Ligaments

- Several ligaments are responsible for maintaining ankle stability and can be divided into four groups: (1) lateral ligaments, (2) lateral subtalar ligaments, (3) medial ligaments, and (4) distal tibiofibular ligaments (Box 22–7, Figure 22–10).
- The lateral ligaments are composed of the anterior talofibular ligament, the posterior talofibular ligament, and the calcaneofibular ligament and attach the lateral malleolus to the talus and calcaneus.
- The anterior talofibular ligament is considered to be the primary restraint to anterior displacement, internal rotation, and inversion of the ankle.
  - It is a flat band that runs anteriomedially from the lateral malleolus to attach to the body of the talus.
  - It is believed to be the weakest of the lateral ligaments, which explains why it is the most commonly injured ligament in ankle sprains.
- The thick and strong posterior talofibular ligament runs from the lateral malleolus medially and posteriorly to attach to the lateral tubercle of the talus.
  - It helps limit internal rotation while the ankle is dorsiflexed.
- The calcaneofibular ligament crosses two joints while traveling posteroinferiorly from the distal margin of the lateral malleolus, under the anterior talofibular ligament, into the lateral aspect of the calcaneus.
  - Provides subtalar stabilization and is only placed under stress with extreme inversion.
- The lateral subtalar ligaments can be divided into three layers (Box 22–7). The cervical ligament serves as the principal restraint to subtalar inversion.
- The strong, fan-shaped medial deltoid ligament is composed of a superficial layer, which resists talar abduction, and a deep layer, which limits external rotation of the talus. This ligament spans out from the tip of the medial malleolus to attach to three tarsal bones (talus, calcaneus, and navicular).
- The distal tibiofibular interosseous ligaments, which stabilize the ankle mortise, consist of the anterior and posterior tibiofibular ligaments and the interosseous membrane.

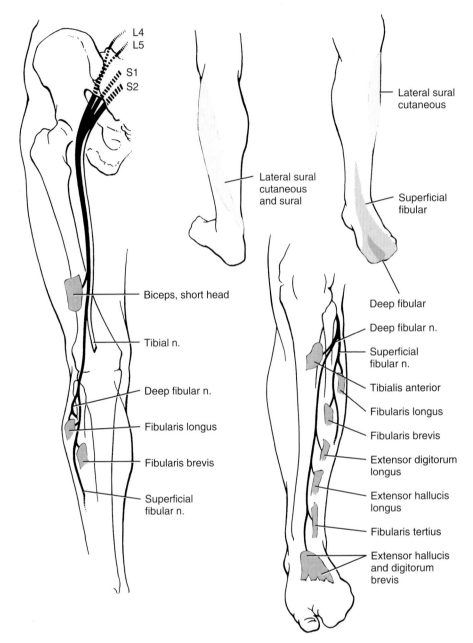

Figure 22–8:
Distribution of the common peroneal nerve. (From Jenkins DB, Hollinshead WH: *Hollinshead's functional anatomy of the limbs and back,* 8th ed. Philadelphia, 2002, Saunders.)

Osteology of the Foot

- The foot is composed of 7 tarsal bones, 5 metatarsals, and 14 phalanges (Figure 22–11).
- The tarsus consists of the talus, calcaneus, cuboid, navicular, and three cuneiforms.
- The head of the talus, which is immediately proximal to the navicular, is usually visible and can be palpated with inversion or eversion of the foot.
  - The head articulates with the navicular and calcaneus.
  - The body of the talus articulates with the tibia, malleoli, and calcaneus.
- The neck of the talus lies between the head and body.
- The calcaneus is the largest and strongest bone of the foot.
  - Its posterior, medial, and lateral sides are easily palpated, but its inferior border lies deep to the plantar aponeurosis and pad of fat.
  - Articulates with the talus via anterior, middle, and posterior surfaces.
  - Articulation with the cuboid occurs distally.
  - The sustentaculum talus is a prominence that can often be palpated distal to the tip of the medial malleolus.

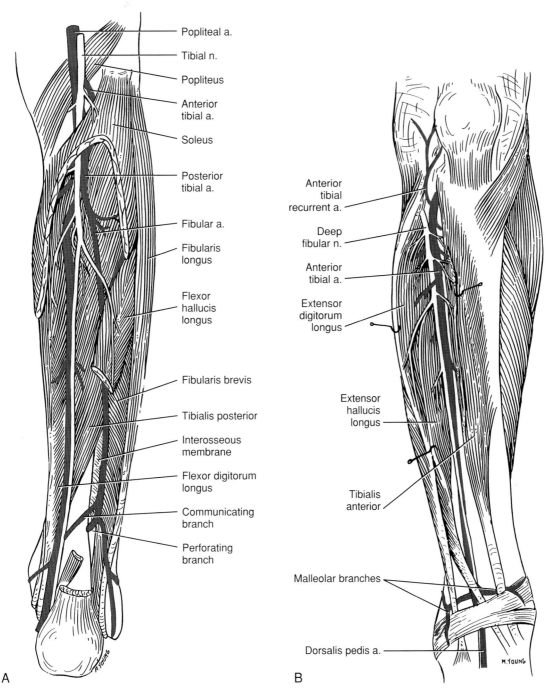

Figure 22–9:
Distribution of arteries and nerves in the leg. **A,** Posterior view. **B,** Anterior view. (From Jenkins DB, Hollinshead WH: *Hollinshead's functional anatomy of the limbs and back,* 8th ed. Philadelphia, 2002, Saunders.)

○ Apart from providing support to the middle articular surface, it creates an overhang under which plantar vessels and nerves can pass.
• The navicular lies along the medial aspect of the foot.
  • Articulates with the talus proximally, the cuboid laterally, and distally with the three cuneiforms.
  • Its tuberosity can be felt anteroinferior to the medial malleolus and serves as an insertion site for the tibialis posterior muscle.

• The cuboid is located along the lateral aspect of the foot and articulates with the calcaneus, lateral cuneiform, and bases of the fourth and fifth metatarsals. It also is distinctly grooved by the peroneus longus.
• The medial, intermediate, and lateral cuneiforms as a group articulate with the navicular, cuboid, and medial three metatarsals.
  • Having the intermediate cuneiform shorter than the others creates a socket between the medial and lateral

cuneiforms, allowing the second metatarsal to key into place.
- The five metatarsals lie between the tarsus and phalanges.
- The great toe is made up of two phalanges. All other digits are composed of three phalanges.

Joints of the Foot

- All bones of the foot are supported by dorsal and plantar ligaments.
- The subtalar, talocalcaneonavicular, and calcaneocuboid joints are the principal intertarsal joints.
- The subtalar joint is a synovial joint between the talus and calcaneus whose principal movements are inversion and eversion.
- The talocalcaneonavicular joint is a ball and socket type synovial joint that makes up part of the transverse tarsal joint.
  - The plantar calcaneonavicular ligament ("spring ligament"), which blends with the deltoid ligament, extends from the sustentaculum tali to the posteroinferior surface of the navicular bone and plays an important role in maintaining the arch of the foot.
- The calcaneocuboid joint is another synovial joint that makes up the remainder of the transverse tarsal joint.
- The transverse tarsal joint (Chopart's joint) is involved in inversion and eversion of the foot.
- The tarsometatarsal joints are synovial, gliding joints.
  - The metatarsals are united with the tarsal bones by plantar, dorsal, and interosseous ligaments.
  - The joint formed by the second metatarsal and intermediate cuneiform makes up the strongest tarsometatarsal joint and has little movement, making it more prone to injury, such as a stress fracture.
- The intermetatarsal joints are created between the bases of the metatarsal bones and are synovial joints that allow some gliding motion, but little individual movement.
  - The heads of the metatarsal bones are connected by the deep transverse ligament that, along with the interosseous ligaments, helps maintain the transverse arch of the foot.
- The metatarsophalangeal joints are knuckle-like synovial joints that permit flexion; extension; and some abduction, adduction, and circumduction.
- The interphalangeal joints are hinge-type synovial joints that only allow flexion and extension.

Muscles and Tendons of the Foot

- The plantar muscles and tendons of the foot can be divided into four layers (Box 22–8, Figure 22–12).
- The dorsal muscles of the foot consist of the extensor digitorum brevis and extensor hallucis brevis.

Box 22–7	**Ligaments of the Ankle**

Lateral ligaments

Anterior talofibular ligament (ATFL)
Posterior talofibular ligament (PTFL)
Calcaneofibular ligament (CFL)

Lateral subtalar ligaments

Superficial layer—calcaneofibular and lateral talocalcaneal ligaments and inferior extensor retinaculum
Intermediate layer—cervical ligament and intermediate portion of the extensor retinaculum
Deep layer—interosseus talocalcaneal ligament and deep portion of extensor retinaculum

Medial ligaments

Superficial deltoid ligament—tibionavicular, tibiocalcaneal, and superficial tibiotalar ligaments
Deep deltoid ligament—anterior and posterior tibiotalar ligaments

Distal tibiofibular ligaments (syndesmosis)

Anterior inferior tibiofibular ligament (AITFL)
Posterior inferior tibiofibular ligament (PITFL)
Interosseous membrane

- The arrangement of tendons and their relationship to surrounding structures are shown (Figure 22–13).

Gait Cycle

- The gait cycle can be divided into the stance phase, the weight-bearing part of the cycle when the foot is on the ground, and the swing phase, when the foot advances forward, each with its own subdivisions.
- The phases can be further subdivided (Figure 22–14).
- The stance phase, making up approximately 62% of the gait cycle, can be described in four parts: (1) heel strike, (2) foot flat, (3) midstance, and (4) push-off or heel-off/toe-off.
- The stance phase is noted to have 12% double limb support, when both feet are on the ground at the start and end of its stage, with 38% of single limb support in between.
- The swing phase, constituting the remaining 38% of the cycle, may be divided into three parts: (1) acceleration, (2) midswing, and (3) deceleration.
- One foot enters the cycle with heel strike shortly after the contralateral foot passes through heel-off.
- When running, there are periods in which neither foot is weight-bearing, and forces on ground contact can increase up to three times a person's body weight.

Text continued on p. 178

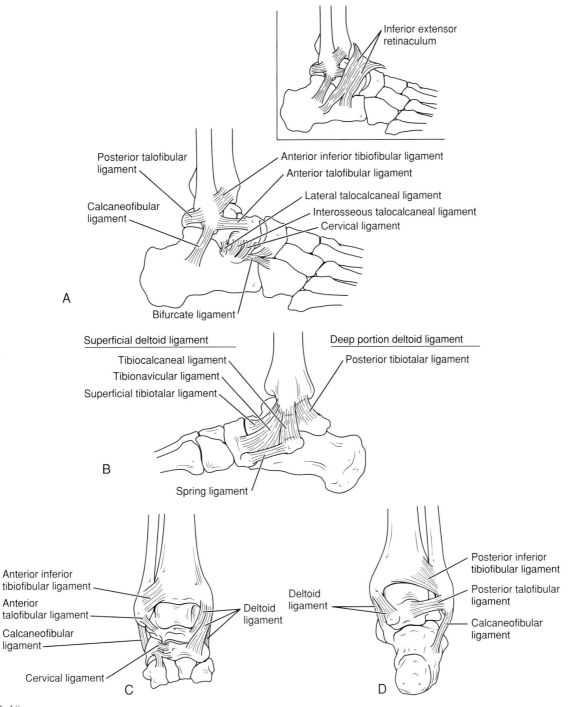

Figure 22–10:
Ligaments of the ankle and subtalar joint. **A,** Lateral view. **B,** Medial view. **C,** Anterior view. **D,** Posterior view. (From DeLee JC, Drez D Jr, Miller MD, editors: *DeLee and Drez's orthopaedic sports medicine: principles and practice,* 2nd ed. Philadelphia, 2003, Saunders.)

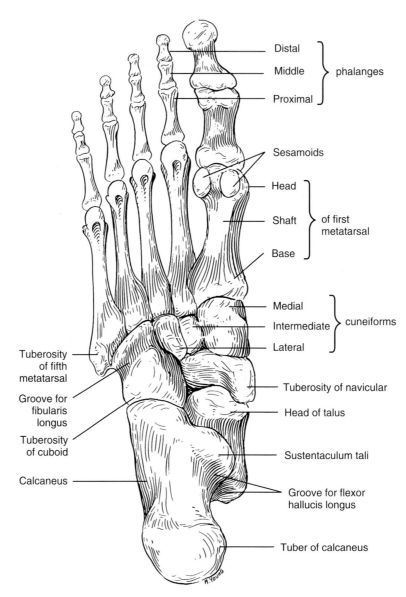

Figure 22–11:
Plantar view of the bones of the foot and ankle. (From Jenkins DB, Hollinshead WH: *Hollinshead's functional anatomy of the limbs and back*, 8th ed. Philadelphia, 2002, Saunders.)

Box 22–8	Muscles of the Ankle and Foot			
Muscle	**Origin**	**Insertion**	**Action**	**Innervation**
Dorsal Layer				
Extensor digitorum brevis (EDB)	Superolateral calcaneus	Base of proximal phalanges	Extend	Deep peroneal
First Plantar Layer				
Abductor hallucis	Calcaneal tuberosity	Base of great toe proximal phalanx	Abduct great toe	Med. plantar
Flexor digitorum brevis (FDB)	Calcaneal tuberosity	Distal phalanges of 2nd–5th toes	Flex toes	Med. plantar
Abductor digiti minimi	Calcaneal tuberosity	Base of 5th toe	Abduct small toe	Lat. plantar
Second Plantar Layer				
Quadratus plantae	Med. and lat. calcaneus	FDL tendon	Helps flex distal phalanges	Lat. planter
Lumbricals	FDL tendon	EDL tendons	Flex MTP, extend IP	Med. and lat. plantar
FDL and FHL	Tibia/fibula	Distal phalanges of digits	Flex toes/invert foot	Tibial
Third Plantar Layer				
Flexor hallucis brevis (FHB)	Cuboid/lat. cuneiform	Proximal phalanx of great toe	Flex great toe	Med. plantar
Adductor hallucis	Oblique: 2nd–4th metatarsals Transverse: MTP	Proximal phalanx of great toe lat.	Adduct great toe	Lat. plantar
Flexor digiti ininimi brevis (FDMB)	Base of 5th metatarsal head	Proximal phalanx of small toe	Flex small toe	Lat. plantar
Fourth Plantar Layer				
Dorsal interosseous	Metatarsal	Dorsal extensors	Abduct	Lat. plantar
Plantar interosseous	3rd–5th Metatarsals	Proximal phalanges medially	Adduct toes	Lat. plantar
(Peroneus longus and tibialis posterior)	Fibula/tibia	Med. cuneiform/navicular	Evert/invert foot	Superficial peroneal/tibial

Note: For abduction and adduction in the foot, the second toe serves as the reference.
EDL, extensor digitorum longus; FDL, flexor digitorum longus; IP, interphalangeal; MTP, metatarsophalangeal.
From Miller MD, editor: *Review of orthopaedics*, 4th ed. Philadelphia, 2004, Saunders.

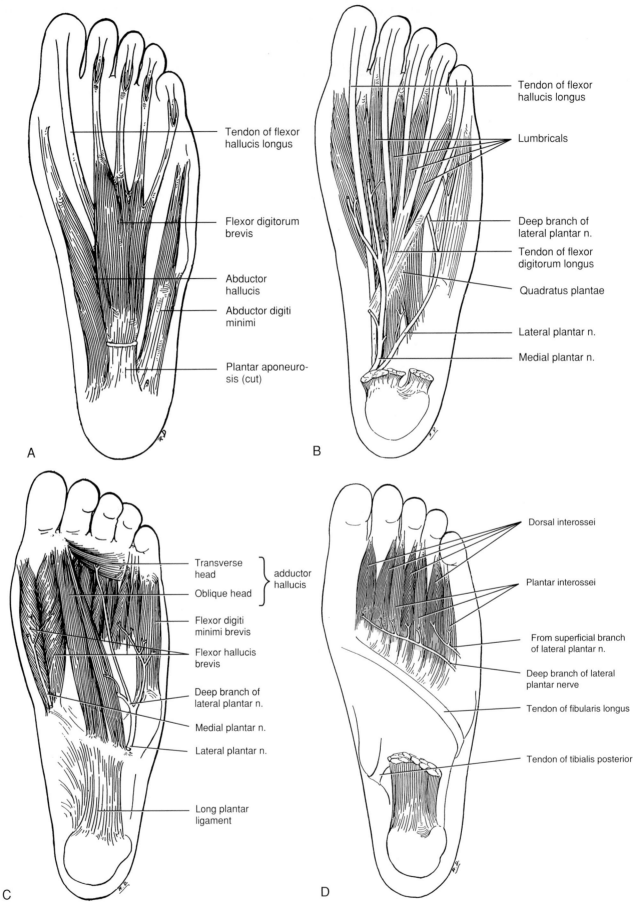

Tendon of flexor hallucis longus

Flexor digitorum brevis

Abductor hallucis

Abductor digiti minimi

Plantar aponeurosis (cut)

A

Tendon of flexor hallucis longus

Lumbricals

Deep branch of lateral plantar n.

Tendon of flexor digitorum longus

Quadratus plantae

Lateral plantar n.

Medial plantar n.

B

Transverse head

Oblique head

} adductor hallucis

Flexor digiti minimi brevis

Flexor hallucis brevis

Deep branch of lateral plantar n.

Medial plantar n.

Lateral plantar n.

Long plantar ligament

C

Dorsal interossei

Plantar interossei

From superficial branch of lateral plantar n.

Deep branch of lateral plantar nerve

Tendon of fibularis longus

Tendon of tibialis posterior

D

Figure 22–12:
Plantar muscles of the foot in layers. **A,** Superficial (first layer). **B,** Second layer. **C,** Third layer. **D,** Deep (fourth layer). (From Jenkins DB, Hollinshead WH: *Hollinshead's functional anatomy of the limbs and back,* 8th ed. Philadelphia, 2002, Saunders.)

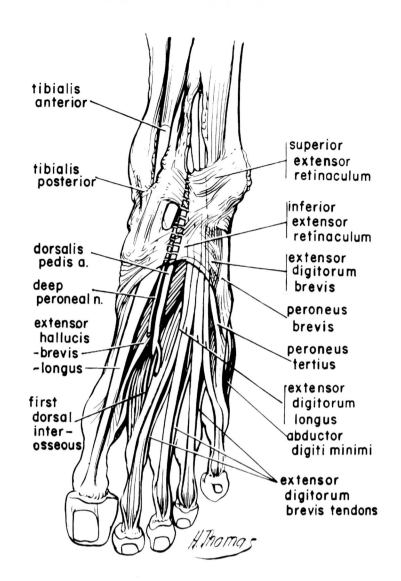

tibialis
anterior

tibialis
posterior

dorsalis
pedis a.

deep
peroneal n.

extensor
hallucis
-brevis
-longus

first
dorsal
inter-
osseous

superior
extensor
retinaculum

inferior
extensor
retinaculum

extensor
digitorum
brevis

peroneus
brevis

peroneus
tertius

extensor
digitorum
longus

abductor
digiti minimi

extensor
digitorum
brevis tendons

A

H.Thomas

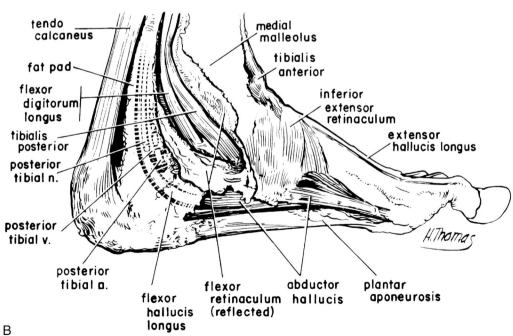

tendo
calcaneus

fat pad

flexor
digitorum
longus

tibialis
posterior

posterior
tibial n.

posterior
tibial v.

posterior
tibial a.

flexor
hallucis
longus

flexor
retinaculum
(reflected)

abductor
hallucis

plantar
aponeurosis

medial
malleolus

tibialis
anterior

inferior
extensor
retinaculum

extensor
hallucis longus

H.Thomas

B

Figure 22–13:

Relationship of the muscles and tendons around the ankle. **A,** Dorsal view. **B,** Medial view.

(*continued*)

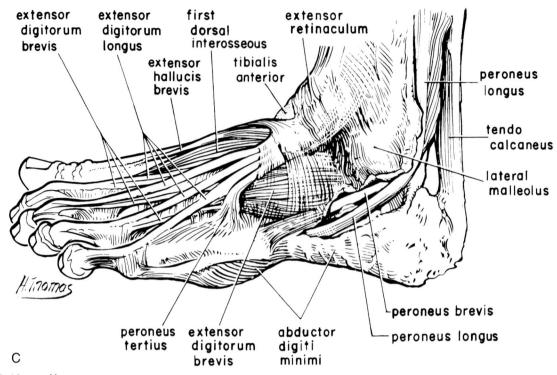

extensor digitorum brevis   extensor digitorum longus   first dorsal interosseous   extensor retinaculum

extensor hallucis brevis   tibialis anterior

peroneus longus

tendo calcaneus

lateral malleolus

peroneus brevis

peroneus longus

peroneus tertius   extensor digitorum brevis   abductor digiti minimi

C

Figure 22–13, cont'd:
C, Lateral view. (From Miller MD, editor: *Review of orthopaedics,* 4th ed. Philadelphia, 2004, Saunders.)

- While walking, the normal base width from heel to heel is between 2 and 4 inches.
- Normal step length is 15 inches.
- The center of gravity oscillates approximately 2 inches vertically during ambulation.
- Approximately 1 inch of lateral displacement of the body occurs with each step.
- Considering the ankle's axes of rotation, when the joint goes through dorsiflexion, some lateral movement of the foot occurs. Likewise, with plantarflexion, medial deviation of the foot is observed.
- At heel strike, the tibia rotates internally as the subtalar hinge joint everts and the calcaneus shifts slightly valgus. Conversely, the tibia rotates externally during toe-off as the subtalar joint inverts and the calcaneus shifts into a varus position.
- The transverse tarsal joint is rigid during push-off, providing the subtalar joint with a lever arm support base as it inverts. During heel strike and midstance, the transverse tarsal joint becomes parallel and flexible, allowing proper foot pronation to occur as the subtalar joint everts and the limb begins its weight-bearing phase.
- The plantar aponeurosis, which runs from the calcaneus to the flexor mechanism of the toes, functions as a windlass mechanism that assists subtalar inversion during heel rise and accentuates the foot arch as the toes dorsiflex at push-off.

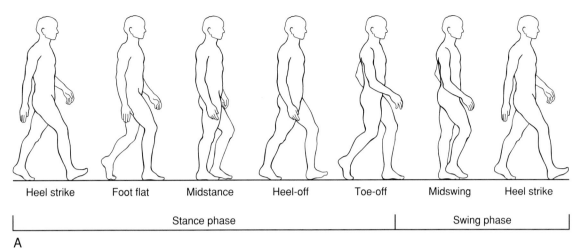

Heel strike   Foot flat   Midstance   Heel-off   Toe-off   Midswing   Heel strike

Stance phase   Swing phase

A

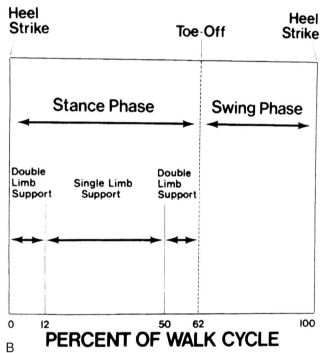

B   **PERCENT OF WALK CYCLE**

Figure 22–14:
The gait cycle. **A,** The normal phases of gait. **B,** Time dimensions of normal gait cycle. (**A** from Jenkins DB, Hollinshead WH: *Hollinshead's functional anatomy of the limbs and back,* 8th ed. Philadelphia, Saunders, 2002; **B** from Miller MD, editor: *Review of orthopaedics,* 3rd ed. Philadelphia, 2000, Saunders.)

References

Brosky T, Nyland J, Nitz A, Caborn DN: The ankle ligaments: consideration of syndesmotic injury and implications for rehabilitation. *J Orthop Sports Phys Ther* 21:197-205, 1995.

Review of syndesmosis injuries and the relevant anatomic and mechanisms of injury. Physical examination maneuvers discussed and rehabilitation issues described.

Hoppenfeld S: Physical examination of the foot and ankle. In *Physical examination of the spine and extremities.* Norwalk, CT, 1976, Appleton & Lange.

Description of the normal anatomy and proper evaluation of the foot and ankle.

Hoppenfeld S: Examination of gait. In *Physical examination of the spine and extremities.* Norwalk, CT, 1976, Appleton & Lange.

Review of the normal gait cycle. Proper methods of evaluation and abnormal findings are discussed.

Hoppenfeld S, deBoer P: The tibia & fibula. In Hoppenfeld S, deBoer P, editors: *Surgical exposures in orthopaedics: the anatomical approach.* Philadelphia, 1994, JB Lippincott.

Anatomy of the tibia and fibula described through useful surgical approaches with special attention to muscle and internervous planes. Descriptions of relevant muscles, osteology, nerves, and vascular blood supply presented.

Hoppenfeld S, deBoer P: The ankle & foot. In Hoppenfeld S, deBoer P, editors: *Surgical exposures in orthopaedics: the anatomical approach.* Philadelphia, 1994, JB Lippincott.

Anatomy of the ankle and foot described through useful surgical approaches with special attention to muscle and internervous planes. Descriptions of relevant muscles, osteology, nerves, and vascular blood supply presented.

Mann RA: Biomechanics of the foot and ankle. In Coughlin MJ, Mann RA, editors: *Surgery of the foot and ankle,* 7th ed. St Louis, 1999, Mosby.

Extensive review of the natural biomechanics of the foot and ankle, particularly how it relates to the walking cycle.

McCrory P, Bell S, Bradshaw C: Nerve entrapments of the lower leg, ankle and foot in sport. *Sports Med* 32:371-391, 2002.

Great review of the anatomy and entrapment conditions of nerves of the lower extremity associated with exercise activity.

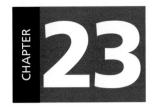

Ankle Arthroscopy

Indications

- Although arthroscopy had historically been performed for diagnostic purposes, it is now recognized as an important therapeutic modality providing simplified access to a wide range of ankle joint pathology.
- Indications for ankle arthroscopy are not as well defined as knee or shoulder arthroscopy but continue to evolve to include many procedures that have historically been performed through an open approach.
- Imaging of the intraarticular space of the ankle is not as well studied as that for other joints and is somewhat limited in delineating pathology that is amenable to arthroscopic treatment.
- More commonly recognized indications include treatment of osteochondral lesions; synovitis; soft tissue and bony impingement; loose bodies; ankle degenerative joint disease (DJD) (fusion); and, in some cases, visualization of intraarticular fractures of the ankle.

Positioning and Portal Placement

- Positioning is largely a matter of surgeon preference; however, the approach to the specific surgical pathology can dictate the option chosen.
  - Supine positioning with or without the end of the table lowered to 90 degrees is commonly used.
  - The use of a "bump" under the ipsilateral hip can assist exposure to the anterolateral and posterolateral portals.
  - The contralateral leg should be secured to the table.
  - If posterior pathology is expected, the patient can be placed in a lateral decubitus or even prone position.
  - The use of a tourniquet is by surgeon preference but can greatly improve visualization.
  - A standard 4-mm arthroscope can be used for easily accessible anterior structures, but a smaller 2.7-mm scope and smaller caliber shaving devices are recommended for most procedures.
- Ankle distraction (Figure 23–1).
  - Procedures involving only the anterior portion of the ankle joint (impinging anterior tibial osteophyte) can be performed without the use of distraction but

prevent adequate visualization during a thorough arthroscopy.
  - Invasive distractors use Steinman pins placed in the calcaneus and anterolateral tibia and provide the best traction but are not as commonly used because of the adequate exposure gained with less invasive techniques.
  - Noninvasive distraction techniques usually allow adequate visualization of all intraarticular structures. These typically clamp to the operating table and provide distraction through soft straps that are placed over the foot and around the heel.
  - Manual traction by an assistant can sometimes be sufficient for temporary distraction but is not recommended for prolonged or complicated therapeutic procedures.
  - A thigh-holder clamped to the table more proximally that flexes the hip and knee can provide countertraction to prevent the patient from migrating down the table and the loss of joint distraction.
- Portals (Figure 23–2).
  - Prior to exsanguination and establishment of portals, the surrounding subcutaneously palpated and visualized anatomy should be marked to avoid injury to these structures. The superficial peroneal nerve can be palpated and sometimes visualized subcutaneously while plantarflexing and inverting the ankle.
  - The ankle joint should be instilled with saline to further distract the joint space and ease the insertion of instrumentation.
  - The *nick and spread* method is used to help avoid neurovascular injury by only incising skin and spreading the soft tissue with a blunt instrument such as a hemostat.
  - Anteromedial portal—placed lateral to the saphenous vein and medial to the anterior tibialis tendon. Usually used as the camera portal but can also be an instrument portal.
  - Anterolateral portal—placed just lateral to the peroneus tertius. Care should be taken to avoid injury to the superficial peroneal nerve, which is in this area.
  - Posterolateral portal—placed just lateral to the Achilles tendon at the level of the joint line. The sural nerve and small saphenous vein are at greatest surgical risk.

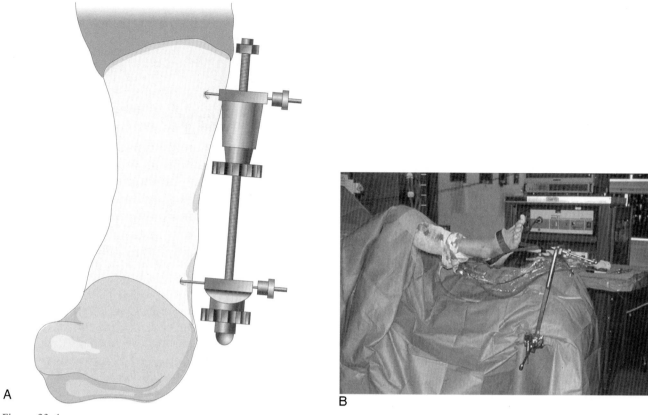

182 SECTION 3 Leg, Ankle, and Foot

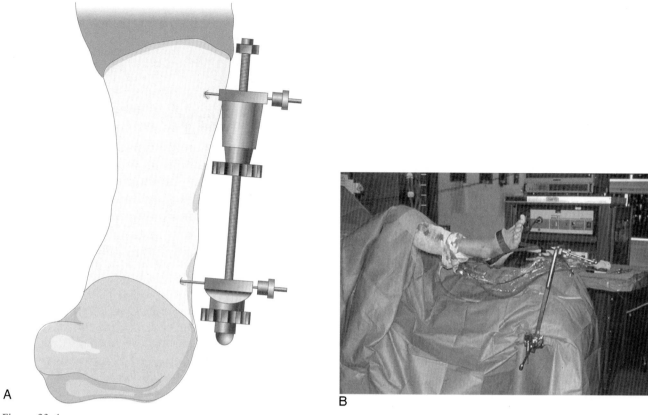

Figure 23–1:
A, Invasive distractors use threaded Steinman pins placed through stab incisions. **B,** Noninvasive distractors include soft ankle holders, an apparatus that is attached to the bed and may include a padded thigh holder. (**B** from Kennedy JG, Slater G, O'Malley MJ: Ankle: patient positioning, portal placement, and diagnostic arthroscopy. In Miller MD, Cole BJ, editors: *Textbook of arthroscopy.* Philadelphia, 2004, WB Saunders.)

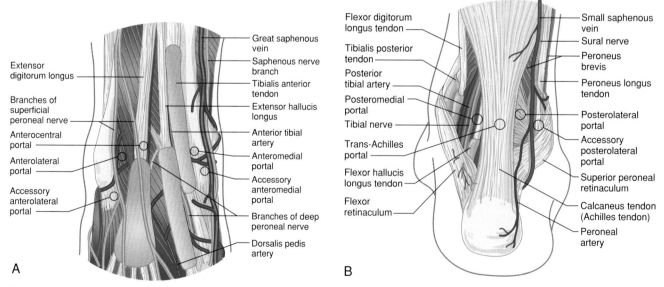

Figure 23–2:
Arthroscopic portals. A, Anterior. **B,** Posterior.

- Posteromedial portal—although some authors do not recommend this portal because of risk to the posterior tibial nerve and artery, this portal can be made safely if it is established adjacent to the border of the Achilles tendon and the *nick and spread* method is used. Frequently required for access and treatment of far posterior osteochondritis dissecans (OCD) lesions.
- Transtendinous portal—if an accessory posterior portal is necessary, a central split through the Achilles tendon is sometimes helpful with less risk of neurovascular injury than the posteromedial portal.
- Accessory portals are made as needed to gain optimal access and orientation to pathology. Neurovascular anatomy must be appreciated with less frequently used approaches.
- Moving the ankle through a range of motion (dorsiflexion, plantarflexion, inversion, eversion) during distraction can reorient talar pathology into closer proximity and assist operative exposure.

Diagnostic Arthroscopy

- A systematic, thorough evaluation of the ankle should be performed. The tibial and talar articular surfaces, medial and lateral gutters, ligaments, tendons, and recesses are visualized. Following a specific sequence on every arthroscopy avoids missing important pathology (loose bodies) (Figure 23–3).
- Dynamic evaluation including stressing of the stabilizing ligaments during arthroscopic visualization can reveal subtle pathology.
- It is important to recognize that the arthroscope and instruments are not directed posteriorly as in knee arthroscopy. These instruments are introduced at an angle almost perpendicular to the tibia (Figure 23–4).

Treatment

- Most osteochondral lesions can be treated through an arthroscopic approach.
  - Posteromedial lesions are usually chronic in nature and can be treated through transmalleolar antegrade or sinus tarsi retrograde approaches with visualization through either a posterolateral or anteromedial portal.
    - Transmalleolar drilling: A Kirchner wire is placed 2 to 3 cm proximal to the tip of the medial malleolus to allow for safer and easier access to posteromedial talar osteochondral lesions that cannot be reached through conventional portals and would otherwise require osteotomy. The ankle can be dorsiflexed and plantarflexed to make multiple drill holes (Figure 23–5).

- Anterolateral lesions are typically acute traumatic lesions and can be easily accessed through standard anterolateral or posterolateral portals.
- Curettage and drilling or microfracture of most lesions results in pain relief.
- Osteochondral plug transfer (OATS, mosaicplasty) using autograft or allograft depending on the size of the lesion can be arthroscopically assisted.
- Some authors recommend diagnostic arthroscopy prior to stabilizing procedures for lateral ankle instability due to the high rate of associated osteochondral pathology.
- Tibiotalar spurs (anterior ankle impingement or footballer's ankle) (Figure 23–6).
  - Commonly encountered in running and cutting sports such as soccer and basketball.
  - Easily debrided with a shaver or burr. Intraoperative fluoroscopy is useful to confirm complete resection.
  - Accelerated recovery time with arthroscopic treatment.
  - Not indicated in globally arthritic tibiotalar joint.
- Tibiotalar arthrodesis.
  - Arthroscopically assisted approach is useful in removing articular cartilage followed by fluoroscopically placed screws that are visualized arthroscopically.
  - Useful in patients with wound healing problems (peripheral vascular disease, venous stasis disease, dermatologic disorders).
  - Cannot be used with angular deformities greater than 15 degrees, significant joint incongruity, or significant bone loss.
- Soft tissue lesions.
  - Posttraumatic fibrous tissue and hypertrophic synovium from recurrent ankle or syndesmotic sprains.
  - The anteroinferior tibiofibular ligament can cause talar impingement with dorsiflexion (Duke lesion) (Figure 23–7).
  - Synovitis not responsive to conservative therapy may be treated with arthroscopic synovectomy (rheumatoid arthritis, pigmented villonodular synovitis, synovial chondromatosis).
- Fracture.
  - Some authors have advocated the use of an arthroscope to confirm anatomic articular reduction of ankle and talar fractures with percutaneous fixation to limit the morbidity associated with open reduction-internal fixation.
  - Extravasation of fluid through the fracture into the surrounding soft tissues can create a compartment syndrome or further soft tissue injury. A fluid pump should not be used and reduction of intraarticular pressure with an egress portal can be used in these scenarios.

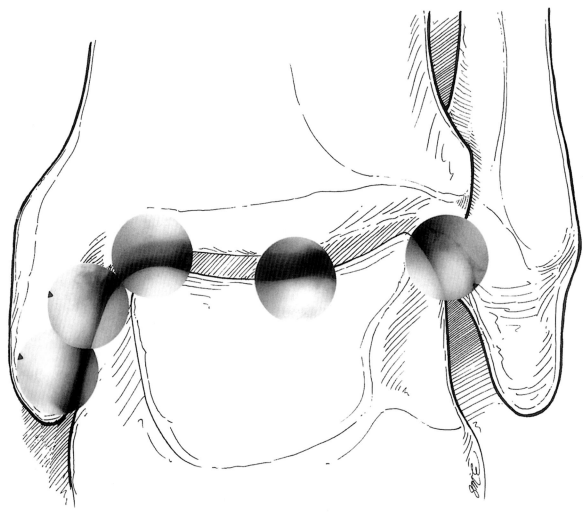

Figure 23–3:
Arthroscopic anatomy of the ankle. (From Miller MD, Osborne JR, Warner JJP, Fu FH: *MRI-arthroscopy correlative atlas.* Philadelphia, 1997, WB Saunders.)

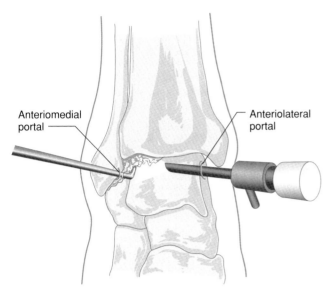

Figure 23–4:
Artist depiction of ankle arthroscopy using the anteromedial (scope) and anterolateral (instrument [probe]) portals. Note the orientation of the arthroscope and probe.

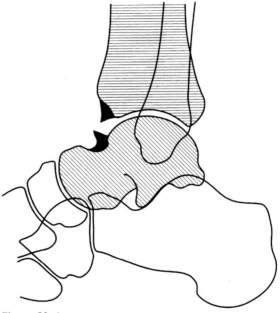

Figure 23–6:
Anterior impingement syndrome. (From Canale ST: Ankle injuries. In Canale ST, editor: *Campbell's operative orthopaedics,* 9th ed. St Louis, 1998, Mosby-Year Book.)

Complications

• Although the reported overall complication rate for ankle arthroscopy is low, the incidence of minor complications (especially iatrogenic chondral injury and superficial peroneal nerve neuropraxia) is probably much higher. This can be greatly reduced by gentle technique with joint distraction and with greater experience (Box 23–1).

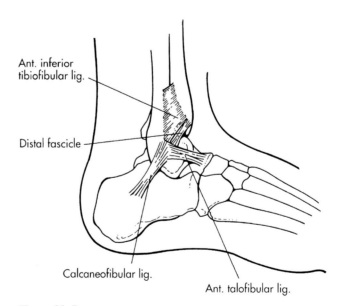

Figure 23–7:
Lateral aspect of the ankle joint. The distal fascicle of the anteroinferior tibiofibular ligament is parallel and distal to the anterior tibiofibular ligament proper and is separated from it by fibrofatty septum. (From Canale ST: Ankle injuries. In Canale ST, editor: *Campbell's operative orthopaedics,* 9th ed. St Louis, 1998, Mosby-Year Book.)

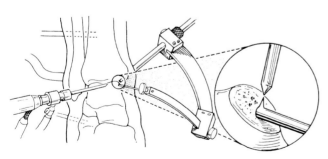

Figure 23–5:
Transmalleolar drilling of an osteochondral lesion. Note the use of an arthroscopic anterior cruciate ligament drill guide. (From Miller MD, Cooper DE, Warner JJP: *Review of sports medicine and arthroscopy.* Philadelphia, 2002, WB Saunders.)

Box 23–1	Complications of Ankle Arthroscopy

Complications include, but are not limited to, the following:
Synovial fistula (reduced with postoperative immobilization for the first postoperative week)
Postoperative hemarthrosis
Infection
Arthrofibrosis
Deep vein thrombosis
Anesthetic complications
Instrument failure
Complex regional pain syndrome
Iatrogenic injury (cartilage, ligaments, fracture)
Neurologic injury

References

Acevedo JI, Busch MT, Ganey TM, et al: Coaxial portals for posterior ankle arthroscopy: an anatomic study with clinical correlation on 29 patients. *Arthroscopy* 16:836-842, 2000.

A cadaveric study shows the safety of anatomic structures with use of a posterolateral portal immediately posterior to the peroneal tendon sheath. The posteromedial portal was established using an "inside-out" technique directly behind the medial malleolus next to the posterior tibial tendon. Risk to anatomic structures is concluded to be equal to that of standard posterior portals.

Carson WG Jr, Andrews JR: Arthroscopy of the ankle. *Clin Sports Med* 6:503-512, 1987.

This is a general overview of indications for ankle arthroscopy and techniques including patient positioning and portal placement. Because ankle conditions such as loose bodies and osteochondral lesions are relatively common, ankle arthroscopy is becoming an increasingly common operative technique.

Casteleyn PP, Handelberg F: Distraction for ankle arthroscopy. *Arthroscopy* 11:633-634, 1995.

Distraction of the ankle joint is an important part of ankle arthroscopy to allow for clear visualization of the anatomic structures. A technique of using a single calcaneal pin with the patient positioned on a fracture table allows for an appropriate level of distraction without causing serious patient complication.

Feiwell LA, Frey C: Anatomic study of arthroscopic portal sites of the ankle. *Foot Ankle* 14:142-147, 1993.

Another cadaveric study to assess the risk to anatomic structures during establishment of arthroscopic ankle portals and distractors. Anteromedial, anterocentral, anterolateral, posteromedial, and posterolateral portals are the most common portals used. The anterocentral is associated with the greatest risk of neurovascular injury, whereas the anteromedial, anterolateral, and posterolateral are considered to have the least risk.

Kennedy JG, Slater G, O'Malley MJ: Ankle: patient positioning, portal placement, and diagnostic arthroscopy. In Miller MD, Cole BJ, editors: *Textbook of arthroscopy.* Philadelphia, 2004, WB Saunders.

This chapter provides the basics of ankle arthroscopy. Figures in this chapter show portal placement in relation to other anatomic structures about the ankle.

Liu SH, Nuccion SL, Finerman G: Diagnosis of anterolateral ankle impingement: comparison between magnetic resonance imaging and clinical examination. *Am J Sports Med* 25:389-393, 1997.

These authors found that clinical examination (swelling, range of motion, and stability) was significantly better than magnetic resonance imaging (MRI) in diagnosing anterolateral ankle impingement. They recommend not obtaining preoperative MRI examination because it is not beneficial or cost-effective.

Miller MD: Ankle arthroscopy. In Miller MD, Howard RF, Plancher KD, editors: *Surgical atlas of sports medicine.* Philadelphia, 2003, WB Saunders.

This succinct chapter provides all of the basics for ankle arthroscopy.

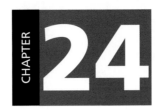

CHAPTER 24

Leg, Ankle, and Foot Overuse Syndromes

History, Physical Examination, and Imaging

- Overuse syndromes are usually the result of abnormal repetitive stress applied to healthy muscles, tendon, or bone, creating damage that exceeds the body's ability to repair itself.
- Injuries resulting from repetitive microtrauma and events characterized by an excessive amount of stress are discussed in this chapter.
- Pathology can be acute (< 2 weeks) or chronic.
- Overuse injuries are commonly seen in "weekend warriors" or well-conditioned athletes who overtrain.
- Extrinsic factors such as inadequate footwear, poor equipment and training techniques and environmental factors may contribute to injury.
- Anatomic factors such as ligament laxity, malalignment, and poor flexibility can make individuals more prone to injury.
- Patients often present with a focal area of pain that can guide the differential diagnosis and the need for special tests.
- Physical examination must take note of any anatomic malalignment, ligamentous laxity, and flexibility.
- Ligament laxity can be assessed by testing (1) passive opposition of the thumb to the flexor aspect of the forearm, (2) passive hyperextension of the fifth metacarpophalangeal joint greater than 90 degrees, (3) hyperextension of the knee, (4) hyperextension of the elbow, and (5) forward flexion of the trunk such that the patient can place the palms on the ground with the knees extended. Presence of three or more of these confirms hyperlaxity.
- Standard imaging should include a standing anteroposterior (AP) and lateral and 45-degree oblique views.

Types

Stress Fractures

- Stress fractures are common in athletes and represent approximately 6% of injuries in runners.
- These fractures result from repetitive stress on bone that exceeds its ability to repair itself.
- Risk factors for stress fractures include increased activity in frequency or intensity, low bone density, improper shoe support, and a history of menstrual irregularities or late menarche.
- The most common sites for stress fractures in the body include the tibia, metatarsals, and fibula. Some locations are more common in certain athletes (Table 24–1).
- Hindfoot stress fractures usually involve the calcaneus.
- Stress fractures are 10 times more likely in the medial sesamoid than the lateral sesamoid and are most common in runners.
- Friedberg infarction, which commonly involves the second metatarsal, is most frequently associated with repetitive stress applied to an adolescent female foot. Radiography often reveals metatarsal head flattening or irregularity.
- History may reveal an increase in training activity or intensity.
- Patients with a low, flexible arch absorb more stress in the foot and are more likely to be affected by metatarsal or tarsal bone stress fractures. Conversely, patients with a high, rigid arch distribute the stress more proximal and have a greater likelihood of developing fractures of the leg bones or femur.
- Patients often request to be evaluated for pain symptoms present during activity and relieved with rest.

Table 24–1: Location of Sport-Specific Stress Fractures	
SPORT	**LOCATION OF MOST COMMON STRESS FRACTURES**
Running	Tibia (distal), fibula, metatarsals
Basketball	Tarsal navicular, tibia (midshaft)
Football	Metatarsals, first metatarsophalangeal sesamoids
Dancing	Metatarsal (base), tibia (midshaft)
Recruits	Metatarsal (distal shaft), calcaneus, tibia (proximal)

From Miller MD, Cooper DE, Warner JJP: *Review of sports medicine and arthroscopy.* Philadelphia, Saunders, 2002.

- Because many of the patients are involved in sports requiring cyclic loading, inadequate shoewear or rigid terrain may contribute to the stress applied to the lower limb.
  - Studies have shown that shoes may lose 70% of shock absorption after being used for 500 miles.
- Classically, there is localized tenderness over the affected area.
- Initial radiographs may not reveal the fracture site for 2 to 6 weeks after onset, if at all.
- Bone scan is most helpful in deriving the diagnosis (detecting changes as early as 24 hours after onset), although it is not as specific as magnetic resonance imaging (MRI). However, both these tests are highly sensitive, allowing one to basically rule out stress fractures when readings are negative.
- A classification system has been proposed to grade stress fractures with imaging studies (Table 24–2).
- The evaluation and treatment of most stress fractures can follow a basic algorithm (Figure 24–1).
- Most stress fractures respond to initial rest and activity modification. Patients may bear weight and are placed on a graduated program. Metatarsal and calcaneal fractures typically resolve after a period of 3 to 4 weeks. Tibial and fibular fractures often require 6 to 8 weeks. Recalcitrant fractures may be considered for surgery.
- Transverse anterior tibial stress fractures that produce a persistent "dreaded black line" on radiographs and a positive bone scan for greater than 6 months may require excision and bone grafting (Figure 24–2).
- Navicular and fifth metatarsal stress fractures (Jones fracture) have a high incidence of nonunion. Therefore they require a period of strict immobilization and non–weight-bearing for 6 to 8 weeks.
  - Some surgeons recommend early consideration for operative treatment, especially in the elite athlete who must return to play as early as possible.
  - Screw fixation of the fifth metatarsal has gained popularity and is usually followed by 2 weeks of

immobilization and weight-bearing for 2 to 4 weeks. Athletes can often return to play as early as 2 months depending on radiographic and clinical evidence of healing.
  - Nonunions will require another fixation procedure with bone graft.
- Great toe sesamoid fractures can be treated with a short-leg walking cast for 6 weeks with a walking heel placed just proximal to the sesamoid to relieve pressure off the area and allow healing to occur.
- Treatment of Friedberg infarctions may involve casting and orthotics. Surgical management is composed of debridement of loose bodies, partial synovectomy, and partial resection of the metatarsal head.

Achilles Tendon Injury

- Achilles tendon injury is common among athletes and can range from tendinitis to complete rupture.
- Tendinitis is the result of overuse and is most frequently seen in runners.
- Injury can occur in the tendon or the peritenon, which surrounds the tendon.
- Achilles tendinitis should be differentiated from peritendinitis. The area of tenderness shifts with the tendon during ankle dorsiflexion and plantarflexion in Achilles tendinitis but is fixed with peritendinitis (Figure 24–3).
- Partial ruptures of the Achilles tendon are associated with long-term morbidity if they do not properly heal with conservative treatment and can produce nodules along the tendon.
- Ruptures of the tendon occur with maximal plantarflexion of the gastrocnemius-soleus muscles, usually during push-off, with the leg extended or after landing on a dorsiflexed foot. It may also occur after a direct blow.
- Ruptures most commonly occur 2 to 6 cm from its insertion site on the calcaneus, which is thought to be the area with its poorest blood supply.

Table 24–2:	Radiologic Grading System for Stress Fractures			
GRADE	RADIOGRAPH	BONE SCAN	MR IMAGING[†]	TREATMENT
1	Normal	Mild uptake confined to one cortex	Positive STIR image	Rest for 3 weeks
2	Normal	Moderate activity; larger lesion confined to unicortical area	Positive STIR and T2-weighted images	Rest for 3-6 weeks
3	Discrete line (+/–), periosteal reaction (+/–)	Increased activity (>50% width of bone)	No definite cortical break; positive T1- and T2-weighted images	Rest for 12-16 weeks
4	Fracture or periosteal reaction	More intense bicortical uptake	Fracture line; positive T1- and T2-weighted images	Rest for 16+ weeks

From Boden BP, Osbahr DC: *J Am Acad Orthop Surg* 8:344-353, 2000. Modified from Arendt EA, Griffiths HJ: *Clin Sports Med* 16:291-306, 1997.
†STIR = short-tau inversion sequence.

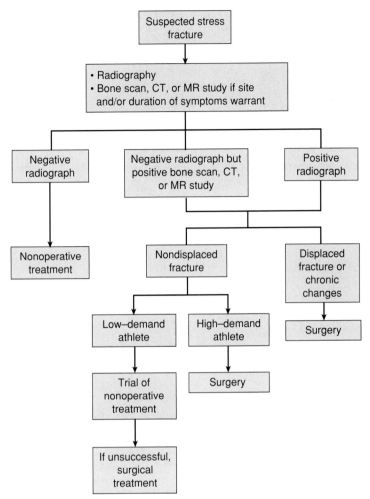

Figure 24–1:
Algorithm for the evaluation and treatment of suspected stress fractures. (From Boden BP, Osbahr DC: *J Am Acad Orthop Surg* 8:344-353, 2000.)

- Patients often present with pain and swelling and may report a "pop" or feeling of being kicked in the heel when the injury occurred.
- The Thompson test is used to evaluate the Achilles tendon. The patient may lay prone or kneel on an elevated surface with the knee and ankle at 90 degrees while the belly of the gastrocnemius-soleus muscle is passively squeezed. Plantarflexion of the foot indicates an intact tendon (Figure 24–4).
- MRI may be helpful in the surgical evaluation of complete tears or suspected partial tears.
  - MRI findings of Achilles tendon injury may be classified as follows: (1) inflammatory reaction, (2) degenerative change, (3) incomplete rupture, and (4) complete rupture.
- Most tendinitis or partial tendon ruptures can be managed with rest, ice, stretching, and nonsteroidal antiinflammatory drugs (NSAIDs) and then gradually returned back to normal level of activity through rehabilitation.

- Orthotic devices may assist in prevention of reinjury by relieving stresses imposed on the affected tendon. A 10- to 15-mm heel wedge for the Achilles tendon assists in decreasing tendon excursion. A molded Achilles pad can prevent irritation.
- Recalcitrant cases of peritendinitis and Achilles tendinitis or chronic cases of partial tears may benefit from tenolysis and debridement, often followed by a period of 3 to 6 weeks in a short-leg cast and a gradual return to activities.
- Treatment for complete ruptures of the Achilles continues to be controversial.
- The patient and surgeon must carefully review the advantages and disadvantages of operative and nonoperative treatment (Table 24–3).
- Surgical repair, however, produces a lower rerupture rate and provides the patient with a quicker and more optimal chance to return to previous sport activity (Box 24–1).
  - Percutaneous repairs that were popular in the past produced relatively high rerupture rates and sural nerve injury.

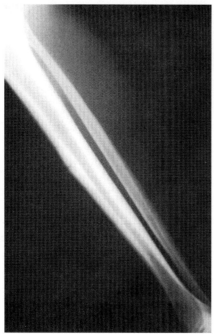

Figure 24–2:
Radiograph illustrating the "dreaded black line" of an anterior tibial stress fracture. (From Miller MD, Cooper DE, Warner JJP: *Review of sports medicine and arthroscopy*. Philadelphia, 2002, Saunders.)

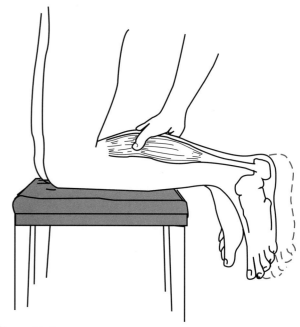

Figure 24–4:
The Thompson test evaluating the Achilles tendon. (Redrawn from Browner BD et al, editors: *Skeletal trauma: basic science, management and reconstruction,* 3rd ed. Philadelphia, 2003, Saunders.)

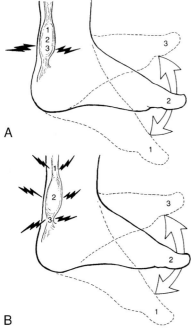

Figure 24–3:
Differentiation between Achilles peritendinitis and tendinitis. **A,** In peritendinitis, the location of tenderness does not vary with foot movement. **B,** In tendinitis, the location of tenderness varies with foot movement. (From Miller MD, Cooper DE, Warner JJP: *Review of sports medicine and arthroscopy*. Philadelphia, 2002, Saunders.)

- Most surgeons today prefer open repair. They have been reported to carry a 10% to 14% complication rate, most often associated with wound healing problems such as necrosis, infection, and scarring (Figure 24–5).
- Conservative measures include various programs using cast immobilization (initially in equinus) and orthotics.
- Chronic Achilles tendon ruptures often result in a substantial gap defect, making repair difficult.
  - Several techniques using the triceps surae, flexor digitorum longus, flexor hallucis longus (FHL), peroneus longus and brevis, fascia lata, plantaris, gracilis, and semitendinosus as free flaps, grafts, or transplants have been proposed for repair and reconstruction. Use

Table 24–3:	Treatment of Achilles tendon rupture	
FACTORS	**NONSURGICAL**	**SURGICAL**
Morbidity	↓	↑
Surgical complications	None	↑
Hospital cost	↓	↑
Physician cost	↓	↑
Strength and endurance	↓	↑
Rerupture rate	18%	2%

From Coughlin MJ, Mann RA, editors: *Surgery of the foot and ankle,* 7th ed. St Louis, 1999, Mosby.

of allografts and synthetic grafts may also be considered (Figures 24–6 to 24–9).
- Small gaps may be repaired using a tendon turndown flap (Figure 24–10).
- Cast immobilization of elderly or sedentary patients with Achilles tendon ruptures is considered appropriate treatment.

Peroneal Tendon Injury

- Tendinitis, subluxation, and dislocation are the most common conditions associated with the peroneal tendon. Rupture is rare.

- Subluxation or dislocation usually results from a violent peroneal reflexive contracture in an everted foot under extreme dorsiflexion, causing the tendon to split through its restraining retinaculum (Figure 24–11).
- This injury is most common in skiers, followed by football players.
- Diagnosis can be made by clinical examination and imaging (Box 24–2).
- Tenderness and swelling about the retromalleolar region overlying the peroneal tendons are typically present on examination.
- Observation of the tendon subluxating when the patient actively everts the foot confirms the diagnosis.
- A fracture from the lateral ridge of the distal fibula (the "fleck sign") indicates an avulsion fracture of the superior peroneal retinaculum from its insertion but is present in less than 50% of cases (Figure 24–12).
- Tenosynovitis, tendinitis, and tendinosis of the peroneal tendon are likely more common than reported and result from repetitive friction within the fibular groove after ankle trauma.
  - Classical findings of longitudinal partial tears on MRI include a chevron-shaped peroneal brevis tendon with a high signal on T2-weighted images (Figure 24–13).
- Habitual peroneal subluxaters typically do not require treatment unless symptoms become significant.
- Conservative treatment for acute peroneal subluxaters involves a short-leg non–weight-bearing cast (in slight plantarflexion and inversion) for 4 weeks or up to 8 weeks in acute dislocations. Primary surgical repair is rarely required.
- Various techniques exist to reconstruct chronically symptomatic subluxating peroneal tendons. All have

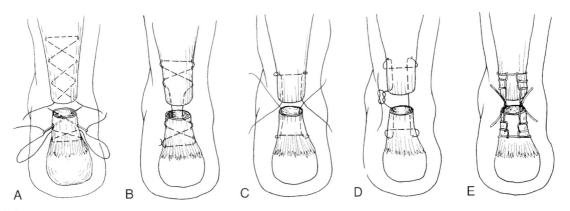

Figure 24–5:
Suture techniques for surgical repair of Achilles tendon ruptures. **A,** Double-suture Bunnell technique. **B,** Single-suture Bunnell technique. **C,** Double-suture Kessler technique. **D,** Single-suture Kessler technique. **E,** Double-suture Krackow technique. (From Coughlin MJ, Mann RA, editors: *Surgery of the foot and ankle,* 7th ed. St Louis, 1999, Mosby.)

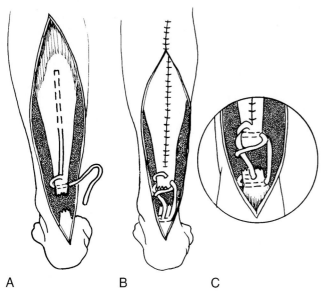

Figure 24–6:
Bosworth technique for Achilles tendon reconstruction using a fascial strip from gastrocnemius-soleus complex. **A**, Fascial strip weaved through proximal stump of Archilles tendon rupture. **B**, Fascial strip then weaved through distal Achilles tendon rupture stump. **C**, Close-up of weave pattern. (From Bosworth D: *J Bone Joint Surg Am* 38:111-114, 1956.)

relatively similar efficacy, although follow-up in studies have been variable (Figure 24–14).

• Decompression, debridement, and primary repair of a partially torn peroneal (brevis) tendon are appropriate for chronic injuries. Extensive tears can be repaired by partial excision of the affected tendon and attachment to the adjoining intact tendon. Similarly, if complete ruptures cannot be repaired primarily because of retraction, tenodesis to the adjacent tendon may be effective (Figure 24–15).

Posterior Tibialis Tendon

• Injury of the posterior tibial tendon is a major cause of medial ankle pain and spans the spectrum of tendonitis to rupture.
• The typical patient is an older, overweight woman.
• Sports requiring abrupt changes in direction such as soccer, tennis, hockey, and basketball are more likely to impose excessive stress on the posterior tibial tendon.
• Repeated stress of the tendon when the foot is pronated during weight-bearing activities is a proposed mechanism of injury.
• Ruptures often occur just posterior to the medial malleolus, where there is little vascularity, and are commonly associated with previous degenerative changes.
• Loss of function results in a collapsed arch and an acquired flatfoot deformity.
• Tenderness and swelling posterior and inferior to the medial malleolus are common examination findings.

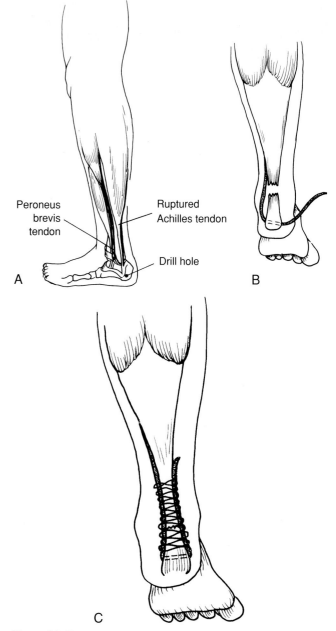

Figure 24–7:
Achilles tendon reconstruction using peroneus brevis tendon transfer. **A**, Peroneus brevis tendon detached from base of fifth metatarsal and a drill hole is placed through the base of the insertion of the Achilles tendon on the calcaneous. **B**, Peroneus brevis tendon is passed through the calcaneal drill hole. **C**, The peroneus brevis tendon is then tensioned and weaved through the Achilles tendon repair. (From Turco V, Spinella A: *Foot Ankle* 7:253-259, 1987.)

• Tenderness along the lateral aspect of the ankle may develop as the hindfoot deformity pushes against the fibula.
• Observation of the ankle often reveals loss of the arch; increased valgus deformity of the heel; and, in advanced cases, forefoot abduction (classic triad).

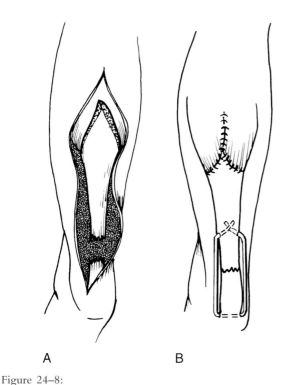

Figure 24–8:
Achilles tendon reconstruction with V-Y gastroplasty. **A,** An inverted V is created through the musculotendinous junction of the gastrocnemius proximally in cases of shortened Achilles tendon ruptures as in chronic cases. **B,** The desired length is achieved and repaired, and the inverted V is closed as an inverted Y. (From Coughlin MJ, Mann RA, editors: *Surgery of the foot and ankle,* 7th ed. St Louis, 1999, Mosby.)

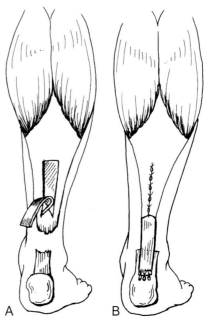

Figure 24–10:
Fascial turn-down flap using the proximal segment for Achilles tendon reconstruction. **A,** A central third fascial strip from proximal Achillies tendon stump is fashioned and turned down distally. **B,** The proximal donor site is closed side to side, and the fascial strip is used to bridge the gap and repaired to the distal stump. (From Coughlin MJ, Mann RA, editors: *Surgery of the foot and ankle,* 7th ed. St Louis, 1999, Mosby.)

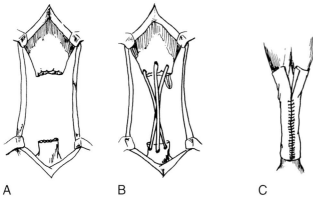

Figure 24–9:
Achilles tendon repair using fascia lata strips. **A,** Achilles tendon rupture defect with tissue loss. **B,** Fascia lata strips are harvested and weaved through the promimal and distal stumps to bridge the defect. **C,** Paratenon is then closed over the bridged defect. (From Coughlin MJ, Mann RA, editors: *Surgery of the foot and ankle,* 7th ed. St Louis, 1999, Mosby.)

This may result in the "too many toes" sign (Figure 24–16).

- Weakness of the tendon will limit the ability to perform a normal heel rise and limit ability to invert the foot against resistance. When the patient stands on the toes with both legs, the affected heel will fail to shift into a varus position (secondary to loss of posterior tibial function). Comparison should be made with the contralateral limb.
- Active inversion of the foot against resistance may elicit pain along the tendon.
- Clinical examination usually suffices to make the diagnosis (Box 24–3).
- MRI, saved for ambiguous cases, will often demonstrate edematous change or other pathology along the tendon.
- Tenosynovitis of the posterior tibial tendon is best managed conservatively with rest, ice, NSAIDs, activity modifications, medial supporting orthotic devices (e.g., heel wedge and longitudinal arch support), and a pronation control athletic shoe.
  - If the tenosynovitis is severe, a period of immobilization in a non–weight-bearing short-leg cast (approximately 4 weeks) with the foot inverted is appropriate.
- Surgical debridement is an option for failed cases.

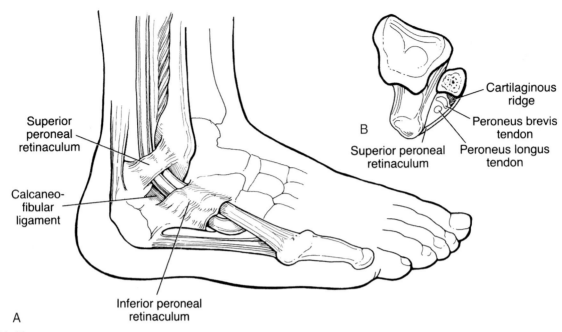

Figure 24–11:
Normal relationship of the peroneal tendons. Note the restraining structures. **A,** Lateral view. **B,** Superior view. (From Miller MD, Cooper DE, Warner JJP: *Review of sports medicine and arthroscopy.* Philadelphia, 2002, Saunders.)

- Debridement and repair of most partial or complete posterior tibial tendon ruptures should be performed in good surgical candidates (Figure 24–17).
  - The flexor digitorum longus tendon can be used for reconstruction.
  - Pure acute avulsions may be directly reattached to the navicular tuberosity.
  - In the presence of significant planovalgus, alignment can be corrected with a medial calcaneal osteotomy, medial column stabilization, or lateral column lengthening procedure.
- Dislocation of the posterior tibialis, although rare, may be repaired similarly to the peroneal tendons, by reconstructing the groove or retinaculum.

Flexor Hallucis Longus

- Injuries to this tendon most commonly occur in athletes performing repetitive push-off activity as found in ballet dancers and runners.

Box 24–2	Findings Associated with Peroneal Tendon Injury

Retromalleolar tenderness and swelling
Subluxation of the tendon with active eversion of the foot
Weakness or reproduction of pain with resisted eversion, or both
Avulsion fracture of the lateral distal fibula (fleck sign)
Chevron sign or edematous changes about the tendon on magnetic resonance imaging

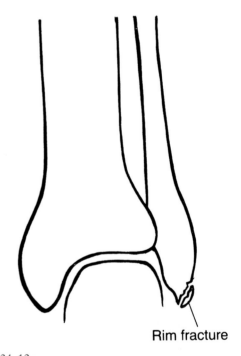

Rim fracture

Figure 24–12:
Rim fracture of the lateral aspect of the distal fibula associated with dislocating peroneal tendons. (From Miller MD, Cooper DE, Warner JJP: *Review of sports medicine and arthroscopy.* Philadelphia, 2002, Saunders.)

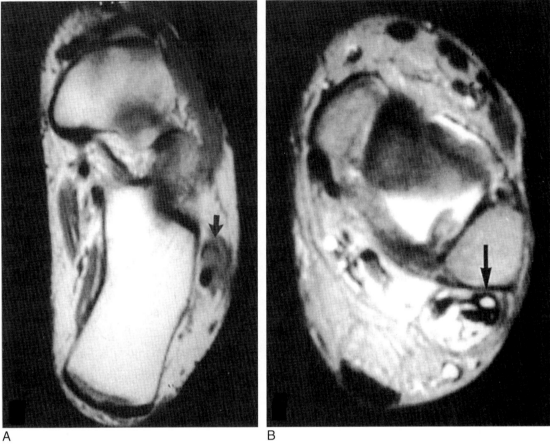

A   B

Figure 24–13:
Magnetic resonance imaging (MRI) of a partially torn peroneal tendon illustrating the chevron sign. **A,** Coronal MRI showing
a partial tear of the peroneal tendon (arrow). **B,** Axial MRI showing the same partial tear (arrow). (From Major NM, Helms CA,
Fritz RC, Speer KP: *Foot Ankle Int* 21:514-519, 2000.)

- Physical examination findings often suggest the diagnosis (Box 24–4).
- Tendon inflammation causing pain and swelling can occur posterior to the medial malleolus where it passes along with the posterior tibial tendon, the knot of Henry; where it crosses with the flexor digitorum longus; or where it passes in between the sesamoids.
- Tenderness will be present at the site of injury, and pain can be reproduced with active or passive motion of the hallux.
- Partial ruptures should be suspected in cases with the previous findings, as well as triggering or clawing of the toe caused by entrapment of the tendon proximal to the flexor retinaculum.
- Complete ruptures, although rare, will reveal loss of interphalangeal flexion.
- Conservative management for FHL tenosynovitis includes rest, ice, NSAIDs, stretching, midsole orthotics (to improve push-off), longitudinal arch support, and heel lift (to reduce tendon excursion) (Box 24–4).
- Tenolysis of chronic FHL tenosynovitis may be considered.

- If an FHL partial tendon tear produces a toe deformity, surgical flexor retinaculum release can be performed to restore the normal glide of the tendon.
  - In ballet dancers, at least 3 months of rehabilitation is required prior to returning to "en pointe" dancing.
- Complete ruptures can be treated with primary end-to-end repair and require postoperative immobilization in a short-leg cast in plantarflexion and slight inversion for 6 weeks.

Anterior Tibialis Tendon

- Tenosynovitis of this tendon occurs with repetitive dorsiflexion and inversion of the foot, which is common in soccer and tennis athletes.
- Complete ruptures are uncommon but have been reported and tend to occur near its insertion site where an underlying bursa exists.
- Typical findings on examination include localized tenderness and swelling and reproducible pain with resisted dorsiflexion and inversion of the foot.
- Dorsiflexion and inversion weakness is present in severe tendinitis or complete ruptures.

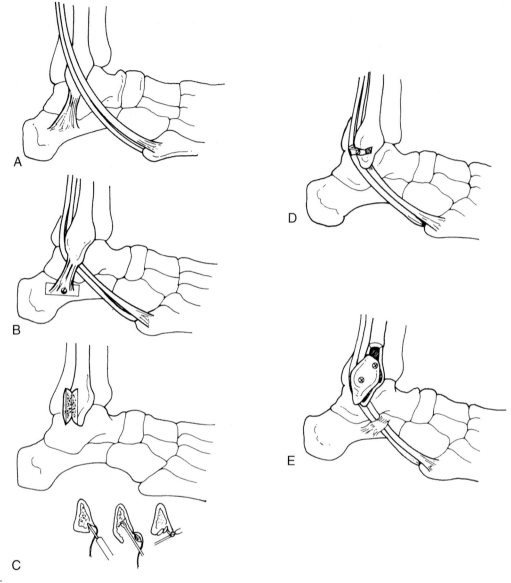

Figure 24–14:
Procedures for correction of peroneal tendon dislocation. **A,** Anterior displacement of the peroneal tendons. **B,** Duijftes bone block method. **C,** Groove-deepening procedure. **D,** DuVries procedure. **E,** Kelly bone block procedure. (From Miller MD, Cooper DE, Warner JJP: *Review of sports medicine and arthroscopy*. Philadelphia, 2002, Saunders.)

- Conservative management of tenosynovitis is generally adequate.
- Anterior tibialis tendon ruptures should be repaired acutely.

Gastrocnemius-Soleus Strains

- Tendinitis of the triceps surae at its insertion site is relatively common and in the past was thought to be caused by rupture of the plantaris muscle.
- Strain is produced with repetitive aggressive plantarflexion of the foot as commonly seen in tennis players (known by many as "tennis leg").
- Often responds to conservative treatment.

Medial Tibial Stress Syndrome

- Commonly referred to as "shin splints," this condition is poorly defined and not well understood.
- Generally, it is thought to derive from overuse of the soleus or tibial posterior muscles that produces undue stress at their fascial insertion along the posteromedial aspect at the middle and distal two thirds of the tibia, respectively.
- Patients often report pain with activity and have tenderness along the middle or distal tibia.
- Any biomechanical abnormalities should be noted and addressed appropriately.

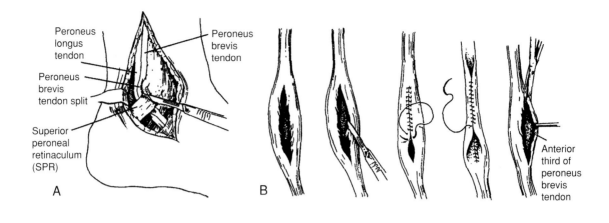

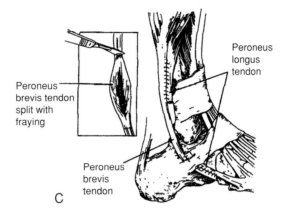

Figure 24–15:
Repair-reconstruction (tenodesis) of a partially torn peroneal tendon. **A,** Drawing showing a split tear of the peroneus brevis tendon. **B,** The intrasubstance degenerative tendinosis is excised and repaired. **C,** If insufficient tendon is remaining following repair, the proximal and distal ends are cut and tenodesed to the adjacent peroneus longus tendon. (From Sobel M, Mizel MS: Peroneal tendon injury. In Pfeffer GB, Frey CC, editors: *Current practice in foot and ankle surgery,* vol 1. New York, 1993, McGraw-Hill.)

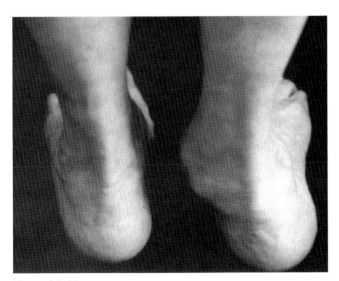

Figure 24–16:
Weight-bearing posterior view illustrating deformity associated with severe posterior tibialis tendon injury. Note the heel valgus, midfoot abduction, and forefoot pronation of the affected right foot and ankle. (From Richardson EG: Disorders of tendons and fascia. In Canale ST, editor: *Campbell's operative orthopaedics,* 9th ed. St Louis, 1998, Mosby-Year Book.)

- Care must be taken to rule out stress fractures, exertional compartment syndrome, and other soft tissue injury.
- Nuclear bone scan may reveal an area of activity consistent with periostitis and rule out stress fractures.
- Medial tibial stress syndrome usually responds to nonoperative management.
- Surgical release of the investing fascia and cauterization of the periosteum have been performed by some surgeons in intractable cases with good success.

Box 24–3	Clinical Findings Associated with Posterior Tibialis Tendon Injury

Posteroinferior malleolar tenderness and swelling
Pain or weakness with resisted inversion, or both
Difficulty performing a normal heel rise (failure of heel to shift into a varus position)
Acquired flatfoot deformity
Valgus deformity
Forefoot adduction
"Too many toes" sign

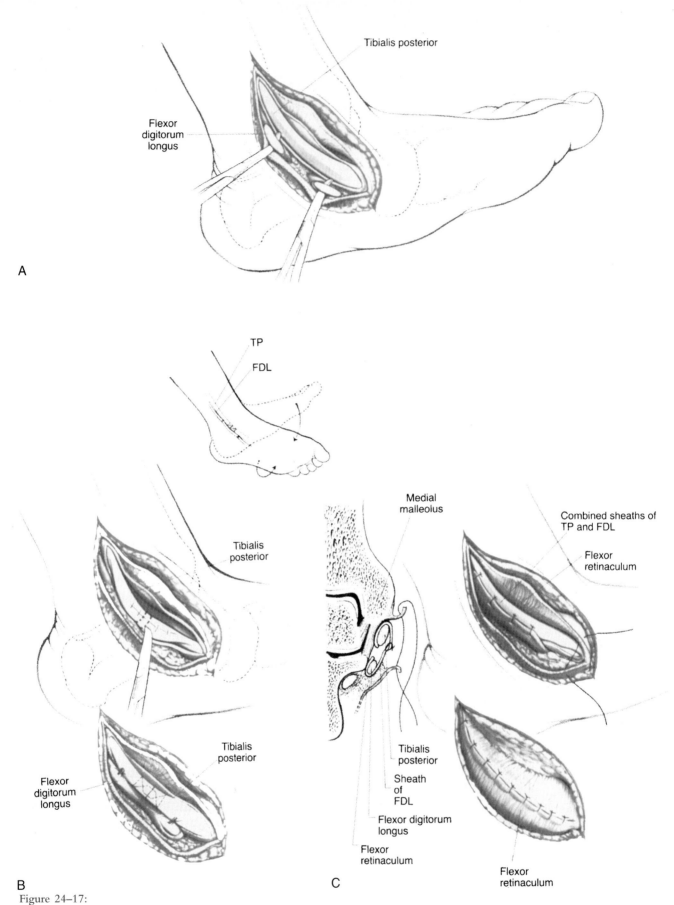

Figure 24–17:

Operative treatment of injured posterior tibialis tendons. **A,** Exposure of the tibialis posterior (TP) and flexor digitorum longus (FDL). **B,** Excision of damaged or redundant tendon and repair with suturing to the flexor tendon proximal and distal. **C,** Repair of the sheaths and retinaculum. (From Jahss MH: *Disorders of the foot and ankle,* 2nd ed. Philadelphia, 1991, Saunders.)

Box 24–4	**Clinical Findings and Conservative Management of Flexor Hallucis Tendon Injury**

Clinical Findings

Tenderness and swelling at site of injury (commonly 1—posterior to medial malleolus, 2—knot of Henry, or 3—between the two hallux sesamoids)
Reproduction of pain with motion of the hallux
Triggering or clawing toe deformity
Loss of or weakened interphalangeal flexion

Conservative Management Measures

Rest, ice, nonsteroidal antiinflammatory drugs
Stretching of affected tendon
Midsole orthotics—improving push-off
Longitudinal arch support
Heel lift—reduces tendon excursion

Box 24–5	**Clinical Examination Findings and Conservative Management of Retrocalcaneal Bursitis**

Clinical Findings

Tenderness/swelling along sides of Achilles tendon
Reproduction of pain with ankle dorsiflexion
Bony calcaneal prominence

Conservative Management

Rest, ice, nonsteroidal antiinflammatory drugs
Heel lifts or wedges
Backless shoes
Short-leg walking cast in recalcitrant cases

Retrocalcaneal Bursitis (Haglund's Deformity)

- The retrocalcaneal bursa lies between the calcaneus and Achilles tendon just superior to its insertion site.
- Inflammation of the bursa can be caused by trauma, pressure from the heel counter of poor fitting shoes, or impingement from calcaneal bony prominences (Figure 24–18).
- Because of its position, it is often difficult to differentiate from Achilles tendinitis, and many times they coexist (Box 24–5).
- On examination, tenderness and swelling along both sides of the Achilles tendon can be appreciated.
- Pain may be reproduced with dorsiflexion of the foot, which compresses the bursa between the calcaneus and tendon.
- Haglund's deformity is characterized by the triad of retrocalcaneal bursitis, Achilles tendinitis, and adventitial bursitis.

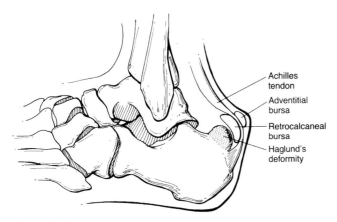

Figure 24–18:
Haglund's deformity. (From DeLee JC, Drez D Jr, Miller MD, editors: *DeLee and Drez's orthopaedic sports medicine: principles and practice,* 2nd ed. Saunders, 2003, Philadelphia.)

- Plain radiographic diagnosis is difficult but may be suggested when the normal wedge-shaped retrocalcaneal recess lucency is lost and replaced with soft tissue density. Furthermore, the presence of a prominent posterior superior calcaneal process (Haglund's process) is frequently present.
- MRI and bursography are both sensitive and specific and can be used in cases in which diagnosis is difficult.
- Retrocalcaneal bursitis usually benefits from heel lifts or wedges (to avoid heel counter pressure over the affected area), backless shoes, and NSAIDs.
- A short-leg walking cast may be used in recalcitrant cases.
- Achilles tendon stretching exercises are recommended once symptoms have resolved.
- Surgical treatment of retrocalcaneal bursitis concentrates on reducing pressure exacted by any bony prominences and removal of the bursa.

Plantar Fasciitis

- Inflammation of the plantar fascia is the most common cause of hindfoot pain.
- Comprises approximately 10% of running injuries.
- Believed to result from repetitive high-impact activities that cause microtears and inflammation of the plantar fascia.
- Reduced ankle dorsiflexion, obesity, and weight-bearing work activity may be risk factors for plantar fasciitis.
- Pain usually occurs at the origination site along the medial calcaneal tuberosity but can certainly extend throughout its course to its insertion site on the metatarsophalangeal joints and proximal phalanges.
- Classically, the pain is greatest when rising out of bed or standing after a prolonged period of sitting.
- Physical examination most often reveals tenderness along the medial calcaneal tuberosity, where the plantar fascia originates.
- Pronation of the foot aggravates the condition.
- Dorsiflexion of the toes can reproduce pain.

- Stress fractures, spinal or radicular pathology, nerve entrapment, and seronegative spondyloarthropathy should be ruled out.
- There is no evidence of a direct relationship between heel spurs and plantar fasciitis.
- Plantar fasciitis is frequently difficult to treat (Box 24–6). Initially, patients are treated with activity modifications, ice, massage, NSAIDs, plantar fasciitis and Achilles tendon stretching, proper shoe cushioning, and medial heel orthotics. Further options include night splinting or even casting to ensure rest for approximately 6 weeks.
- Extracorporeal shock wave treatment (both high- and low-energy modalities) has been studied and implemented with mixed results.
- Release of the plantar fascia is saved for intractable plantar fasciitis after all conservative options have been exhausted (Figure 24–19).
  - Can be performed either open or endoscopically.
  - Open release is performed through an incision overlying the first branch of the lateral plantar nerve (look up extent).
  - Endoscopic technique involves using two portals with the cannula inserted across the plantar aspect of the fascia.
  - Many recommend only releasing the medial third of the plantar fascia.

Turf Toe

- Turf toe describes the injury that results from extreme dorsiflexion of the first metatarsophalangeal joint (Figure 24–20).
- This is most commonly seen in football offensive linemen who squat down with their heels raised and push off their toes during the start of play.
- Examination will reveal tenderness and swelling over the joint and reproduction of pain with passive flexion.
- Diminished push-off strength, joint subluxation, and deformities such as hammering, clawing, and hallux rigidus may occur in chronic cases.
- Radiographs should be ordered to evaluate possible disruption of the plantar-plate of the flexor hallucis brevis or a bipartite sesamoid.

Box 24–6	**Management Options for Plantar Fasciitis**

Activity modifications
Rest, ice, nonsteroidal antiinflammatory drugs
Stretching exercises for the plantar fascia
Orthotics
Steroid injections
Night splinting
Casting
Extracorporeal shock wave treatment
Surgical release for recalcitrant cases

- Avulsion fractures off the plantar aspect of the proximal phalanx or sesamoids should be noted.
- Proximal migration of the sesamoid (compared with the contralateral foot) suggests disruption of the plantar complex.
- MRI is useful in patients with abnormal radiographs or severe injury to define the degree of injury and any associated damage.
- Sand toe describes injury incurred by severe plantarflexion of the toe, as seen in beach volleyball players, and has a similar presentation and course of treatment as turf toe.
- A classification system for turf toe and sand toe has been devised and expanded (Table 24–4).
- Turf and sand toe should be treated with ice, NSAIDs, taping, and rehabilitation. Shoe modification (or special turf shoes) may help prevent reinjury (Figure 24–21).
- Severe cases may require the use of a walking boot, crutches, or casting.
- Acute tears of the plantar complex rarely occur but should be surgically repaired.

Rehabilitation

- Rest, ice, and pain control are required in many cases prior to beginning rehabilitation.
- It is important to send all patients treated with immobilization to rehabilitative stretching and strengthening because atrophy of muscles and weakness commonly occur.
- Care must be taken not to return athletes to sporting activities prior to full rehabilitation.
- Taping is effective in providing ankle stability during rehabilitation and can help prevent reinjury when returning to sport participation.
- Proper shoe wear and support should be stressed to the patient.

Complications

- Nonunion of stress fractures often requires operative fixation or bone grafting, or both.
- If no healing occurs after 6 months of a sesamoid fracture, partial or complete excision of the sesamoid is acceptable, although bone grafting techniques can also be considered.
- Steroid injections into tendon can cause weakening or rupture of the tendon and are therefore usually not recommended for treatment of tendinitis or tenosynovitis.
- Steroid injection of bursa about the ankle should also be avoided because leakage can occur and cause disruption of adjacent tendons.
- Use of steroid injections for plantar fasciitis may provide relief of symptoms, but reports of subsequent rupture

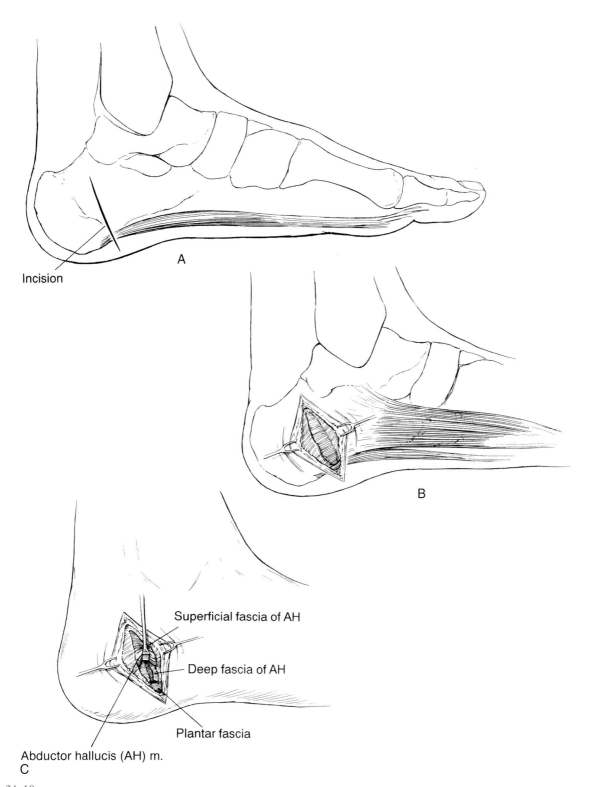

Figure 24–19:
Plantar fascia release. A, Initial incision location. **B,** Release of the abductor hallucis muscle fascia. **C,** Abductor hallucis is reflected promimally. (From Miller MD, Cooper DE, Warner JJP: *Review of sports medicine and arthroscopy.* Philadelphia, 2002, Saunders.)

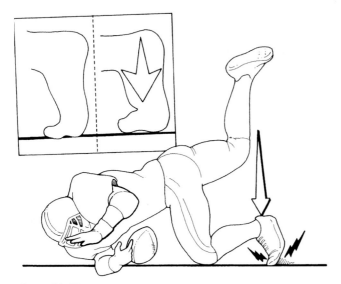

Figure 24–20:
Mechanism of injury for turf toe is acute dorsiflexion of the
first metatarsophalangeal joint. (From Miller MD, Cooper DE,
Warner JJP: *Review of sports medicine and arthroscopy.*
Philadelphia, 2002, Saunders.)

have occurred in up to one third of patients.
Furthermore, injections should be performed from the
medial aspect of the heel, avoiding the fat pad where
atrophy can occur.

- Recovery after plantar fascia release may be long and
require additional treatment. Abnormal foot function may
also result.
- Complete plantar fascia release may be complicated by a
fallen arch and persistent pain.
- Turf toe commonly is complicated by decreased range of
motion and chronic pain of the metatarsophalangeal
joint.

Table 24–4: Classification of Turf Toe and Sand Toe Injuries

TYPE OF INJURY	CLASSIFICATION	CHARACTERISTICS	ACTIVITY LEVEL	TREATMENT
Hyperextension (turf toe)	Grade 1–Stretching of the plantar complex	Localized plantar or medial tenderness, minimal swelling, no ecchymosis	Continued athletic participation	Symptomatic
	Grade 2–Partial tear	Diffuse and intense tenderness, mild to moderate swelling, ecchymosis, restricted movement with pain	Loss of playing time for 3 to 14 days	Walking boot and crutches as needed
	*Grade 3–Frank tear	Severe and diffuse tenderness to palpation, marked swelling and ecchymosis; limited movement with pain; positive vertical Lachman's test, if pain allows	Loss of playing time for at least 4 to 6 weeks	Long-term immobilization in boot or cast versus surgical repair
	Associated injuries	Medial or lateral injury; sesamoid fracture with bipartite diastasis; articular cartilage and subchondral bone bruise		
Hyperflexion (sand toe)	Dislocation–Type I	Dislocation of the hallux with the sesamoids		
		No disruption of the intersesamoid ligament; usually irreducible		
	Type II	Associated disruption of intersesamoid ligament; usually reducible		
	II A			
	II B	Associated transverse fracture of one of the sesamoids; usually reducible		
	II C	Complete disruption of intersesamoid ligament fracture of one of the sesamoids; usually reducible		

*Grade 3 injuries may represent spontaneously reduced dislocations.
Data combined from Coughlin MJ, Mann RA, editor. *Surgery of the foot and ankle*, 7th ed. St Louis, 1999, Mosby; and-OKU Sports Medicine 3, American Academy of Orthopaedic Surgeons.

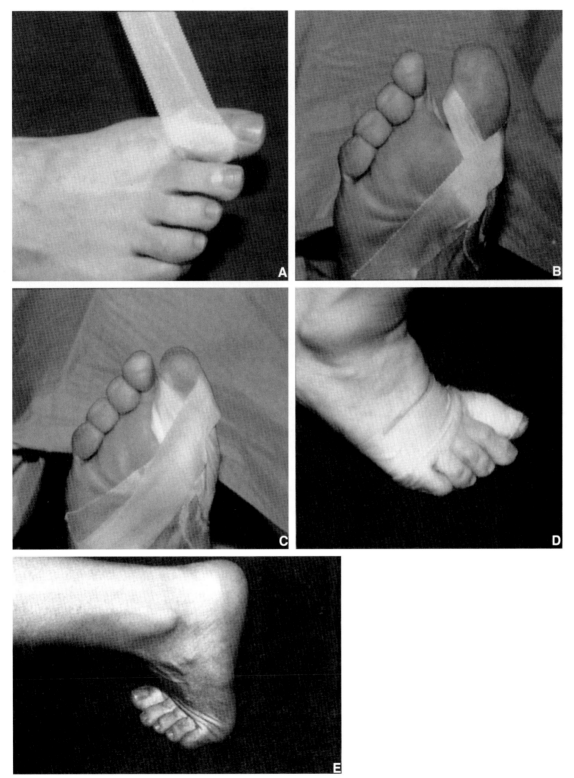

Figure 24–21:
Taping of turf toe. **A,** Apply spica strips over great toe metatarsophalangeal (MTP) joint. **B,** Strips cross and intersect on the plantar aspect to support the MTP joint, **C,** Repeat strips and apply supportive strips to limit great toe extension (**D**) compared with normal great toe hyperextension (**E**). (From Sammarco GJ: *Physician Sports Med* 169:115, 1998.)

References

Alfredson H, Lorentzon R: Chronic Achilles tendinosis recommendations for treatment and prevention. *Sports Med* 29:135-146, 2000.

Review of conservative and operative management and preventive measures for Achilles tendinitis. Authors also discuss their results of a prospective study in 15 athletes with chronic Achilles tendinosis (who failed conventional treatment) treated with a heavy load eccentric calf muscle training program. All these patients reported resolution of their symptoms during running 12 weeks after starting the program. After 2 years, only one patient required surgery. The use of this technique was continued on 66 patients with great success and only 4 required surgery. Authors also discuss the preliminary results of a randomized study comparing concentric and eccentric training regimens with the latter demonstrating better outcomes and reinforcing their previous results. This regimen may obviate the need for surgery in patients who fail general conservative treatment.

Boden BP, Osbahr DC: High risk stress fractures: evaluation and treatment. *J Am Acad Orthop Surg* 8:344-353, 2000.

General review of the evaluation methods and treatment options of stress fractures of the lower extremity. Specific injuries of the femoral neck, patella, tibia, medial malleolus, talus, tarsal navicular, fifth metatarsal, and great toe sesamoid are discussed. An MRI grading system and evaluation/treatment algorithm for stress fractures are also reviewed.

Buchbinder R: Plantar fasciitis. *N Engl J Med* 350:2159-2166, 2004.

Good general review of plantar fasciitis. An excellent table of the differential diagnosis of pain in the inferior heel with distinguishing clinical features is provided. Operative and nonoperative treatment options are reviewed, and guidelines set forth by the American College of Foot and Ankle surgeons are briefly discussed.

Dombek MF, Lamm BM, Saltrick K, et al: Peroneal tendon tears: a retrospective review. *J Foot Ankle Surg* 42:250-258, 2003.

Retrospective review of 40 patients with peroneal tendon tears. Eighty-eight percent of patients had peroneus brevis tears, 13% had isolated peroneus longus tears, and 37% had combined peroneus brevis and longus tears. Presentation, findings, mechanism of injury, and management are reviewed. All patients in this study received surgical repair with 98% of the patients returning to full activity without pain at an average follow-up of 13 months. The authors comment that, although these injuries may initially be treated conservatively, surgical correction is usually required and provides good, reliable results.

Gill LH: Plantar fasciitis: diagnosis and conservative management. *J Am Acad Orthop Surg* 5:109-117, 1997.

Comprehensive review of plantar fasciitis, including anatomy, etiology, differential diagnosis, risk factors, and treatment. Although this condition is difficult to treat, with a wide variety of treatment options, the authors note that up to 90% of cases can be managed nonoperatively.

Haake M, Buch M, Schoellner C, et al: Extracorporeal shock wave therapy for plantar fasciitis: randomized controlled multicenter trial. *BMJ* 327:75-80, 2003.

Randomized, blinded, multicenter study with 272 patients studying the effectiveness of extracorporeal shock wave therapy for the management of plantar fasciitis. After 12 weeks of intervention, success was demonstrated in 34% of the treated group and 30% in the placebo group with no significant difference. After 1 year, 81% of the therapy group and 76% of the placebo group demonstrated good outcomes. In summary, the authors concluded that extracorporeal shock wave therapy is ineffective in the treatment of plantar fasciitis.

Kocher MS, Bishop J, Marshall R, et al: Operative versus nonoperative management of acute Achilles tendon rupture. *Am J Sports Med* 30:783-790, 2002.

Cross-sectional study with results favoring operative management. The principal advantage of operative management was a lower rerupture rate, whereas nonoperative management avoided the potential for wound complications. As a result, the authors recommend joint decision making by the physician and patient after considering the risks of the different treatment modalities and the desired activity level of the patient.

Mosier SM, Pomeroy G, Manoli A: Pathoanatomy and etiology of posterior tibial tendon dysfunction. *Clin Orthop* 1(365):12-22, 1999.

Authors describe histopathologic findings supporting degenerative tendinosis (and not an inflammatory process) as the principal disease process associated with posterior tibialis dysfunction. Nevertheless, it is not clear whether the changes precede or postdate the tendon dysfunction. Several possible etiologies are reviewed including traumatic, anatomic, mechanical, inflammatory, and ischemic factors that may lead to tendon degeneration and an insufficient repair response. Authors note that the disease is most likely multifactorial and further research is necessary for more definitive answers and insight into best possible treatments.

Riddle DL, Pulisis M, Pidcoe P, Johnson RE: Risk factors for plantar fasciitis: a matched case-control study. *J Bone Joint Surg Am* 85:872-877, 2003.

Case control study demonstrating reduced ankle dorsiflexion (odds ratio 23.3), obesity (odds ratio 5.6), and work-related weight-bearing (odds ratio 3.6) as independent risk factors for plantar fasciitis, with reduced ankle dorsiflexion as the most significant factor. Authors also report a positive dose response relationship of limited dorsiflexion and body mass index with plantar fasciitis. Nevertheless, the study does not meet the criterion of temporal progression and therefore cannot provide causality for the previously listed risk factors.

Sorosky B, Press J, Plastaras C, Rittenberg J: The practical management of Achilles tendinopathy. *Clin J Sport Med* 14:40-44, 2004.

Review of Achilles tendinopathy with emphasis on treatment and rehabilitation. Authors stress and describe the importance of the heel drop exercise during rehabilitation targeting both the soleus (with the knee flexed) and gastrocnemius (with the knee extended) muscles. Eccentric exercises are favored. An Achilles tendinopathy treatment algorithm is provided.

Wallace RGH, Traynor IER, Kernohan WG, Eames MHA: Combined conservative and orthotic management of acute ruptures of the Achilles tendon. *J Bone Joint Surg Am* 86:1198-1202, 2004.

Authors study the use of cast immobilization in equinus for 4 weeks (non–weight-bearing) followed by a removable orthosis for another 4 weeks and physiotherapy in 140 consecutive patients with acute Achilles tendon rupture. Subjective results demonstrated 116 patients (83%) satisfied with their outcome, 21 (15%) satisfied with minor reservations, 2 (1%) satisfied with major reservations, and only 1 (1%) dissatisfied completely. Objectively there were small but significant differences in active ranges of dorsiflexion (22 vs. 21.1); plantarflexion (26.4 vs. 27.1; calf circumference (35.4 vs. 36.6); and plantarflexion peak torques at 30, 90, and 60 degrees per second (137.9, 91.2, 60.3 v. 158.7, 101.2, 64.3) between the injured and uninjured legs, respectively. Overall results were better than the surgically treated group in the study by Leppilahti et al. used as comparison: (nonoperative vs. operative) excellent (56% vs. 34%), good (30% vs. 46%), fair (12% vs. 17%), and poor (2% vs. 3%).

Wong J, Barrass V, Maffulli N: Quantitative review of operative and nonoperative management of Achilles tendon ruptures. *Am J Sports Med* 30:565-574, 2002.

Authors performed a retrospective review analysis of data from 125 articles on the management of Achilles tendon rupture. Study revealed that open repair and early mobilization is most likely the superior method of management, limiting the risk of rerupture and showing a decline in the complication rate in recent years. However, conservative management may be preferred in older individuals or those who do not desire to undergo the risks of surgery. The authors note that although the quality of studies appear to be improving, the majority of the studies used were retrospective and only four were randomized controlled trials.

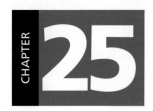

Exertional Compartment Syndrome

Introduction

- Exertional compartment syndrome is defined as the development of pain and neurologic symptoms in the lower extremity with exertion.
  - Deep, cramping pain is characteristic.
- Muscle bulk increases up to 20% during exercise and may contribute to a transient elevation in intracompartmental pressure.
  - Less compliant fascia may be contributory.
- Symptom onset occurs with exercise, and symptoms improve with rest.
  - Symptoms occur within 10 to 30 minutes of exertion.
  - Symptoms resolve within 1 hour after stopping exercise.
  - Players are unable to play through the pain.

- There are four compartments in the lower leg (anterior, lateral, superficial posterior, and deep posterior), and one or all may be affected in cases of exertional compartment syndrome (Figure 25–1).
- The anterior compartment is the most commonly affected and has the best prognosis.
- The cause is an abnormal elevation of the intracompartmental pressure, which leads to hypoperfusion of the muscle and therefore ischemic pain.
- Neurologic symptoms develop with direct compression of the nerves as they pass through the affected compartment (Box 25–1).
- Documentation of elevated compartment pressure after exertion is diagnostic.
- Exertional compartment syndrome may be associated with a muscle hernia in 30% to 40% of cases, which may

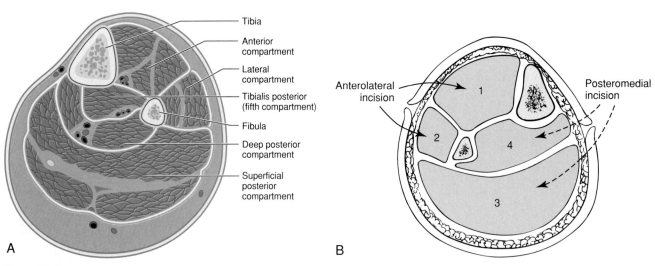

A

B

Figure 25-1:

A, Cross-sectional anatomy of the lower extremity. **B,** Cross-sectional view of the lower extremity compartments showing a position of anterolateral and posteromedial incisions that allows access to the anterior and lateral compartments (1 and 2) and the superficial and deep posterior compartments (3 and 4). (B from Amendola A, Twaddle BC: Compartment syndromes. In Browner BD, Jupiter JB, Levine AM, Trafton PG, editors: *Skeletal trauma,* 3rd ed. Philadelphia, 2003, WB Saunders.)

Box 25–1	**Four Factors Contributing to Exertional Compartment Syndrome**

Enclosure of muscles in an inelastic fascial sheath
Increased volume of skeletal muscle with exercise resulting from blood flow and edema
Muscle hypertrophy from exercise
Dynamic contractions due to the gait cycle

itself be an aggravating factor. It often occurs at the site where the superficial peroneal nerve exits the lateral compartment. When the muscle enlarges during exercise, the portion that herniates may apply direct pressure to this nerve.

Anatomy

- Four compartments located in the lower leg may be involved in exertional compartment syndrome: anterior, lateral, superficial posterior, and deep posterior.
- The anterior compartment contains the deep peroneal nerve and the anterior tibial artery.
- The lateral compartment contains the superficial peroneal nerve.
- The superficial posterior compartment contains the sural nerve.
- The deep posterior compartment contains the posterior tibial nerve, the posterior tibial artery, and the peroneal artery.
- Some authors have suggested that a subcompartment of the deep posterior compartment may be created by a variation in the attachment of the flexor digitorum longus.

Diagnostic Testing

- Measurement of the intracompartmental pressure after a period of exercise is the most common method of diagnosing exertional compartment syndrome (Figure 25–2).
- Positive if resting pressure is greater than 15 mm Hg or return to baseline takes more than 5 to 10 minutes.
- Some authors have advocated the use of near infrared spectroscopy (NIRS) to measure tissue oxygen saturation.
- This provides a noninvasive method for diagnosing exertional compartment syndrome.

Differential Diagnosis

- Tibial stress fracture.
  - Bone scan helpful.
- Venous thrombosis.
  - Noninvasive monitoring helpful such as ultrasound.
- Local nerve compressions.

- Electrodiagnostic testing helpful.
- Periostitis.
  - Bone scan/magnetic resonance imaging (MRI) may be helpful.
- Intermittent claudication.
  - In older patients.
  - Vascular studies may be helpful.

Treatment

- Conservative.
  - The first step in conservative management of exertional compartment syndrome is activity modification.
  - The use of custom orthotics may be beneficial.
- Surgical.
  - Fasciotomy of one or more compartments is the surgical treatment of choice for this condition (Figure 25–3).

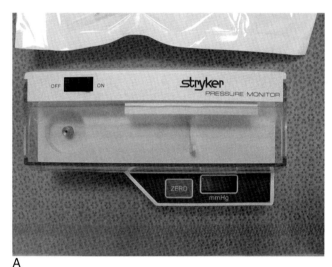

A

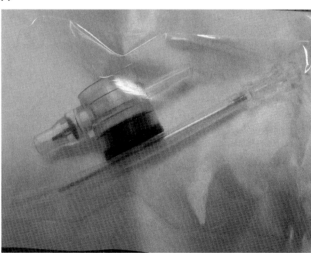

B

Figure 25-2:
A and B, Device for measuring compartment pressure.

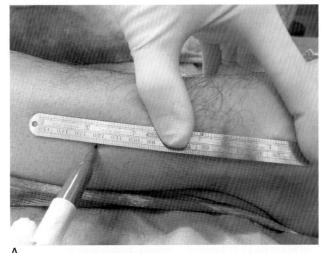

A

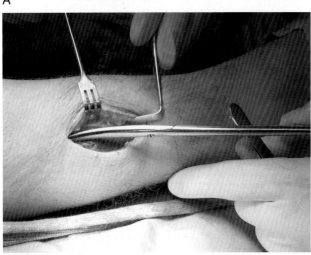

B

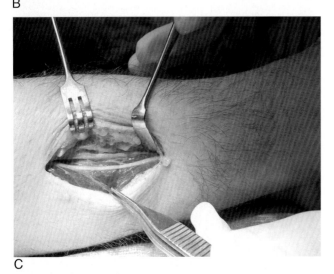

C

Figure 25-3:
Surgical procedure for exertional compartment release. **A,** The superficial peroneal nerve exits the deep fascia approximately 12 cm from the tip of the lateral malleolus. **B,** After blunt dissection, a long pair of Metzenbaum scissors is used to release the fascia subcutaneously. **C,** The superficial peroneal nerve (shown here) is protected throughout the release of the anterior and lateral compartments.

- The primary concern is the possibility of injuring neurovascular structures secondary to lack of direct visualization of the anatomy.
- The structures at greatest risk include the peroneal nerve and saphenous vein.

References

Brennan FH Jr, Kane SF: Diagnosis, treatment options, and rehabilitation of chronic lower leg exertional compartment syndrome *Curr Sports Med Rep* 2:247-250, 2003.

Runners are one of the foremost groups associated with the development of exertional compartment syndrome. Because of the prevalence of running as part of military training and conditioning, this can be a serious problem in this group. Conservative treatment is rarely beneficial, and surgery often becomes the most successful treatment option.

Fraipont MJ, Adamson GJ: Chronic exertional compartment syndrome. *J Am Acad Orthop Surg* 11:268-276, 2003.

An overview of exertional compartment syndrome shows that the key to diagnosis really lies in taking a good history of exactly what the patient's symptoms are and what exacerbates them followed by performing compartment pressure testing. Although most people respond to a period of rest, most will not get prolonged symptom relief without surgical intervention.

Hislop M, Tierney P, Murray P, et al: Chronic exertional compartment syndrome: the controversial "fifth" compartment of the leg. *Am J Sports Med* 31:770-776, 2003.

Cadaveric analysis demonstrates that the flexor digitorum longus tendon may have normal anatomic variants in its attachment that may divide the deep posterior compartment into subcompartments. This could have implications on testing of compartment pressures and surgical release of the deep posterior compartment.

Hutchinson MR, Bederka B, Kopplin M: Anatomic structures at risk during minimal-incision endoscopically assisted fascial compartment releases in the leg. *Am J Sports Med* 31:764-769, 2003.

By performing endoscopic lower extremity compartment release in cadaver models, we learn that a significant risk to the saphenous vein exists with this smaller incision approach.

Van den Brand JG, Verleisdonk EJ, van der Werken C: Near infrared spectroscopy in the diagnosis of chronic exertional compartment syndrome. *Am J Sports Med* 32:452-456, 2004.

These authors demonstrate that NIRS can be a useful tool in the diagnosis of exertional compartment syndrome. Significant differences in the control group, as well as in the experimental group presurgery and postsurgery, demonstrate the potential for this to be a useful noninvasive test.

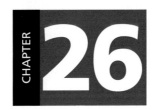

CHAPTER 26

Ankle Instability

History, Physical Examination, and Imaging

- Ankle injuries are perhaps the most common joint condition seen in primary care offices and orthopaedics.
- Ankle sprains usually result in damage to the lateral ligaments, with the anterior talofibular ligament (ATFL) being the most common (Box 26–1).
- The ATFL provides stability to the ankle in plantarflexion, and the calcaneofibular ligament (CFL) is believed to provide stability in all positions.
- The most common mechanism of injury is a forced inversion of a foot that is in plantarflexion. Anatomically, this greatly stresses and stretches the weak ATFL, explaining its frequent association with ankle sprains (Figure 26–1).
- Forced inversion of a foot in dorsiflexion would place greater stress on the CFL.
- It is important to ask the patient if he or she can recall the position of the foot and ankle when injury occurred because this can help direct diagnosis and examination findings.
- Many patients have a history of recurrent ankle sprains and instability, usually indicating poor rehabilitative results or efforts.
- If the patient presents within a few hours of injury, an area of swelling and tenderness may localize the site of injury (Box 26–2).
- Palpation of individual ligaments is recommended to help specify injury. This may not be possible in delayed

presentations in which moderate to severe swelling, ecchymosis, and diffuse tenderness obscure findings.

- The anterior drawer test, which evaluates the ATFL, is performed with the patient's foot slightly plantarflexed (recall that this position places the greatest stress on the ATFL) and while stabilizing the tibia with one hand, pulling the hindfoot anteriorly with the other hand cupped around the calcaneus. Increased translation when compared with the other side is indicative of an ATFL rupture. Extreme translation may suggest a combined ATFL/CFL tear (Figure 26–2A and B).
- The talar tilt test evaluates the integrity of the CFL and is performed by inverting the affected foot while stabilizing the tibia and palpating the lateral aspect of the joint to estimate the degree of tilt. Positive findings should be documented only after comparison with the contralateral ankle (Figure 26–2C and D).
- Two tests are available to evaluate the syndesmosis (Figure 26–3).
  - The squeeze test is considered positive if simultaneous compression of the tibia and fibula at the midcalf produces ankle pain.
  - The external rotation test is performed with the knee in 90 degrees of flexion and the ankle in neutral position. Pain in the syndesmosis region when external rotation of the foot is executed indicates possible injury.
- Standard radiographic evaluation usually consists of anteroposterior (AP), lateral, and mortise views of the ankle.
- Fractures of the fibula or talus may be present on ankle radiographs.
- An AP view of the foot is appropriate if a fracture of the fifth metatarsal or anterior process of the calcaneus is suspected.
- Stress views can be used to confirm ATFL and CFL disruption (Figure 26–4).
  - Anterior translation (while performing the anterior drawer test) 3 mm greater than the opposite ankle or 5- to 10-mm translation of the affected ankle are considered to be abnormal and indicate ATFL rupture.

Box 26–1	Approximate Incidence of Ligaments Damaged in Ankle Sprains

Isolated ATFL injury occurs in 66% of sprains
ATFL + CFL occurs in 20%
Isolated CFL is rare
Deltoid injury in approximately 2.5%
Syndesmotic injury in 1% to 10%

ATFL, anterior talofibular ligament; CFL, calcaneofibular ligament.

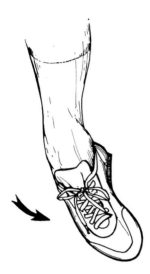

Figure 26–1:
Common mechanism injury of ankle sprains involves inversion of the plantarflexed ankle, often resulting in anterior talofibular ligament injury. (From DeLee JC, Drez D Jr, Miller MD, editors: *DeLee and Drez's orthopaedic sports medicine: principles and practice.* Philadelphia, 1994, Saunders.)

- A positive talar tilt is reproduced radiographically when there is more than 5 degrees of variance when compared with the opposite side or an absolute value greater than 15 mm, suggesting injury to the CFL.
- Syndesmotic injury is indicated by a clear space (measured from the medial aspect of the fibula and the lateral border of the posterior tibia, 1 cm above the tibiotalar joint) greater than 5 mm or a tibiofibular overlap less than 6 mm or 42% of fibular width on AP view or less than 1 mm on mortise view (Figure 26–5).

Types

- Classically, ankle sprains have been classified into three grades.
  - Grade I indicates stretching of the ATFL with minimal loss of function and no evidence of mechanical instability.
  - Grade II indicates a partial tear of the ATFL with moderate swelling and tenderness and mild to moderate instability and loss of function.

Box 26–2	Area of Tenderness/Swelling and Most Probable Site of Injury

Inferior to lateral malleolus—injury to lateral ligaments
Sinus tarsi/midfoot—injury to subtalar joint, midfoot, and/or anterior calcaneus
Supramalleolar—possible rupture of syndesmosis or fracture of fibula

- Grade III indicates a complete tear of the ATFL ± CFL with severe ankle swelling, ecchymosis, loss of function, and usually an inability to bear weight. These injuries demonstrate significant instability, and a positive anterior drawer test ± a positive talar tilt test.
- Another similar classification system based on pathology and instability has been devised by Trevino et al. (Table 26–1).
- Subtalar instability can frequently occur simultaneously with ankle instability, particularly when the CFL, a lateral stabilizer of the subtalar joint, is torn. Tenderness over the sinus tarsi and loss of parallelism between the posterior aspect of the talus and the calcaneus on stress Broden's view (performed with the heel in varus and foot internally rotated with the beam pointed 20 degrees caudally) are classic findings (Figure 26–6).
- Syndesmotic injuries/high ankle sprains are rare but most commonly occur in professional athletes.
  - It is believed to result from hyperdorsiflexion and excessive external rotation of the ankle and foot.
  - Indicative findings include a positive squeeze test and external rotation stress test, as well as diastasis on radiographs.
- Syndesmotic injuries can be classified into three types (Box 26–3).
- Medial ankle instability, although rare, is associated with eversion type trauma that typically occurs when running down stairs or on uneven ground.
  - Patients may report their ankle "giving way," recurrent injuries, and pain along the anteromedial ankle.
  - Examination findings include tenderness over the medial gutter and a valgus and pronation deformity that is corrected with recruitment of the posterior tibialis.
  - Arthroscopy helps confirm the diagnosis and allows for the evaluation of medial and lateral instability and assessment of surrounding structures for any associated damage.
  - Hintermann et al. proposed a classification system of medial ankle instability on the basis of clinical and intraoperative findings that helps guide treatment (Table 26–2).

Treatment

- Grade I and II ankle sprains should be managed nonoperatively with rest, ice, elevation, and compression.
- Ankle support with several types of braces and casts that limit inversion and eversion and initial ambulatory assistance with crutches or a cane may be appropriate (Table 26–3).

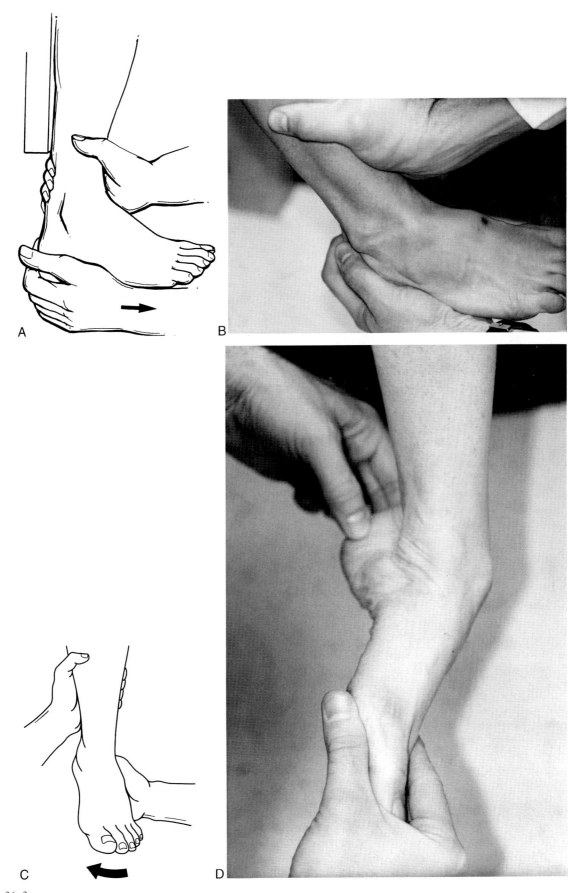

Figure 26–2:
A and **B,** Anterior drawer test. **C** and **D,** Talar tilt test assessing ankle instability. (From DeLee JC, Drez D Jr, Miller MD, editors: *DeLee and Drez's orthopaedic sports medicine: principles and practice,* 2nd ed. Philadelphia, 2003, Saunders.)

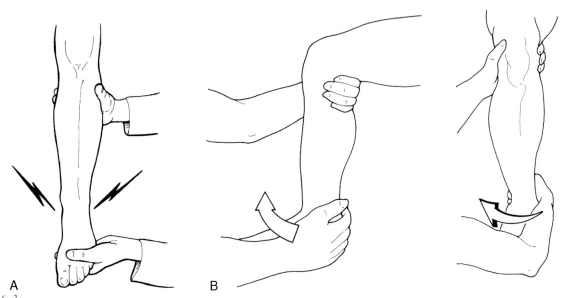

Figure 26–3:
Clinical evaluation for syndesmotic injury. **A**, Squeeze test. **B**, Abduction-external rotation stress test. (From Miller MD, Cooper DE, Warner JJP: *Review of sports medicine and arthroscopy*. Philadelphia, 2002, Saunders.)

- Patients should be placed on a protocol of weight-bearing as tolerated and physical therapy to strengthen the ankle and prevent reinjury.
  - It is reported that patients placed on a regimen of protected weight-bearing were found to have less pain and decreased atrophy and returned to sports earlier than those treated with immobilization.
- Many surgeons have recommended acute repairs for grade III ankle sprains in elite athletes. However, several studies have shown similar end results between patients treated nonoperatively with functional bracing and patients treated surgically. Furthermore, other studies concluded that patients treated conservatively avoided surgical complications and returned to activity earlier than the surgical group. Nevertheless, approximately 10% to 20% of those treated nonoperatively will require surgical repair.

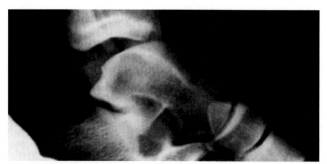

Figure 26–4:
Positive anterior drawer stress radiograph. (From Canale ST: Ankle injuries. In Canale ST, editor: *Campbell's operative orthopaedics,* 9th ed. St Louis, 1998, Mosby-Year Book.)

- Delayed anatomic repair has also been reported to produce equal results to reconstruction performed acutely.
- After conservative measures fail, several techniques for repair can be used for definitive treatment and can generally be divided into anatomic or augmented nonanatomic procedures.
- The Brostrom procedure, which consists of anatomically tightening the lateral ligaments, is favored among orthopaedists. Reinforcement can be supplemented using the extensor retinaculum, or in severe cases, a peroneus brevis graft. The Gould modification includes shortening and anatomic reinsertion of the ATFL and CFL, reinforced by suturing the extensor retinaculum to the distal fibula (Figure 26–7).
- Augmentation procedures have been described using several graft options including the peroneus brevis, peroneus longus, extensor retinaculum, plantaris, extensor digitorum brevis, Achilles tendon, fascia lata, patellar tendon-bone, and allografts (Figure 26–8).
- Subtalar instability is initially managed nonoperatively in a similar fashion to ankle sprains, with the additional use of a heel cup to stabilize the subtalar joint.
- When surgical repair is considered for subtalar instability, attention is focused on carefully reconstructing the CFL. In severe cases, some surgeons recommend reconstructing the ATFL, CFL, lateral talocalcaneal ligament (LTCL), interosseous talocalcaneal ligament, and cervical ligament, using the peroneus brevis, plantaris, or Achilles tendon. Although some of the previously mentioned procedures for lateral instability have been used to

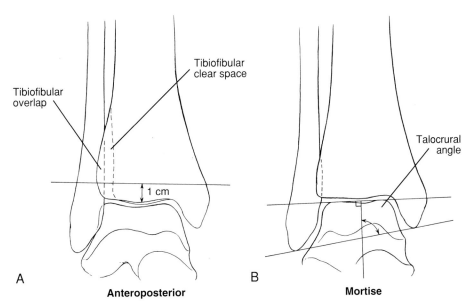

Figure 26–5:
Normal relationship of the distal tibia and fibula and talus. **A,** Anteroposterior view. **B,** Mortise view. (From Scioli M: Injuries about the ankle. Instability of the ankle and subtalar joint. In Myerson MS, editor: *Foot and ankle disorders.* Philadelphia, 2000, Saunders.)

correct subtalar instability, several newer procedures have been studied that focus on reconstructing the more important stabilizing ligaments of the subtalar joint (Figure 26–9).

- Surgical techniques for ankle and subtalar instability continue to be studied as new anchoring techniques develop and anatomic and biomechanical understanding improves.
- Syndesmotic injuries usually require a recovery period that is twice as long as ankle sprains.
- Syndesmotic injuries are generally treated according to type.

- Type 1—ankle supporting brace with weight-bearing as tolerated. Patients usually return to sport activity by 6 weeks.
- Type 2—long- or short-leg non–weight-bearing cast for 4 weeks followed by a weight-bearing cast or walking boot for another 4 weeks. Frequent radiographic evaluation of the syndesmosis should be performed throughout treatment. Return to sport activity occurs between 8 to 10 weeks.
- Type 3 and types 1 and 2 refractory to conservative management—closed reduction and surgical fixation

Table 26–1: Ankle Injury Classification System

GRADE	PATHOLOGY	INSTABILITY
I	Stretch	None
II	Partial tear	Mild to moderate
IIIa	Complete tear of ATFL	Positive anterior drawer test
IIIb	Complete tear of ATFL and CFL	Positive anterior drawer and talar tilt tests
IIIc1	Complete tear of ATFL and CFL, tear of peroneal tendon	Positive anterior drawer and talar tilt tests; peroneal tendon stable in groove but tender to palpation
IIIc2	Complete tear of ATFL and CFL, peroneal tendon subluxation or dislocation	Positive anterior drawer and talar tilt tests, peroneal tendon subluxation or dislocation with resisted eversion and dorsiflexion
IVa	Complete tear of ATFL and CFL, avulsion fracture of the fibula	Positive anterior drawer and talar tilt tests
IVb	Complete tear of ATFL and CFL, osteochondral fracture of the talus	Positive anterior drawer and talar tilt tests
IVc	Complete tear of ATFL and CFL, lateral process fracture of the talus	Positive anterior drawer and talar tilt tests

ATFL, anterior talofibular ligament; CFL, calcaneofibular ligament.
From Miller MD, Cooper DE, Warner JJP: *Review of sports medicine and arthroscopy.* Philadelphia, 2002, Saunders.

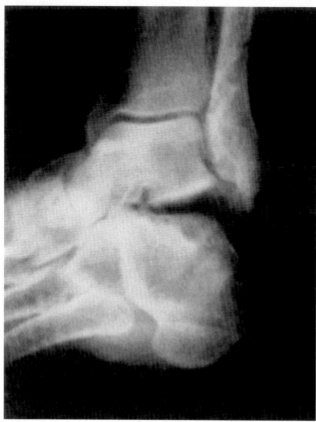

Figure 26–6:
Broden's stress view demonstrating subtalar instability. (From Keefe DT, Haddad SL: *Foot Ankle Clin North Am* 7:577-609, 2002.)

- Rehabilitation can last 2 to 8 weeks depending on injury severity and should follow three phases sequentially (Box 26–4).
- Studies have demonstrated that up to 50% of patients with recurrent ankle instability have peroneal weakness and no ligament laxity.
- There is no absolute evidence that taping or high-top shoes assist with ankle instability.
- Semirigid braces may provide stability to the ankle after reconstruction procedures and some support when the patient returns to sports.
- Patients with grade I sprains can usually return to sports by 3 weeks, whereas those with grade III injuries require at least 6 weeks of therapy.

Complications

- Improper or incomplete rehabilitation may result in chronic instability and recurrent sprains.
- Late complications of joint injury may result in arthritis and chronic pain.
- Anterolateral impingement syndrome and sinus tarsi syndrome may develop after inversion injuries.
  - Patients report pain with activity and demonstrate tenderness over the affected area.
  - Radiographic evaluation is usually not helpful.
  - An intraarticular injection of lidocaine with subsequent relief may be more diagnostic.
  - Initial treatment is conservative, reserving surgical debridement for recalcitrant cases.
- Nonanatomic augmented reconstructions of the lateral ligaments may be complicated by loss of subtalar motion and lead to significant morbidity.
- Syndesmotic injuries may be complicated by heterotropic ossification formation, which may delay recovery and increase the risk of recurrent sprains.
  - Excision of heterotropic ossification has been shown to relieve symptoms and allow athletes to return to play in a more timely manner.

with syndesmotic screws. Weight-bearing is protected for 6 to 8 weeks, and the screws are commonly removed after 8 to 12 weeks. Athletes can expect to return to previous activity in approximately 6 months.

- Symptomatic medial ankle instability may be treated by repairing or reconstructing the affected ligaments, including those on the lateral aspect of the ankle if indicated.

Rehabilitation

- Contrast baths can help reduce swelling 2 days after the injury.

Table 26–2:   Classification of Medial Ankle Instability

TYPE	LOCALIZATION	INVOLVED LIGAMENTS	N	(%)	SURGICAL PROCEDURE	AFTER TREATMENT
I	Proximal "interval"	Tibionavicular ligament, tibiospring ligament (spring ligament)	39	72%	Repair, reattachment	Stabilizing shoe
II	Intermediate	Tibionavicular ligament, tibiospring ligament (spring ligament)	5	9%	Repair, reattachment (two flap technique)	Plaster
III	Distal	Tibionavicular ligament, spring ligament	10	19%	Repair, reattachment	Plaster

From Hintermann B: *Foot Ankle Clinic North Am* 8: 723-738, 2003.

Table 26–3:   Immobilization Methods for Foot and Ankle Injuries

IMMOBILIZATION METHOD	COMMON APPLICATION	ADVANTAGE	DISADVANTAGE
Short-leg nonwalking cast	Initial treatment for severe ankle and midfoot sprains: definitive treatment of stable syndesmosis and Lisfranc injuries	Excellent protection for all foot injuries and most ankle injuries: effective edema management	Poor rotational control for ankle syndesmosis: rapid deconditioning; inconvenient for dressing, showering, and sleeping
Short-leg walking cast	Initial treatment for severe ankle and moderate foot sprains	Excellent protection for most foot and ankle injuries; improved ability to bear weight; effective edema management: effective pain management	Poor rotational control for the ankle syndesmosis; rapid deconditioning; inconvenient for dressing, showering, and sleeping
Removable cast boot (3D Walker, Bledsoe Boot [Bledsoe Brace Systems, Grand Prairie, TX], CAM boot)	Initial treatment for moderate ankle and foot sprains	Removable protection for ankle and foot injuries; improved ability to bear weight; continuous rehabilitation provided; self-applied device	No rotational control through ankle; poor edema control; athletic participation restricted
Semirigid pneumatic ankle brace (Air-Stirrup, Aircast, Summit, NJ)	Functional treatment for hindfoot and ankle injuries at various recovery phases, including acute ankle sprains, prevention of recurrent ankle sprains, and bifurcate ligament injuries	Rigid support for hindfoot and ankle injuries—allows ankle range of motion,[92] allows continued athletic participation, assists resolution of edema (air cell systems); self-applied device; device used within shoe; low cost	No rotational control through ankle; bulky within shoe
Nonrigid functional ankle brace (lace-up or Velcro closures)	Functional treatment for hindfoot and ankle injuries at various recovery phases, including chronic injuries	Nonrigid support for hindfoot and ankle injuries—allows ankle range of motion, allows continued athletic participation; self-applied device; device used within shoe	No rotational control through ankle
Ankle and foot taping	Functional treatment for foot and ankle injuries at various recovery phases, including chronic injuries	Custom-applied support for foot and ankle injuries; provides resistance to inversion, provides biofeedback, allows continued athletic participation	Rapid loosening with time-limited effectiveness; requires trained personnel for application; high cost over the course of a regular season

From DeLee JC, Drez D Jr, Miller MD, editors: *DeLee and Drez's orthopaedic sports medicine: principles and practice*, 2nd ed. Philadelphia, 2003, Saunders.

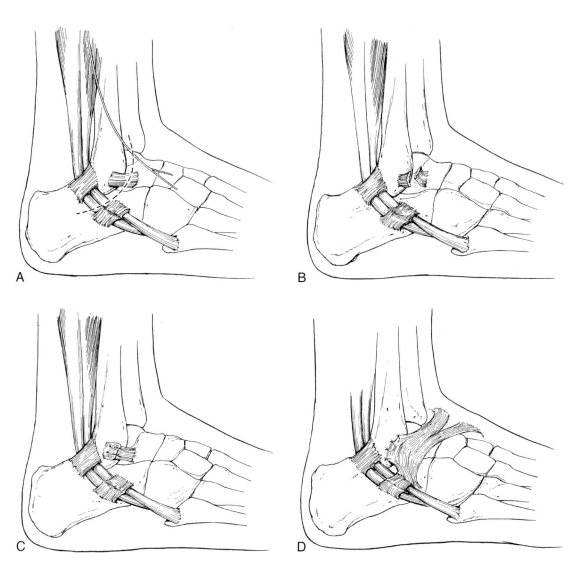

Figure 26–7:
Gould modification of Brostrom reconstruction procedure for lateral ankle instability. **A,** Curvilinear incision centered on the anterior talofibular ligament with care to avoid the superficial peroneal nerve. **B,** Torn anterior talofibular ligament is identified and the end freshened. **C,** The anterior talofibular ligament is then anatomically repaired. **D,** The adjacent inferior extensor retinaculum is then used to reinforce the repair. (From Scioli M: Injuries about the ankle. Instability of the ankle and subtalar joint. In Myerson MS, editor: *Foot and ankle disorders.* Philadelphia, 2000, Saunders.)

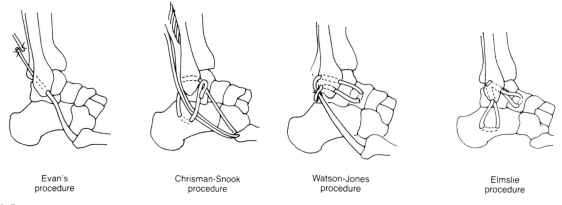

Evan's
procedure

Chrisman-Snook
procedure

Watson-Jones
procedure

Elmslie
procedure

Figure 26–8:
Augmented reconstructions for lateral ankle instability. (From Miller MD, Cooper DE, Warner JJP: *Review of sports medicine and arthroscopy.* Philadelphia, 2002, Saunders.)

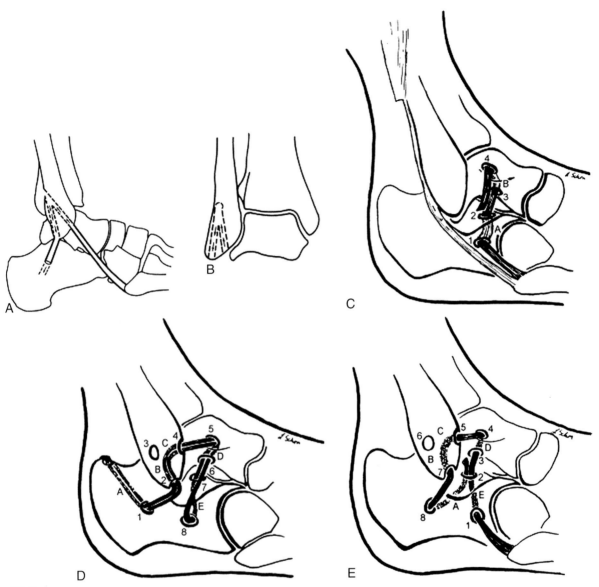

Figure 26–9:
Ligament reconstruction procedures for subtalar instability. **A** and **B,** Larsen reconstruction using a whole peroneus brevis graft. **C,** Schon cervical reconstruction using a half peroneus brevis tendon graft. **D,** Schon triligamentous reconstruction using a plantaris tendon graft. **E,** Schon triligamentous reconstruction using a peroneus brevis graft.

(continued)

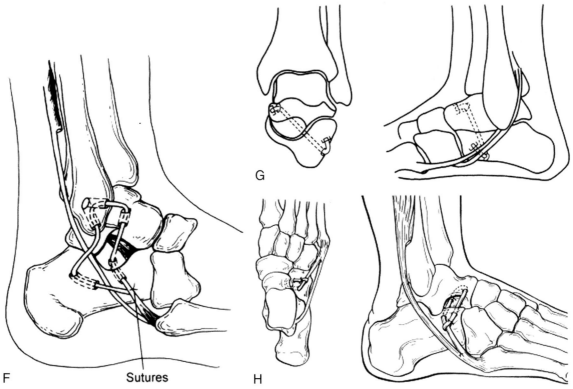

Figure 26–9, cont'd:
F, Mann triligamentous reconstruction using a half peroneus tendon graft. **G**, Kato interosseous talocalcaneal ligament reconstruction using a partial Achilles tendon graft. **H**, Pisani interosseous talocalcaneal ligament reconstruction using a half peroneus brevis tendon graft. (From Keefe DT, Haddad SL: *Foot Ankle Clin North Am* 7:577-609, 2002.)

Box 26–4	**Rehabilitation Regimen Proposed Following Ankle Sprains**

Phase I—RICE, NSAIDs, weight-bear as tolerated with ambulatory support if necessary, ankle braces or stirrups. Walking boot for severe sprain may assist with healing and ambulation. Once pain-free, patient may advance to phase II.

Phase II—Work on peroneal and dorsiflexion strengthening and Achilles tendon stretching. Use of brace, is usually continued. Plantar flexion exercises place the joint in a vulnerable position for injury and should be avoided in this phase. Advancement to next stage requires recovery of full range of motion and 80% return of strength.

Phase III—concentration on proprioception, agility, and endurance exercises and return of full strength. Use of brace may be slowly discontinued.

NSAIDs, Nonsteroidal antiinflammatory drugs; RICE, rest, ice.

References

Barnum MJ, Ehrlich MG, Zaleske DJ: Long-term patient-oriented outcome study of a modified Evans procedure. *J Pediatr Orthop* 18:783–788, 1998.

Authors report their long-term results on 20 patients who were surgically treated for ankle instability using a modified Evans procedure. Satisfactory results were found in 95% of patients 1 year after surgery and 85% of patients during a long-term follow-up (range 7 to 20 years).

Colville MR: Surgical treatment of the unstable ankle. *J Am Acad Orthop Surg* 6:368–377, 1998.

Good review of several available reconstruction procedures to treat ankle instability, most with greater than 80% success rates. Author notes that nonanatomic reconstructions using tendon grafts may limit ankle and subtalar motion. Important anatomy, biomechanics, and diagnostic techniques are reviewed.

Hintermann B: Biomechanics of the unstable ankle joint and clinical implications. *Med Sci Sports Exerc* 31:S459-S469, 1999.

Author reviews the anatomy and biomechanics of the normal and unstable ankle joint, as well as associated clinical manifestations and differential diagnosis of ankle instability. Author comments that chronic functional instability frequently results from impaired ankle proprioception. Furthermore, when surgery is considered, anatomic reconstruction is preferred to limit alterations to the ankle biomechanics. Most tenodesis or augmented procedures limit subtalar motion and thus affect the normal biomechanics of the ankle.

Hintermann B: Medial ankle instability. *Foot Ankle Clin North Am* 8:723-738, 2003.

Good review of the anatomy and function of the medial ligaments of the ankle and clinical findings associated with medial instability. A classification system is provided and surgical treatment is described for each type, including postoperative management.

Karlsson J, Lansinger O: Chronic lateral instability of the ankle in athletes. *Sports Med* 16:355-365, 1993.

> *Review of acute and chronic lateral ligament injury. Authors provide good descriptions of several available surgical repair techniques (with study results) that can be performed if conservative measures fail. Authors prefer anatomic reconstructions, facile to perform.*

Kato T: The diagnosis and treatment of instability of the subtalar joint. *J Bone Joint Surg Br* 77:400-406, 1995.

> *Author describes radiographic technique and measurements to assess subtalar instability. Conservative and operative treatment is reviewed. Author stresses the importance of reconstructing the talocalcaneal interosseus ligament for subtalar instability and describes his technique using a segmented Achilles tendon graft. He further describes his modified Chrisman-Snook procedure that reconstructs the ATFL, CFL, and LTCL, which can be used concomitantly when severe ankle instability is also present. All 14 patients that he surgically treated had excellent results.*

Keefe DT, Haddad SL: Subtalar instability etiology, diagnosis, and management. *Foot Ankle Clin North Am* 7:577-609, 2002.

> *Comprehensive review of subtalar instability, including anatomy, potential mechanisms, diagnostic techniques, and both acute and chronic management. Older and newer surgical techniques are reviewed with detailed descriptions and specific study results.*

Kitaoka HB, Lee MD, Morrey BF, Cass JR: Acute repair and delayed reconstruction for lateral ankle instability: twenty-year follow up study. *J Orthop Trauma* 11:530-535, 1997.

> *Retrospective study comparing long-term outcomes of 22 acute primary ligament repairs (within 2 weeks) and 31 delayed reconstruction (18 Evans, 13 Watson-Jones) for lateral ankle instability. Average follow-up was 22 years after the procedure and demonstrated similar clinical and radiologic results in both groups. In addition, no significant differences were found between the two reconstructive procedures. Authors comment that the majority of patients with grade III sprains can successfully be treated with conservative management. Reconstructive procedures may be reserved for those patients with persistent instability. Authors also note that there were slightly better clinical results in the primary repair group, suggesting acute repair may benefit selected patients such as elite athletes.*

Krips R, Niek van Dijk C, Lehtonen H, et al: Sports activity level after surgical treatment for chronic anterolateral ankle instability. *Am J Sports Med* 30:13-19, 2002.

> *Retrospective multicenter study comparing results of anatomic reconstruction with tenodesis procedures for lateral ankle instability. Forty-one patients underwent a Brostrom procedure (13 with periosteal flap reinforcement), and 36 patients underwent various tenodesis procedures (14 Evans, 1 Watson-Jones, 9 modified Castaing, and 12 Viernstein). Thirty-six patients in the anatomic reconstruction group had good or excellent results compared with only 21 in the tenodesis group. Furthermore, the tenodesis group had significantly more patients with limited ankle dorsiflexion (15 vs. 3 in the anatomic reconstruction group) and more frequent medial osteophytes (suggesting a higher risk of medially located degenerative changes in the ankle joint). As a result, the authors conclude that anatomic reconstruction should be the procedure of choice when surgical management of lateral ankle instability is indicated.*

Sammarco GJ, Iduusuyi OB: Reconstruction of the lateral ankle ligaments using a split peroneus brevis tendon graft. *Foot Ankle Int* 20:97-103, 1999.

> *Authors describe a modified Chrisman-Snook surgical technique using a slotted tendon stripper to harvest half of the peroneus brevis tendon and bone anchors to secure the graft. The authors report a 94% good to excellent clinical result and 97% mechanical instability in 31 consecutive ankles they treated. The authors believe their technique is simple, reliable, and can provide stable reconstruction in patients with high-demand ankles with minimal morbidity.*

Sugimoto K, Takakuura Y, Kumai T, et al: Reconstruction of the lateral ankle ligaments with bone-patellar tendon graft in patients with chronic ankle instability. *Am J Sports Med* 30:340-346, 2002.

> *Authors describe a new procedure for the surgical management of chronic lateral ankle instability using a bone-split patellar tendon graft. The procedure allows bone-to-bone fixation in the fibula rather than tendon-to-bone healing required by other tenodesis techniques. Authors report successful outcomes in 13 patients with a low complication rate. A controlled study is necessary to further support the technique.*

Westlin NE, Vogler HW, Albertsson MP, et al: Treatment of lateral ankle instability with transfer of the extensor digitorum brevis muscle. *J Foot Ankle Surg* 42:183-192, 2003.

> *Authors describe their surgical technique of lateral ankle instability correction using the extensor digitorum brevis muscle. Authors retrospectively review results in 10 patients (13 ankles). All patients considered their results as either excellent or good.*

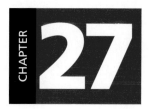
Lower Extremity Fractures

Introduction

- Although there are obviously a variety of fractures of the lower extremity, this chapter concentrates on common sports medicine-related fractures. Many of these are stress fractures. It is important to understand the diagnosis and treatment for these injuries.

Hip Fractures

- Although proximal femoral fractures are common in the elderly population, younger active adults can sustain these fractures as well.
- Typically a more violent force is necessary to sustain injuries in the younger adults.
- Younger adults have a higher incident of soft tissue trauma and complications such as avascular necrosis and nonunion.
- Anatomic reduction and rigid fixation of these fractures is critical to achieving a good outcome.

Stress Fractures of the Hip

- Typically related to overuse, especially in running athletes.
- May present with groin or thigh pain and may demonstrate painful or reduced hip range of motion.
- Classification is based on the location of the fracture.
  - Superior or tension side fractures have a worse prognosis and higher chance to go onto a complete fracture.
  - Compression or inferior fractures have less propensity for completion and can often be managed nonoperatively.
- Magnetic resonance imaging (MRI) has been helpful in the diagnosis and treatment of these injuries (Figure 27–1).
- Compression side fractures or those that radiographically show only minimal early change may be treated conservatively with a period of very gradual return to activity over a period of several months.
- Fractures that involve the superior cortex or significantly involve more than 50% of the femoral neck in a linear pattern should be prophylactically fixed with large cannulated screws.

Femur Fractures

- Less commonly seen in athletic populations because it usually involves a high-energy injury mechanism.
- Should consider the possibility of a pathologic fracture, especially when the mechanism is of lower energy than is typically seen in femur fractures of young adults.
- Surgical treatment indicated, which involves open reduction and internal fixation (ORIF) with plating or intermedullary fixation.
- Open fractures or those associated with other significant injury may require initial treatment with a spanning external fixator prior to consideration of more definitive treatment.

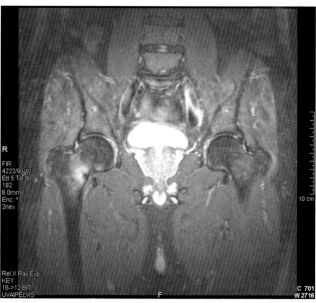

Figure 27-1:

Magnetic resonance imaging appearance of stress fracture of the hip.

Bony Avulsion Fractures About the Knee

- These typically include avulsion fractures associated with anterior cruciate ligament (ACL), posterior cruciate ligament (PCL), and lateral collateral ligament (LCL) injuries. Some controversy exists about proper treatment (Figure 27–2).
- These require primary ORIF and may require supplemental graft reinforcement.
- If the ligaments are significantly attenuated, ligament reconstruction should be considered as an alternative.

Patella Fractures

- These may occur as a result of direct trauma to the knee or as a stress reaction, especially in sports that require repetitive jumping.

- Patella fracture can also occur as a rare complication of surgical ACL reconstruction using a patella tendon autograft.
- The integrity of the extensor mechanism should be evaluated in all cases of suspected patella fracture.
- Patella fractures are classified as transverse, vertical, or comminuted.
- A displaced fracture is one that exhibits greater than 3 mm of fragment separation or greater than 2 mm of articular step-off.
- Nondisplaced fractures may be treated nonoperatively if the extensor mechanism remains intact.
  - Initially these are managed with a hinged knee brace locked into extension.
  - As healing occurs, motion may be slowly advanced in the brace.
  - In the brace, patients may bear weight as tolerated.
- Surgical treatment for displaced fractures may be done with tension band wiring or fixation with K-wires or cannulated screws.

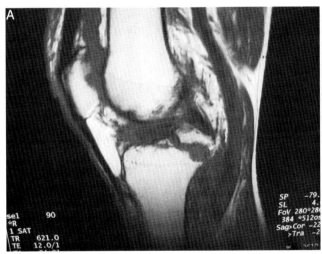

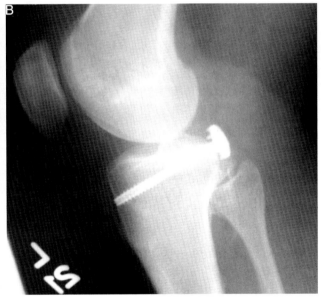

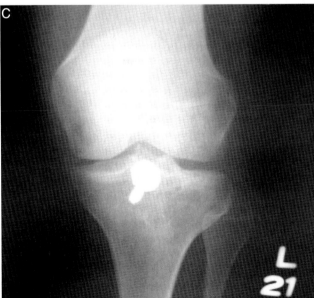

Figure 27-2:
A, Magnetic resonance imaging appearance of posterior cruciate ligament (PCL) avulsion. **B,** Lateral radiograph after open reduction and internal fixation (ORIF) of PCL avulsion. **C,** Posteroanterior radiograph after ORIF of PCL avulsion.

Tibia Fractures

- Traumatic midshaft tibia fractures can occur with any contact sport and typically result from a direct blow.
- Treatment typically involves intermedullary fixation of the tibia.

- Open fractures require initial surgical debridement and consideration of external fixation versus intermedullary fixation (Figure 27–3).
- Tibial plateau fractures may also occur in the athletic population.
  - Schatzker classification
    - 1: Split (nondepressed) lateral tibial plateau.
    - 2: Split (depressed) lateral tibial plateau.

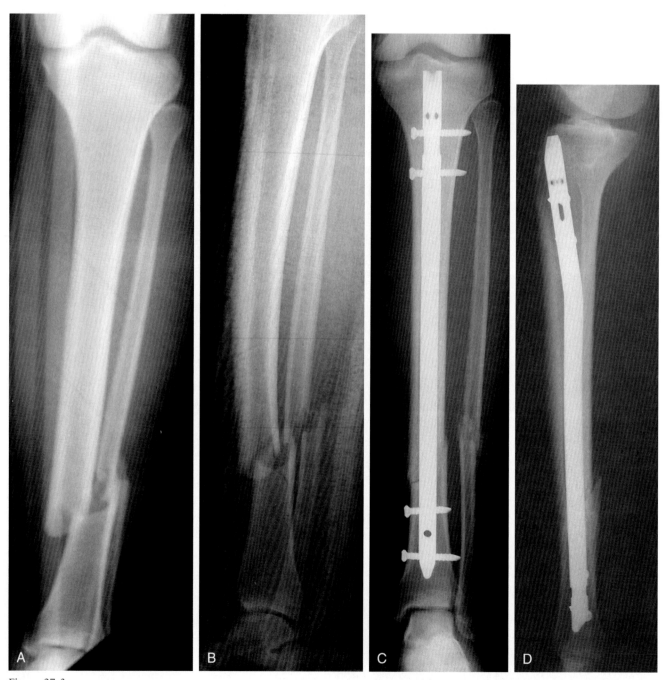

Figure 27-3:
Intermedullary nailing of a tibial fracture at the junction of the distal and middle thirds. **A,** Anteroposterior (AP) radiograph of injury. **B,** Lateral radiograph of injury. **C,** AP radiograph following intramedullary (IM) nailing. **D,** Lateral radiograph following IM nailing.(From Trafton PG: Tibial shaft fractures. In Browner BD, Jupiter JB, Levine AM, Trafton PG: *Skeletal trauma,* 3rd ed. Philadelphia, WB Saunders, 2003.)

- 3: Depressed lateral tibial plateau.
- 4: Medial tibial plateau.
- 5: Bicondylar involvement.
- 6: Bicondylar involvement with metaphyseal/diaphyseal disassociation.
- Nondisplaced tibial plateau fractures may be treated conservatively with a non–weight-bearing status.
- Displaced tibial plateau fractures should undergo ORIF and the menisci evaluated for possible entrapment in the fracture site.

Tibial Stress Reactions/Fractures

- Stress reactions of the tibia are commonly seen in athletes, especially those involved in endurance sports such as distance running.
- Pain is usually insidious in onset, worsens with activity, and improves with rest.
- Athletes are focally tender over the site of injury.
- The most common site of stress reaction in the tibia is the posteromedial cortex.
- Anterior cortex injuries, on the tension side, are less common and are associated with longer recovery and increased rate of progression.
- Plain radiographs are typically negative at the early stage but may demonstrate cortical thickening as the condition resolves or go on to demonstrate linear lucency if the condition is left untreated and begins to develop into an actual fracture.
- Bone scan or MRI is often a more helpful diagnostic tool in these cases.
- In the absence of a frank fracture line, the treatment of tibial stress reaction is conservative.
- The athlete must refrain from any activities that reproduce the pain. This means that if normal daily walking is painful, the athlete should be made non-weight-bearing for a period of 2 to 3 weeks and then reexamined.
- Activity is generally advanced slowly as tolerated as long as symptoms do not reappear.

Ankle Fractures

- Ankle fractures are common in the sports population.
- The Ottawa ankle rules help determine when to get radiographs in the training room (Box 27–1).
  - Criteria for radiographs include the following:
    - Distal posterior tenderness
    - Fifth metatarsal base tenderness
    - Navicular tenderness
    - Inability to bear weight
- Classification.
  - The Danis-Weber classification system describes the level of the fracture of the lateral malleolus.

Box 27–1 **The Ottawa Ankle Rules**
Distal posterior tenderness
Fifth metatarsal base tenderness
Navicular tenderness
Inability to bear weight

- A: Below the level of the mortise
- B: At the level of the mortise
- C: Above the level of the mortise
- It is also important to describe involvement of the medial malleolus or the medial soft tissue stabilizers (deltoid ligament), or both because injury here results in a rotary instability of the fracture, which will require surgical intervention.
- ORIF remains the mainstay of treatment of treatment for ankle fractures with displaced mortise (Figure 27–4).
- Sixty percent of ankle fractures have a tibiotalar articular injury associated with them.

Lateral Process of the Talus Fracture

- This has been termed "snowboarder's ankle" because of an increased incidence in this type of fracture in this particular athletic population.
- The injury results from a dorsiflexion and inversion mechanism and also involves a degree of axial loading, which occurs as the result of some jumping maneuvers.
- The clinical picture is similar to that seen with a simple ankle sprain but a fracture of the lateral talus may be noted on radiograph.
- Computed tomography (CT) scan may be useful in making this diagnosis as well (Figure 27–5).
- May require ORIF.

Calcaneus Fractures

- Calcaneus fractures also may occur as a result of direct trauma or as a stress reaction to overuse.
- Athletes exhibit localized tenderness that is increased with a calcaneal squeeze test.
- As with most stress reactions, plain radiographs are often initially negative but may show increased bony sclerosis over time as the condition improves.
- Again, treatment is typically conservative with slow progression back to normal activities as indicated by the athlete's symptoms.

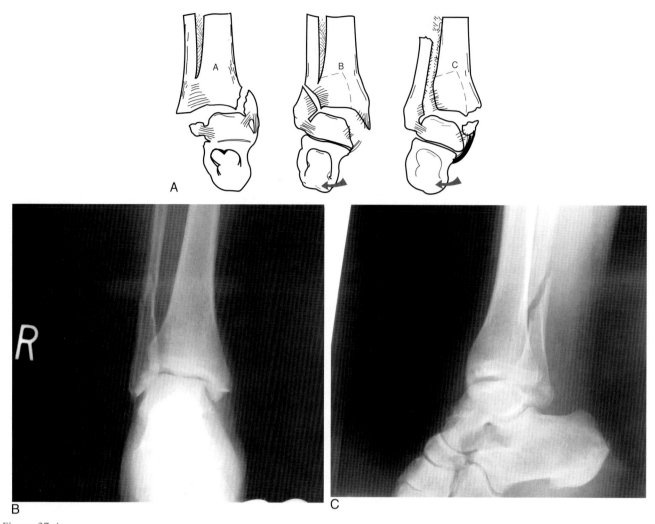

Figure 27-4:
Weber classification of ankle fractures. **A,** Danis-Weber (AO/ASIF) classification of ankle fractures. **B,** Weber C ankle fracture—note the fracture is above the level of the mortise. C, Lateral view of Weber C ankle fracture. (**A** redrawn from Carr JB, Trafton PG: In Browner BD, Jupiter JB, Levine AM, Trafton PG, editors: *Skeletal trauma,* 2nd ed. Philadelphia, 1998, WB Saunders.)

Fifth Metatarsal Base Fractures (Jones Fracture)

- This is common in the athletic population.
- It may be related to stress injuries.
- The mechanism of injury for Jones fracture is forefoot adduction.
- Internal fixation with an intramedullary screw can result in earlier return to training for competitive athletes (Figure 27–6).

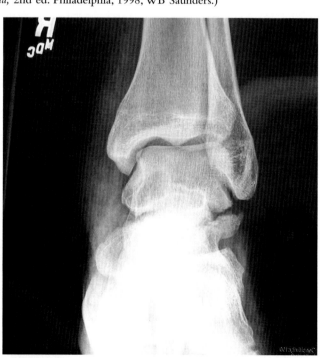

Figure 27-5:
Snowboarder's ankle (fracture of the lateral process of the talus).

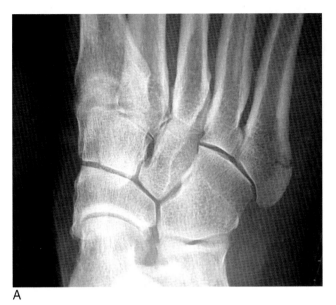

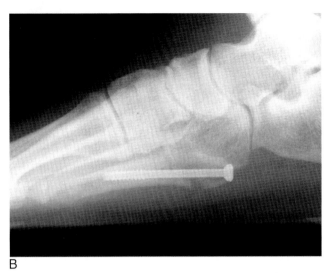

Figure 27-6:
A, Radiographic appearance of Jones fracture. **B,** Lateral radiograph of Jones fracture open reduction and internal fixation.

References

Arendt E, Agel J, Heikes C, Griffiths H: Stress injuries to bone in college athletes. *Am J Sports Med* 31:959-968, 2003.

> *This retrospective review of Division I college athletes identified those factors related to stress injuries to bone that have the greatest effect on return to play. The authors formulate their own grading system of stress reaction to demonstrate their findings.*

Boon AJ, Smith J, Zobitz ME, Amrami KM: Snowboarder's talus fracture. *Am J Sports Med* 29:333-338, 2001.

> *These authors discuss "snowboarder's ankle." It is thought that these injuries result from a dorsiflexion and inversion mechanism. The axial loading that occurs as a result of jumping maneuvers may also play a role. The clinical picture resembles a simple ankle sprain, but radiographs often demonstrate a fracture of the lateral process of the talus.*

Clough TM: Femoral neck stress fracture: the importance of clinical suspicion and early review. *Br J Sports Med* 36:308-309, 2002.

> *This author reviews the clinical presentation of stress fractures of the femoral neck and emphasizes that these fractures are often missed initially, but keeping a high index of suspicion can lead to earlier diagnosis and treatment.*

Korpelainen R, Orava S, Karpakka J, et al: Risk factors for recurrent stress fractures in athletes. *Am J Sports Med* 29:304-310, 2001.

> *These authors identify the risk factors leading to the development of stress fractures by questioning and examining athletes with the diagnosis. They discover factors such as high training mileage, high arch, leg-length discrepancy, and irregular menses in females all play a role in the development of this condition.*

Reese K, Litsky A, Kaeding C, et al: Cannulated screw fixation of Jones fractures. *Am J Sports Med* 32:1736-1742, 2004.

> *These authors address the problem of the Jones fracture, which is known for a high incidence of delayed union and refracture. They retrospectively review their own cases, as well as perform an in vitro biomechanical study to determine cannulated screw strength.*

Shin AY, Morin WD, Gorman JD, et al: The superiority of magnetic resonance imaging in differentiating the cause of hip pain in endurance athletes. *Am J Sports Med* 24:168-176, 1996.

> *These authors advocate that MRI is markedly superior to other imaging studies, specifically plain radiography and bone scan, in identifying femoral neck stress fractures. They cite a sensitivity of only 68% for bone scan and 100% for MRI in evaluating this particular disorder.*

Stanish WD: Lower leg, foot, and ankle injuries in young athletes. *Clin Sports Med* 14:651-668, 1995.

> *This is a review of common lower extremity injuries that occur in sports including compartment syndrome, tendonitis, ankle sprains, and fractures.*

Leg, Ankle, and Foot Nerve Entrapment Syndromes

History, Physical Examination, and Imaging

- Although pathology may exist anywhere along the course of a particular nerve, several nerve entrapment conditions occur as a result of nerve compression along typical anatomic sites (Box 28–1).
- The superficial peroneal nerve is most commonly affected in athletes.
- Symptoms are most often produced with certain activities, and a good history can aid in directing the diagnosis. However, patients may also present with nonspecific and poorly localized symptoms.
- Similar symptoms may be produced by compartment syndrome, muscular injury, and vascular or nerve root pathology and should be ruled out. Occasionally, more than one condition coexists.
- A complete examination and electrodiagnostic studies may suffice to derive at the appropriate diagnosis.
- A good understanding of the neural anatomy of the lower extremity and motor and sensory distributions is essential for proper evaluation (Table 28–1).
- The patient may need to be examined after a period of exercise for diagnostic purposes.
- Commonly, there is tenderness along the affected nerve and a positive Tinel's sign can be elicited.
- Occasionally, electrodiagnostic studies may be negative, requiring the physician to make the diagnosis solely on clinical examination.
- Positive electromyography or nerve conduction studies may not correlate with surgical findings or outcomes.
- Radiographs should be ordered to rule out any bony pathology.
- Occasionally, magnetic resonance imaging (MRI) and ultrasound may be useful adjuncts for diagnosis and preoperative assessment.

Types

Saphenous Nerve

- Impingement can occur at the site of Hunter's (adductor) canal or as it pierces the fascia lata between the sartorius and gracilis muscles.
- Injury of its infrapatellar branch during knee surgery may result in a symptomatic neuroma.
- Patients may complain of medial knee or leg pain when exercising.

Common Peroneal Nerve

- Entrapment takes place as it travels between the biceps tendon and lateral head of the gastrocnemius muscle or posterior to the fibular neck between the heads of the peroneus muscle (peroneal tunnel) (Figure 28–1).
- Injury to the nerve may occur by a direct blow to the lateral knee or a genu varus deformity.
- Plantar flexion or inversion of the ankle tightens the peroneus longus, which may compress the nerve against the proximal fibula. Activities that require these

---

Box 28–1 | Common Sites of Nerve Entrapment

Saphenous n.—Hunter's canal or between the sartorius and gracilis muscles as it passes through the fascia lata

Common peroneal n.—Between the biceps tendon and lateral head of the gastrocnemius or between the heads of the peroneus muscle (peroneal tunnel), posterior to the fibular neck

Superficial peroneal n.—8-12 cm superior to the lateral malleolus as it pierces the fascia

Deep peroneal n.—Inferior extensor retinaculum

Tibial n.—Flexor retinaculum

Lateral plantar n.—Between the fascia of the abductor hallucis longus and quadratus plantae muscle

Medial plantar n.—At the intersection of the digitorum longus and flexor hallucis longus

Sural n.—Distal to the lateral malleolus

Interdigital n.—Between the third and fourth digits

Table 28–1:   Motor and Sensory Distribution of Nerves of the Lower Leg

NERVE	MOTOR	SENSORY
Saphenous		Anteromedial knee Medial leg and foot
Common peroneal	Divides into superficial and deep peroneal nerves	Provides lateral sural cutaneous nerves
Superficial peroneal (branch off common peroneal)	Peroneus longus Peroneus brevis	Inferior anterolateral leg Dorsum of foot Dorsum of great, second, third, and fourth toes
Deep peroneal (branch off common peroneal)	Tibialis anterior Extensor digitorum longus Extensor digitorum brevis Peroneus tertius Extensor hallucis longus Extensor hallucis brevis	Skin between great and second toe (first web space)
Tibial	Gastrocnemius Soleus Plantaris Popliteus Tibialis posterior Flexor digitorum longus Flexor digitorum brevis	Provides medial sural cutaneous nerve and cutaneous calcaneal branches
Sural		Lateral calf, heel, and foot
Lateral plantar	Three lateral lumbricals Quadratus plantae Flexor digiti minimi brevis Abductor digiti minimi Adductor hallucis Plantar interossei Dorsal interossei	Plantar skin of about 1½ of the lateral digits
Medial plantar	Abductor hallucis Flexor hallucis brevis Flexor digitorum brevis First lumbrical	Plantar skin of about 3½ of the medial digits
Interdigital nerves—Formed from the medial and lateral plantar nerves		

movements repetitively, such as running and bicycling, may explain symptoms.

- Postexercise examination may reveal weak ankle dorsiflexion and inversion.
- Other possible examination findings include a positive Tinel's sign at the fibular neck and increase of pain symptoms when the peroneus longus is put on stretch with ankle inversion.

Superficial Peroneal Nerve

- Supplies innervation to the peroneus brevis and longus.
- Usually entrapped 8 to 12 cm above the lateral malleolus where it pierces the fascia of the anterolateral compartment (Figure 28–2).
- Entrapment may be caused by fascial defects, fibrous strands, and muscle herniation.
- Patients most commonly complain of pain along the lateral, distal aspect of their calf and dorsum of the

foot that is aggravated by activity and often relieved with rest.

- Improper shoe wear and activities requiring quick turns and frequent contraction of the peroneals, such as in skiing and skating, are common extrinsic factors.
- Passive plantar flexion and eversion or active dorsiflexion and eversion against resistance may reproduce tenderness at the site of entrapment.

Deep Peroneal Nerve

- Also known as anterior tarsal tunnel syndrome.
- Most common site of impingement occurs under the inferior extensor retinaculum.
- Compression along the superior edge of the retinaculum where the extensor hallucis longus crosses over the nerve is proposed to be the primary cause (Figure 28–3).

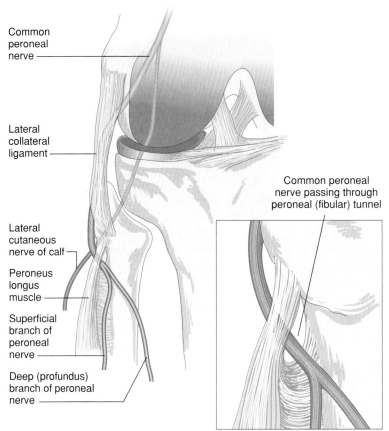

Figure 28–1:
Anatomy of the common peroneal nerve and peroneal tunnel. (From McCrory P, Bell S, Bradshaw C: *Sports Med* 32:371-391, 2002.)

- Symptoms of dorsal foot pain, occasionally radiating to the first web space, are often present.
- Examination is notable for localized tenderness, reduced sensation in the first web space, and extensor digitorum brevis weakness.

Tibial Nerve

- Also known as tarsal tunnel syndrome.
- Impingement occurs under the flexor retinaculum, posterior to the medial malleolus, and can occasionally be associated with compression from space-occupying lesions such as ganglia or varicosities (Figure 28–4).
- Other possible etiologies include trauma and foot or ankle deformity.
- Patients may report diffuse pain along the medial malleolus, which is greater with activity, and paresthesias along the medial ankle that may radiate to the arch of the foot.
- Examination may uncover tenderness posterior to the medial malleolus, a positive Tinel's sign, and decreased sensation along the nerve distribution.
- A dorsiflexion-eversion test has been described as an effective provocative diagnostic maneuver. The ankle is

maximally everted and dorsiflexed while all the toes are dorsiflexed, causing further compression of the tibial nerve, often resulting in an intensification of symptoms (Figure 28–5).

Sural Nerve

- Compression may be produced anywhere along its course but is most prone to damage distal to the lateral malleolus.
- Inversion ankle injuries may lead to symptoms (Figure 28–2).
- Contributing extrinsic factors include ganglia, postsurgical scars, and inflammation of the Achilles tendon. Tight ski boots and casts may also aggravate the nerve.

Lateral Plantar Nerve

- As a branch of the tibial nerve, entrapment occurs distal to the medial malleolus, usually between the fascia of the abductor hallucis longus and the quadratus plantae muscle.
- Symptoms include pain and paresthesias along the distribution of the nerve.

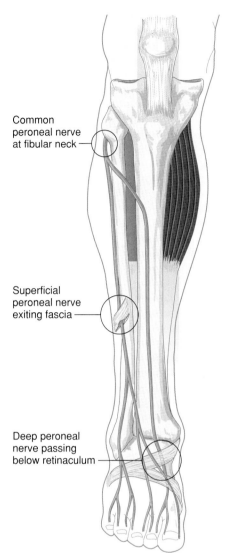

Figure 28–2:
The peroneal nerve can be trapped at the neck of the fibula (common peroneal nerve) as it exits the fascia (superficial peroneal nerve) or as it passes below the retinaculum (deep peroneal nerve).

- Examination may demonstrate abduction weakness of the small toe, secondary to the compromised innervation of the abductor digit quinti, and decreased sensation along the lateral 1½ digits.

Medial Plantar Nerve

- Entrapment of the nerve usually occurs near the knot of Henry, where the flexor digitorum longus intersects with the flexor hallucis longus tendon.
- Nicknamed "jogger's foot," this condition often results from arch supports or calluses or by a hallux valgus deformity that places tension on the nerve.
- Patients often complain of pain and paresthesias radiating to the medial toes.
- Examination may reveal localized tenderness and decreased sensation of the medial digits.

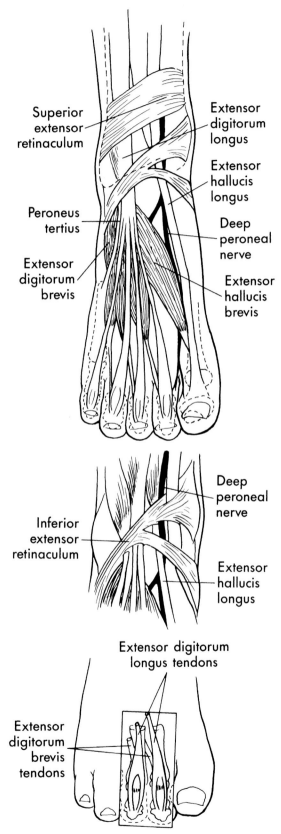

Figure 28–3:
Anatomy of the anterior tarsal tunnel. (From Richardson EG: Neurogenic disorders. In Canale ST, editor: *Campbell's operative orthopaedics,* 9th ed. St Louis, 1998, Mosby-Year Book.)

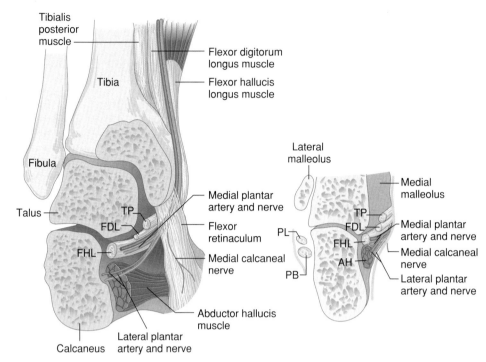

Figure 28–4:
Anatomy of the tarsal tunnel. AH, abductor hallucis; FDL, flexor digitorum longus; FHL, flexor hallucis longus; PB, peroneus brevis; PL, peroneus longus; TP, tibialis posterior. (From McCrory P, Bell S, Bradshaw C: *Sports Med* 32:371-391, 2002.)

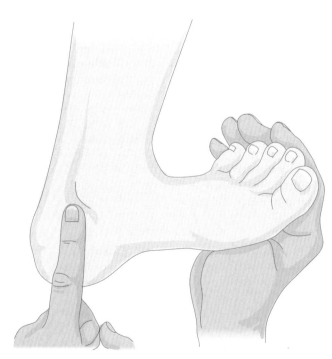

Figure 28–5:
Dorsiflexion–eversion test for the diagnosis of tarsal tunnel syndrome. The ankle is maximally dorsiflexed and everted while all the toes are maximally dorsiflexed.

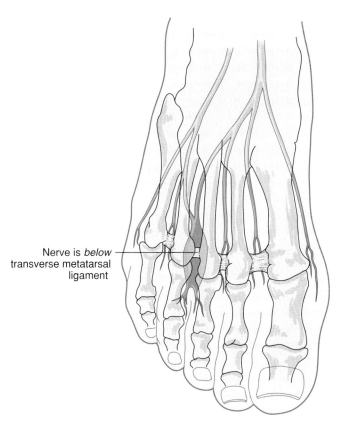

Nerve is *below* transverse metatarsal ligament

Figure 28–6:
Resection of interdigital neuroma. (Redrawn from Mann RA, Baxter DE: Diseases of the nerves. In Coughlin MJ, Mann RA, editors: *Surgery of the foot and ankle,* 6th ed. St Louis, 1993, Mosby.)

Interdigital Nerve

- Classically referred to by its misnomer, Morton's neuroma, this condition is produced by perineural fibrosis from repetitive nerve irritation of the common digital nerve between the metatarsal heads (Figure 28–6).
- Can occur between any of the toes but most commonly arises between the third and fourth digits.
- It is most common in women and is associated with compression from tight-fitting shoes.
- Patients most frequently complain of localized plantar pain, aggravated with activity or high-heeled shoes, and feel as though they have a marble or rock in their shoe. They may also report paresthesias of adjacent toes and relief at rest with their shoes off.
- Stress fractures, metatarsalgia, and arthritis should be ruled out.

Treatment

- Many of these conditions resolve over time or can be controlled by nonoperative management.
- Patients should be instructed on possible extrinsic factors that may be modified, such as shoe wear, training techniques, and aggravating activities.

- Orthotics and pads may reduce stresses imposed on the nerve.
- Nonsteroidal antiinflammatory drugs (NSAIDs), stretching, and warm baths may also provide relief.
- Steroid injection of Morton's neuroma may be considered during treatment.
- Surgical exploration and release of impingement sites or resection of neuromas and ganglia, or both, following failure of conservative techniques, is often successful. (Figures 28–6 and 28–7).

Rehabilitation

- Patients should be instructed on appropriate stretching exercises that may relieve muscular tension.
- Patients should be advised that, after surgical treatment, recovery of nerve function may be delayed.

Complications

- Complex regional pain syndrome may develop from nerve entrapment syndromes.
- Chronic paresthesias and pain may lead to plantar ulcers.
- Neuromas may recur or become more symptomatic after excision.
- Surgical release may result in scarring and persistent pain.

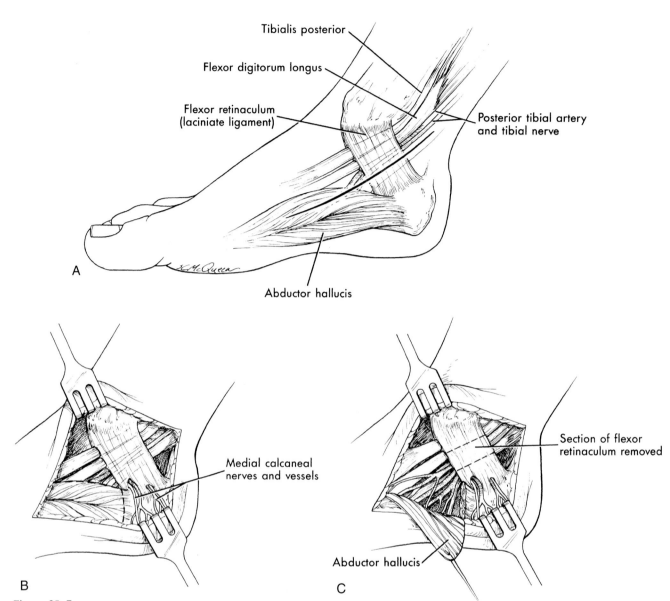

Figure 28–7:

A-C, Tarsal tunnel release. (From Richardson EG: Neurogenic disorders. In Canale ST, editor: *Campbell's operative orthopaedics*, 9th ed. St Louis, 1998, Mosby-Year Book.)

References

Bailie DS, Kelikian AS: Tarsal tunnel syndrome: diagnosis, surgical technique, and functional outcome. *Foot Ankle Int* 19:65-72, 1998.

Authors review the diagnosis and surgical treatment of tarsal tunnel syndrome in 47 patients. Authors comment that diagnosis is best made clinically after demonstrating a positive Tinel's sign and nerve compression test in all their patients. Electrodiagnostic studies were abnormal in 81% of the cases. Authors stress the importance of also dividing part of the abductor hallucis fascia during surgical release of the tarsal tunnel. Overall, 72% of the patients were satisfied after surgery.

Delfaut EM, Demondion X, Bieganski A, et al: Imaging of foot and ankle nerve entrapment syndromes: from well-demonstrated to unfamiliar sites. *Radiographics* 23:613–623, 2003.

Authors review the anatomy of nerve entrapment syndromes in the foot and ankle. MRI findings and predisposing factors of nerve entrapment are also discussed. Several MRI images are provided.

Kinoshita M, Okuda R, Morikawa J, et al: The dorsiflexion-eversion test for diagnosis of tarsal tunnel syndrome. *J Bone Joint Surg Am* 83:1835-1839, 2001.

Authors describe a provocative maneuver to diagnose tarsal tunnel syndrome. The dorsiflexion-eversion test was noted to intensify symptoms in 82% of the 44 feet with tarsal tunnel syndrome.

Lau JTC, Daniels TR: Tarsal tunnel syndrome: a review of the literature. *Foot Ankle Int* 20:201-209, 1999.

Authors provide a good review of tarsal tunnel syndrome. Anatomy, etiologies, clinical presentation, diagnosis, and nonoperative and operative treatment with results are discussed. Diagnostic and treatment algorithms are provided. Revision of tarsal tunnel release is also reviewed.

McCrory P, Bell S, Bradshaw C: Nerve entrapments of the lower leg, ankle and foot in sport. *Sports Med* 32:371-391, 2002.
Great review of the anatomy and entrapment conditions of nerves of the lower extremity associated with exercise activity. Etiologies, clinical presentation, diagnosis, and treatment of each nerve are discussed individually, including surgical techniques for operative management.

Mitra A, Stern JD, Perrotta VJ, Moyer RA: Peroneal nerve entrapment in athletes. *Ann Plast Surg* 35:366-368, 1995.
Authors review findings of 12 patients with exercise-induced peroneal nerve entrapment and 7 cadaveric dissections. All patients complained of exertional leg pain and impaired performance and demonstrated weakness on foot dorsiflexion and positive electroneuromyographic studies. Cadaveric dissection demonstrated that common sites of entrapment include the proximal origin of the peroneus longus (fibular tunnel) and the intermuscular septum, both of which must be divided for successful nerve decompression.

Oh SJ, Meyer RD: Entrapment neuropathies of the tibial (posterior tibial) nerve. *Neurol Clin* 17:593-615, 1999.
Comprehensive review of entrapment neuropathies of the tibial nerve including proximal tibial neuropathy, tarsal tunnel syndrome, medial plantar neuropathy, lateral plantar neuropathy, calcaneal neuropathy, interdigital neuropathy, and sural neuropathy. Anatomy with a focus on sites of entrapment is well covered.

Sharp RJ, Wade CM, Hennessy MS, Saxby TS: The role of MRI and ultrasound imaging in Morton's neuroma and the effect of size of lesion on symptoms. *J Bone Joint Surg Br* 85:999-1005, 2003.
Prospective study comparing the accuracy of clinical examination, MRI, and ultrasound in correctly diagnosing Morton's neuroma. Results demonstrated that clinical assessment was the most sensitive and specific modality, even when compared with the use of both MRI and ultrasound. Authors also report that neuroma size does not predict severity of symptoms or correlate with postoperative outcomes. Neurectomy performed on the 29 cases studied produced excellent to good results in 89% of the patients.

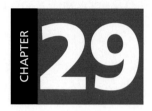

Toe Injuries/Disorders

Turf Toe

- The term *turf toe* refers to injury to the first metatarsophalangeal joint.
- Mechanism is forced hyperextension to the plantar plate (Figure 29–1).
- Grades of turf toe (Table 29–1).
- Dorsiflexion stress radiograph may detect disruption of the plantar plate by evaluating the sesamoids (Figure 29–2).
- Magnetic resonance imaging (MRI) is recommended for any patient with radiographic abnormalities and all grade 2 and 3 sprains.
- Conservative treatment is generally indicated.
  - Rest.
  - Ice.
  - Nonsteroidal antiinflammatory drugs (NSAIDS).
  - Taping.
  - Rigid orthoses.
- Surgical intervention is usually not necessary but may be indicated in cases of osteochondral injury or instability of the first metatarsophalangeal joint (Box 29–1).
  - Primary repair of the plantar plate complex is indicated whenever possible.
  - The abductor hallucis can be used to reinforce the plantar plate.
- Primary repair of the plantar plate may be indicated in elite athletes.
- The long-term sequela of turf toe includes hallux rigidus.

Fractures

- The most common mechanism of sports-related phalangeal fracture is direct trauma (being stepped on by another player).
- Most common in the proximal phalanx.
- Fifth toe most commonly affected.
- Treatment is generally conservative with buddy taping and use of rigid soled shoes.

Dislocations

- Complex dislocations occur when the plantar plate and deep transverse metatarsal ligament are displaced over the head of the metatarsals and become trapped between the flexor tendons laterally and the lumbricals medially.
- Treatment may require open reduction with division of the transverse metatarsal ligament and plantar plate.
- Interphalangeal joint dislocations are rare.
- Closed reduction and buddy taping is usually successful.
- Hallux interphalangeal dislocations are often irreducible and may require open reduction with removal of trapped plantar plate.

Sesamoiditis

- Sesamoiditis refers to the general inflammation associated with tendinitis of the flexor hallucis longus.

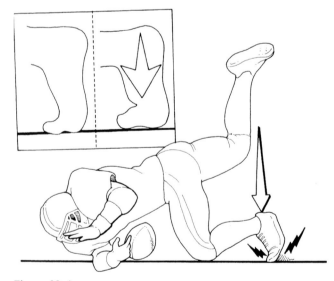

Figure 29–1:
The mechanism of injury of turf toe involves acute dorsiflexion of the first metatarsophalangeal joint. (From Miller MD, Cooper DE, Warner JJP: *Review of sports medicine and arthroscopy*. Philadelphia, 2000, WB Saunders.)

GRADE	INJURY	SYMPTOMS	RETURN TO PLAY
1	Stretching of capsulo-ligamentous complex	Localized tenderness Minimal swelling	May return but uncomfortable
2	Partial tear of capsule.	Intense tenderness Diffuse swelling Ecchymosis Decreased ROM (guarding)	Unable to play at normal level
3	Tearing of plantar plate and joint impaction +/- sesamoid injury	Severe pain Marked swelling Marked ecchymosis Tender plantar and dorsal	Unable to bear weight

Table 29–1:   Grades of Turf Toe

ROM, range of motion.

- The medial sesamoid is the most commonly involved.
- Generally there is no specific injury reported but rather a gradual onset of pain.
- Pain on weight-bearing is the most common complaint.
- May result in significant disabling pain to the athlete.
- Physical examination reveals tenderness over the area of the sesamoids and increased pain with active great toe flexion.
- Radiographs are typically normal, although this condition may lead to sesamoid chondromalacia.
- Bone scan may show increased signal to the sesamoids but is relatively nonspecific.
- Treatment is generally conservative.
  - Rest.
  - Ice.

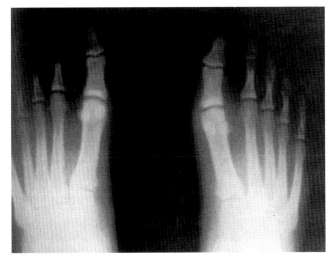

Figure 29–2:
Anteroposterior radiograph demonstrating proximal migration of the sesamoids (right) following plantar plate rupture. (From Mullen JE, O'Malley MJ: *Clin Sports Med* **23:97-121, 2004.)**

- NSAIDs.
- Metatarsal bars to unload the area of the metatarsal heads.
- In rare cases, surgical treatment with sesamoidectomy may be warranted.
  - In these cases, only one sesamoid should be excised to avoid a claw toe deformity.

Sesamoid Fracture

- Fractures of the sesamoid may occur as a result of direct trauma or forced great toe hyperextension.
- Medial sesamoid fractures are the most common.
- Diagnosis is made by history of trauma, tenderness over the sesamoid bones, and radiographic images.
  - Images should include anteroposterior (AP), lateral, and oblique views. An axial view may also be helpful.
- The history and physical examination should be able to distinguish between true sesamoid fracture and bipartite sesamoids.
- Treatment is generally conservative with hard-soled shoes, although symptoms may be prolonged.
- Sesamoidectomy may be necessary if there is persistent pain despite appropriate conservative treatment.
- Other surgical indications include nonunion and posttraumatic degenerative changes.
- Stress fracture of the sesamoids may also occur.
  - These should be treated in a short-leg cast with a toe plate for up to 6 weeks.

Nail Bed Disorders

- Subungual hematoma.
  - Hemorrhage beneath the nail bed.
  - Drilling or burning through the nail plate may relieve pressure.
- Paronychia.

Box 29–1	Surgical Indications for Turf Toe

Large capsular avulsions with unstable joint.
Diastasis of a bipartite or sesamoid fracture
Traumatic bunion
Retraction of sesamoids
Loose body

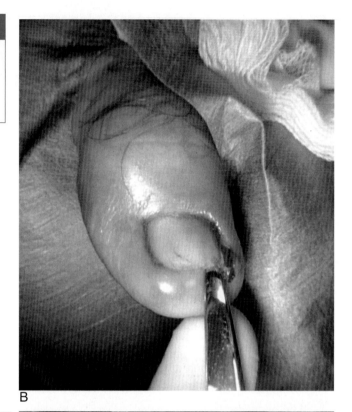

- Inflammation of the nail groove.
- May extend to the nail matrix (onychia).
- May be related to an ingrown toenail.
- Treatment involves excising a linear portion of the nail margin (Figure 29–3).
- For more extensive infection, complete toenail removal may be required (Figure 29–4).

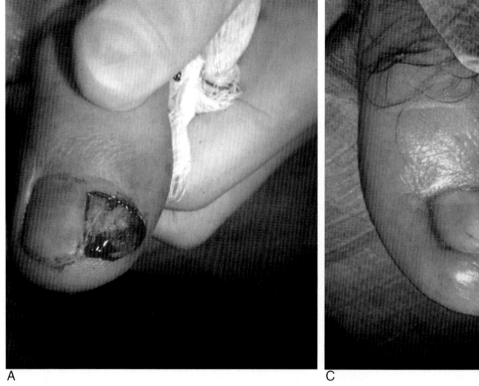

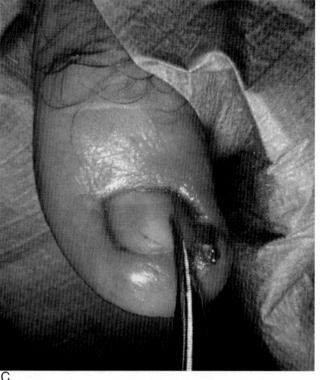

Figure 29–3:
A, Excision of a linear portion of the nail after freeing the undersurface of the nail. The lateral edge is longitudinally sectioned. **B,** The free edge of the nail is grasped and elevated with the hemostat. **C,** The nail is longitudinally resected.

(*continued*)

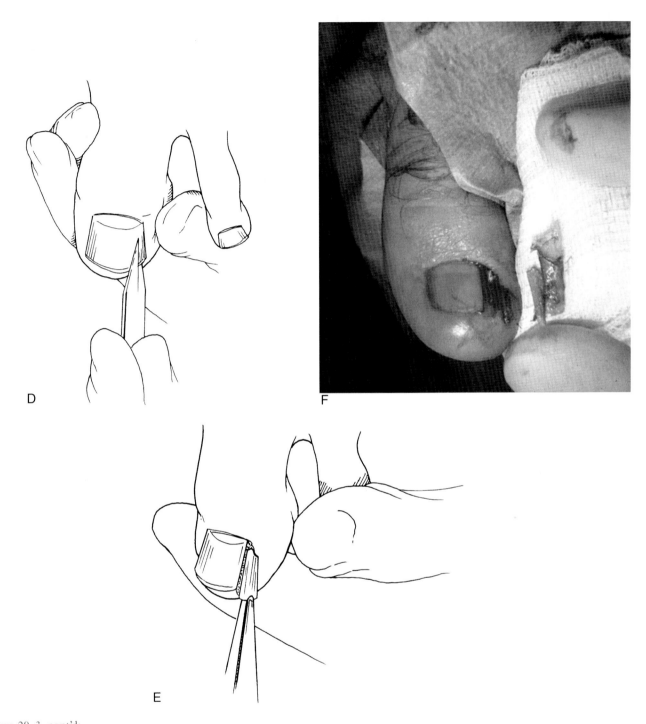

Figure 29–3, cont'd:
D, The nail is longitudinally resected. **E,** The edge is grasped with a hemostat. **F,** The free edge is removed. (**A, B, C,** and **F** from Mann RA, Coughlin MJ: *The video textbook of foot and ankle surgery.* St Louis, 1990, Medical Video Productions; **D** and **E** from Coughlin MJ: Toenail abnormalities. In Coughlin RJ, Mann RA, editors: *Surgery of the foot and ankle,* 7th ed. St Louis, 1999, Mosby.)

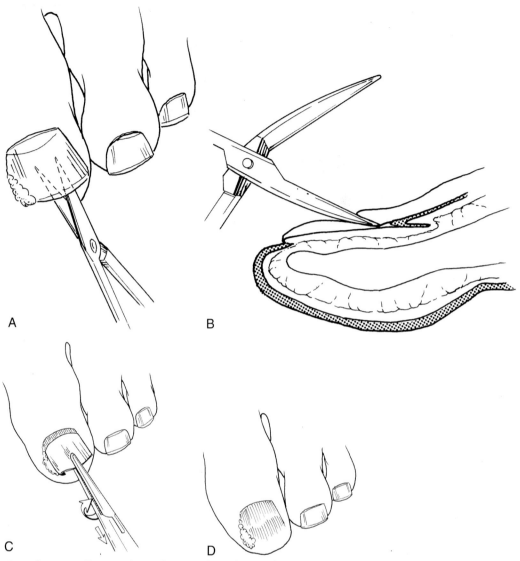

Figure 29–4: Complete toenail removal. **A,** Elevation from the nail bed. **B,** Removal of dorsal soft tissue attachments of the nail plate. **C,** The nail plate is grasped with the hemostat and removed. **D,** Toenail completely removed. (From Coughlin MJ: Toenail abnormalities. In Coughlin RJ, Mann RA, editors: *Surgery of the foot and ankle,* 7th ed. St Louis, 1999, Mosby.)

References

Biedert R, Hintemann B: Stress fractures of the medial great toe and sesamoids. *Foot Ankle Int* 24:137-141, 2003.
> *The authors look at the common signs and symptoms associated with stress fractures of the medial great toe and sesamoids. Bone scan and sagittal CT scan were the most useful tests. They also recommend surgical excision of the fragments if conservative treatment fails.*

Bowers KD Jr, Martin RB: Turf-toe: a shoe surface related football injury. *Med Sci Exer* 8:81-83, 1976.
> *This is the original description of turf toe. They found that this was an injury related to hard play surface and the use of flexible shoewear.*

Clanton TO, Ford JJ: Turf toe injury. *Clin Sports Med* 13:731-741:1994.
> *This article reviews the diagnosis especially in athletic populations. They discuss the long-term complications of this injury and review the incidence and treatment options.*

Clanton TO, Schon LW: Athletic injuries to the soft tissues of the foot and ankle. In Mann RA, Coughlin MJ, editors: *Surgery of the Foot and Ankle,* 6th ed. St Louis, 1993, Mosby Yearbook.
> *This chapter provides an excellent review of sports-related injuries to the foot and ankle. Discussion includes turf toe, fractures, dislocations, and other common injuries.*

Coughlin MJ: Toenail abnormalities. In Mann RA, Coughlin RJ, editors: *Surgery of the Foot and Ankle,* 6th ed. St Louis, 1993, Mosby-Year Book.
> *An excellent overview of toenail disorders including nail bed injuries, fractures, and dislocations and the treatment option for each type of injury.*

Grace DL: Sesamoid problems. *Foot Ankle Clin* 5:609-627, 2000.
> *This article provides a reivew o the newest imaging techniques and innovations in treatment of common sesamoid problems.*

Mullen JE, O'Malley MJ: Sprains—residual instability of subtalar Lisfranc joints and turf toe. *Clin Sports Med* 23:97-121, 1994.
> *A review of foot injuries in athletics with discussion specifically of turf toe including treatment recommendations.*

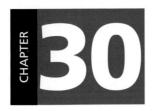
Shoulder Anatomy and Biomechanics

Introduction

- The shoulder is composed of three bones (clavicle, scapula, humerus) that form four joints (glenohumeral, acromioclavicular [AC], scapulothoracic [not truly a joint], and sternoclavicular) (Figure 30–1).
- The shoulder girdle, composed of the clavicle and scapula, serves to connect the trunk and upper limb.
- The shoulder has a great range of mobility when compared with its lower extremity counterpart (the hip) at the expense of decreased stability.
- The shoulder can be divided into four supporting layers (Figure 30–2, Box 30–1).

Osteology

Clavicle

- A horizontally S-shaped extension from the manubrium to the acromion, serving to attach the upper extremity to the axial skeleton.
- Has a double curvature where anteriorly it is convex along the medial two thirds of its body and then flattens out and becomes concave at its lateral one-third portion. This is believed to provide increased resiliency.
- It is the first bone in the body to ossify at 5 weeks of fetal gestation and the last to fuse at approximately 25 years of age.
- It derives from medial and lateral primary ossification centers and a sternal secondary ossification center.
- Attachment to the scapula is secured through AC and coracoclavicular (CC) ligaments (Figure 30–3).
- AC ligaments provide anteroposterior stability to the joint, and the CC ligaments prevent inferior migration of the acromion and coracoid from the clavicle.
- Has three primary functions.
  - Serves as a fulcrum on which the upper limb is held free from the trunk, allowing a maximum range of motion.
  - Provides attachment sites for muscles.
  - Transmits forces from the upper extremity to the trunk.

Scapula

- Triangular-shaped bone that spans the second through seventh ribs and connects the clavicle to the humerus via the AC and glenohumeral joints.
- Its surfaces provide attachment sites for several muscles (Figure 30–4).
- Anteriorly the bone is concave, allowing better contact with the underlying rib cage, and posteriorly it is convex.
- The spine of the scapula projects from the posterior surface and serves as a division between the smaller supraspinous and larger infraspinous fossas.
- Anterior projections include the acromion ("point of the shoulder") and the coracoid, which help form and stabilize the AC joint.
- The acromion serves as a site of origination for most of the deltoid muscle and one of the insertion sites for the trapezius and an area of attachment for the AC ligaments.

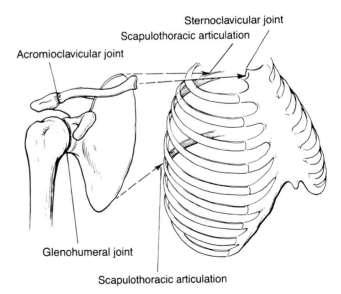

Figure 30–1:
Anatomy of the shoulder girdle and associated joints. (From Warner JJP, Caborn DN: *Crit Rev Phys Rehabil Med* 4:145-198, 1992.)

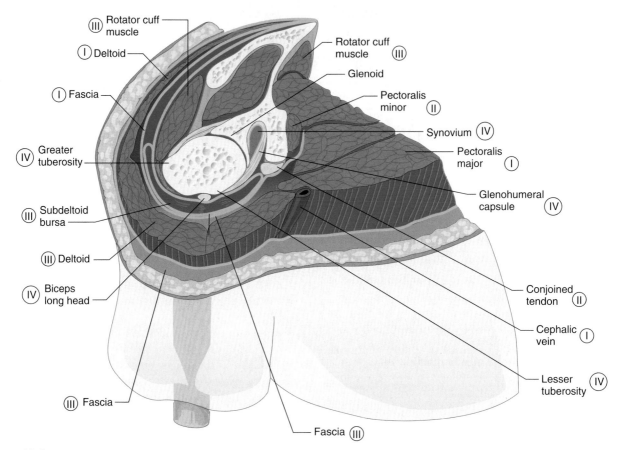

Figure 30–2:
Cross-sectional view of the right shoulder demonstrating the four layers.

- The coracoid provides a surface for the origin of the short head of the biceps and coracobrachialis (conjoined tendon) and attachment sites for the pectoralis minor muscle and CC ligament.
- Composed of three angles: superior (at level of T2 vertebra), inferior (at level of T7 vertebra), and lateral.

Box 30–1   Supporting Layers of the Shoulder

I	Deltoid
	Pectoralis major
II	Clavipectoral fascia
	Conjoined tendon, short head biceps and coracobrachialis
	Coracoacromial ligament
III	Deep layer of subdeltoid bursa
	Rotator cuff muscle (subscapularis, supraspinatus, infraspinatus, teres minor)
IV	Glenohumeral joint capsule
	Coracohumeral ligament

From Miller MD, editor: *Review of orthopaedics*, 3rd ed. Philadelphia, 2000, Saunders.

- The glenoid fossa, at the superolateral end of the scapula, is a pear-shaped socket that is narrower superiorly and averages a vertical diameter of 35 mm and transverse diameter of 25 mm.
- Version of the glenoid may range from 7 degrees retroversion to 10 degrees anteversion and with a 5-degree upward tilt.

Humeral Head

- This relatively smooth, spheroidal-shaped bone averages a diameter of 43 mm.
- It is normally positioned in 30 degrees of retroversion, and its articulating surface tilts approximately 130 degrees superiorly relative to the shaft (Figure 30–5).
- Its two major prominences, the greater and lesser tuberosities, are divided by the bicipital groove and provide attachment sites for the rotator cuff muscles.
- The greater tuberosity serves as the attachment site for the supraspinatus, infraspinatus, and teres minor tendons, whereas the lesser tuberosity is the attachment site for the subscapularis muscle.

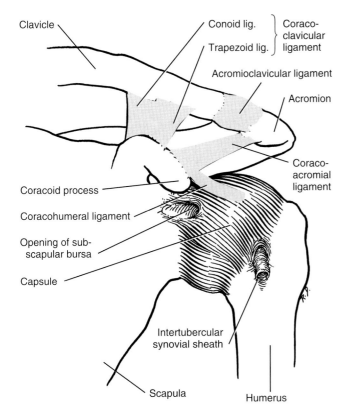

Figure 30–3:
Ligaments about the shoulder. (From Jenkins DB, Hollinshead WH: *Hollinshead's functional anatomy of the limbs and back,* 8th ed. Philadelphia, 2002, Saunders.)

Joints

Glenohumeral Joint

- "Ball and socket" joint that provides greater freedom of motion than any other joint in the body at the expense of stability.
- Movement occurs mainly along three axes allowing flexion-extension, abduction-adduction, circumduction, and rotation.
- The shallow, smaller, pear-shaped glenoid cavity accepts a third of the larger spheroidal head of the humerus, producing a relatively unstable glenohumeral joint.
- The glenoid labrum is a fibrocartilaginous ring that increases the articulation surface area and deepens the joint cavity (Figure 30–6).
- The labrum is well fixed inferiorly but its superior aspect, which is more mobile and less vascular, may predispose this area to a greater risk of injury.
- Studies have demonstrated that excision of the labrum reduces socket depth by 50% and stability by 20%.
- Strength and stability of the joint are highly dependent on both static and dynamic restraints (Box 30–2).

- Static restraints
  - Articular version—deviation from the normal 30 to 40 degrees of retroversion can be associated with increased instability.
  - Glenoid labrum—provides increased surface area and attachment sites for capsuloligamentous structures. Damage to this fibrous structure compromises shoulder stability (Figure 30–6).
  - Articular conformity—less than 30% of articular contact will likely result in greater instability. Conditions such as glenoid dysplasia, fractures, and labral tears may affect the contact area (Figure 30–7).
  - Negative intraarticular pressure—effective only with low load, some stabilization of the joint occurs through a vacuumlike effect produced within the closed shoulder compartment and an adhesion-cohesion effect produced by the viscous synovial fluid (Figure 30–8).
  - Capsuloligamentous structures—several thickenings of the fibrous capsule that assist in preventing excessive translation (when the particular ligament is put in stretch) in various extreme positions of the shoulder joint. They are described by their origins and insert onto the lesser tuberosity (Figure 30–9).
    - Superior glenohumeral ligament and coracohumeral ligament (rotator interval)—limit inferior translation and external rotation in adduction and posterior translation in an arm that is flexed, adducted, and internally rotated. Also prevent anterosuperior displacement of the humeral head (Figure 30–10).
    - Middle glenohumeral ligament—limits external rotation in adduction; inferior translation of an adducted, externally rotated arm; and anterior/posterior translation when the arm is externally rotated and partially abducted (Figure 30–10).
    - Inferior glenohumeral ligament—limits anterior, posterior, and inferior translation between 45 and 90 degrees of elevation (Figure 30–11).
  - Posterior capsule—restrains posterior translation in a humerus that is flexed, adducted, and internally rotated. Is the thinnest portion of the articular capsule.
  - Rotator interval—area in the shoulder joint bordered by the supraspinatus superiorly, subscapularis inferiorly, coracoid process medially, and the biceps and humerus laterally (Figure 30–12).
    - A deficient rotator interval may contribute to inferior instability with the arm in adduction.
    - A tight interval may result in decreased range of motion and stiffness.
- Dynamic restraints—enhanced stability during midrange positions of the joint.
  - Joint compression—rotator cuff and biceps muscles force the humeral head onto the glenoid cavity throughout the range of motion (enhance concavity-compression effect).

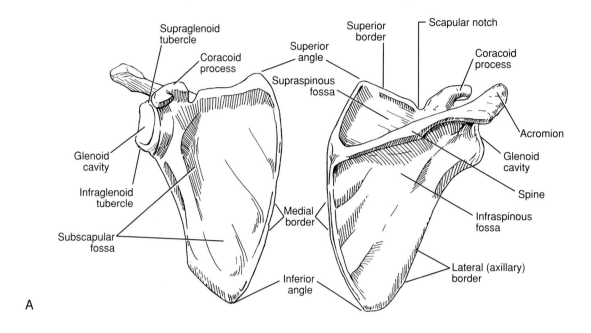

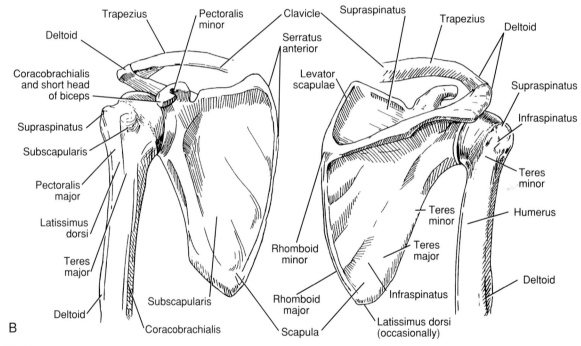

Figure 30–4:

Osteology of the shoulder region and origins and insertions of muscles about the shoulder. **A,** Anterior and posterior views of the bony landmarks of the scapula. **B,** Anterior and posterior view of shoulder muscle insertions. (From Jenkins DB, Hollinshead WH: *Hollinshead's functional anatomy of the limbs and back,* 8th ed. Philadelphia, 2002, Saunders.)

- Rotator cuff—direct attachments to the capsule allow these muscles to increase articular capsule tension, reinforcing joint stability. Furthermore, compression from the musculotendinous units on the joint provides additional support (Figure 30–13).
- Scapular rotators—trapezius, rhomboids, latissimus dorsi, serratus anterior, and levator scapulae ensure that the humerus and scapula harmonize to maintain normal joint articulation throughout range of

motion. There is a 2:1 ratio of humeral-to-scapular elevation. Scapular rotation raises the acromion away from the humeral head, preventing impingement of the rotator cuff muscles (Figures 30–14 and 30–15).

- Long head of the biceps—prevents excessive torsion of the joint when the shoulder is rotating and the elbow is flexing. In addition, it serves to depress the humeral head (Figure 30–16).

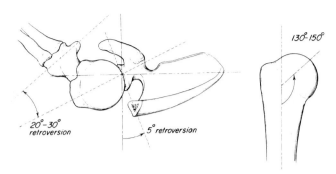

Figure 30–5:
Normal orientation of the humeral head and glenohumeral joint. (From Warner JJP, Caborn DN: *Crit Rev Phys Rehabil Med* 4:145-198, 1992.)

- Proprioception—a muscular reflex response counters capsular stretch and shoulder motion detected by sense receptors.
- Rotator cuff muscles help depress the head of the humerus within the glenoid cavity.
- The supraspinatus and coracoacromial arch (coracoid + CC ligament + acromion) guard the joint superiorly, the infraspinatus and teres minor stabilize it

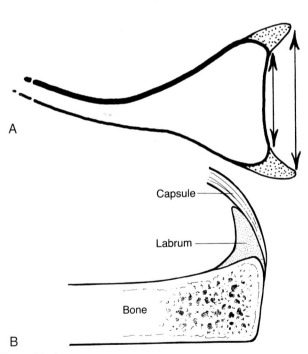

Figure 30–6:
A, Superior view of the scapula and glenoid. Note the glenoid labrum extends the edges of the glenoid, increasing the surface area and depth of the glenoid fossa. **B,** Transverse section through the glenoid demonstrating the association of the labrum and capsule. (A from Warner JJP, Caborn DN: *Crit Rev Phys Rehabil Med* 4:145-198, 1992; B from Miller MD, Cooper DE, Warner JJP: *Review of sports medicine and arthroscopy.* Philadelphia, 2002, Saunders.)

Box 30–2	Static and Dynamic Restraints of the Glenohumeral Joint

Static Restraints

Articular version
Articular conformity
Glenoid labrum
Negative intraarticular pressure
Superior, middle, and inferior glenohumeral ligaments
Capsule
Coracoacromial arch (coracoid + CC ligament + acromion)

Dynamic Restraints

Joint compression
Rotator cuff complex
Scapular rotators
Long head of the biceps
Proprioceptive receptors

CC, Coracoclavicular.

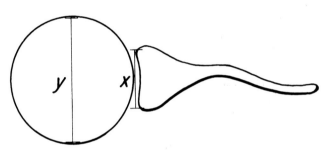

Figure 30–7:
Relationship of humeral head and glenoid. Glenohumeral index (GH) = x/y. (From Warner JJP, Caborn DN: *Crit Rev Phys Rehabil Med* 4:145-198, 1992.)

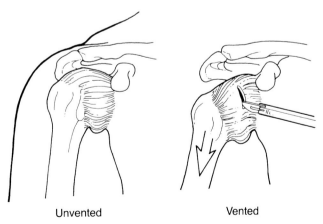

Unvented   Vented

Figure 30–8:
Demonstration of normal negative intraarticular pressure. Note that when the joint is vented, there is inferior subluxation of the humerus. (From Miller MD, Cooper DE, Warner JJP: *Review of sports medicine and arthroscopy.* Philadelphia, 2002, Saunders.)

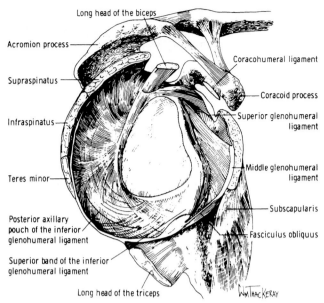

Figure 30–9:
Glenohumeral ligaments and rotator cuff muscles. (From Turkel SJ, Panio MW, Marshall JL, et al: *J Bone Joint Surg Am* 63:1209, 1981.)

posteriorly, and the subscapularis protects the shoulder anteriorly.

- The thin and lax articular capsule connects medially to the glenoid cavity, envelopes the long head of the biceps superiorly, and attaches to the anatomic neck of the humerus laterally.
  - The capsule is weakest inferiorly.

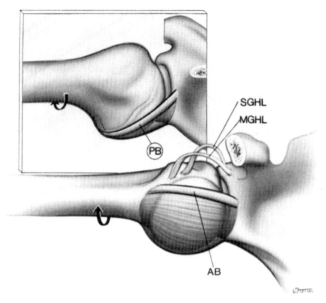

Figure 30–11:
Inferior glenohumeral ligament tightens with abduction and external rotation. (From Warner JJP, Deng X-H, Warren RF, Tozilli AP: *Am J Sports Med* 20:675-685, 1992.)

- Passage of the biceps brachii muscle and connection of the subscapular bursa to the synovial joint inferior to the coracoid create openings in the capsule (Figure 30–3).
- The transverse humeral ligament, which bridges the intertubercular groove, helps maintain the long head of the biceps within its groove as it emerges out from the articular capsule.

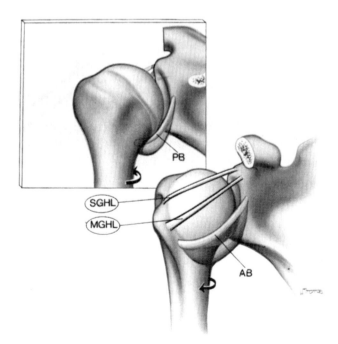

Figure 30–10:
Superior and middle glenohumeral ligaments tighten with adduction and external rotation. (From Warner JJP, Deng X-H, Warren RF, Tozilli AP: *Am J Sports Med* 20:675-685, 1992.)

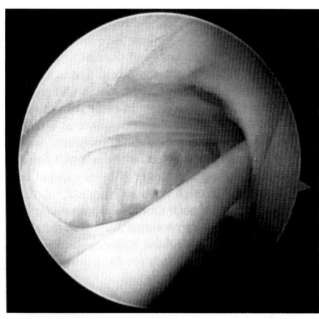

Figure 30–12:
Anatomy of the rotator interval. (From DeLee JC, Drez D Jr, Miller MD, editors: *DeLee and Drez's orthopaedic sports medicine: principles and practice,* 2nd ed. Philadelphia, 2003, Saunders.)

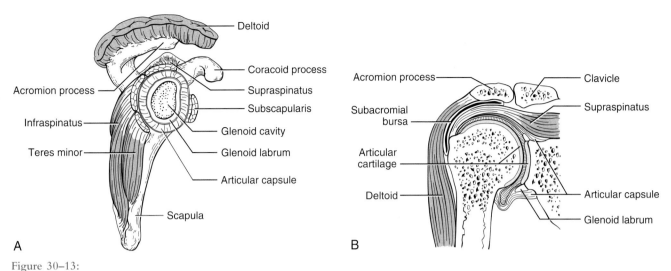

Figure 30–13:
Anatomy of the glenohumeral joint and surrounding structures. Note the relationship of the rotator cuff muscles, the joint, and articular capsule. **A,** Lateral view. **B,** Anterior view. (From Jenkins DB, Hollinshead WH: *Hollinshead's functional anatomy of the limbs and back,* 8th ed. Philadelphia, 2002, Saunders.)

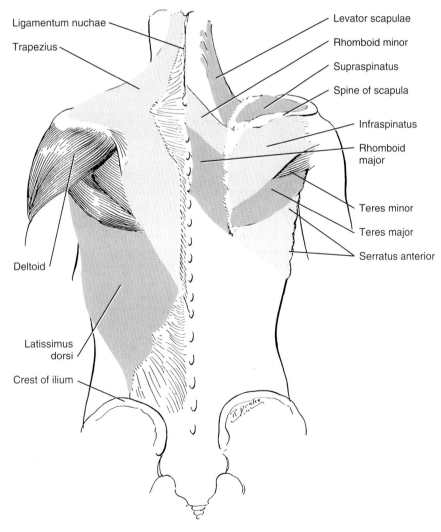

Figure 30–14:
Musculature of the shoulder, posterior view. (From Jenkins DB, Hollinshead WH: *Hollinshead's functional anatomy of the limbs and back,* 8th ed. Philadelphia, 2002, Saunders.)

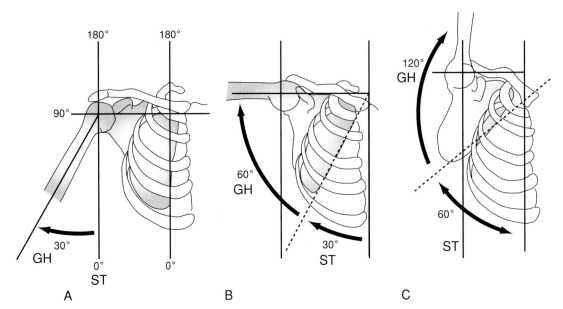

Figure 30–15:
A, Average ratio of glenohumeral (GH) to scapulothoracic (ST) motion is 2:1. **B** and **C,** For the first 30 degrees of abduction it is all glenohumeral motion. In the last 60 degrees of elevation there is almost equal contribution between the glenohumeral and scapulothoracic joints. (From DeLee JC, Drez D Jr, Miller MD, editors: *DeLee and Drez's orthopaedic sports medicine: principles and practice,* 2nd ed. Philadelphia, 2003, Saunders.)

- The coracohumeral ligament helps reinforce the superior portion of the capsule.
- Blood supply is derived from articular branches of the anterior and posterior circumflex humeral arteries.
- Articular nerves branch from the suprascapular, axillary, and lateral pectoral nerves.

Acromioclavicular Joint

- Plane, gliding synovial joint formed by the lateral end of the clavicle and acromion approximately 2 to 3 cm medially from the lateral border of the acromion (Figure 30–3).
- Both articular surfaces are enveloped with fibrocartilage and slope inferomedially.
- An incomplete articular disc sits primarily at the superior portion of the joint.
- The AC ligament provides anteroposterior stability to the distal clavicle.
- The CC ligament, composed of the trapezoid ligament anterolaterally and the stronger conoid ligament posteromedially, limits superior translation of the distal clavicle.
- The CC ligament is the strongest and primary stabilizing attachment of the scapula to the clavicle.
- Rotation and anterior-posterior motion of the acromion relative to the clavicle are associated with movement of the scapula and sternoclavicular joint.
- A fibrous capsule encloses the articular surface but provides only minimal support, which is reinforced by

the previously mentioned ligaments and the trapezius muscle.
- The joint receives its blood supply from branches of the suprascapular and thoracoacromial arteries.
- Innervation to the joint derives from branches of the supraclavicular, lateral pectoral, and axillary nerves.

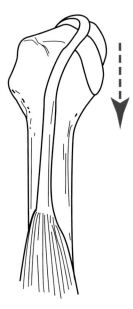

Figure 30–16:
The long head of biceps tendon assists in depressing the humeral head. (From DeLee JC, Drez D Jr, Miller MD, editors: *DeLee and Drez's orthopaedic sports medicine: principles and practice,* 2nd ed. Philadelphia, 2003, Saunders.)

Sternoclavicular Joint

- Double, gliding, saddle-type synovial joint formed by the medial end of the clavicle, first costal cartilage, and the superolateral aspect of the manubrium.
- Only joint in the body connecting the axial skeleton and upper limb.
- An articular disc, dividing the two synovial cavities, has firm attachments superiorly and inferiorly and is continuous with the anterior and posterior sternoclavicular ligaments.
- The posterior sternoclavicular ligament/capsule is the primary stabilizer to the sternoclavicular joint.
- The articular disc serves as a shock absorber of forces transmitted from the upper limb to the axial skeleton and prevents medial translation of the clavicle.
- Thickenings of the capsule surrounding the joint form the anterior and posterior sternoclavicular ligaments and the interclavicular ligaments (Figure 30–17).
- The extracapsular costoclavicular ligament is the strongest stabilizing ligament that ascends from the first rib and costal cartilage to the medial end of the clavicle, limiting superior translation of the medial clavicle.
- This joint rotates approximately 30 degrees with shoulder motion.
- Branches of the internal thoracic and suprascapular arteries provide vascularity to the joint.
- The nerve to the subclavius muscle and medial supraclavicular nerve provide branches that innervate the joint.

Scapulothoracic Joint

- Permits movement of the scapula in relation to the rib cage.
- Not a true joint.

Muscles

- The muscles that act on the shoulder have several functions but can be grouped into three general categories (Table 30–1, Box 30–3).

Bursae

- Subscapular bursa—lies between the subscapularis tendon and neck of the scapula, protecting the tendon as it travels over the neck of the scapula and inferior to the coracoid. It communicates with the shoulder joint cavity, forming one of the two openings in the capsule (Figure 30–3).
- Subacromial bursa—large bursa, inferior to the acromion, between the deltoid muscle, supraspinatus muscle, and joint capsule, assisting movement of the deltoid above the shoulder joint.
- Several bursae about the scapula have been defined (Figure 30–18, Box 30–4).

Vessels

- The subclavian artery, a continuation of the aorta on the left and the brachiocephalic trunk on the right, accompanies the brachial plexus through the scalenus anterior and medius muscles of the neck.
- At the lateral border of the first rib, the subclavian artery turns into the axillary artery, which divides into three parts in relation to the pectoralis minor muscle (Figure 30–19).
  - The first part passes medial to the muscle, at its superior border, and gives off the supreme thoracic branch.
  - The second part, deep to the muscle, gives off the thoracoacromial and lateral thoracic arteries. The

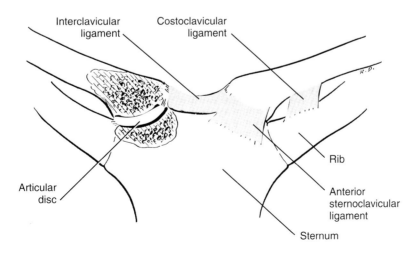

Figure 30–17:
The sternoclavicular joint and surrounding ligaments. The joint on the left has been sectioned to expose the articular disc. (From Jenkins DB, Hollinshead WH: *Hollinshead's functional anatomy of the limbs and back,* 8th ed. Philadelphia, 2002, Saunders.)

Table 30–1: Muscles of the Shoulder

MUSCLE	ORIGIN	INSERTION	ACTION	INNERVATION
Trapezius	Spin. proc. C7–T12	Clavicle, scapula (AC, SP)	Rotate scapula	CN XI
Lat. dorsii	Spin. proc. T6–S5, ilium	Humerus (ITG)	Ex., add., IR humerus	Thoracodorsal
Rhomboid maj.	Spin. proc. T2–T5	Scapula (med. border)	Adduct scapula	Dorsal scapular
Rhomboid min.	Spin. proc. C7–T1	Scapula (med. spine)	Adduct scapula	Dorsal scapular
Lev. scapulae	T. proc. C1–C4	Scapula (sup. med.)	Elevate, rotate scapula	C3, C4
Pectoralis maj.	Sternum, ribs, clavicle	Humerus (L-ITG)	Add., IR arm	M and L PN
Pectoralis min.	Ribs 3–5	Scapula (coracoid)	Protract scapula	MPN
Subclavius	Rib 1	Inf. clavicle	Depress clavicle	U trunk
Serratus ant.	Ribs 1–9	Scapula (vent. med.)	Prevent winging	Long thoracic
Deltoid	Lateral clavicle, scapula	Humerus (deltoid tub.)	Abduct arm (2)	Axillary
Teres major	Inf. scapula	Humerus (M-ITG)	Add., IR, ext.	L subscapular
Subscapularis	Ventral scapula	Humerus (LT)	IR arm, ant. stability	U and L subscapular
Supraspinatus	Sup. scapula	Humerus (GT)	Abd. (1), ER arm stability	Suprascapular
Infraspinatus	Dorsal scapula	Humerus (GT)	Stability, ER arm	Suprascapular
Teres minor	Scapula (dorsolateral)	Humerus (GT)	Stability, ER arm	Axillary

AC, Acromion; GT, greater tuberosity; ITG, intertubercular groove; LT, lesser tuberosity; SP, spinous process.
From Miller MD, editor: *Review of orthopaedics*, 4th ed. Philadelphia, 2004, Saunders.

thoracoacromial branch further divides into four branches: acromial, deltoid, pectoral, and clavicular.

- The third part passes lateral to the muscle, at its inferior border, and gives off the subscapular artery (which further divides into the circumflex scapular and thoracodorsal arteries); anterior circumflex artery, which encircles the humerus anteriorly; and the larger posterior circumflex artery, which passes through the quadrangular space along with the axillary nerve at the posterior wall of the axilla.

Nerves

- The brachial plexus, derived from the ventral rami of C5 through T1 and extending from the neck to the axilla, provides innervation to the upper extremity (Figure 30–20).
- The plexus can be divided into five sections: rami, trunks, divisions, cords, and branches (remembered by the mnemonic Rob Taylor Drinks Cold Beer).
- The five rami enter the posterior triangle of the neck between the anterior scalene and medius to form the upper, middle, and lower trunks, which lie above the clavicle.

- Four preclavicular nerve branches derive from the rami and trunks: dorsal scapular, long thoracic, suprascapular nerves, and the nerve to the subclavius.
- Each trunk divides into anterior and posterior divisions under the clavicle, which supply the flexor and extensor muscles of the upper limb, respectively.
- At the axilla, the divisions form the posterior, lateral, and medial cords, which in turn provide the branches that innervate the upper extremity.

Box 30–4 Bursae around the Scapula

Major/Anatomic Bursae

Infraserratus bursae—Between serratus anterior and chest wall
Supraserratus bursae—Between subscapularis and serratus anterior muscles
Scapulotrapezial bursae—Between superomedial scapula and the trapezius

Minor/Adventitial Bursae

Superomedial Angle of the Scapula

Infraserratus bursae—Between serratus anterior and chest wall
Supraserratus bursae—Between supscapularis and serratus anterior

Inferior Angle of the Scapula

Infraserratus bursae—Between serratus anterior and chest wall

Spine of Scapula

Trapezoid bursae—Between medial spine of scapula and trapezius

From Kuhn JE, Hawkins RJ: Evaluation and treatment of scapular disorders. In Warner JJP, Iannotti JP, Gerber C (editors): *Complex and revision problems in shoulder surgery*. Philadelphia, 1997, Lippincott-Raven.

Box 30–3 General Categories of Muscles about the Shoulder

Connect upper limb to axial skeleton—Trapezius, latissimus, rhomboid major and minor, and levator scapulae
Connect upper limb to thorax—Pectoralis major and minor, subclavius, and serratus anterior
Act on shoulder joint—Deltoid, teres major, supraspinatus, infraspinatus, teres minor, and subscapularis (last four make up the rotator cuff)

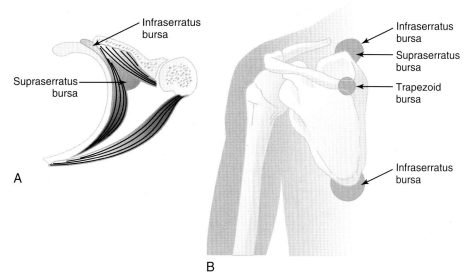

Figure 30–18:
Bursae about the scapula. (From Miller MD, Cole BJ, editors: *Textbook of arthroscopy.* Philadelphia, 2004, Saunders.)

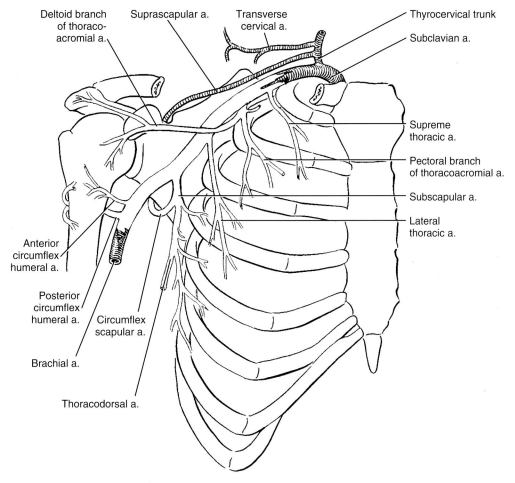

Figure 30–19:
Arteries of the upper thorax and shoulder. Axillary artery and its branches are shaded black. Other vessels are striped. (From Jenkins DB, Hollinshead WH: *Hollinshead's functional anatomy of the limbs and back,* 8th ed. Philadelphia, 2002, Saunders.)

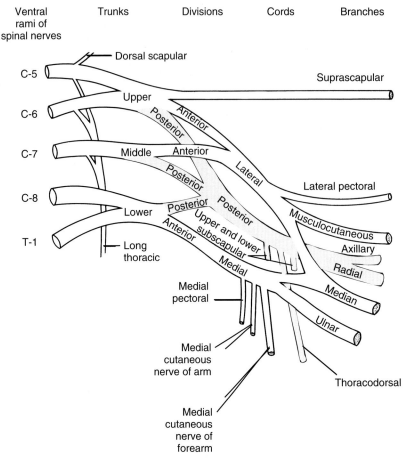

Figure 30–20:
The brachial plexus. (From Jenkins DB, Hollinshead WH: *Hollinshead's functional anatomy of the limbs and back,* 8th ed. Philadelphia, 2002, Saunders.)

References

Halder AM, Itoi E, An K: Anatomy and biomechanics of the shoulder. *Orthop Clinic North Am* 31:159-176, 2000.
Extensive and detailed review of shoulder anatomy and biomechanics. Scapulothoracic joint is also discussed. 106 references.

Kibler WB: Normal shoulder mechanics and function. *Instr Course Lect* 46:39-42, 1997.
Brief general review of shoulder biomechanics. The joint is considered as part of a kinetic chain that transfers forces from the legs to the hand. Bony, ligamentous, and muscular constraints are discussed. Furthermore, the importance of force couples about the shoulder controlling shoulder motion is addressed.

Kibler WB: The role of the scapula in athletic shoulder function. *Am J Sports Med* 26:325-337, 1998.
Focused review on scapular anatomy and biomechanics. Abnormalities, evaluation, and management of certain conditions are briefly discussed.

Ruotolo C, Penna J, Namkoong S, Meinhard BP: Shoulder pain and the overhand athlete. *Am J Orthop* 32:248-258, 2003.
Review article discussing the biomechanics involved in the five phases of throwing and how it may relate to common overuse injuries. The authors state that the late cocking and early deceleration phases of throwing are most commonly associated with the development of injuries. Several conditions, including their pathophysiology, diagnosis, and treatment are discussed. A good understanding of the normal biomechanics allows proper evaluation of patients and may assist with diagnosis and therapeutic regimens.

Valadie AL, Jobe CM, Pink MM, et al: Anatomy of provocative tests for impingement syndrome of the shoulder. *J Shoulder Elbow Surg* 9:36-46, 2000.
Authors study the anatomic relationship of shoulder structure during the performance of the Neer and Hawkins tests for the diagnosis of shoulder impingement. Fresh-frozen cadaver shoulders were used in the study. Authors determined that the Neer test created soft tissue contact with the medial acromion. The Hawkins test produced contact between the soft tissues and the coracoacromial ligament. Both tests demonstrated contact between the articular surface of the rotator cuff tendons and anterosuperior glenoid rim.

Volk AG, Vangsness CT: An anatomic study of the supraspinatus muscle and tendon. *Clin Orthop Related Res* 384:280-285, 2001.
Anatomic study of the myotendinous portion of the supraspinatus is performed using coronal and sagittal dissections from 20 shoulder specimens. Findings and measurements are discussed. The authors note the

anterior portion of the muscle consisted of a more prominent tendinous area than its posterior portion, which they propose offers an ideal area for suture repairs. Furthermore, their findings may improve our interpretations seen on magnetic resonance imaging and shoulder evaluation during open or arthroscopic procedures.

Wiedmer M, Mukherjee DP, Ogden AL, et al: A biomechanical evaluation of the role of labrum on anterior/posterior translation of shoulders at different degrees of abduction. *J Long Term Effects Med Implants* 13:309-318, 2003.

Authors study the roles of the anterior and posterior labrums on anterior and posterior translation of the shoulder. Thirteen cadavers with no evidence of pathology were evaluated intact, vented, and after arthroscopic incision of the anterior and posterior labrums. Results demonstrated no significant increases in anterior or posterior shoulder translation in any tested positions after incising the anterior and posterior labrums.

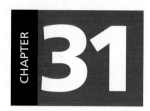

Shoulder History, Physical Examination, and Imaging

Introduction

- The shoulder evaluation should begin with a thorough history of the presenting complaint.
- Throughout the history and physical examination, information regarding the surrounding anatomy (neck, elbow, chest, diaphragm) should be included with emphasis on the cervical spine and associated nerves.
- Imaging should be selected on the basis of clinical suspicion from the examination and not simply as a way to "make the diagnosis."

History

- The age of the patient and the chief complaint should be recognized first with subsequent questions structured to decipher the pathology specific to that patient population.
  - Young patients: acute injuries, instability, acromioclavicular (AC) joint injury.
  - Middle-aged: inflammatory conditions, impingement, adhesive capsulitis.
  - Older: arthritis, impingement, rotator cuff pathology.
- A history of injury, either acute or chronic, should be obtained in detail including the specific mechanism of injury and any association with secondary gain (litigation, workers' compensation, or psychiatric illness).
- Information regarding the pain should include the character, location, intensity, duration, radiation, aggravating or alleviating factors, and interference with work or activities of daily life (ADLs).
- Objective measures of pain: visual analog scale (VAS), validated shoulder scoring systems, quantity of pain medication required.
- Frequently missed associated symptoms may include numbness, tingling, weakness, or altered perception of heat/cold.
- The patient's activity level both at work and in athletics should be determined to assess the relative level of disability.
- Response to previous attempts at treatment either acutely (emergency room [ER]) or chronically

(nonsteroidal antiinflammatory drugs [NSAIDs], physical therapy, injections, surgery).

Physical Examination

Inspection/Palpation

- A brief general overview of the patient's physical appearance and gross anatomy should be performed first.
- Observation of simple tasks performed outside the specific shoulder examination (disrobing) can reveal subtle or misrepresented pathology.
- General muscle tone and symmetry should be observed.
- Bony prominences may be visualized and palpated for tenderness.
- Skin coloration may be abnormal with conditions such as Raynaud's or complex regional pain syndrome (formerly reflex sympathetic dystrophy [RSD]).
- Evaluate for systemic laxity (thumb-to-forearm flexibility, knee/elbow recurvatum) as a predisposing factor for the pathology and the possible failure of its treatment (Figure 31–1).

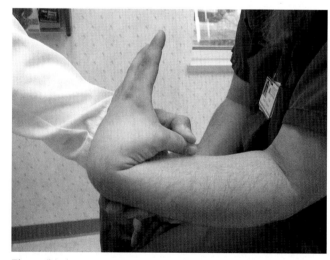

Figure 31–1:
Congenital hyperlaxity associated with thumb-to-forearm flexibility.

Range of Motion

- Range of motion must be assessed both passively and actively because a discrepancy may be indicative of a certain disease process (Box 31–1).
  - With adhesive capsulitis, both passive and active motion are restricted.
  - With rotator cuff pathology, active range of motion may be limited but passive range of motion is typically unrestricted.
- Measured arcs as recommended by the Society of American Shoulder and Elbow Surgeons.
  - Forward elevation (comfortably).
  - External rotation (in both adduction and abduction).
  - Internal rotation (highest vertebral level reached).
- Normal shoulder motion combines that achieved through both the glenohumeral joint and the scapulothoracic articulation in a 2:1 ratio.
- The pathologic shoulder should be compared with the contralateral shoulder to establish relative levels of function.

Strength

- The graded system of manual muscle testing provides an objective description of strength (Box 31–2).
- In cases of shoulder impingement, resisted abduction can reproduce the patient's pain and cause a false decrease in strength on examination. In these patients, it is helpful to test for external rotation strength with the elbows "tucked into" the patient's side to eliminate the painful position.
- It is important to remember that loss of strength may be due to a neurologic problem, as well as to an injury to the muscle, so isolating each muscle is an important part of the examination.

Special Testing

Impingement

- Neer's impingement sign (Figure 31–2A).
  - Evaluates for subacromial impingement.
  - Passive forward elevation of the arm causes impingement of the supraspinatus tendon under the coracoacromial arch.
  - A positive test is indicated by reproduction of the pain.

Box 31–1	Normal Shoulder Range of Motion

Abduction: 180 degrees
Adduction: 45 degrees
Flexion: 180 degrees
Extension: 45 degrees
Internal rotation: 55 degrees
External rotation: 45 degrees

Box 31–2	Manual Muscle Testing
5/5	Full range of motion against gravity and against *full* resistance
4/5	Full range of motion against gravity and against *some* resistance
3/5	Full range of motion against gravity but *no* resistance
2/5	Full range of motion at gravity neutral
1/5	Muscle contracts but unable to produce motion
0/5	Muscle unable to contract

- Neer's impingement *test* is not to be confused with Neer's impingement *sign*.
- This test is performed by giving a subacromial injection with a local anesthetic.
- A positive test is indicated by pain relief after the injection.
- The test is the most sensitive and specific evaluation for impingement.
- Hawkin's impingement sign (Figure 31–2B).
  - Another technique to assess for subacromial impingement.
  - Performed by having the adducted shoulder flexed forward to 90 degrees with internal rotation.
  - A positive test is indicated by reproduction of the pain.

Rotator Cuff

- Supraspinatus stress test (Figure 31–3A).
  - Resisted abduction of the internally rotated and forward flexed arm (in the plane of the scapula) produces pain and weakness with a supraspinatus tendon tear.
  - Also referred to as the "empty (beer/soda) can sign."
  - Can also be performed in supination to eliminate symptoms associated with concomitant impingement.
- Drop arm test.
  - This is used to determine the presence of a rotator cuff tear and typically represents a larger tear.
  - The test is performed by passively abducting the shoulder to 90 degrees and asking the patient to hold it in that position and then slowly lower it to his or her side.
  - A positive test is indicated by an inability to hold the arm up or an inability to lower it slowly and smoothly.
- Lift-off test (Figure 31–3B).
  - Indicates a possible subscapularis tear.
  - The patient is unable to lift the internally rotated arm away from the lower back.
  - Eliminates the pectoralis muscle as an internal rotator.
  - Similar to "belly-push test" with the patient's hand pressed against the abdomen while attempting to maintain the elbow positioned anterior to the midaxillary line (Figure 31–3C).

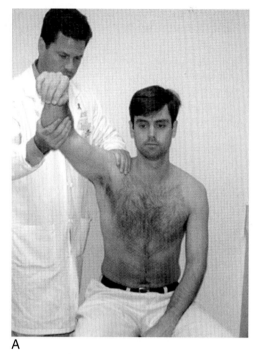

A

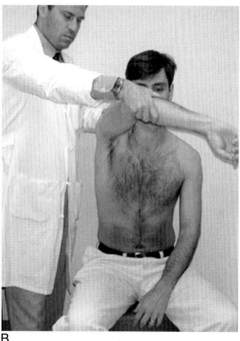

B

Figure 31–2:
Impingement tests. A, Neer's impingement sign. **B,** Hawkin's impingement sign. (From Miller MD, Cooper DE, Warner JJP: *Review of Sports Medicine and Orthroscopy.* Philadelphia, 2002, Saunders.)

Instability

- Apprehension test (Figure 31–4*A*).
  - This is used to determine the presence of shoulder instability.
- This test is performed by placing the shoulder in the "unstable" position of abduction and external rotation.
- A positive test is indicated by resistance and "apprehension" on the part of the patient as the humeral head subluxates anteriorly.
- May also produce posterior shoulder pain with "internal impingement" (interposition of the rotator cuff between the greater tuberosity and the posterior labrum).
- Best performed in the supine position to stabilize the scapula.
- Relocation test (Figure 31–4*B*).
  - This is an extension of the apprehension test for instability.
  - The test is performed by placing the patient in the apprehensive position and then applying a posteriorly directed force to the proximal humerus.
  - A positive test is indicated by relief of the apprehension and a greater degree of obtainable external rotation.
- Load and shift test.
  - This is also used to determine the presence of shoulder instability.
  - This can be performed with the patient in the seated position with the arm adducted while the examiner holds the proximal humerus and attempts to translate anteriorly and posteriorly (Figure 31–4*C*).
  - Can also be performed with the arm abducted to position in the scapular plane with an axial load applied to the elbow to concentrically reduce the humeral head. This is followed by attempted translation anteriorly and posteriorly (Figure 31–4*D*).
  - The amount of translation is graded on the degree of translation.
- Sulcus sign (Figure 31–4*E*).
  - Determines the presence of inferior shoulder laxity.
  - This test is performed by placing downward traction on the arm as it hangs at the patient's side (neutral rotation and neutral flexion-extension).
  - A positive test is indicated by inferior translation of the humerus, which produces a gap between the humeral head and the acromion and can be graded by the size of the gap.
- Jerk test (Figure 31–4*F*).
  - Determines presence of posterior instability.
  - Posteriorly directed force on the forward flexed and adducted arm produces posterior subluxation.
  - Placement of the arm in the coronal plane may relocate the subluxated humeral head with an audible or palpable "clunk."

Biceps Tendon

- O'Brien's test (active compression test) (Figure 31–5).
  - This is used to test for labral pathology (superior labral anterior and posterior [SLAP] tears) but is relatively nonspecific.

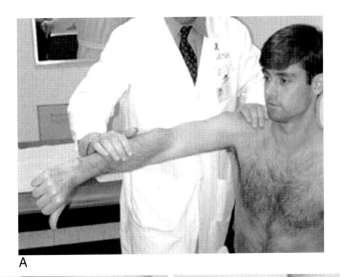

A

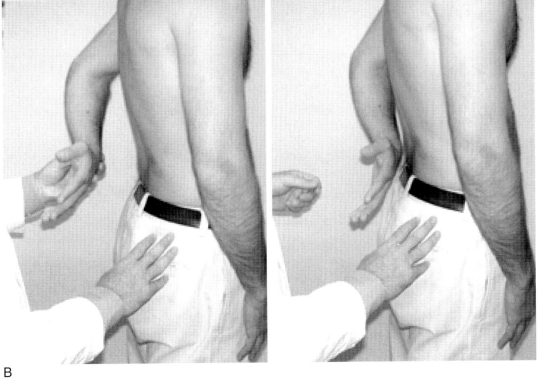

B

Figure 31–3:
Rotator cuff tests. **A,** Supraspinatus stress test. **B,** (*left*) Lift-off test and (*right*) failure to maintain the maximally internally rotated arm away from the small of the back.

(*continued*)

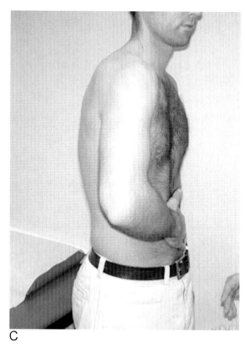

C

Figure 31–3, cont'd:

C, Belly-push test. (From Miller MD, Cooper DE, Warner JJP: *Review of sports medicine and arthroscopy,* **2nd ed. Philadelphia, 2002, Saunders.)**

- This test is performed with the shoulder forward flexed to 90 degrees and slightly adducted across the body. The elbow is kept straight and the arm is internally rotated. The patient resists the examiner as a downward force is placed on the arm.
- A positive test is indicated by reproduction of pain and relative relief with supination.
- Yergason's test.
  - This is used to test for bicipital tendinitis.
  - Resisted forearm supination with the elbow slightly flexed.

- Positive test reproduces pain.
- Speed's test
- This is also used to test for biceps tendinitis.
  - The test is performed with the elbow extended as the patient forward flexes the shoulder against resistance.
  - A positive test is indicated by the reproduction of pain.
- Cross-body adduction test.
  - This is used to test for AC joint degeneration.
  - The test is performed by passively adducting the arm across the patient's chest while palpating the AC joint.
  - A positive test is pain in the area of the AC joint.

Imaging Studies
Plain Radiography

- Standard trauma series.
  - True anteroposterior (AP) view (in the plane of the scapula) (Figure 31–6*A* and *B*).
  - Axillary lateral view (Figure 31–6*C*).
    - Arm abducted 70 to 90 degrees with beam into axilla.
  - Alternatives to axillary lateral view (not equivalent substitutes—should always obtain an axillary radiograph).
    - Velpeau view—patient leaning backward over cassette with superior to inferior directed beam.
    - Trauma axillary lateral view—arm forward flexed 20 degrees with beam directed cephalad in supine patient.
    - Scapular Y view (Figure 31–6*D*)—beam directed parallel to scapular spine (posteromedial to anterolateral).
  - Used to visualize the glenohumeral joint and confirm reduction.
- Internal/external rotation views.

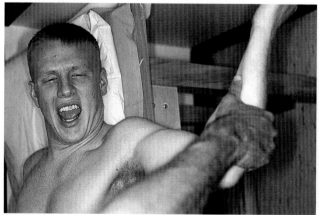
A
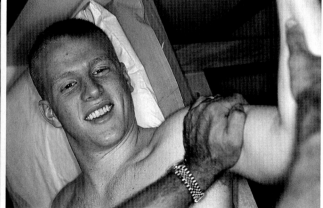
B

Figure 31–4:

Instability tests. A, Apprehension test. B, Relocation test.

(continued)

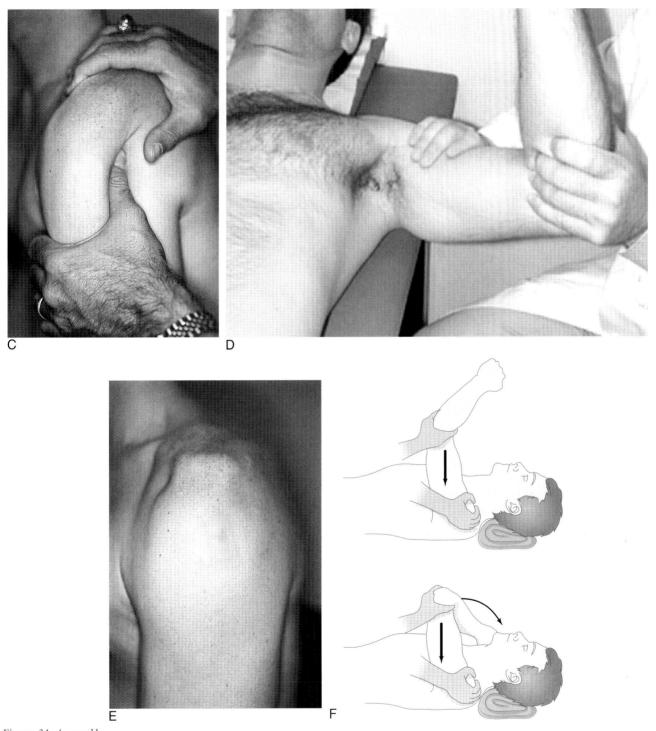

Figure 31–4, cont'd:
C, Load-and-shift test (seated). **D,** Load-and-shift test (supine). **E,** Sulcus sign. **F,** Jerk test. (**A, B, C,** and **E** from Miller MD, Howard RF, Plancher KD: *Surgical atlas of sports medicine.* Philadelphia, 2003, Saunders; **D** from Miller MD, Cooper DE, Warner JJP: *Review of sports medicine and arthroscopy.* Philadelphia, 2002, Saunders.)

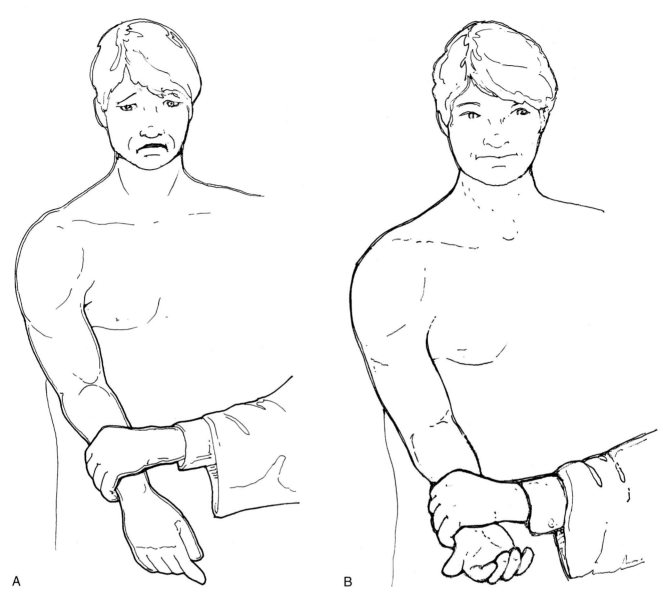

A   B

Figure 31–5:
O'Brien's test. Deep anterior pain with (**A**) resisted downward force of the adducted, 90-degree forward elevated, and fully inter-
nally rotated arm that is (**B**) relieved with external rotation is consistent with a superior labral anterior and posterior lesion.
(From Miller MD, Howard RF, Plancher KD: *Surgical atlas of sports medicine.* Philadelphia, 2003, Saunders.)

- Evaluate for presence of Hill-Sachs or reverse Hill-Sachs lesions associated with dislocations.
- Also useful in the evaluation of possible proximal humeral growth plate injury in young throwing athletes (Little League shoulder).
  - Comparison views of the contralateral side may be necessary.
- Clavicle/AC joint.
  - Zanca view (Figure 31–7).
  - 10 degrees cephalic tilt centered on AC joint.
  - Voltage reduced to avoid overpenetration.
  - Sometimes incidental finding on standard trauma chest film.

- 30-degree caudal tilt view.
  - Demonstrate anteroinferior acromial spurring.
  - Also useful to determine adequacy of a previous acromioplasty.
- Scapular outlet or supraspinatus outlet view.
  - Lateral scapula view with beam directed 10 degrees caudally.
  - Demonstrates acromial morphology.
    - Bigliani types I to III (flat, curved, hooked) (Figure 31–8).
- West Point view (Figure 31–9A).
  - Useful in evaluating anteroinferior glenoid rim in cases of instability.

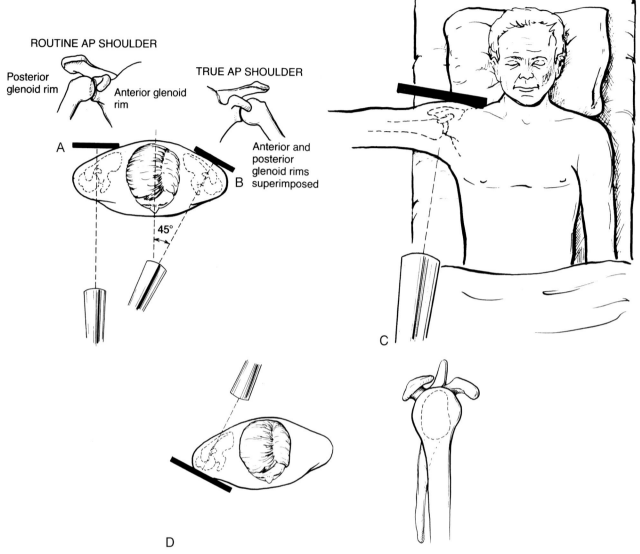

Figure 31–6:
Standard shoulder radiographs. A, Routine anteroposterior (AP) view of shoulder. **B,** True AP view of shoulder. **C,** Axillary lateral radiograph. **D,** Scapular Y radiograph. (From Warner JJP, Caborn DN: *Crit Rev Phys Rehabil Med* 4:145-198, 1992.)

- Similar to axillary lateral view but with patient positioned prone and beam directed 25 degrees inferiorly and medially.
- Same visualization but opposite technique of the Garth view, which is true AP view with the beam angled 45 degrees inferiorly and the arm internally rotated.
- Stryker notch view (Figure 31–9B).
  - Allows visualization of Hill-Sachs defect.
  - Supine shoulder AP centered on coracoid with 10 degrees of cephalic tilt while the patient's hand is placed on the top of the head.
- Sternoclavicular (SC) joint.
- Hobbs view.
  - Posteroanterior (PA) chest film with patient leaning over cassette.
- Serendipity view.
  - Supine AP chest film with beam directed 40 degrees cephalad.
  - Comparison made with contralateral medial clavicle.
    - Superior displacement on film indicates anterior dislocation.
    - Inferior displacement on film indicates posterior dislocation.
- Computed tomography (CT) most sensitive and specific test.

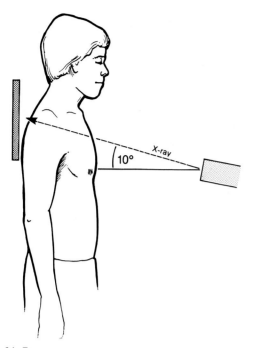

Figure 31–7:
Zanca view. (From Rockwood CA Jr, Szalay EA, Curtis RJ Jr, et al: X-ray evaluation of shoulder problems. In Rockwood CA Jr, Matsen FA III, editors: *The shoulder.* **Philadelphia, 1990, WB Saunders.)**

Arthrogram

- Dye is injected into the glenohumeral joint, and images are obtained at intervals following the injection to determine whether or not dye will extravasate outside of the joint capsule into the subacromial space.
- Historically used to diagnose rotator cuff tears.
- Does not allow determination of size, degree of retraction, or muscle quality of rotator cuff.
- Has been replaced for the most part by arthrogram CT or magnetic resonance imaging (MRI).
- Useful for patients for whom an MRI is contraindicated (implanted defibrillator, implant, metal foreign body) or in evaluation for revision.

Magnetic Resonance Imaging

- MRI is the most useful test for examining soft tissue injury (rotator cuff, labrum, capsule) in the shoulder (Figure 31–10).
- This is also useful for evaluating conditions such as avascular necrosis and some tumors of the proximal humerus.
- Arthrogram MRI may be more useful for evaluating rotator cuff and labral tears.

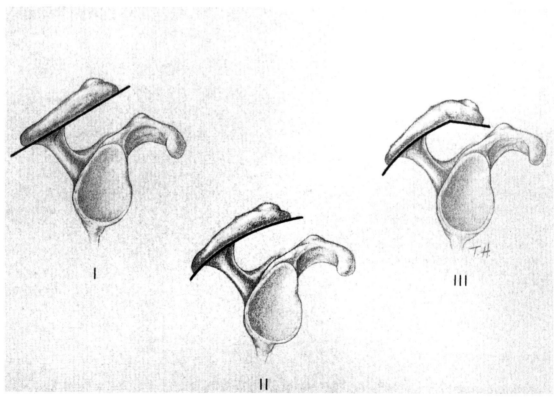

Figure 31–8:
Acromion morphology. (From Esch JC: *Op Tech Orthop* **1:200, 1991.)**

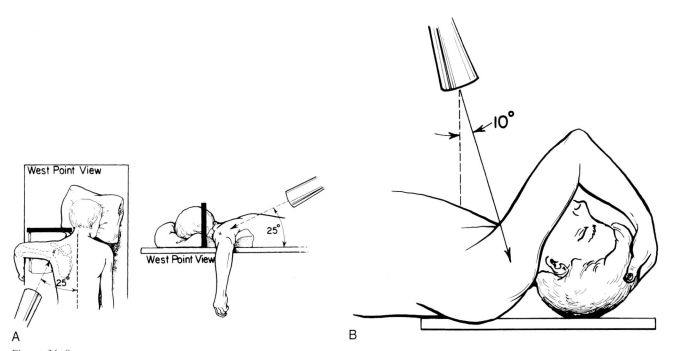

Figure 31–9:
A, West Point view. **B,** Stryker Notch view. (From Warner JJP, Caborn DN: *Crit Rev Phys Rehabil Med* 4:145-198, 1992.)

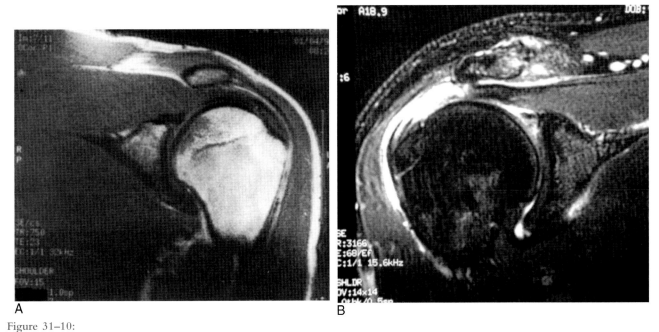

Figure 31–10:
A, Coronal magnetic resonance imaging (MRI) of normal rotator cuff. **B,** Coronal MRI of torn rotator cuff. (From Miller MD, Cooper DE, Warner JJP: *Review of sports medicine and arthroscopy,* 2nd ed. Philadelphia, 2002, Saunders.)

Computed Tomography

- Most helpful in evaluating complex multipart fractures of the proximal humerus or scapula, bony tumors, arthritic architectural changes, and glenoid abnormalities for preoperative planning.
- This test is also helpful in assessing the degree of bony union in delayed unions or nonunions of the humerus.
- CT-guided aspirations and biopsies as minimally invasive diagnostic procedures.

Ultrasound

- Emerging as reliable technique for evaluation of possible rotator cuff tears.
- Highly operator dependent and requires specific training in this imaging technique.
- Most useful with full-thickness tears and less reliable with partial-thickness pathology.

References

Byers GE, Berquist TH: Radiology of sports-related injuries. *Curr Prob Diagn Radiol* 25:1-49, 1996.

This is a review article that addresses the proper imaging studies to evaluate sports-related trauma to the shoulder. The authors address the shoulder by anatomic "part" and by mechanism of injury being studied.

Chronopoulos E, Kim TK, Park HB, et al: Diagnostic value of physical tests for isolated chronic acromioclavicular lesions. *Am J Sports Med* 32:655-661, 2004.

This is a retrospective analysis that shows the reliability of three common physical examination indicators of AC pathology: the cross-body adduction stress test, the AC resisted extension test, and the active compression test. This shows that the cross-body adduction stress test is the most sensitive, whereas the active compression test is the most specific of the three.

Cole B, Katolik L: Shoulder. In Miller MD, Cooper DE, Warner JP, editors: *Review of arthroscopy and sports medicine.* Philadelphia, 2002, Saunders.

This chapter provides a complete and concise outline of the physical examination of the shoulder including photographs demonstrating the examination maneuvers.

Hoppenfeld S: *Physical examination of the spine and extremities.* Norwalk, CT, 1976, Appleton-Century-Crofts.

This is a concise and extremely well-illustrated guide to the orthopaedic examination. It includes a systematic review of the anatomy, nerve innervation, joint range of motion, and special testing for all of the extremities and spine.

Levy AS, Lintner S, Kenter K, Speer KP: Intra- and interobserver reproducibility of the shoulder laxity examination. *Am J Sports Med* 27:460-463, 1999.

This study examines the reproducibility of common physical examination findings to diagnose shoulder instability in Division I college athletes.

Lo IKY, Nonweiler B, Woolfrey M, et al: An evaluation of the apprehension, relocation, and surprise tests for anterior shoulder instability. *Am J Sports Med* 32:301-307, 2004.

In looking at these three common tests for anterior shoulder instability, the authors evaluate for predictive value and intertester reliability (0.83). They show the surprise test to be the most accurate of the three with a sensitivity of almost 64% and a specificity of almost 99%.

McFarland EG, Kim TK, Savino RM: Clinical assessment of three common tests for superior labral anterior-posterior lesions. *Am J Sports Med* 30:810-815, 2002.

This article provides a good review of three commonly used tests for evaluating SLAP tears: active compression test, anterior slide, and compression-rotation test. The most sensitive test is the active-compression test with the anterior slide being the most specific.

Nicholson DA, Lang I, Hughes P, Driscoll PA: ABC of emergency radiology. The shoulder. *BMJ* 307:1129-1134, 1993.

Another review article that addresses the proper imaging studies of the shoulder for injury-related diagnoses. This includes discussion of plain radiographs appropriate to examine these conditions and when the examiner should perform special tests such as MRI or CT scan.

Tennent TD, Beach WR, Meyers JF: Clinical sports medicine update. A review of the special test associated with shoulder examination. Part 1: the rotator cuff tests. *Am J Sports Med* 31:154-160, 2003.

This is a good review of special tests of the shoulder to diagnosis rotator cuff pathology. The authors are careful to present descriptions of the test to indicate how they were intended to be performed by the authors who first described them.

Tennent TD, Beach WR, Meyers JF: Clinical sports medicine update. A review of the special test associated with shoulder examination. Part II: Laxity, instability, and superior labral anterior and posterior (SLAP) lesions. *Am J Sports Med* 31:301-307, 2003.

This is the second part of the authors' review of physical examination of the shoulder. In this article, they discuss the special tests used to evaluate SLAP tears and shoulder instability.

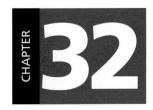

CHAPTER 32

Shoulder Arthroscopy

Introduction

- Advances in equipment and technique have refined shoulder arthroscopy and expanded its use.
- Shoulder arthroscopy allows effective treatment for several shoulder conditions with minimal complications and recovery time.
- Indications (Box 32–1).
- Contraindications (Box 32–2).

Surgical Technique

- Lateral decubitus (Figure 32–3) or beach chair position (Figure 32–4).
- Beach chair position does not require traction on the arm and assists conversion to an open procedure.
- Lateral decubitus position requires positioning the patient on a beanbag or similar device with the torso angled posteriorly approximately 25 to 30 degrees to align the glenoid parallel to the floor. The arm is abducted and placed in a traction device with the arm in neutral.
- General endotracheal anesthesia and interscalene block can be used individually or combined.
- Using epinephrine in the arthroscopic fluid helps maintain hemostasis and improves visualization during the procedure.
- After the patient has been properly anesthetized, the shoulder joint is examined and any instability is noted.

Box 32–1 | Indications

Diagnostic
Rotator cuff repair
Labral tears (Figure 32–1)
Subacromial decompression
Capsular plication
Intraarticular debridement and lysis of adhesions
Distal clavicle excision
Paralabral cyst decompression
Biceps pathology (Figure 32–2)

- Outlining the acromion, acromioclavicular (AC) joint, and distal clavicle with marker assists in portal placement (Figure 32–5).
- Routine arthroscopy relies on an anterior and posterior portal, with several other available portal sites for specific needs (Figure 32–6).
- The site of the posterior portal is approximately 2 cm inferior and 1 to 2 cm medial to the posterolateral border of the acromion (Figures 32–5 and 32–6).
  - Site should be injected with local anesthesia and followed up by injecting 30 to 60 mL of saline into the joint using a spinal needle to distend the joint and reduce the risk of articular cartilage damage with portal insertion.
  - A trocar and cannula are then inserted into the joint, via a small incision, parallel to the lateral acromial border and floor and aiming toward the coracoid process.
  - The suprascapular nerve is at risk medially while the axillary nerve and posterior humeral circumflex artery are at risk inferiorly.
- The anterior portal site is marked 2 cm medial and 1 cm inferior to the anterolateral rim of the acromion (Figures 32–5 and 32–6).
  - Injury to the musculocutaneous nerve can be avoided by placing the arm in adduction.
  - The port is inserted under arthroscopic visualization within the rotator interval after confirming the proper location with a spinal needle. (This portal can alternatively be placed from the inside-out.)
- Additional portals are available to assist with certain procedures.
  - Lateral portal—slightly distal and approximately 2 cm posterior to the anterolateral corner of the acromion. Used for subacromial decompression and rotator cuff repair (visualization). Axillary nerve is at risk for injury inferiorly (Figures 32–5 and 32–6).
  - Anteroinferior (5 o'clock) portal—2 cm distal to site of anterior portal. Valuable for Bankart repairs and anterior stabilization procedures. The musculocutaneous nerve is at risk medially, and the axillary nerve is at risk inferomedially (Figures 32–5 and 32–6).

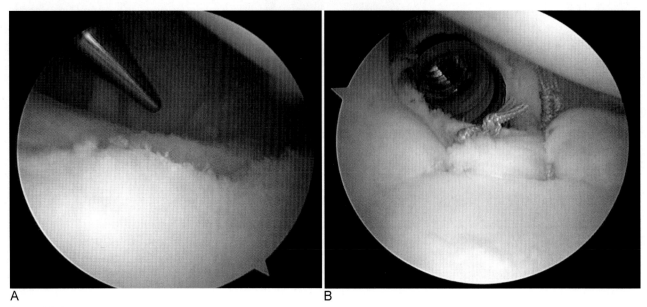

A   B

Figure 32–1:
A, Bankart labral tear that has healed medially to the glenoid rim (anterior labral periosteal sleeve avulsion [ALPSA] lesion).
B, Bankart tear repaired to the glenoid rim anatomically.

- Posteroinferior (7 o'clock) portal—2 cm distal to site of posterior portal. Useful when additional posterior access is required during instability repairs, particularly for the placement of sutures or anchors into the posteroinferior glenoid.
- Posterolateral portal—approximately 1 cm lateral and 1 cm anterior to the posterolateral corner of the acromion, posterior to lateral portal site. Ideal for superior labral anterior to posterior (SLAP) repairs.
- Anterolateral (superolateral) portal—1 to 2 cm anterior to lateral portal, just lateral to the anterolateral corner of the acromion. Practical in rotator cuff repairs (particularly for anchor and suture techniques) and anterior shoulder procedures.
- Supraspinatus (Neviaser) portal—placed in corner of supraspinatus fossa. Can provide additional visualization and instrumentation during rotator cuff repairs (particularly anterior supraspinatus injuries) and useful in distal clavicle resections. The suprascapular nerve and artery are at risk medially (Figures 32–5 and 32–6).
- Port of Wilmington—1 cm lateral and 1 cm anterior to the posterolateral corner of the acromion. Generally

functions as a fixation device portal for SLAP repairs. Cannulas are not used at this site to prevent injuries to the infraspinatus tendon (Figure 32–7).

- After portal placement, examination of the joint should be performed in an orderly, thorough manner. The biceps tendon, rotator cuff, labrum, capsuloligamentous structures, and articular cartilage and surfaces should be evaluated for any fraying, tears, deformity, and erythema (Figure 32–8).

Box 32–2	**Contraindications**

Local skin pathology
Potential spread of infection from remote site
Patient with significant medical risks

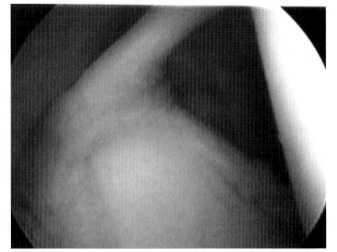

Figure 32–2:
Arthroscopic view of the biceps and biceps anchor (superior labrum).

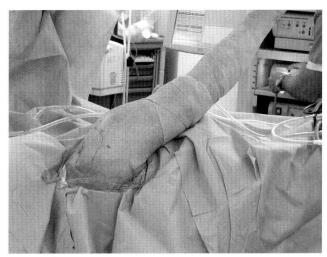

Figure 32–3:
Lateral decubitus position with the patient on a beanbag and the arm angled 30 degrees and in traction.

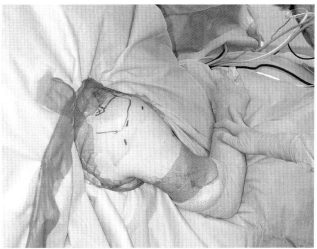

Figure 32–4:
Beach chair position with the arm positioned at the side.

Arthroscopic Shoulder Stabilization

- Arthroscopic treatment of glenohumeral instability has become increasingly popular with several well-designed clinical studies documenting efficacy (Figure 32–9).

- Thermal capsulorrhaphy, although initially very popular due to its ease of use, has lost favor due to high recurrence rates and complications.
- The use of thermal energy may still have a role as an adjunct to suture capsulorrhaphy or with subtle microinstability and internal impingement.

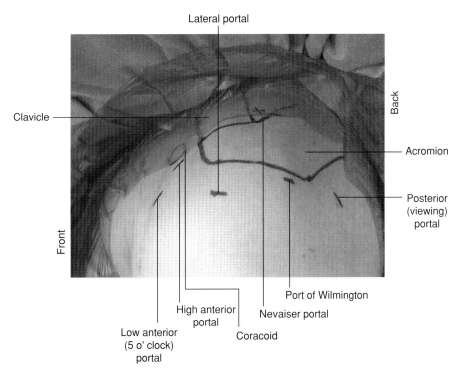

Figure 32–5:
Bony landmarks and portal sites outlined for shoulder arthroscopy in the beach chair position.

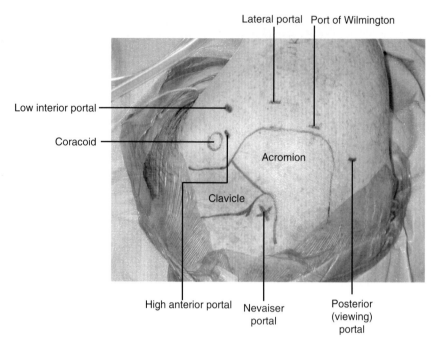

Figure 32–6:
Bony landmarks and portal sites outlined for shoulder arthroscopy in the lateral position.

- Contraindications to arthroscopic stabilization include large bony defects of the glenoid and humeral head and inexperience with the technique because it is technically demanding.

Rehabilitation

- Most surgical repairs require a period of sling immobilization for 4 to 6 weeks.

- Pendulum exercises and active hand, wrist, and elbow range of motion exercises are essential in the immediate postoperative period.
- Limited shoulder range of motion exercises can begin as early as 2 weeks and are advanced gradually.
- After pain-free full range of motion is restored, resisted strength training can be initiated.
- Patients should be aware that they will not be able to return to full sport activity for 4 to 8 months.

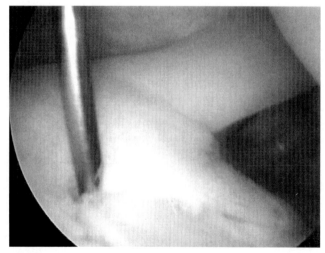

Figure 32–7:
Spinal needle through the accessory Port of Wilmington to be used for superior labral anterior to posterior (SLAP) anchor placement.

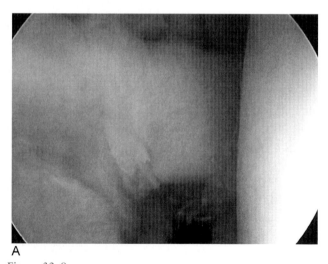

A

Figure 32–8:
Intraarticular joint structures. **A,** Biceps tendon in a patient with continued pain following a previous shoulder arthroscopy.

(continued)

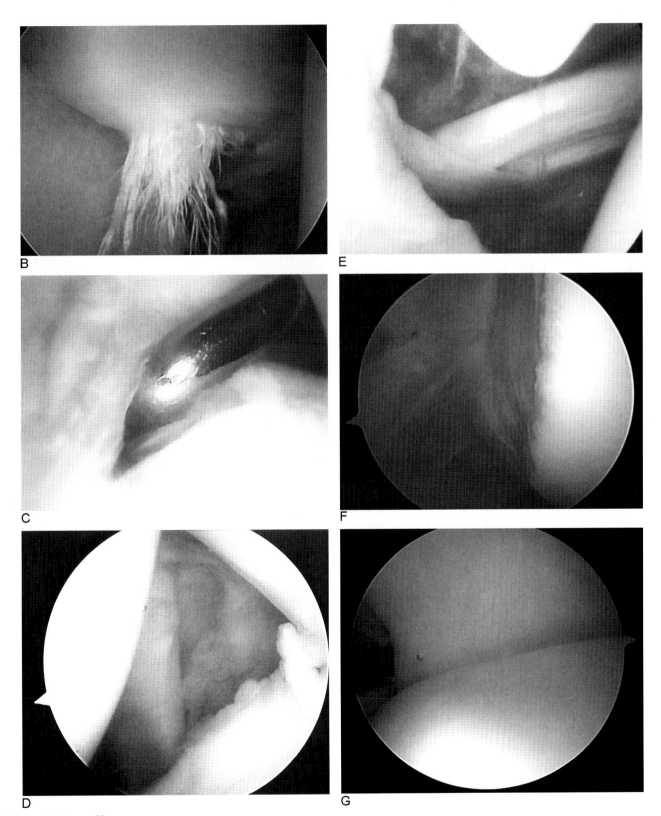

Figure 32–8, cont'd:
B, The source of pain became obvious when the biceps tendon was pulled interarticularly into the glenohumeral joint. **C,** Always probe lesions to determine whether they are intact or not as in this superior labral anterior to posterior (SLAP) tear. **D,** View of the rotator interval identified between the borders of the subscapularis, biceps, and anterior superior labrum. **E,** The middle glenohumeral ligament crosses the rolled border of the subscapularis tendon at 45 degrees. **F,** A large Hill-Sachs lesion is seen in this patient with recurrent, traumatic, anterior shoulder instability. **G,** Articular-sided view of the supraspinatus tendon.

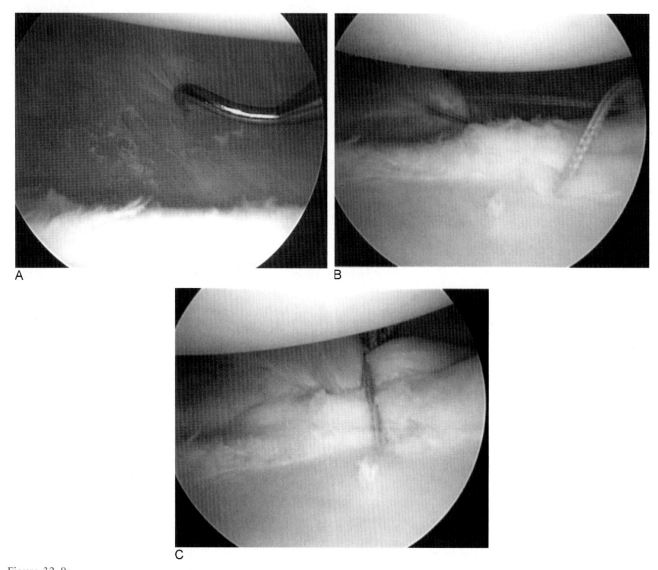

Figure 32–9:
Arthroscopic capsular plication. **A,** Soft tissue penetrator takes a tuck of capsule at the 6 o'clock position in a right shoulder. **B,** The suture on the anchor is shuttled through this tuck of capsule after it was passed through the labrum at the 7 o'clock position posteriorly. **C,** The suture is then tied, repairing the labrum anatomically and plicating the inferior and posterior-inferior capsule.

- Simple debridement or diagnostic procedures may follow a similar protocol in a much shorter period of time.

Complications

- Greater incidence of complications than arthroscopic knee surgery, although still low.
- Nerve damage (most common complication).
  - Anterior portals risk damage to the musculocutaneous nerve, which runs 2 cm inferior and 1 cm medial to the coracoid process.
  - The axillary nerve lies approximately 5 cm below the acromion and is at greatest risk with posteroinferior portal placement.

- Neurapraxia from traction (associated with the lateral decubitus position) or positioning errors.
- Fluid extravasation.
- Iatrogenic tendon injury, fractures, and articular damage.
- Stiffness.
- Equipment failure.
- Implant failure.
- Capsular necrosis.

References

Buuck DA, Davidson MR: Rehabilitation of the athlete after shoulder arthroscopy. *Clin Sports Med* 15:655-672, 1996.

Authors review the importance of rehabilitation to provide the shoulder with the greatest functionality following arthroscopic surgery. Modalities and rehabilitation protocols are reviewed in general terms and for specific arthroscopic procedures.

Craig EV: Shoulder arthroscopy in the throwing athlete. *Clin Sports Med* 15:673-700, 1996.

Author reviews the benefits of using shoulder arthroscopy as a diagnostic tool to confirm suspected pathology, assess associated conditions, and provide therapeutic options in the throwing athlete with shoulder problems. Anatomy and biomechanics of the shoulder are discussed. Several shoulder conditions are reviewed in detail, with an emphasis on arthroscopic findings and treatment possibilities.

Hulstyn MJ, Fadale PD: Arthroscopic anatomy of the shoulder. *Orthop Clinic North Am* 26:597-612, 1995.

Detailed, extensive review of arthroscopic anatomy of the shoulder. Portal placement and associated neurovascular structures at risk are discussed. Surface, bone, muscle, ligament, synovial, capsular, and joint anatomy are all addressed.

Jahnke AH, Greis PE, Hawkins RJ: Arthroscopic evaluation and treatment of shoulder instability. *Orthop Clin North Am* 26:613-630, 1995.

Authors review the use of arthroscopy in evaluating and treating the unstable shoulder. Normal anatomy is discussed and contrasted with pathologic findings associated with shoulder instability. Several therapeutic arthroscopic techniques are reviewed and compared.

Khan AM, Fanton GS: Electrothermal assisted shoulder capsulorraphy-monopolar. *Clin Sports Med* 21:599-618, 2002.

Indications, rationale, and techniques for monopolar electrothermal capsulorraphy are discussed. The authors describe its use in arthroscopic treatment of anterior, posterior, multidirectional, and traumatic shoulder instabilities. Postoperative rehabilitation and complications are reviewed. The authors report good results after 1- to 3-year follow-up in patients (overall satisfaction of approximately 90%), particularly in those with only unidirectional instability. Its ease of use and low complication rate make this an appealing therapeutic technique.

McFarland EG, O'Neill OR, Hsu CY: Complications of shoulder arthroscopy. *J Southern Orthop Assoc* 6:190-196, 1997.

General review of complications associated with shoulder arthroscopy. The authors report that neurovascular injury is the most common complication and often associated with the use of traction and the lateral decubitus position. The authors also mention some less common complications such as tension pneumothorax, deep venous thrombosis, and iatrogenic rotator cuff and chondral damage.

Nord KD, Mauck BM: The new subclavian portal and modified Neviaser portal for arthroscopic rotator cuff repair. *Arthroscopy* 19:1030-1034, 2003.

Authors describe two new portals (subclavian and modified Neviaser portals) that they have developed to improve on arthroscopic rotator cuff repairs. The authors study and review the portal anatomy using 20 cadaveric dissections and conclude that they offer optimal approaches to the rotator cuff tendons while reducing the risk of injury to surrounding structures.

Sekiya JK, Ong BC, Bradley JP: Thermal capsulorrhaphy for shoulder instability. *AAOS Instruct Course Lect* 52:65-80, 2003.

General review of thermal capsulorrhaphy and its use in shoulder instability. Techniques and results reviewed for anterior, posterior, multidirectional instability, and internal impingement. Thermal energy should only be used as an adjunct to suture capsulorrhaphy or plication.

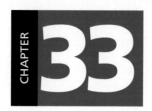
Anterior Shoulder Instability

Introduction

- One of the most common shoulder injuries in athletes.
- Anterior shoulder instability can occur in overhead throwing athletes (chronic, overuse injuries) but more commonly occurs in contact athletes (acute traumatic dislocations).
- Conceptually thought of as a continuum of pathology with possible contributions from many of the intraarticular shoulder structures (anterior labrum, superior labrum, biceps tendon, rotator interval, subscapularis).

Classification

Traumatic

Mechanism

- Most often associated with a posteriorly directed force applied to the anterior aspect of an abducted, externally rotated arm.
- A direct blow (from posterior) can also cause a traumatic anterior shoulder dislocation.
- Commonly includes a Bankart lesion, which is an avulsion of the labrum and anterior band of the inferior glenohumeral ligament from the anterior inferior glenoid (Figure 33–1).
- Considered essential lesion secondary to association with 90% of cases of anterior instability.
- If left untreated, there is an age-related recurrence rate of anterior instability.
- Active patients younger than 20 years may have recurrent instability rates approaching 80% to 90%.
- Recent studies have suggested that early splinting in external rotation may reduce this recurrence rate in first-time dislocators (Figure 33–2).
- Matsen has coined the term "TUBS" (traumatic unidirectional, Bankart lesion [often requiring] surgery) to characterize this problem.
- Traumatic subluxation (anterior displacement without complete dislocation of the glenohumeral joint) can occur as initial or recurrent injuries.

Associated Pathology

- Hill-Sachs lesion (Figure 33–3).
  - Chondral impaction injury in posterosuperior humeral head secondary to traumatic contact with glenoid rim.
  - 80% of cases of traumatic dislocation.
  - 25% of subluxations.
- Rotator cuff tears.
  - Older patients (>40 years).
- Nerve injury.
  - Usually temporary neuropraxia of the axillary nerve.
- Glenoid labral articular defect (GLAD).
  - Shearing off portion of articular cartilage along with labrum (repaired labrum must fill defect).
- Anterior labral periosteal sleeve avulsion (ALPSA).

Atraumatic

- Most often associated with underlying ligamentous laxity or overuse injury (can also be associated with traumatic injury bringing subacute injury to clinical attention).
- Usually responds to a nonoperative approach (rotator cuff strengthening and rehabilitation).

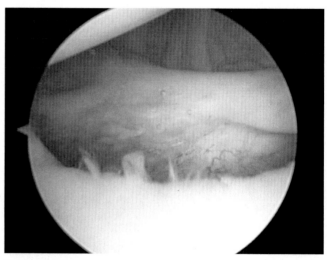

Figure 33–1:
Bankart lesion. (From Gartsman GM: *Shoulder arthroscopy.* Philadelphia, 2003, Saunders.)

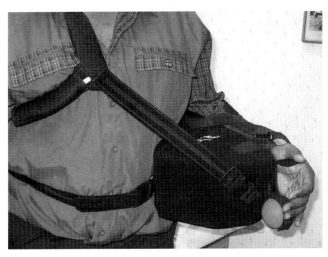

Figure 33–2:
External rotation splint.

- Surgery, when indicated, should include a capsulorraphy (classically an inferior capsular shift, but arthroscopic placation procedures are becoming popular).
- Matsen has coined the term "AMBRI" (atraumatic, multidirectional, bilateral, rehabilitation, [rarely requiring] inferior capsular shift) to characterize this condition.

Physical Examination

- Usually present with arm in a fixed, slightly externally rotated and abducted position.
  - The displaced humeral head may be observed or palpated (asymmetric to contralateral side).
  - Subacromial sulcus can be palpated.
  - Patient may splint affected arm with unaffected arm.
  - Neurologic evaluation should be performed before and after reduction attempts.

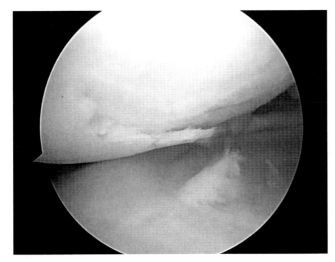

Figure 33–3:
Hill-Sachs lesion seen during shoulder arthroscopy in lateral decubitus position (left shoulder). (From Gartsman GM: *Shoulder arthroscopy.* **Philadelphia, 2003, Saunders.)**

- Range of motion and provocative testing including the apprehension, relocation, and load and shift testing should be performed at follow-up visit.
  - Comparison of examination to contralateral shoulder for reference.

Imaging

- Orthogonal views are mandatory.
  - True anteroposterior (AP) (in the plane of the scapula) and axillary lateral radiographs are preferred (Figure 33–4*A* and *B*).
  - "Scapular Y" view does not rule out a dislocation.
- Hill-Sachs lesions are best visualized with a Stryker notch view or an AP in internal rotation.
- Bony Bankart lesions can be visualized with a West Point (modified axillary lateral) view.
- Magnetic resonance imaging (MRI) can be helpful in identifying labral tears (the addition of intraarticular contrast [MR arthrogram] increases the sensitivity and specificity of the test) (Figure 33–4*C*).

Treatment

Reduction

- A variety of techniques have been described, but simple traction-countertraction is most commonly used.
- Prone positioning with gravity-assisted reduction has also been found to be effective.
- Relaxation of the patient is essential (sedation as necessary).

Immobilization

- Conventional immobilization has not proven to be beneficial; however, newer studies have suggested that immobilization in external rotation may reduce recurrent instability. More studies need to be done to validate this approach, which is still not popular due to noncompliance.

Physical Therapy

- Strengthening of dynamic stabilizers (rotator cuff and periscapular musculature).
- This has also been largely unsuccessful in TUBS patients but is the mainstay of treatment for AMBRI patients.
- Improving neuromuscular function and proprioceptive feedback.

Surgical Treatment

- Approached by treatment of specific causative etiology (Table 33–1).
- Early repair of first-time dislocators remains controversial.
  - Advocates propose that early repair prevents inevitable recurrence in young patients and also prevents propagation of pathology.

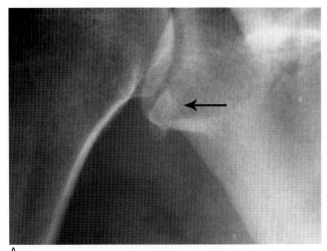

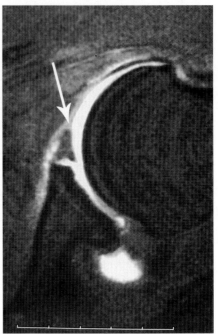

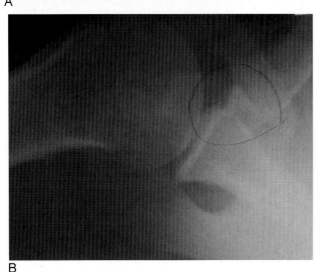

Figure 33–4:

A, Bony Bankart on anteroposterior radiograph. **B,** Bony Bankart on axillary lateral radiograph. **C,** Bankart lesion on magnetic resonance imaging. (**A** and **B** from Gartsman GM: *Shoulder arthroscopy.* Philadelphia, 2003, Saunders; **C** from Miller MD, Howard RF, Plancher KD: *Surgical atlas of sports medicine.* Philadelphia, 2003, Saunders.)

TABLE 33–1:	**Anatomic Considerations in Shoulder Stabilization**
POSITION OF ABNORMAL TRANSLATION	**DEFICIENT ANATOMIC STRUCTURE**
Inferior subluxation (in adduction)	Rotator interval
Translation at 45 degrees	Middle glenohumeral ligament
Translation at 90 degrees	Anterior, inferior glenohumeral ligament
Inferior subluxation (in abduction)	Axillary recess
Posterior translation at 90 degrees	Posterior, inferior glenohumeral ligament
Posterior translation at 45 degrees	Mid-posterior capsule

From Guanche CA: *Oper Tech Sports Med* 10:19, 2002.

- Repair of the Bankart lesion can be accomplished using arthroscopic or open techniques.
- Capsulorraphy (open or arthroscopic) is favored for refractory AMBRI cases and recurrent dislocators.
  ○ Open approaches are the gold standard and most appropriate for recurrent dislocators requiring a larger capsular shift (Figure 33–5).

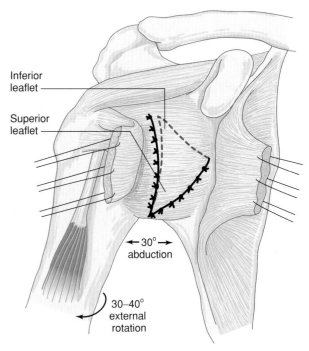

Figure 33–5:

Open capsular shift. (From Ortiguerra CJ, Brodersen MP: *Oper Tech Sports Med* 10:54, 2002.)

○ Complications of open capsulorraphy include subscapularis rupture, axillary nerve injury (risk can be reduced by abducting and externally rotating the arm during the inferior shift), and capsular overtightening (may require late capsular release or subscapularis Z-plasty, or both).

○ Arthroscopic approaches are advocated in first-time dislocators with Bankart tears and have less morbidity but are associated with a steeper learning curve (Table 33–2).

○ Complications of arthroscopic procedures can include a greater incidence of recurrence and neurologic injury.

• Thermal capsulorraphy.
  • Using heat to cause disruption of the intermolecular bonds through denaturation of the collagen.
  • Has been associated with high recurrence rates (10% to 50% failure rates) and other complications such as capsular necrosis.

• Largely operator dependent due to technique-dependent depth of penetration.
• Requires close patient compliance.
• Bone grafting may be necessary for cases with inferior glenoid deficiencies (inverted pear) (Figure 33–6).
  • Greater than 30% of glenoid articular surface considered unstable.
• Rotator interval closure (open or arthroscopic) is indicated in multi-directional instability (MDI) or persistent inferior or inferoposterior translation (Figure 33–7).
• Nonanatomic procedures such as the Bristow (coracoid transfer), Putti-Platt (medial subscapularis tenodesis), and Magnussen-Stack (lateral subscapularis tenodesis) have largely fallen out of favor because of associated complications (recurrence, loss of external rotation, and late arthrosis [posterior glenoid wear]).

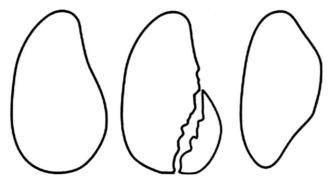

Figure 33–6:
Inverted pear concept. (From Douoguih WA, Shaffer BS: *Oper Tech Sports Med* 12:94, 2004.)

Table 33–2:	Arthroscopic Stabilization Techniques	
TECHNIQUE	**ADVANTAGES**	**DISADVANTAGES**
Staple capsulorrhaphy		High failure (30%)
		Staple migration/breakage
		Does not address capsular laxity
Transglenoid sutures	Multiple fixation points address capsular laxity	High failure rate
		Suture loosening with time
		Sutures cannot be tied arthroscopically
		Suprascapular nerve injury
Cannulated bioabsorbable implants	Avoids transscapular drilling	Does not address capsular laxity
	Short learning curve	Possible synovial reaction to polyglyconate
Suture anchors	Low failure rate (10%)	Technical difficulty
	Arthroscopic knot tying	Suture breakage
		Screw migration

From Miller MD, Cooper DE, Warner JJP: *Review of sports medicine and arthroscopy.* Philadelphia, 2002, Saunders. Adapted from Cole BJ, Warner JJP: *Clin Sports Med* 19:19–48, 2000.

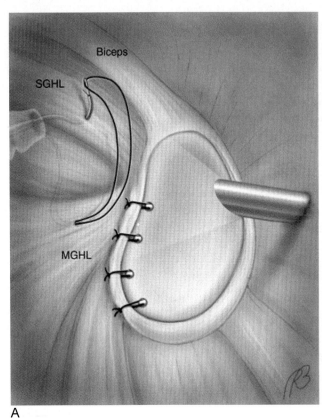
A

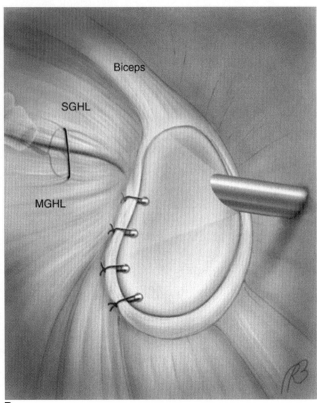
B

Figure 33–7:

Rotator interval closure. A, Before closure. **B,** After closure. MGHL, Superior glenohumeral ligament; SGHL, middle glenohumeral ligament. (From Miles JW, Tasto JP: *Oper Tech Sports Med* 12:132-133, 2004.)

References

Fleega BA: Arthroscopic reinforced capsular shift of anterior shoulder instability. *Arthroscopy* 20:543-546, 2004.

This author describes a technique of using standard shoulder arthroscopy to make an inverted L-shaped incision in the capsule, passing a suture through the flap and mobilizing it to tie over the upper subscapularis. Benefits described using this technique may include fewer operative steps and operating room time, complete lack of retained hardware, and faster rehabilitation schedule and return to sport.

Freedman KB, Smith AP, Romeo AA, et al: Open Bankart repair versus arthroscopic repair with transglenoid sutures or bioabsorbable tacks for recurrent anterior instability. *Am J Sports Med* 32:1520-1527, 2004.

This is a meta-analysis of literature to date on comparison between arthroscopic and open repair of Bankart lesions. Traditionally, the open technique is thought to provide a more stable repair. The authors suggest that more research on newer arthroscopic Bankart repair techniques is necessary.

Gaunche CA: Arthroscopic shoulder stabilization. *Oper Tech Sports Med* 10:18-24, 2002.

Useful resource in providing a quick, high-yield overview of the operative technique in arthroscopy anterior labral repair.

Gill TJ, Zarins B: Open repairs for the treatment of anterior shoulder instability. *Am J Sports Med* 31:142-153, 2003.

These authors discuss all of the pathologic lesions that are associated with shoulder instability, emphasizing that no one particular lesion is solely responsible for the instability. Surgical technique and rehabilitation plan should be tailored to each individual case.

Itoi E, Hatakeyama Y, Kido T, et al: A new method of immobilization after traumatic anterior dislocation of the shoulder: a preliminary study. *J Shoulder Elbow Surg* 12:413-415, 2003.

This is a prospective randomized study that demonstrates that treating first-time dislocators in an external rotation brace rather than the traditional internal rotation brace may reduce the risk of recurrence.

McCarty ED, Ritchie P, Gill HS, McFarland EG: Shoulder instability: return to play. *Clin Sports Med* 23:335-351, 2004.

This is a review article that addresses the problem of determining the appropriate criteria for return to play for competitive athletes. The article includes discussion of rehabilitation goals after dislocation/subluxation events treated conservatively and those for athletes who undergo surgical treatment of shoulder instability.

Nelson BJ, Arciero RA: Arthroscopic management of glenohumeral instability. *Am J Sports Med* 28:602-614, 2000.

This is a review of the arthroscopic treatment option for patients with shoulder instability. Current techniques for first-time dislocators, those with multidirectional instability, and recurrent unidirectional dislocators are discussed.

Robinson CM, Dobson RJ: Anterior instability of the shoulder after trauma. *J Bone Joint Surg Br* 86:469-479, 2004.

A review article discussing traumatic unidirectional shoulder instability. The authors address issues of initial treatment, rehabilitation, surgical options and indications, and return to play.

Sanders TG, Morrison WB, Miller MD: Imaging techniques for the evaluation of glenohumeral instability. *Am J Sports Med* 28:414-434, 2000.

This article serves as a review of all imaging techniques for the evaluation of shoulder instability. A discussion of proper plain radiographic views, computed tomography, plain MRI, and arthrogram MRI are all included.

Walton J, Paxinos A, Tzannes A, et al: The unstable shoulder in the adolescent athlete. *Am J Sports Med* 30:758-767, 2002.

There is such a high rate of recurrence of shoulder dislocation in young athletes that there is concern regarding the appropriate way to treat this patient population. This article discusses treatment and rehabilitation goals for this special group of athletes.

CHAPTER **34**

Posterior Shoulder Instability

Introduction

- Posterior shoulder instability is much less common than anterior instability with a reported incidence of 2% to 12% of all shoulder instability cases.
- Underlying pathology is predominantly attributed to capsular stretch, injury or deformation of capsuloligamentous structures, and/or damage to the glenolabral socket.
- Increased humeral or glenoid retroversion or glenoid hypoplasia are possible underlying bony abnormalities leading to posterior instability.
- Because posterior instability usually occurs during shoulder midrange motion, when the capsule and ligaments are lax, it has been postulated that capsular or ligament pathology alone cannot explain the presence of posterior instability.
- Primary stabilizers during midrange motion include orientation of the articular surfaces, the rotator cuff complex, and the deepening of the glenoid fossa produced by the labrum.
- Studies have demonstrated that the subscapularis muscle is the primary dynamic restraint to posterior translation. Furthermore, the coracohumeral ligament was noted to be an essential structure with the humerus in neutral position, and the inferior glenohumeral ligament was a significant contributor when the humerus underwent extreme internal rotation.

History, Physical Examination, and Imaging

- Posterior instability can be unidirectional, bidirectional (e.g., posteroinferior), or multidirectional with prevalent posterior instability symptoms.
- Posterior instability can result from trauma, overuse, or atraumatic mechanisms.
- Posterior dislocations may result after seizures or electrical shocks.
- The shoulder is vulnerable to posterior subluxation or dislocation in the flexed, adducted, and maximally

internally rotated arm. Posterior instability is most commonly the result of a traumatic injury with the arm in this position.
- Weight lifters, throwers, gymnasts, swimmers, racquet sports players, and football players are the most common athletes at risk (sports involving repetitive overhead activities or contact sports).
- Patients often report pain with activities that place their arm in a position of posterior vulnerability (adduction, flexion, internal rotation).
- Patients with an acute or missed posterior dislocation may present with a prominent posterior shoulder and anterior coracoid and have limited external rotation and elevation. The arm may be internally rotated and adducted.
- Posterior dislocations are missed in up to 50% of cases on initial evaluation.
- Mechanism of injury and specific symptoms should be elicited from all patients.
- Most posterior dislocations reduce spontaneously.
- Acute subluxations are often associated with avulsions of the posterior band of the inferior glenohumeral ligament.
- Posterior Bankart lesions are characterized by the detachment of the posterior inferior capsulolabral complex (Figure 34–1). Chronic reverse Bankart lesions may develop a paralabral cyst (Figure 34–2).
- Patients with recurrent subluxation often develop a large capsular pouch into which the humerus can sublux. Tears and detachment of the capsule occur in traumatic cases.
- Dislocations that do not readily reduce are often associated with humeral impression (reverse Hill-Sachs) fractures that keep the humerus locked posteriorly.
- Differentiation between laxity and instability must be made. Laxity refers to a shoulder with capsular or ligamentous stretch that can allow up to 2+ translation without symptoms (Lintner). In comparison, instability produces symptoms.
- Examination must carefully evaluate motion, laxity, and stability (Box 34–1).
- Stability and laxity may be evaluated under anesthesia and should be documented when surgical repair is performed.

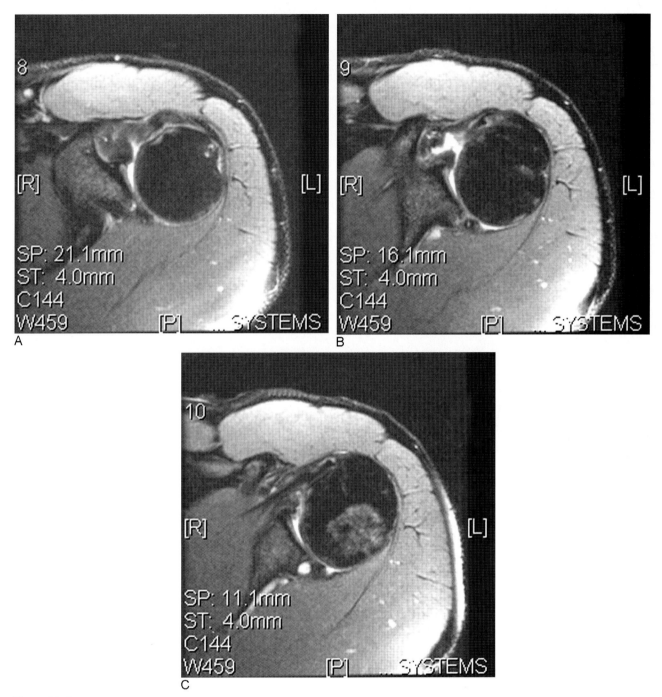

Figure 34–1:
A-C, Magnetic resonance imaging arthrogram showing a posterior labral tear (reverse Bankart lesion).

- Neurologic evaluation of the brachial plexus should be included in every examination.
- Associated pathology should also be evaluated, such as scapular winging, and corrected before any surgical intervention is entertained (Figure 34–3).
- It should be noted that overhead athletes (pitchers) that develop laxity secondary to their activity demands and are asymptomatic do not require treatment unless symptoms develop.
- Laxity can be graded according to the amount of translation (Box 34–2).
- Jerk test is often positive. This test is performed with the arm elevated 90 degrees and internally rotated. Posterior pressure is applied while stabilizing the scapula and

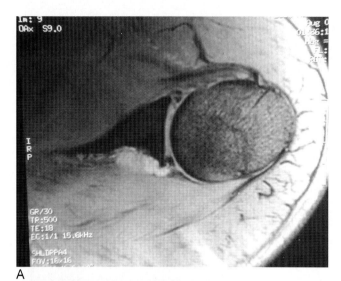

A

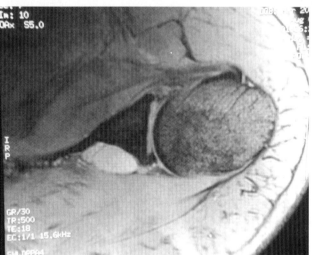

B

Figure 34–2:

A and B, Magnetic resonance imaging arthrogram showing a chronic posterior labral tear with paralabral cyst formation.

translation is noted. If the humerus is posteriorly subluxated, a palpable reduction with a "clunk" or jerk is produced when the arm is abducted (Figure 34–4). The posterior apprehension test is performed in a similar fashion and considered positive if the patient demonstrates significant guarding or apprehension.

- Anterior and posterior load-shift tests, the crank test, and sulcus tests should also be incorporated into the instability portion of the examination (Figure 34–5).
- It is important to test for bidirectional or multidirectional instability patterns.
- Standard radiographs should include anteroposterior (AP), axillary, and apical oblique (Garth) views.
  - The Garth view, taken as an AP view with the radiograph directed 45 degrees caudad, provides a coronal view of the glenohumeral joint that is sensitive

to anterior or posterior translation, Hill-Sachs lesions, and anteroinferior glenoid rim pathology.
- Velpeau views should be performed on patients unable to abduct the arm for traditional axillary views (Figure 34–6).
- Reverse Hill-Sachs lesions (anteromedial humeral head impaction fractures) and posterior glenoid rim fractures suggest posterior shoulder pathology.

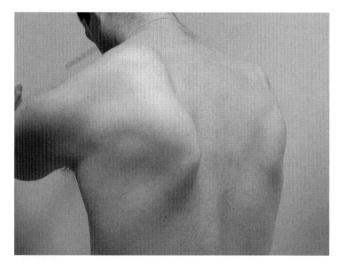

Figure 34–3:

Severe scapular winging in this patient may contribute to shoulder instability.

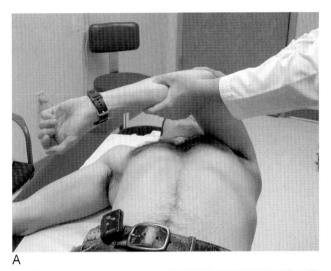
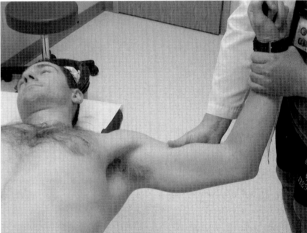
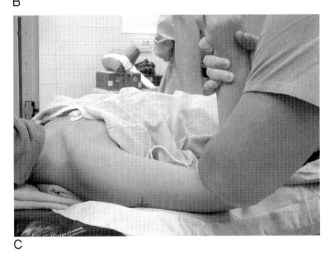

A

B

C

Figure 34–5:
A, Jerk test with arm brought into maximal adduction, internal rotation, and 90 degrees of forward flexion with the humeral head posteriorly subluxated. **B,** Arm gently brought into horizontal abduction and external rotation reduces the humeral head anteriorly, producing a characteristic "jerk."
C, Inferior sulcus testing during the examination under anesthesia evaluates inferior instability.

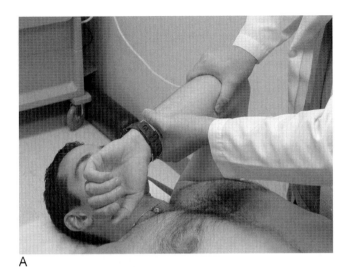

A

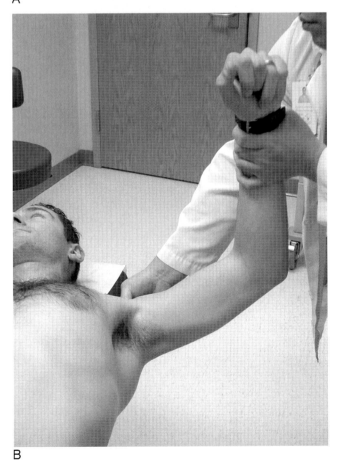

B

Figure 34–4:
A, Posterior apprehension testing. **B,** Modified posterior load and shift test.

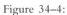

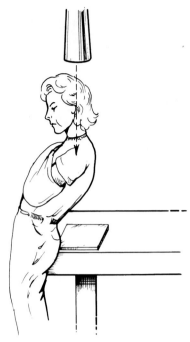

Figure 34–6:
Technique for Velpeau view, a modified axillary view. (From Warner JJP, Caborn DN: *Crit Rev Phys Rehabil Med* 4:145-198, 1992.)

- Observation of glenoid hypoplasia, humeral or glenoid retroversion, ossific lesions (Bennett lesions), and glenoid or humeral fractures should be noted.
- Computed tomography (CT) is recommended in cases where glenoid hypoplasia, occult fractures, or abnormal version of the humerus or glenoid is suspected.
- Magnetic resonance imaging (MRI) arthrography is extremely useful and is used by many surgeons (see Figures 34–1 and 34–2).

Types

- Classification of shoulder instability is generally divided among acute and chronic dislocations and traumatic and atraumatic injuries (Box 34–3).

Box 34–3	**Classification of Posterior Dislocations**

Acute posterior dislocation: <6 weeks
Chronic posterior dislocation: >6 weeks
Recurrent subluxation
   Traumatic
   Atraumatic
      Voluntary
      Involuntary

From Miller MD, Cole BJ, editors: *Textbook of arthroscopy.* Philadelphia, 2004, Saunders.

- Atraumatic injuries are further subdivided into voluntary and involuntary types.
- Voluntary dislocation/subluxation can be further subdivided.
  - Habitual dislocators may have an underlying personality disorder that must be ruled out.
  - Dislocations that can willfully be reproduced by muscular control when asked but not performed for any personal gain.
- Posterior instability may also be part of bidirectional or multidirectional patterns.

Treatment

- Initial treatment consists of physical therapy and rehabilitation and avoidance of activities that impose stress on the posterior capsule.
- Acute dislocations should be reduced and immobilized in neutral position for a period of 4 to 6 weeks. The presence of instability or significant articular damage may further direct management (Box 34–4).
- Atraumatic instability responds significantly better to nonoperative management than instability resulting from trauma (80% vs. 16%—Rockwood). Conversely, patients with traumatic instability and minimal ligamentous laxity have the best surgical prognosis.
- Open or arthroscopic surgical repairs are reserved for patients who fail nonoperative treatment, are chronic dislocators, or have associated glenoid or displaced lesser tuberosity fractures.
- Restoring the glenolabral concavity, reducing capsular redundancy, and repairing damaged intrinsic stabilizers are key elements in surgical repair.
- Arthroscopic repairs are best suited in patients requiring only soft tissue repairs (Figure 34–7).
- Patients with bony abnormalities, fractures, or congenital anomalies often require an open approach.

Box 34–4	**Management of Posterior Dislocations**

<40% articular surface
Reduce
Evaluate stability
   Stable
      Splint in 10 degrees of external rotation
   Unstable
      Arthroscopy
      Repair capsule and labral avulsion
      Splint in 10 degrees external rotation
>40% articular surface
Reduce
Hemiarthroplasty

From Miller MD, Cole BJ, editors: *Textbook of arthroscopy.* Philadelphia, 2004, Saunders.

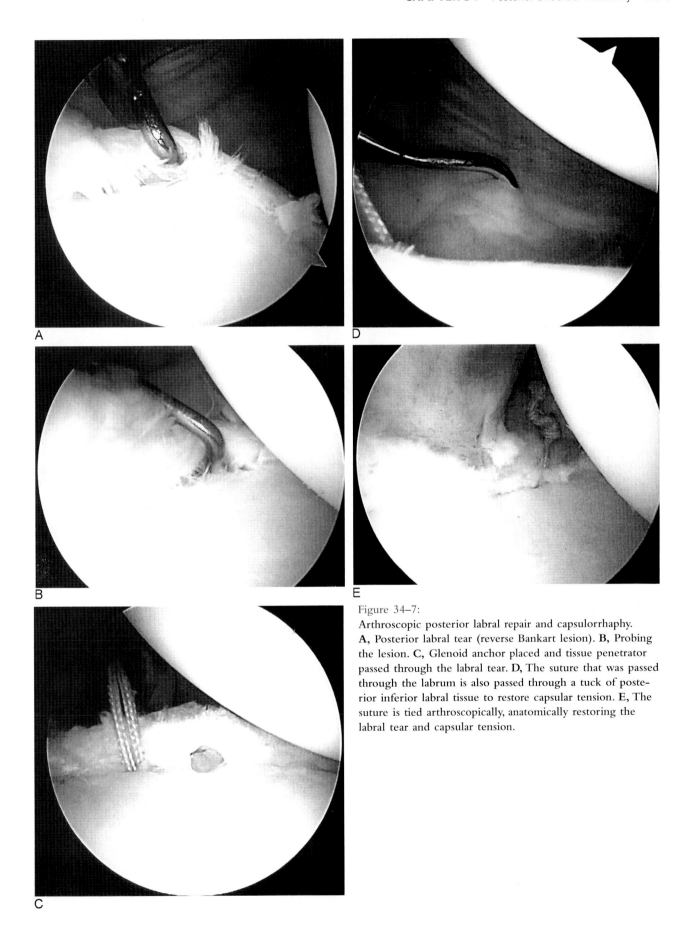

Figure 34–7:
Arthroscopic posterior labral repair and capsulorrhaphy.
A, Posterior labral tear (reverse Bankart lesion). **B,** Probing the lesion. **C,** Glenoid anchor placed and tissue penetrator passed through the labral tear. **D,** The suture that was passed through the labrum is also passed through a tuck of posterior inferior labral tissue to restore capsular tension. **E,** The suture is tied arthroscopically, anatomically restoring the labral tear and capsular tension.

- Patients with involuntary instability generally have better surgical outcomes than those with voluntary instability and general ligamentous laxity.
- Several surgical procedures have been developed to correct the soft tissue lesions associated with posterior instability: posterior labral repair (reverse Bankart repair), posterior or staple capsulorrhaphy, posterior inferior capsular shift, infraspinatus imbrication (reverse Putti-Platt), and posterior bone block.
- Reducing the rotator interval may augment repairs and reduce posteroinferior translation in an adducted shoulder (Figure 34–8).
- When increased humeral or glenoid version is present, opening-wedge glenoplasty and external rotational

humeral osteotomy can be used in conjunction with soft tissue repairs.
- Several arthroscopic techniques have also been developed and are becoming more and more popular. Many recent studies demonstrate outcomes comparable to open procedures.
- Thermal capsulorrhaphy is recommended by some as an adjunct to further shrink and tighten the posterior capsule following suture plication or capsulorrhaphy.

Rehabilitation

- Rehabilitation protocols for traumatic (Box 34–5) and atraumatic posterior instability (Box 34–6).

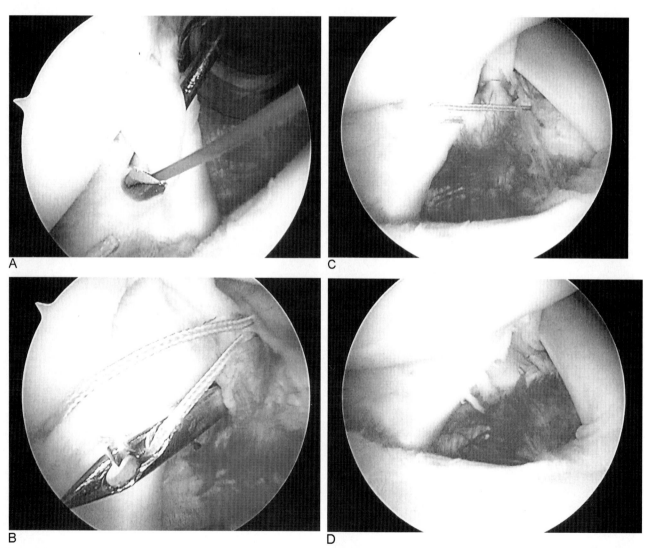

Figure 34–8:
Arthroscopic rotator interval closure. **A,** Suture penetrator is passed through the middle glenohumeral ligament as it crosses the subscapularis tendon. **B,** A soft tissue penetrator is then passed through the superior portion of the rotator interval and pulled through extraarticularly. **C,** The suture is tightened and then tied arthroscopically on the external portal of the anterior capsule. **D,** The contracted rotator interval following arthroscopic closure.

- Conservative management should focus on strengthening the rotator cuff, posterior deltoid, and scapular stabilizers.
- Initial rehabilitation should use closed-chain exercises that do not create shear forces across the shoulder joint.
- Early on, attention should be given to the entire kinetic chain, which includes the legs, hip, and trunk, specific to the athlete's sport and normal activity.
- After surgical stabilization procedures, the extremity can be placed in a pillow sling, rigid "handshake," or gunslinger orthosis with the arm in neutral position. Depending on the surgery, amount of laxity, and speed of recovery, this may last 4 to 8 weeks.
- While the extremity is immobilized, patients should be instructed on range-of-motion exercises of the wrist and elbow and Codman exercises.
- Adduction, flexion, and internal rotation are to be avoided during the early part of rehabilitation to allow proper healing of the posterior capsule.
- External rotation exercises can be incorporated during initial rehabilitation.
- Range-of-motion exercises are also prohibited until 6 to 8 weeks, when the capsule has regained approximately 80% of its strength.

Box 34–6 Rehabilitation Protocol for Atraumatic Posterior Instability

Weeks 0–3

No motion! Patient in handshake orthosis (gunslinger brace) at all times
Grip strengthening and supination, pronation of forearm

Weeks 3–8

Active ROM only to regain FF and ER at side as tolerated
IR-ADD limited to stomach or active cross-body ADD without pain
IR in ABD permitted if active only
Begin isometrics with arm at side—ER, IR, ABD, ADD; no resisted FF or biceps motion
Start strengthening scapular stabilizers (trapezoids, rhomboids, levator scapulae)
No passive motion of posterior capsule

Weeks 8–12

Increase posterior capsule ROM gently (active ROM)
Advance strengthening as tolerated: isometrics → bands → weights; 10 repetitions/1 set per rotator cuff, deltoid, and scapular stabilizers; no resisted FF or biceps motion yet
Do strengthening only 3 times/wk to avoid rotator cuff tendinitis

Months 3–12

Advance to full ROM as tolerated
Begin eccentrically resisted motions, plyometrics, proprioception, body blade, and closed chain exercises at 16 wk
Resume sports, throwing at 6 mo postop

ABD, Abduction; ADD, adduction; ER, external rotation; FF, forward flexion; IR, internal rotation; ROM, range of motion.
From Miller MD, Cole BJ, editors: *Textbook of arthroscopy.* Philadelphia, 2004, Saunders.

- Range-of-motion exercises are then started, but internal rotation should be limited to 15 degrees less than the opposite side to prevent stretching of the capsular repair. Cross-arm adduction is also limited at this time. These last degrees of motion can usually be recovered by the patient on his or her own when a self-directed exercise program is instituted.
- After range of motion is recovered, strengthening of the surrounding musculature is advanced through closed chain exercises, plyometrics, interval sports training, and finally to preinjury sport activities.
- Patients usually do not return to sports earlier than 6 to 8 months after surgery.
- Postoperative rehabilitation follows a similar pattern to conservative management, with initial focus on regaining full range of motion. Strengthening exercises against progressive resistance are then initiated in all planes of motion until the patient returns to preinjury levels. Patients with hyperlaxity should receive further strengthening of the dynamic stabilizers.

Complications

- Failure rates up to 50% have been reported in posterior stabilization procedures.
- Adhesive capsulitis.
- Suprascapular nerve injury is possible with excessive retraction or instrumentation medial to the posterior glenoid rim.
- Axillary nerve injury can occur with inferior dissection that encroaches the quadrangular space or with poor portal placement.
- Returning patients to sport activities too early may place them at risk of reinjury and recurrent subluxations or dislocations.
- Staple migration, loosening, and impaction (with staple capsulorrhaphy).
- Glenoplasty, osteotomy, and infraspinatus imbrication procedures have a higher rate of limited motion and accelerated degenerative changes.
- Osteonecrosis, arthritis, and impingement of the humeral head on the coracoid have been reported with glenoid opening-wedge osteotomies.
- Rotational osteotomies may be complicated by nonunion and loss of external rotation.

References

Abrams JS: Arthroscopic repair of posterior instability and reverse glenohumeral ligament avulsion lesions. *Orthop Clin North Am* 34:475-483, 2003.
Pathology and surgical correction of posterior instability is reviewed. Author stresses the importance of repairing reverse humeral glenohumeral ligament avulsions (RHAGL) when present. Surgical technique is described, including RHAGL repair, capsular shift, suture anchor repair, and closure of the rotator capsular interval.

Antoniou J, Harryman II DT: Repair of athletic shoulder injuries: Posterior instability. *Orthop Clin North Am* 32:463-473, 2001.

> *Review of the pathophysiology, evaluation, and treatment of posterior shoulder instability. Authors' preferred operative technique is described with postoperative management. Authors stress the importance of restoring the glenolabral cavity and reducing capsular redundancy. Authors report on findings and results in 41 consecutive patients with primary posteroinferior instability. Results demonstrated improved stability on examination in 86% of patients, although only 59% of patients reported complete resolution of their instability. Only 25% of the nine revision patients stated they had no instability postoperatively.*

Goubier JN, Iserin A, Duranthon LD, et al: A 4-portal arthroscopic stabilization in posterior shoulder instability. *J Shoulder Elbow Surg* 12:337-341, 2003.

> *Authors describe a four-portal posterior stabilization procedure with capsular plication and suture anchors. Authors comment that the four portals allow greater visualization and access to the injured glenoid, allowing good repair of posterior glenoid lesions that extend anteriorly. Capsular plication is emphasized to reduce the glenohumeral volume. This technique used on 13 shoulders resulted in postoperative satisfaction in all patients at a mean follow-up of 34 months. However, four shoulders had a loss of range of motion and two shoulders reported moderate pain symptoms. None of the shoulders treated experienced recurrent posterior shoulder instability.*

McIntyre LF, Caspari RB, Savoie FH: The arthroscopic treatment of posterior shoulder instability: two-year results of a multiple suture technique. *Arthroscopy* 13:426-432, 1997.

> *Authors describe and perform an arthroscopic posterior capsular shift in 20 symptomatic shoulders. Twelve of the shoulders had posterior Bankart lesions, and 10 had anterior Hill-Sachs lesions. At an average 31-month follow-up, there were 15 excellent, 2 good, 1 fair, and 3 poor results. There was an overall 25% recurrence rate that included two dislocations and three subluxations, all in patients with posterior Bankart lesions, and four in patients with a voluntary component to their insta-bility. After a review of previous literature, the authors contend that patients with voluntary posterior instability may receive better outcomes from open capsulorrhaphy procedures.*

Petersen SA: Conservative management of shoulder injuries: posterior shoulder instability. *Orthop Clin North Am* 31:263-274, 2000.

> *Review of posterior shoulder instability, including both dislocation and subluxation. Classification and anatomic constraints are discussed. Nonoperative treatment is emphasized and extensively covered.*

Sekiya JK, Ong BC, Bradley JP: Thermal capsulorrhaphy for shoulder instability. *Instruct Course Lect* 52:65-80, 2003.

> *General review of thermal capsulorrhaphy and its use in shoulder instability. Techniques and results reviewed for anterior, posterior, multidirectional instability, and internal impingement. Thermal energy should only be used as an adjunct to suture capsulorrhaphy or plication.*

Steinmann SP: Posterior shoulder instability. *Arthroscopy* 19:102-105, 2003.

> *Good brief review of current concepts regarding posterior shoulder instability. Classification, presentation, evaluation, and treatment of posterior dislocations and recurrent posterior instability are discussed.*

Williams RJ, Strickland S, Cohen M, et al: Arthroscopic repair for traumatic posterior shoulder instability. *Am J Sports Med* 31:203-209, 2003.

> *Retrospective study of arthroscopic repair of posterior Bankart lesions in 27 shoulders using bioabsorbable tack fixation. All patients (26) had a preceding traumatic episode and had minimal to no posterior capsular laxity on examination. Mean follow-up was 5.1 years. Results demonstrated relief of symptoms in 92% of patients with 8% (two patients) requiring additional surgery for persistent symptoms and muscle weakness. No patients had a limited range of motion. Authors comment on the importance of reconstructing the posterior labral complex and recreating proper tension on the posterior band of the inferior glenohumeral ligament, a static restraint to posterior translation when the arm is abducted between 30 and 90 degrees.*

SLAP Tears and Internal Impingement

Introduction

- Superior labrum anterior to posterior (SLAP) tears and internal impingement are part of a continuum of shoulder pathology that the overhead athlete, particularly pitchers, frequently suffers from.
- Forces generated in the shoulder during throwing can exceed two to three times body weight and can lead to overuse injuries with repetitive activity.
- During the pitching cycle, hand velocity approaches 7000 degrees/second.
- SLAP lesions were originally recognized by Andrews in 1985 and later described as "SLAP" by Snyder and Walsh in 1991 when they noted pathologic changes to the superior labrum in 6% of their shoulder arthroscopies.
- Internal impingement (impingement of the supraspinatus tendon on the posterosuperior glenoid rim with late cocking) was initially described in the early 1990s by surgeons including Walsh and Jobe.
- Both these entities have been associated with anterior instability and rotator cuff disease.

Superior Labrum Anterior to Posterior Lesions

History

- Patients may complain of vague deep shoulder pain that is sometimes associated with catching, popping, or locking of their shoulder with overhead activities.
- Pain is secondary to interposition of the labrum between the humeral head and the glenoid.

Mechanism

- Described as either a traction or compression injury related to a fall on an outstretched arm.
- The pathophysiology begins with contracture of the posteroinferior glenohumeral ligament, which shifts the glenohumeral contact point posterosuperiorly. This increases shear forces on the posterosuperior labrum creating a peel-back effect and finally, a SLAP.

Physical Examination

- Patients, particularly baseball pitchers, commonly have a glenohumeral internal rotation deficit (GIRD) in comparison with their nondominant shoulder (Figure 35-1).
- A variety of examinations have been described.
- Tenderness at the rotator interval.
- The "crank" test—pain or "click" with varying positions within the axial plane while passively internally rotating and axially loading the abducted shoulder.
- O'Brien test—pain with resisted forward flexion of the slightly adducted and pronated arm (with the elbow straight) that improves with supination.
- 85% of patients with pathology have a positive apprehension test, and 86% have a positive relocation test.

Imaging

- Radiographs are usually not helpful.

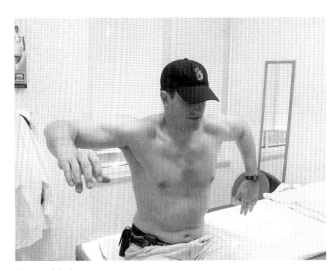

Figure 35-1:
Glenohumeral internal rotation deficit. Right shoulder is affected side.

- Magnetic resonance imaging (MRI) is sometimes helpful but is not highly sensitive or specific. Sensitivity and specificity increase with the addition of an arthrogram (Figure 35–2).
- Posterior subtype can be associated with a spinoglenoid perilabral cyst.

Arthroscopy

- The diagnosis is commonly made incidentally during arthroscopy, but there is not complete consensus regarding diagnostic criteria.
- Anatomic variation sometimes confused with pathology.
  - Pathology frequently associated with hemorrhage or other signs of trauma (fraying).
  - Manipulation with a probe essential for complete evaluation.
  - Dynamic peel-back test (Figure 35–3) to confirm SLAP tear—arm brought from resting position to 90 degrees external rotation and 90 degrees abduction with observation of biceps anchor peeling off superior glenoid rim.
  - Common normal variants (Figure 35–4A).
    ○ Sublabral foramen (Figure 35–4B).
    ○ Meniscoid appearance.
    ○ Buford complex-cordlike middle glenohumeral ligament with attachment to base of biceps anchor

and complete absence of anterosuperior labrum (Figure 35–4C).
- Associated pathology.
  - Older patients.
    ○ Partial rotator cuff tear (29%).
    ○ Complete rotator cuff tear (11%).
  - Younger patients.
    ○ Bankart lesion (22%).
    ○ Signs of instability (widened rotator interval, drive-through sign).

Classification

- Originally described by Snyder with four types (Figures 35–5 and 35–6).
  - Type I: Labral fraying (rarely clinically symptomatic).
  - Type II: Detachment of biceps anchor from supraglenoid tubercle.
  - Type III: Bucket-handle tear with displacement into joint (anchor intact).
  - Type IV: Bucket-handle tear with propagation into biceps tendon.
- Types V to VII described by Maffett, involve anterior instability and inferior labrum.
- Types VIII to X described by Nord and Ryu.
- Importance is integrity of biceps anchor.

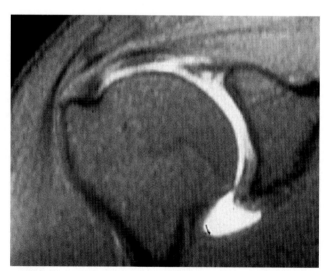

Figure 35–2:
Magnetic resonance arthrogram of superior labrum anterior to posterior tear.

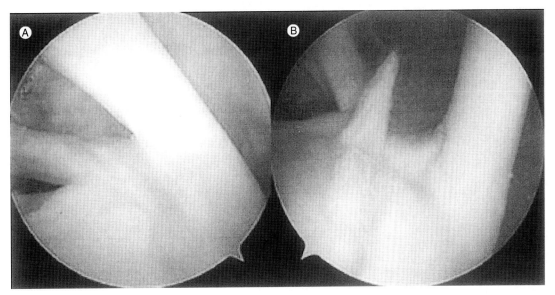

Figure 35–3:
Peel-back test. **A,** With arm in 90° external rotation and 90° abduction. **B,** The "peel back" off the superior glenoid. (From Parten PM, Burkhart SS: *Oper Tech Sports Med* 10:1, 2002.)

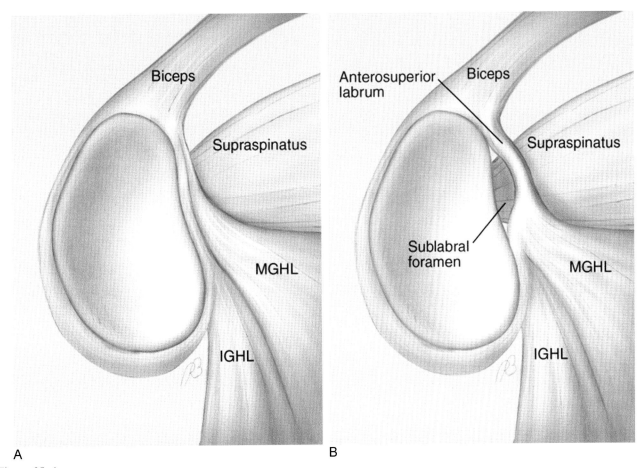

Figure 35–4:
Labral normal anatomic variation. A, Normal anatomy. **B,** Isolated sublabral foramen.

(continued)

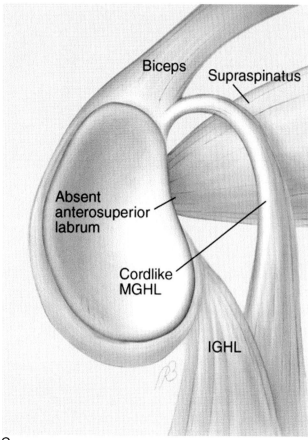

C

Figure 35–4, cont'd:
**C, Buford complex. IGHL, middle glenohumeral ligament.
MGHL, Middle glenohumeral ligament.** (From Powell SE,
Nord KD, Ryu RKN: *Op Tech Sports Med* 12:100-101, 2004.)

Treatment

Principles

- Type I: Debridement of flaps.
- Type II: Debridement with reattachment of biceps anchor.
- Type III: Debridement of flaps with possible repair depending on extent.
- Type IV: If tendon propagation less than $\frac{1}{3}$ diameter, then excise; otherwise repair.
- Type V to X: Stabilization of large labral tears and detachment of the biceps anchor.
- Bankart repair for lesions that extend inferiorly.
- Correct GIRD if present with posterior capsular release.

Technique

- Must have appropriate angle to glenoid rim for proper seating of suture anchor.
- Anterosuperior portal (rotator interval) used for anterior portion of tear.

- Port of Wilmington (posterolateral portal) used for posterior tear (Figure 35–7).
- Neviaser portal as accessory portal.

Rehabilitation

- Sling for 3 weeks with passive forward elevation; full elbow, wrist, and hand range of motion; avoidance of abduction and external rotation.
- Weeks 4 to 6: passive and active range of motion to 90 degrees of flexion.
- Before week 6: avoid flexion past 90 degrees and active biceps contraction.
- Sleeper stretch (posterior capsule) if capsulotomy performed.

Internal Impingement

Introduction

- Also referred to as posterosuperior glenoid impingement.
- Initially recognized during arthroscopies of athletes with partial articular-sided rotator cuff tears (treatment with debridement—85% of patients returned to preinjury level of activity).
- Mechanism: mechanical impingement of the greater tuberosity (with its attached supraspinatus) on the posterosuperior aspect of the glenoid rim during shoulder abduction, external rotation, and extension (Figure 35–8).
- Controversial subject including mechanism (overuse, acute), diagnosis (MRI, scope), associated pathology (instability, SLAP, rotator cuff tear), and treatment (debridement, labral repair, humeral osteotomy).
  - Jobe suggested the underlying cause to be microinstability allowing anterior translation, resulting in impingement of the supraspinatus tendon between the glenoid rim and greater tuberosity. Recommended treatment with capsular procedure to address microinstability.
  - Morgan and Burkhart suggested a mechanism of posterosuperior instability as opposed to anterior instability and recognized the association of the partial rotator cuff tear with the posterior subtype of type II SLAP lesions.

History

- Occurs commonly in pitchers as an overuse injury.
- Symptoms occur in the late cocking/early acceleration phase of throwing.

Examination

- Patients may present with lack of internal rotation as compared with the opposite side (GIRD).

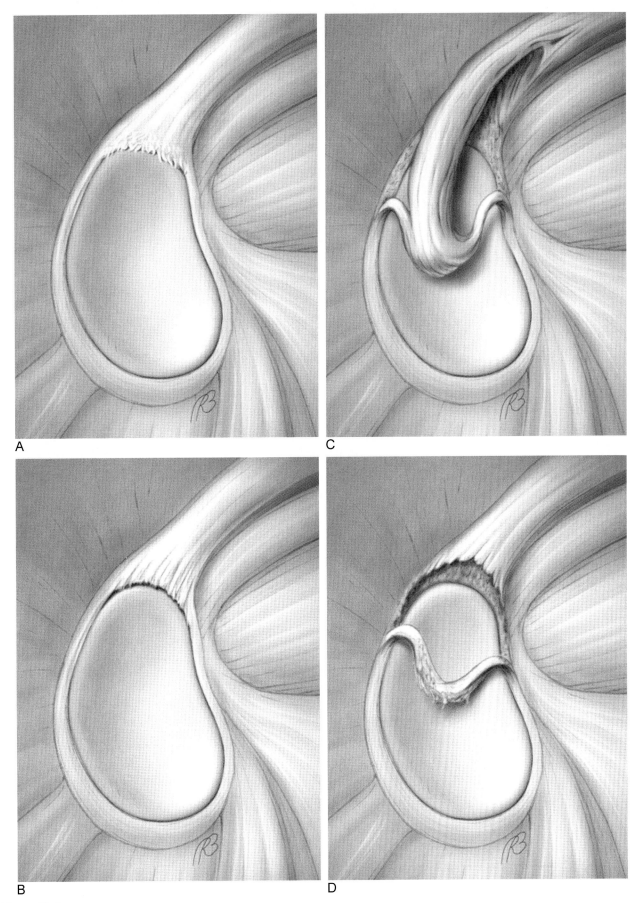

Figure 35–5:
Superior labrum anterior to posterior lesion classification. **A,** Type I. **B,** Type II. **C,** Type III. **D,** Type IV. (From Powell SE, Nord KD, Ryu RKN: *Oper Tech Sports Med* 12:101-102, 2004.)

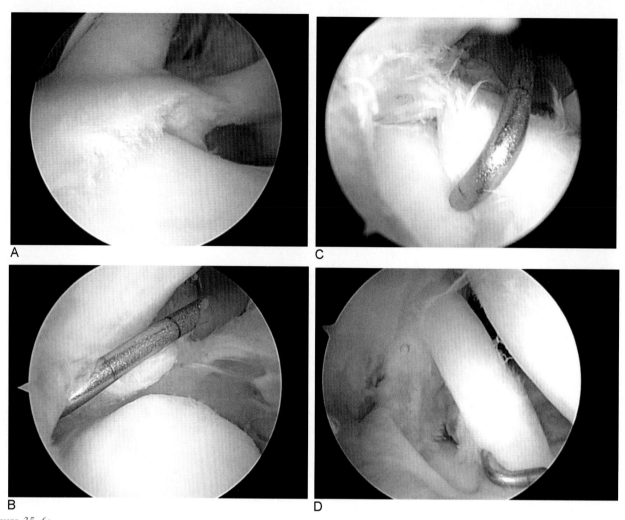

Figure 35–6:
Arthroscopic views of superior labrum anterior to posterior classification. **A,** Type I. **B,** Type II. **C,** Type III. **D,** Type IV. (From Gartsman GM: *Shoulder arthroscopy.* Philadelphia, 2003, Saunders.)

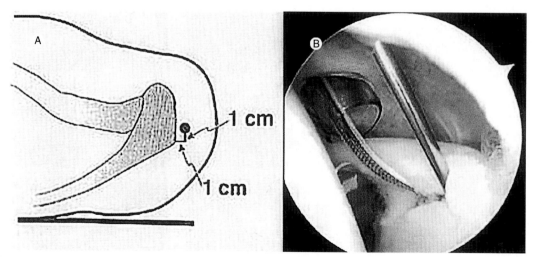

Figure 35–7:
Port of Wilmington. **A,** Portal is located off the anterolateral tip of the acromion. **B,** Establish portal with a spinal needle with 45 degree angle to the superior glenoid. (From Parten PM, Burkhart SS: *Oper Tech Sports Med* 10:15, 2002.)

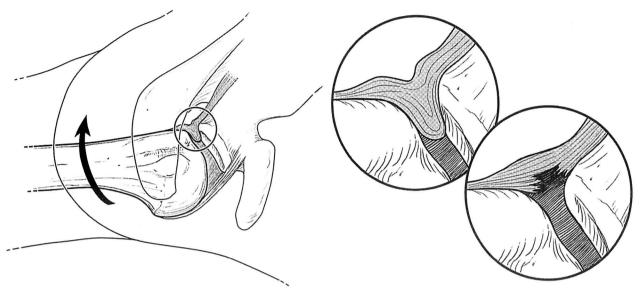

Figure 35–8:
Internal impingement. (From Edwards TB, Walch G: *Oper Tech Sports Med* 10:41, 2002.)

- Interestingly, these patients will have the same total arc of motion, but they sacrifice internal rotation for external rotation.
- Typically have pain posteriorly with apprehension test that is relieved with relocation test (no apprehension with apprehension test).
- Evaluate for common associated pathology (SLAP, rotator cuff tear, posterior capsular tightness, instability).
- Radiographs are often normal, but a posterior capsule exostosis (Bennett's lesion) may be present.

Treatment

Nonoperative

- Changing mechanics of throwing to avoid position of impingement.
  - Prevent extension beyond the plane of the scapula during cocking and acceleration.
- Rotator cuff strengthening (focus on internal rotation strengthening).
- Posterior capsular stretching ("sleeper stretch"—passive internal rotation of abducted down shoulder in the lateral decubitus position).

Operative

- Although most agree that debridement of the posterior superior labrum and posterosuperior rotator cuff is appropriate, treatment of associated GIRD or anterior microinstability, or both, is a hotly debated topic.
- Refractory GIRD can be treated with a posterior capsulotomy or humeral derotation osteotomy.
- Anterior microinstability may be treated with plication or selective thermal capsulorraphy.

References

Andrews JR, Broussard TS, Carson WG: Arthroscopy of the shoulder in the management of partial tears of the rotator cuff: a preliminary report. *Arthroscopy* 1:117-122, 1985.

Presented 36 patients with partial tears of the supraspinatus portion of the rotator cuff having undergone arthroscopic examination and debridement of the lesion. All patients, whose average age was 22 years, were involved in competitive athletics; 64% were baseball pitchers. Associated pathology included tears of the glenoid labrum and partial tearing or tendinitis of the long head of the biceps tendon. Of the 34 patients available for follow-up, 26 (76%) had excellent results, 3 (9%) had good results, and 5 (15%) had poor results. Eighty-five percent of the patients returned satisfactorily to their preoperative athletic activity.

Andrews JR, Carson WG, McLeod WD: Glenoid labral tears related to the long head of the biceps. *Am J Sports Med* 13:337-341, 1985.

First article to recognize the pathology later referred to as a "SLAP lesion." Tears of the glenoid labrum were observed in 73 baseball pitchers and other throwing athletes who underwent arthroscopic examination of the dominant shoulder. Also highlights the importance of the biceps with deceleration during the follow-through phase of throwing.

Andrews JR, Levitz C, Dugus J: Current concepts: internal impingement in the shoulder. Presented at the 26th annual meeting of AOSSM, Sun Valley, Idaho, June 2000.

Presented findings initially recognized during arthroscopies of athletes with partial articular-sided rotator cuff tears. First to describe the pathologic process as "internal impingement." The authors' treatment with debridement of the partial tears resulted in 85% of patients returning to their preinjury level of activity.

Cooper DE, Arnoczky SP, O'Brien SJ, et al: Anatomy, histology, and vascularity of the glenoid labrum. An anatomical study. *J Bone Joint Surg Am* 74:46-52, 1992.

Study of the gross, histologic, and vascular anatomy of the glenoid labrum in shoulders from cadavers. Findings included that the superior and anterosuperior portions of the labrum are loosely attached to the glenoid, and the macro-anatomy of those portions is similar to that of the meniscus of the knee. Also, the superior and anterosuperior parts of the labrum have less vascularity than do the posterosuperior and inferior parts, and the vascularity is limited to the periphery of the labrum.

Edwards TB, Walsh G: Posterosuperior glenoid impingement: is microinstability really the problem? *Oper Tech Sports Med* 10:1 40-46, 2002.

Addresses the controversy of the etiologic factors involved in the development of internal impingement. Presents both camps of thought and develops an argument supporting posterosuperior instability and refuting anterior instability.

Maffett MW, Gartsman GM, Moselet B: Superior labrum-biceps tendon complex lesions of the shoulder. *Am J Sports Med* 23:93-98, 1995.

The authors further classified SLAP tears that did not fit into the standard four types described by Snyder. They collected data over a 5-year period and found that 11.8% of patients had significant labral abnormalities, 6.2% had lesions that fit within the four-type classification system (Type II, 55%; III 4%; IV, 4%), but 38% had significant findings that could not be classified. These unclassifiable lesions fit into three distinct categories. They also recognized that examined under anesthesia, 43% of the shoulders were considered to have increased humeral head translation when compared with the other shoulder and should prompt the surgeon to investigate glenohumeral instability as the source of a patient's complaints.

Morgan CD, Burkhart SS, Palmeri M, et al: Type II SLAP lesions: three subtypes and their relationships to superior instability and rotator tears. *Arthroscopy* 14:553-565, 1998.

Investigated 102 type II SLAP lesions without associated pathology and found three distinct subtypes based on anatomic location: anterior (37%), posterior (31%), and combined anterior and posterior (31%). They also found that SLAP lesions with a posterior component develop posterior-superior instability that manifests itself by a secondary anterior-inferior pseudolaxity (drive-through sign) and that chronic superior instability leads to secondary lesion-location-specific rotator cuff tears that begin as partial thickness tears from inside the joint.

Morgan CD, Burkhart SS, Palmari M, et al: The peel-back mechanism: its role in producing and extending posterior type II SLAP lesions and its effect on SLAP repair rehabilitation. *Arthroscopy* 14:637-640, 1998.

Describes a mechanism of injury for posterior type II SLAP lesions with the primary feature of this mechanism as a torsional peel-back of the posterosuperior labrum. Article suggests fixation by posterior-superior placement of suture anchors into the posterosuperior corner of the glenoid is essential. Also advocates the repair being protected against torsional peel-back forces by avoiding external rotation beyond 0 degrees for 3 weeks.

Nord KD, Ryu RKN: 2004). *Further refinement of SLAP classification.* E-poster, AANA annual meeting, Orlando, Florida, April 22-25, 2004.

Further classification of SLAP lesions into types VIII to X based on associated pathology.

Powell SE, Nord KD, Ryu RKN: The diagnosis, classification, and treatment of SLAP lesions. *Oper Tech Sports Med* 12:2 99-110, 2004.

Thorough review of SLAP lesions with clear illustrations of the 10 described types. Provides a review of the literature and specific operative techniques used in the treatment of each type of lesion.

Snyder SJ, Karzel RP, DelPizzo W, et al: SLAP lesions of the shoulder. *Arthroscopy* 6:274-279, 1990.

A retrospective review of more than 700 shoulder arthroscopies performed at the authors' institution. Described arthroscopically recognized injury as a "SLAP lesion." The most common mechanism of injury was a compression force to the shoulder, usually as the result of a fall onto an outstretched arm, with the shoulder positioned in abduction and slight forward flexion at the time of the impact. The most common clinical complaints were pain, greater with overhead activity, and a painful "catching" or "popping" in the shoulder. The authors divided the superior labrum pathology into four distinct types.

Rotator Cuff Injuries

Introduction

- The rotator cuff complex is considered the major dynamic stabilizer of the glenohumeral joint.
- The rotator cuff muscles provide a concavity-compression effect and mechanically depress the humeral head within the glenohumeral joint, counteracting the superiorly directed force produced by deltoid activity. This function predominates in midrange shoulder motion, when the capsuloligamentous restraints are lax (Figure 36–1).
- The rotator cuff also acts to depress the humeral head, particularly when the arm is elevated above 90 degrees, reducing humeral head impingement.
- The rotator cuff muscles contribute to shoulder abduction and external rotation strength.
- The subscapularis functions as an internal rotator.
- Poor blood supply, further compromised with the arm in abduction, is believed to be the reason why the supraspinatus is the rotator cuff muscle most commonly injured.
- It is believed that rotator cuff pathology results from a combination of several possible intrinsic and extrinsic factors (Box 36–1).
- A tight posterior capsule may result in humeral head elevation and the development of impingement.
- Rotator cuff tendinitis often is most often a result of impingement, chronic overuse, acute overload, or degeneration.
- Studies have demonstrated that rotator cuff pathology is not an inflammatory response but closely resembles a degenerative process. As a result, the term tendinosis (rather than tendinitis) is a more appropriate pathologic term. Without a definitive etiology, such pathology can clinically be described as a tendinopathy.
- Impingement refers to a specific common condition whereby the anterior third of the acromion undersurface causes irritation of the underlying rotator cuff tendons (usually the supraspinatus), producing symptoms.

- Normal scapular rotation is required to raise the acromion away from the humeral head when the arm is elevated and to maintain a clear space for the rotator cuff complex.
- There is very little clear space between the rotator cuff and acromion. Normally, the space between the greater tuberosity and acromion is 6 to 7 mm, and rotator cuff thickness is approximately 5 to 6 mm. However, in a normal shoulder with properly functioning shoulder girdle musculature, scapula, and humeral motion, it is sufficient enough to limit irritation of the tendons underlying the acromion.

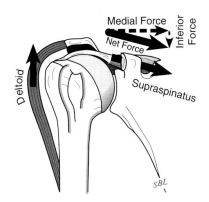
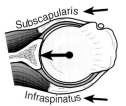

Figure 36–1:

The inferior force component of the supraspinatus is too small to counteract the upward pull of the deltoid. However, the compression effect of the rotator cuff complex stabilizes the humeral head within the glenoid socket. (From Rockwood CA Jr, Matsen FA III, Wirth MA, Lippitt SB: *The shoulder,* **3rd ed. Philadelphia, 2004, Saunders. Modified from Matsen FA III, Lippitt SB, Sidles JA, Harryman DT II:** *Practical evaluation and management of the shoulder.* **Philadelphia, 1994, Saunders.)**

Box 36–1	Intrinsic and Extrinsic Factors Believed To Be Associated with Rotator Cuff Pathology

Intrinsic Factors

Rotator cuff muscle imbalance
Rotator cuff muscle inflexibility
Internal tensile overload
Poor blood supply
Degenerative tissue

Extrinsic Factors

Subacromial impingement
Acromioclavicular morphology
Acromioclavicular arthritis or injury
Bone spurs
Scapular dyskinesis
Imbalance, inflexibility, or weakness of surrounding musculature
Intraarticular injury or pathology
Tensile overload
Repetitive stress

History, Physical Examination, and Imaging

- Athletes involved in repetitive overhead activities are the most common young patients afflicted with impingement and rotator cuff disease.

- Tears of the rotator cuff muscle are usually found in the older population and often associated with impingement.
- Tears associated with impingement frequently occur along the bursal surface in the older population and at the articular surface in young overhead athletes.
- Rotator cuff tears can have associated superior labral anterior to posterior (SLAP) lesions, subacromial and distal clavicle spurs, and rotator cuff arthropathy in advanced cases.
- It is often difficult to distinguish between true impingement, rotator cuff tears, and underlying pathology, such as arthritis, instability, and acromioclavicular disease or fractures, which may produce similar symptoms and secondary impingement (Table 36–1).
- A good history can help direct further evaluation and concentrates on identifying patient age, onset, chronicity of symptoms, and aggravating and alleviating activities.
- Most frequent complaint is shoulder pain with overhead activity, which can radiate to the deltoid and midarm.
- Traditionally, rotator cuff disease was associated with a patient's age. However, given the increased participation in sports and recreational activities, these conditions have begun to overlap in the different age groups.
  - 15 to 25 years old—usually aggressively active athletes involved in repetitive overhead sports or labor. Pain is associated with the overhead activity and normally

Table 36–1: **History and Physical Examination Features of Conditions Associated with and Commonly Confused with Rotator Cuff Tears**

	ROTATOR CUFF TENDINOSIS		AC JOINT DERANGEMENT	SLAP LESION	PRIMARY GLENOHUMERAL OA
	IMPINGEMENT	**CUFF TEAR**			
History					
Trauma	+/−	+/−	+/−	+	−
Pain	Anterior, superior, lateral ↑ with overhead use	Anterior, superior, lateral ↑ with overhead use	Superior ↑ with cross-body use	Posterior, superior ↑ with overhead, throwing	Anterior, posterior ↑ at extremes of motion
Disability	Overhead activities	Overhead activities, ADLs	Cross-body activities, weight lifting	Overhead activities, overhead sports	ADLs
Physical Examination					
Tenderness	Anterior, superior, lateral	Anterior, superior, lateral	Over AC joint	Posterior, superior	Anterior, posterior
Crepitus	Subacromial	Subacromial	Acromioclavicular	—	Glenohumeral
ROM	PROM = AROM	PROM > AROM	PROM = AROM	PROM = AROM	PROM = AROM
	May have ↓ IR	May have ↓ IR	Full ROM	Full ROM	↓ ROM, especially IR
		AROM ↓ in ER and FE		Overhead athletes may have ↑ ER and ↓ IR in abduction	
Strength	Normal	Weakness in ER, FE	Normal	Normal, unless with spinoglenoid cyst	Normal
Special tests	+ Impingement signs	+ Impingement signs	+ Cross-body abduction	+ Jobe relocation test	
		+ Painful arc			
	+ Painful arc	+ Impingement test		+ O'Brien test	
	+ Impingement test	+ Drop arm		+ Biceps load test	
		+/− Liftoff test			
		+/− Napoleon test			

AC, Acromioclavicular; ADLs, activities of daily living; AROM, active range of motion; ER, external rotation; FE, forward elevation; IR, internal rotation; OA, osteoarthritis; PROM, passive range of motion; ROM, range of motion; SLAP, superior labral anterior to posterior.
From Miller MD, Cole BJ, editors: *Textbook of arthroscopy.* Philadelphia, 2004, Saunders.

disappears with rest. Persisting pain that intensifies at night could suggest a partial rotator cuff tear.

- 25 to 50 years old—normally afflicted with tendinitis resulting from overuse. Partial tears are more common than in the younger group. Full-thickness tears are frequently associated with a superimposed traumatic event and usually do not affect the entire tendon width. These patients will present with weakness and commonly complain of nighttime pain.
- >50 years old—often affected with true bony impingement and chronic rotator cuff pathology. Many patients develop subacromial spurs, which further wear away the rotator cuff and biceps tendon and can cause pain that affects sleep and overhead daily activities. Complete tears in this age group are commonly associated with a fall or strenuous lifting activity. These patients often present with significant weakness in abduction and external rotation.

- Inspection should document any swelling, bony deformity, scars, and atrophy of the shoulder musculature.
- Electromyography (EMG) should be performed in young individuals with severe atrophy to rule out suprascapular nerve dysfunction and cervical radiculopathy.
- Palpation of the clavicle, scapula, and proximal humerus should note any localized tenderness.
- Several examination findings and tests may suggest rotator cuff pathology (Box 36–2).
- Range-of-motion testing may produce a "painful arc" that classically occurs between 60 and 140 degrees, when the greater tuberosity border moves under the acromion.
- Muscle testing may reveal weakness in abduction, flexion, and external rotation, with the latter being the most sensitive for rotator cuff tears.
- The supraspinatus can be tested with the arm in approximately 60 degrees abduction, 45 degrees flexion, and internally rotated with the thumb pointing downward (Jobe's test). The patient is then asked to counter applied downward resistance (Figure 36–2).
- Patients with a significant tear will demonstrate a positive drop arm test and may appear to shrug or "hike" the shoulder when asked to lift the arm.

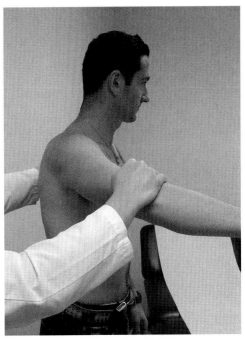

Figure 36–2:
Jobe's test. The tested arm is abducted, flexed, and maximally internally rotated with the thumb pointing downward. With resisted downward force, supraspinatus strength is evaluated.

- The lift-off test or the belly-press test is performed to evaluate the subscapularis (Figure 36–3).
- The infraspinatus is best evaluated by resisting external rotation with the arm adducted and elbow flexed at 90 degrees (Figure 36–4).
- A positive Neer's impingement test can be supplemented with a diagnostic injection of lidocaine (Xylocaine) into the subacromial space. Relief of pain supports the diagnosis of impingement. Furthermore, increase in muscular strength after injection may help distinguish between tears and impingement (Figure 36–5).
- The Hawkins sign further substantiates an impingement condition (Figure 36–6).
- Appropriate tests to rule out cervical disease and thoracic outlet syndrome should be incorporated into the examination (Figure 36–7).
- Standard radiographs are taken and can be supplemented with Zanca, 30 degrees caudal, and supraspinatus outlet views to examine bone morphology and pathology.
- A morphologic classification system described by Bigliani and Morrison can be used to describe the acromion using the supraspinatus outlet view (Figure 36–8, Box 36–3).
- A modification of the acromion classification (by Snyder) based on thickness, which can be combined with the previous system, can guide the surgeon on the amount of bone that can be safely removed during decompression to avoid iatrogenic acromial fractures (Figure 36–9, Box 36–3).

Box 36–2	Clinical Findings and Tests Associated with Rotator Cuff Pathology

Weakness in abduction, flexion, and particularly external rotation
Painful arc (pain between 60 and 140 degrees of abduction)
Neer's impingement test
Hawkins sign
Lift-off/belly-press test (evaluates subscapularis)
Jobe's test (evaluates supraspinatus)
External rotation weakness against resistance with the arm adducted and elbow at 90 degrees flexion (evaluates infraspinatus)
Drop arm test

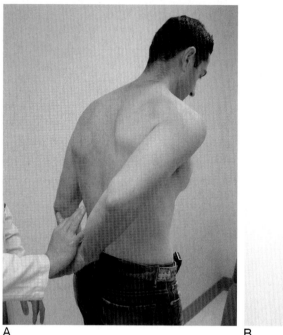

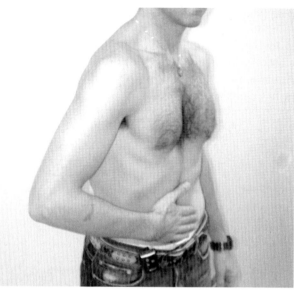

A   B

Figure 36–3:

Subscapularis muscle testing. **A,** Lift-off test. Inability to maintain the maximally internally rotated arm away from the lower back suggests a subscapularis tendon tear. **B,** For patients with decreased internal rotation or the inability to move their hand behind their back, or both, the belly-press sign can also evaluate subscapularis function. The inability to press down on their abdomen and/or flare their elbow forward, or both, is indicative of subscapularis weakness.

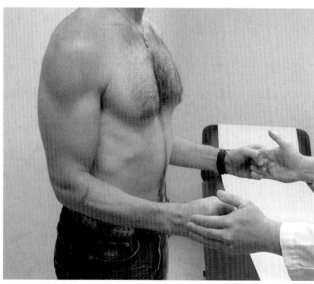

Figure 36–4:

Evaluation of the infraspinatus muscle is performed by resisting external rotation of the adducted arm flexed 90 degrees at the elbow.

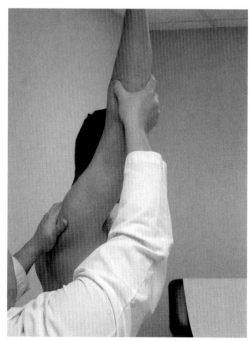

Figure 36–5:

Neer's impingement sign. Pain elicited with forward flexion of the affected arm is consistent with impingement. Relief of pain after an anesthetic injection into the subacromial space further supports the diagnosis.

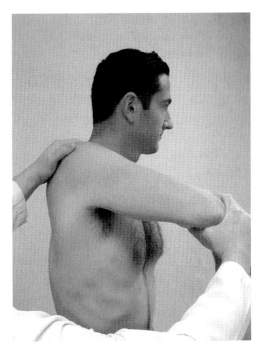

Figure 36–6:
Hawkins impingement sign. Adducting and internally rotating the flexed arm enhances the sensitivity for the diagnosis of impingement syndrome.

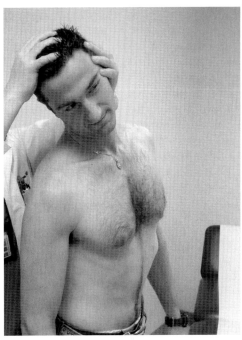

Figure 36–7:
Sperling's test for cervical nerve root impingement. The head is compressed, extended, and rotated toward the affected shoulder. A sensation of radicular pain and reproduction of symptoms is considered positive.

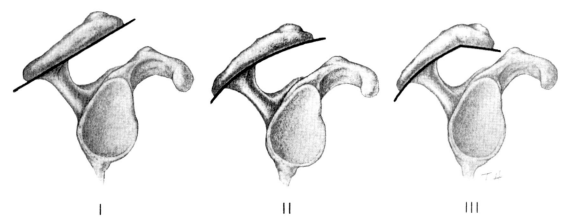

I   II   III

Figure 36–8:
Bigliani classification of acromion morphology. (From Esch JC: *Op Tech Orthop* 1:200, 1991.)

- Findings suggestive of rotator cuff or impingement pathology on radiography include superior humeral migration, greater tuberosity sclerosis or cystic changes, narrowing of the acromiohumeral space (<7 mm), and inferior acromial spurs (Figure 36–10).
- With its high sensitivity and specificity, magnetic resonance imaging (MRI) is now the gold standard for further evaluation of rotator cuff conditions and can be enhanced with gadolinium if the initial readings are ambiguous or negative and pathology is still suspected (Figure 36–11).
- Aside from demonstrating rotator cuff tear size, configuration, location, and chronicity, MRI also allows evaluation of the surrounding bone, cartilage, and labrum.

Box 36–3	Acromion Classification

Bigliani and Morrison

Type I: Flat undersurface that extends away from the humeral head
Type II: Gently curved, convex undersurface that parallels the contour of the humeral head
Type III: Anterior osteophyte, or "beak," that narrows the arc of the supraspinatus outlet

Snyder Modification

Type A: Thin acromion, < 8 mm
Type B: Average acromial thickness, 8–12 mm
Type C: Thick acromion, > 12 mm

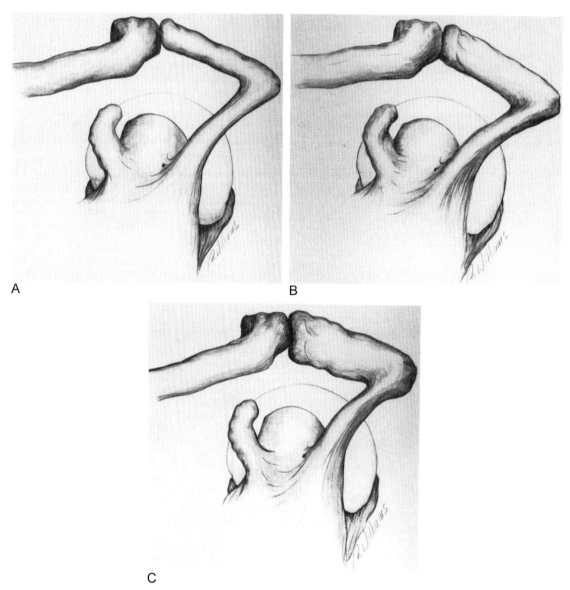

A

B

C

Figure 36–9:
Classification of acromion based on thickness. A, Less than 8 mm. **B,** 8 to 12 mm. **C,** Greater than 12 mm. (From Snyder SJ, Wuh HCK: *Op Tech Orthop* 1:212-213, 1991.)

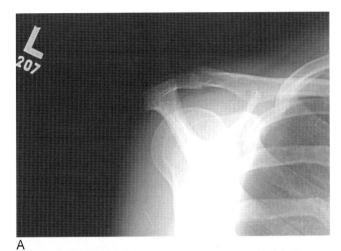

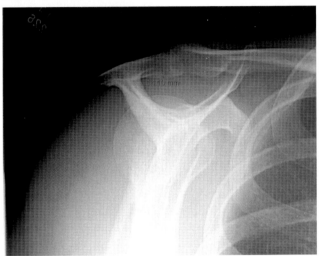

Figure 36–10:
Supraspinatus outlet views depicting a Bigliani type III acromion (**A**) and a Snyder type C acromion (**B**).

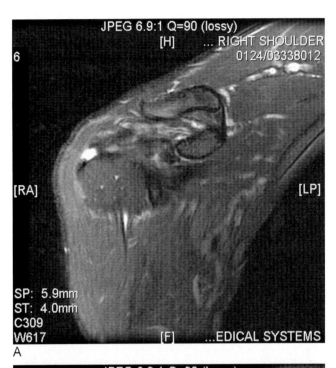

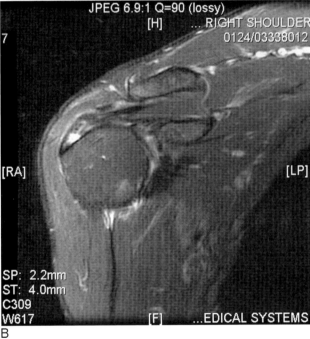

Figure 36–11:
A and B, Magnetic resonance imaging demonstrating a full-thickness rotator cuff tear of the supraspinatus.

Type

- Subacromial impingement.
  - Specific extrinsic condition within the subacromial space that classically has been described to advance in stages, increasing in severity with age, ranging from edema to rotator cuff tears and arthropathy (Table 36–2).
  - Impingement often results from rotator cuff fatigue or disease, allowing the humeral head to elevate superiorly and cause impingement.
  - A hooked acromion, os acromiale, and a thickened coracoacromial ligament may be independent risk factors for rotator cuff disease, limiting the area within the subacromial space.
  - It is believed by some that spurs result from chronic impingement rather than causing primary compression.
  - Symptoms most commonly occur with arm elevation.
  - Examination often reveals rotator cuff weakness, Neer's impingement, and Hawkins signs. Relief of symptoms after a subacromial local injection suggests a bursal etiology, although it is not specific.

Table 36–2:	Stages of Subacromial Impingement Syndrome			
STAGE	AGE (YEARS)	PATHOLOGY	CLINICAL COURSE	TREATMENT
I	<25	Edema and hemorrhage	Reversible	Conservative
II	25–40	Fibrosis and tendinitis	Activity-related pain	Therapy/operative
III	>40	AC spur and cuff tear	Progressive disability	Acromioplasty/repair

AC, Acromioclavicular.
From Miller MD, editor: *Review of orthopaedics*, 3rd ed. Philadelphia, 2000, Saunders.

- Supraspinatus outlet view can help evaluate acromial morphology and spurs.
- Rotator cuff tendinitis/tendinosis.
  - Can result from extrinsic or intrinsic impingement, overload, overuse, or trauma.
  - Most commonly associated with impingement.
  - Anterior microinstability may result in internal impingement of the rotator cuff on the rim of the posterior superior glenoid and can produce posterolateral shoulder pain.
  - Frequently seen in repetitive throwers.
  - Calcific tendinitis is a specific kind of tendinitis with painful calcific deposits within the rotator cuff tendon. If conservative management fails, surgical excision of the deposit with rotator cuff repair of the defect is usually curative (Figure 36–12).
- Rotator cuff tears.
  - Usually results from trauma or the progression of rotator cuff pathology.
  - More commonly seen in the older population with tears occurring along the bursal side.
  - Articular side tears are more common in young athletes with glenohumeral instability.
  - Can be classified according to tear pattern: (1) crescent-shaped tears, (2) U-shaped tears, (3) L-shaped tears, and (4) massive, contracted, immobile tears (Figure 36–13).

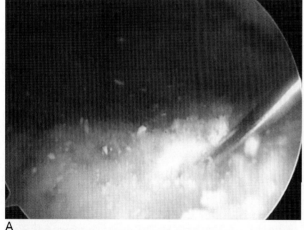

A

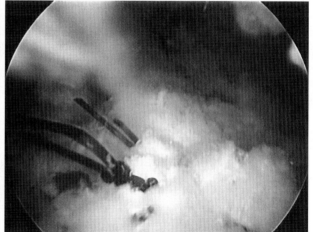

C

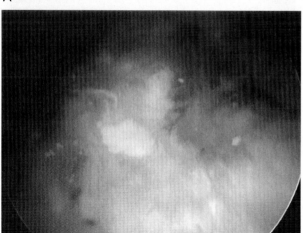

B

Figure 36–12:
Calcific rotator cuff tendinitis. **A,** Needle localization of calcific deposits within the supraspinatus tendon. **B,** Note the large calcium deposit that was eluted from the supraspinatus tendon during debridement. **C,** Arthroscopic closure of the rotator cuff tendon defect following calcium deposit removal.

Treatment

- Initial management of rotator cuff conditions includes a period of rest; nonsteroidal antiinflammatory drugs (NSAIDs); activity modifications; rehabilitation; therapeutic modalities; and, occasionally, subacromial injections.
- The period of rest should be adequate enough to reduce the inflammation and pain and averages 1 to 2 weeks.

- Judicious use of steroid injections can provide relief and enable the patient to successfully follow rehabilitation protocols. Subsequent injections can be performed after 2 to 3 months with a maximum total of three injections. It should be noted that steroid injections can lead to tendon weakening and rupture.
- Patients younger than the age of 60 who sustain complete rotator cuff tears after a specific event are best managed with surgical repair within 6 weeks of the injury.

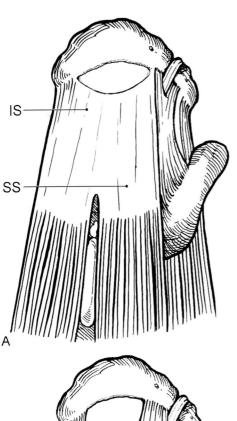

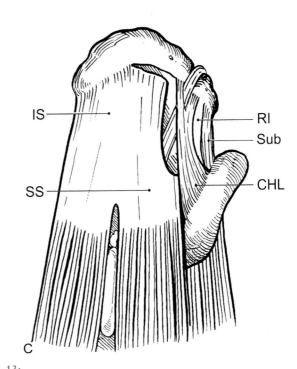

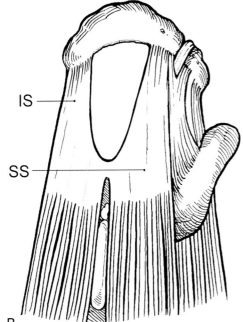

Figure 36–13:
Rotator cuff tear patterns. **A**, Crescent-shaped tear. **B**, U-shaped tear. **C**, L-shaped tear. CHL, Coracohumeral ligament; IS, infraspinatus; RI, rotator interval; SS, supraspinatus; Sub, subscapularis. (From Miller MD, Cole BJ, editors: *Textbook of arthroscopy*. Philadelphia, 2004, Saunders.)

- Patients who remain symptomatic after 6 or more months of nonoperative management of chronic tears should be considered for surgical treatment.
- Arthroscopic techniques for the treatment of rotator cuff tears are becoming increasingly popular with several advantages (Box 36–4). However, particularly with regard to large and massive tears, the current literature suggests a high rate of recurrent re-tears with arthroscopic treatment.
- Subacromial decompression is used in patients with impingement syndrome without rotator cuff tears and as an adjunct in many tendon repair procedures.
  - Diagnostic arthroscopy and release of adhesions of the subacromial space may be performed via a posterior and anterior portal.
  - A lateral portal should allow the cannula to enter between the humeral head and acromion and can be located using a spinal needle.
  - A shaver is introduced through the lateral portal and used to open the bursa tissue, release the coracoacromial ligament, and inspect the undersurface of the acromion and coracoacromial ligament.
  - The acromial branch of the thoracoacromial trunk passes in proximity to the anteromedial acromion and should be avoided.
  - Acromioplasty, performed with a bur, should proceed from lateral to medial and anterior to posterior until a uniplanar, flat surface is created. The spine of the scapula is used to perform a cutting block technique and care is taken not to remove too much bone (Figure 14A to C).
  - After decompression is performed, better visualization of surrounding anatomy may reveal concomitant pathology.
  - Distal clavicle resection may be performed if indicated (Figure 36–15).
  - In cases of large rotator cuff tears in which the repair may be questionable, a more limited decompression should be performed with preservation of the coracoacromial ligament to avoid anterior superior instability.
- Rotator cuff repair can be performed using an open or mini-open approach or arthroscopically.

| Box 36–4 | **Advantages of Arthroscopic Rotator Cuff Treatment** |

Smaller skin incisions
No deltoid detachment
Ability to perform complete glenohumeral inspection
Treatment of associated intraarticular pathology
Less soft tissue dissection
Minimal pain
Quicker recovery period

- Partial-thickness tears with a normal subacromial space respond well to anatomic repair.
- Partial tears that are less than 50% of the thickness and associated with impingement may have good results with debridement and subacromial decompression.
- Treatment decision of tears can be difficult and should consider the patient's age; activity level; quality of tissues; and acuity, location, configuration, and degree of tear.
- Classification describing tears is based on degree of tear and location (articular or bursal surface) and can guide treatment decisions.
- Open repair can occur through an anterior deltopectoral approach, requiring an extensive incision, or a mini-open approach with a smaller incision made along Langers' lines over the anterior half of the lateral acromion that spares deltoid detachment (and usually follows arthroscopic evaluation and decompression) (Figure 36–16).
  - After acromioplasty is performed, the torn muscle is mobilized.
  - Chronically retracted tears may require rotator interval release and releases deep to the muscle belly. Care must be taken not to proceed deeper than 2 cm superiorly over the glenoid and 1 cm posterior to the glenoid to avoid damaging the suprascapular nerve.
  - A cancellous bed for the tendon is produced by decortication of the anatomic footprint just lateral to the articular surface border until bleeding is produced.
  - Certain techniques are recommended for specific tear configurations (Table 36–3 and Figure 36–17).
  - The injured tendon can be repaired anatomically using a modified Mason-Allen stitch and osseous tunnels or suture anchors (discouraged in osteoporotic bone) (Figures 36–18 and 36–19).
  - Subscapularis repairs often require mobilization of the axillary nerve.
- Arthroscopic repair is followed after a careful glenohumeral examination (Figure 36–20).
  - Debridement and lysis of adhesions may be required for improved visualization.
  - When appropriate, subacromial decompression or selective subacromial shaping is performed.
  - When a tear is identified, no. 1 PDS suture passed through a spinal needle to mark the area assists with further evaluation from all angles.
  - The tendon is debrided and the rotator cuff footprint decorticated.
  - Side-to-side sutures are used to repair the vertical component of tears, realigning the tendon and relieving stress from the laterally anchored component to bone.
  - Two to three anchors are recommended when attaching the torn tendon to the prepared footprint, often using a shuttle technique.
- Massive, irreparable rotator cuffs are a difficult clinical problem.
  - Conservative management is the mainstay of treatment.

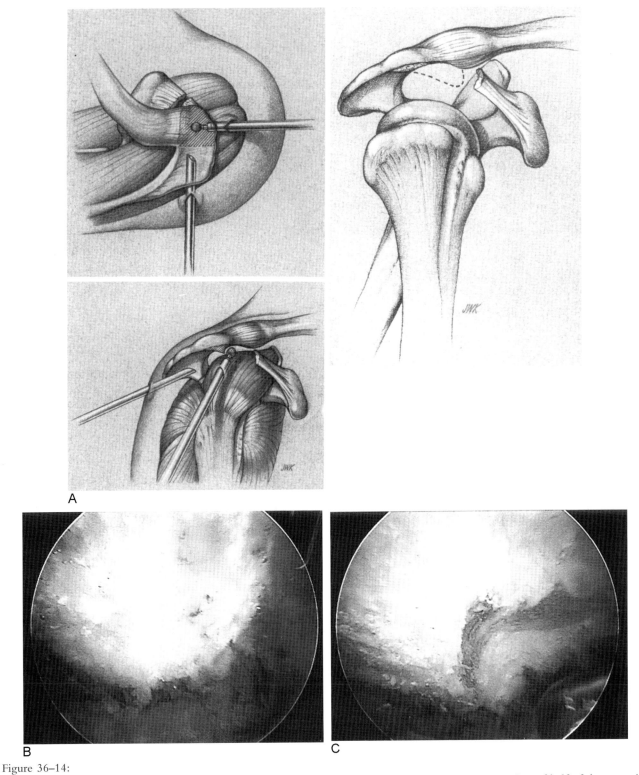

Figure 36–14:
A, Technique for arthroscopic acromioplasty. **B,** Arthroscopic view of the acromial spur. **C,** Decompression of half of the acromial spur. (**A** from Harner CD: *Op Tech Orthop* 1:229-234, 1991.)

(*continued*)

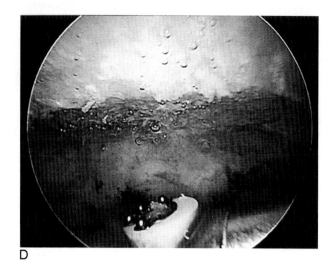

D

Figure 36–14, cont'd:

D, Removal of the entire acromial spur.

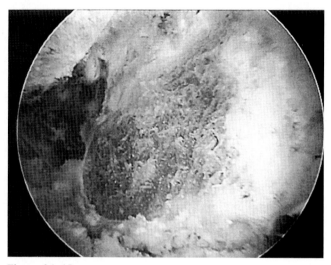

Figure 36–15:

Arthroscopic distal clavicle excision.

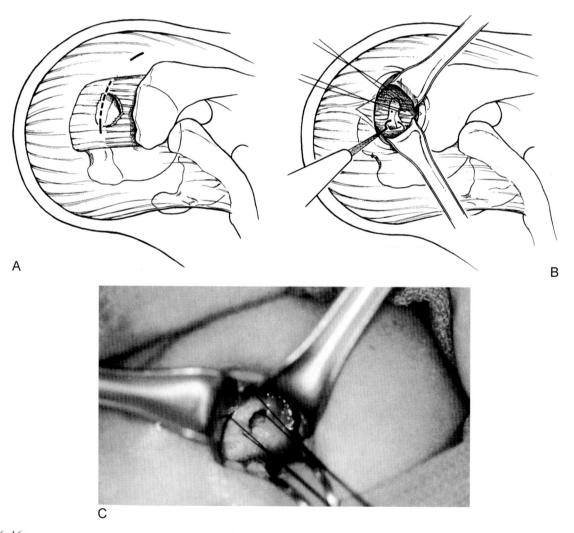

A

B

C

Figure 36–16:

Mini-open repair of rotator cuff tears. **A,** Dashed line showing the planned incision placed in Langer's lines parallel to the acromial edge and centered over the rotator cuff tear. **B,** The rotator cuff is repaired through a split in the deltoid muscle in line with its fibers. **C,** Refractors are placed to improve visualization. (From Pollock RG, Flatow EL: *Orthop Clin North Am* 28:169-177, 1997.)

Table 36–3: Arthroscopic Repair According to Rotator Cuff Tear Configuration

TEAR CONFIGURATION	REPAIR TECHNIQUE
Crescent	Repair of free margin of cuff tendon directly to bone with suture from suture anchors
U-shaped	Side-to-side repair of medial to lateral extent of tear leading to tear margin convergence, then repair of the free lateral margin of the cuff tendon directly to the bone with sutures from the anchor
L-shaped/reverse L-shaped	Anchor placement corresponding to the elbow of the L followed by repair of the soft tissue component of the elbow of the L to that point; then, side-to-side repair followed by repair of the remaining lateral margin to bone with suture from suture anchors

From Romeo AA, Cohen B, Cole BJ. Arthroscopic repair of full-thickness rotator cuff tears. Surgical technique and available instrumentation. *Orthopaedic Special Edition* 7:25–30, 2001.

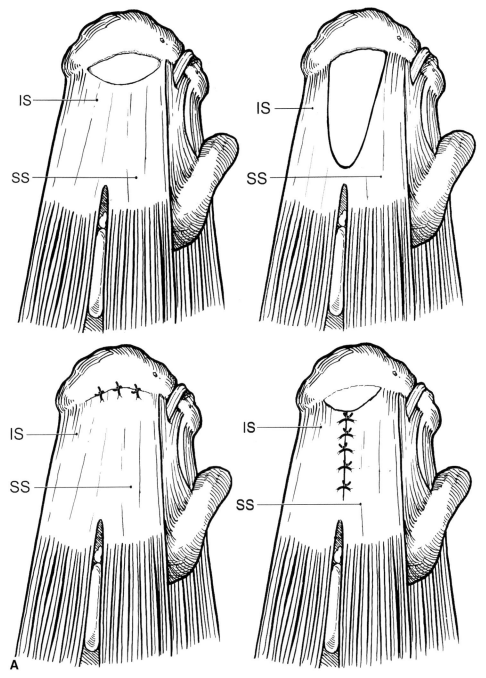

Figure 36–17:
Rotator cuff repairs according to tear pattern. A, Crescent-shaped tear repair. IS, Infraspinatus; SS, supraspinatus.

(continued)

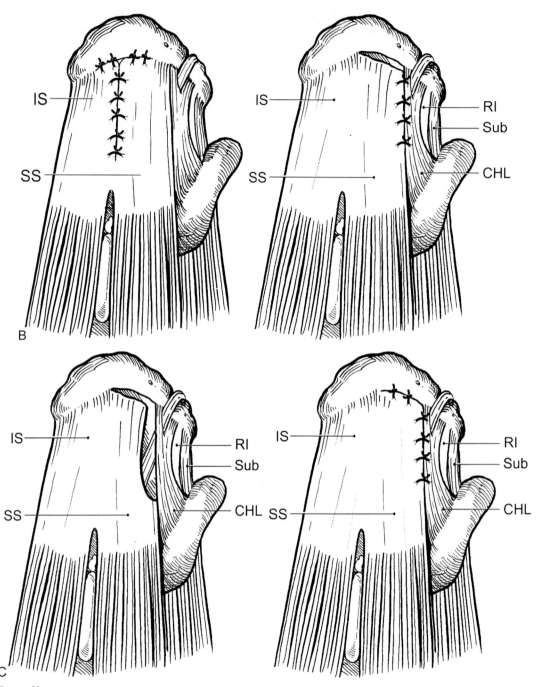

Figure 36–17, cont'd:
B, U-shaped tear repair. **C,** Acute L-shaped tear repair. *CHL,* Coracohumeral ligament; *IS,* infraspinatus; *RI,* rotator internal; *SS,* supraspinatus; *Sub,* subscapular.

(continued)

- Arthroscopic debridement may be helpful in select cases. However, care should be exercised not to perform an exuberant decompression and to preserve the coracoacromial ligament because loss of this structure may lead to anterior superior humeral head escape.
- For massive, irreparable supraspinatus and infraspinatus tendon tears with an intact subscapularis, latissimus dorsi transfer has had some success with improving

external rotation and aiding with humeral head depression during shoulder elevation (Figure 36–21).

Rehabilitation

- Rehabilitation is an essential component to both conservative and postoperative management and should begin as early as possible.

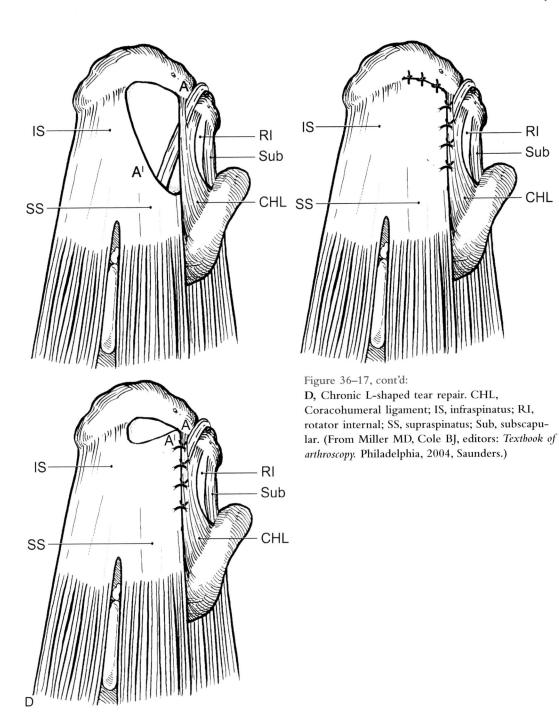

Figure 36–17, cont'd:
D, Chronic L-shaped tear repair. CHL, Coracohumeral ligament; IS, infraspinatus; RI, rotator internal; SS, supraspinatus; Sub, subscapular. (From Miller MD, Cole BJ, editors: *Textbook of arthroscopy.* Philadelphia, 2004, Saunders.)

- Heat before exercise and ice after assists in patient comfort.
- Physical therapy programs usually involve three phases.
  - Phase I—control pain and begin stretching exercises with passive assistance to restore/maintain range of motion.
    - Stretching can be performed using stick and pulley exercises.
    - Additional exercises include Codman's/pendulum exercises, wall walking, posterior capsular stretches, and door hanging.
    - It can take 4 to 6 weeks to regain a functional range of motion.
  - Phase II—after pain-free range of motion is recovered, a regimen for strengthening the scapular stabilizers, rotator cuff, and deltoid is followed.
    - Usually begins with isometric exercises and advances to isotonic and isokinetic exercises.
    - Rotator cuff strengthening can be achieved with the use of therabands, light weights, or pulleys.

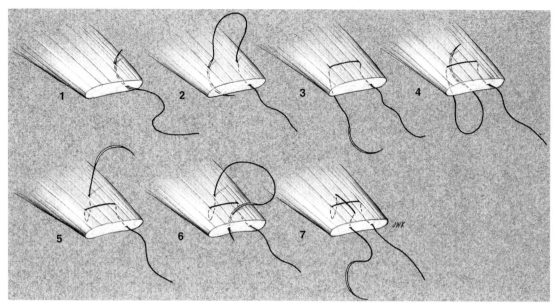

Figure 36–18:
Modified Mason-Allen stitch. (From Griggs S, Williams GR, Iannotti JP: *Op Tech Orthop* 8:205-217, 1998.)

○ Scapular stabilizers benefit from wall, knee, or military pushups; shoulder shrugs; and shoulder pressups.
○ Patients should be given specific guidelines for home therapy.
○ Keeping the routines short, and spread throughout the day, will prevent overuse injury.
○ This phase takes a minimum of 3 months to complete.

• Phase III—aimed at returning the patient to preinjury strength and functional activity that can be tailored to specific sports or needs of the patient.
○ Patients are gradually returned to preinjury activities and advanced with care.
○ Patient must be instructed to continue a maintenance program of stretching and strengthening.

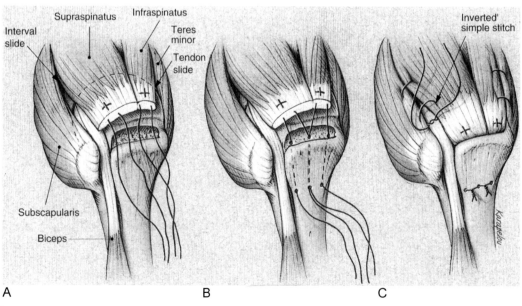

Figure 36–19:
Rotator cuff repair using modified Mason-Allen stitches and bone tunnels for the passage of sutures to attach the torn muscle to bone. A, Modified Mason-Allen stitches placed through the freshened edge of the rotator cuff tear. B, Sutures are passed through bone funnels passed through a bone trough. C, Sutures are tied, reducing the rotator cuff into the prepared bony trough. (From Griggs S, Williams GR, Iannotti JP: *Op Tech Orthop* 8:205-217, 1998.)

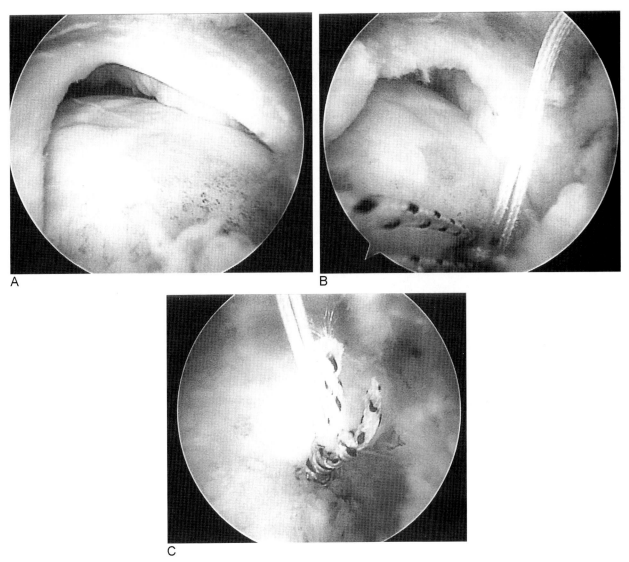

Figure 36–20:
Arthroscopic repair of a rotator cuff tear. A, Crescent-shaped rotator cuff tear. B, Arthroscopic anchor placement in the footprint of the rotator cuff. C, Arthroscopic rotator cuff repair.

- The basis for rehabilitation is to reestablish the normal muscle balance and force couples about the shoulder and scapula and ensure that the entire kinetic chain is properly reinforced.
- Focus is usually concentrated on three muscle groups.
  - Humeral head depressors—subscapularis, infraspinatus, and teres minor.
  - Scapula stabilizers—trapezius, serratus anterior, and rhomboids.
  - Prime humeral positioners—deltoid, pectoralis major, and latissimus dorsi.
- Impingement often responds best to rehabilitation programs that strengthen the humeral head depressors and scapula stabilizers, both of which help maintain the subacromial clear space and prevent irritation of the rotator cuff as the arm is elevated.

- In the past, rehabilitation efforts concentrated on isolating the supraspinatus muscle, which is counteractive because it acts together with the deltoid to elevate the head of the humerus.
- Postoperatively, the cuff is usually protected for 4 to 6 weeks but allowing passive range of motion of the wrist and elbow and Codman's/pendulum exercises.
- The postoperative rehabilitation program must be tailored to the individual's needs but follows a basic protocol.
- Rehabilitation after arthroscopic repair of rotator cuff tears can follow early or delayed programs (Table 36–4). Early rehabilitation aims at reducing the risk of postoperative stiffness, whereas delayed rehabilitation minimizes the risk of failure of the rotator cuff repair.

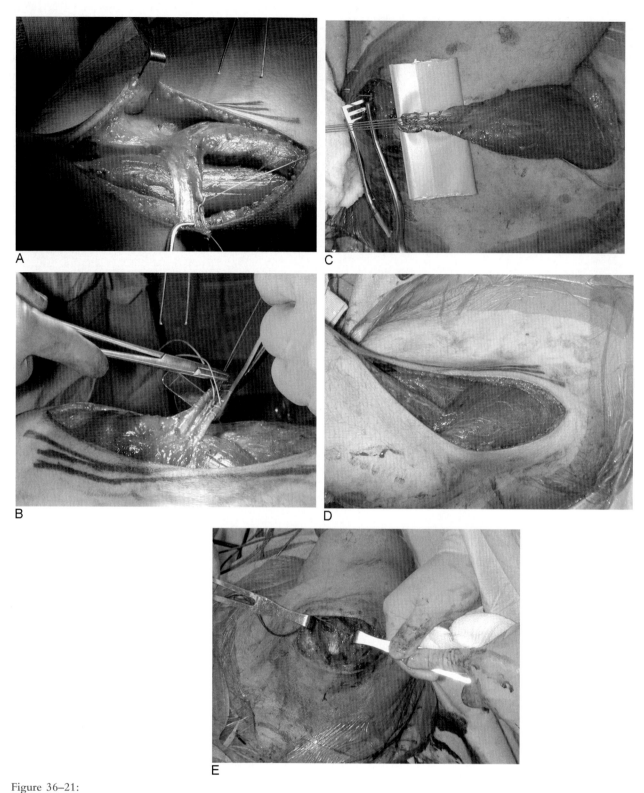

Figure 36–21:
Latissimus dorsi transfer for irreparable, massive supraspinatus/infraspinatus tendon tears. **A,** Latissimus dorsi tendon insertion on the humerus is identified and sectioned. **B,** The tendon is secured with no. 2 braided, nonabsorbable suture. **C,** The neurovascular pedicle is carefully dissected to avoid tension, and then tendon excursion is determined. **D,** The latissimus dorsi tendon is passed under the posterior deltoid. **E,** The tendon is repaired to the greater tuberosity at the anatomic insertion of the supraspinatus and infraspinatus tendons.

Table 36–4: Early and Delayed Rehabilitation Protocols Following Arthroscopic Rotator Cuff Repair

EARLY REHABILITATION	DELAYED REHABILITATION
Immobilizer for 3 wk	Immobilizer for 6 wk
Elbow/wrist ROM immediately	Elbow/wrist ROM immediately
Pendulum exercises immediately	Passive ER exercises with arm in adduction only
Shoulder shrugs immediately	
Active assisted ROM at 3–4 wk	Active and active assisted ROM at 6 wk
Pool exercises at 3–4 wk	Stretching at 6 wk
Formal physical therapy at 3–4 wk	
Rotator cuff strengthening at 7 wk	Strengthening at 12 wk (rotator cuff, deltoid, biceps, scapular stabilizers)
Deltoid strengthening after 12 wk	Consider formal physical therapy at 12 wk if necessary

ER, External rotation; ROM, range of motion.
From Miller MD, Cole BJ, editors: *Textbook of arthroscopy.* Philadelphia, 2004, Saunders.

Complications of Surgery

- Progression of rotator cuff pathology that may ultimately result in tears.
- Chronic pain.
- Adhesive capsulitis.
- Joint degeneration.
- Neurovascular injury with portal placement or rotator cuff repair procedures.
- Inadequate or excessive acromial resection.
- Acromial fracture.
- Rotator cuff repair failure.
- Loose hardware.

References

Bryant L, Shnier R, Bryant C, Murrell GAC: A comparison of clinical estimation, ultrasonography, magnetic resonance imaging, and arthroscopy in determining the size of rotator cuff tears. *J Shoulder Elbow Surg* 11:219-224, 2002.

Authors study the accuracy of clinical examination, ultrasound, MRI, and arthroscopy in determining the size of rotator cuff tears in 33 consecutive patients. Results demonstrated that arthroscopy best correlated with actual tear size (Pearson correlation coefficient r = 0.92). MRI (r = 0.74) and ultrasound (r = 0.73) estimations were similar, whereas clinical assessment showed poor estimates (r = 0.41). All of the previously mentioned methods underestimated the size of the tear by 12%, 30%, 33%, and 38%, respectively, which the authors note may affect treatment recommendations.

Gartsman GM: Repair of athletic shoulder injuries: all arthroscopic rotator cuff repairs. *Orthop Clin North Am* 32:501-510, 2001.

Author provides a detailed description of the operative technique in arthroscopic repair of both partial and complete rotator cuff tears. Author reports a 90% satisfaction rate among his patient population who have undergone arthroscopic repair. He also comments on the advantages of arthroscopic repair over open procedures, including the ability to evaluate and treat concomitant intraarticular lesions and allowing a more rapid recovery.

Gartsman GM, Brinker MR, Khan M: Early effectiveness of arthroscopic repair for full-thickness tears of the rotator cuff. *J Bone Joint Surg Am* 80:33-46, 1998.

Authors report on the results of 50 patients with chronic rotator cuff tears treated by arthroscopic repair using standardized questionnaires. At an average 13-month follow-up, scores taken from the Short Form 36 (SF-36) General Health Survey, University of California of Los Angeles (UCLA) Shoulder Score, and the American Shoulder and Elbow Surgeons (ASES) Shoulder Index all showed significant improvement in general health and shoulder function. The authors discuss the use of standardized questionnaires and the need for improved region-specific questionnaires and evaluation for better representation of a patient's condition.

MacDonald PB, Clark P, Sutherland K: An analysis of the diagnostic accuracy of the Hawkins and Neer subacromial impingement signs. *J Shoulder Elbow Surg* 9:299-301, 2000.

Authors study the accuracy of the Neer's and Hawkins signs in diagnosing subacromial bursitis and rotator cuff pathology. Results demonstrated sensitivities of 75% and 85% for the Neer's sign and 92% and 88% for the Hawkins sign for subacromial bursitis and rotator cuff tearing, respectively. The two signs also were found to have high negative predictive values. However, specificity and positive predictive values of either sign were low (51% or less).

Mantone JK, Burkhhead WZ, Noonan J Jr: Conservative management of shoulder injuries: Nonoperative treatment of rotator cuff tears. *Orthop Clin North Am* 31:295-311, 2000.

Authors discuss the rationale and biomechanics of conservative treatment for rotator cuff tears. The authors note that certain patients, based on age and activity level, have greater outcomes with surgical treatment. A rehabilitation protocol as described by Rockwood is reviewed.

Millstein ES, Snyder SJ: Arthroscopic evaluation and management of rotator cuff tears. *Orthop Clin North Am* 34:507-520, 2003.

Authors provide a good review of the history, physical examination, imaging, and classification of rotator cuff tears. Authors also describe their technique of arthroscopic rotator cuff repair using suture anchor fixation (and side-to-side suture repairs when indicated) that has resulted in great outcomes at their institution. Authors also comment on the difficulties of treating massive rotator cuff tears and offer therapeutic recommendations.

Morrison DS, Greenbaum BS, Einhorn A: Conservative management of shoulder injuries: shoulder impingement. *Orthop Clin North Am* 31:285-293, 2003.

Authors review the anatomy, pathology, and considerations involved when treating shoulder impingement nonoperatively. Authors stress the importance of initially concentrating rehabilitation efforts on strengthening the humeral head depressors. Rehabilitation then continues with strengthening the scapular stabilizers and prime humeral positioners. Authors discuss their protocol in detail, as well as specific treatment by cause. Authors indicate that up to 70% of patients can achieve resolution of symptoms using their conservative approach.

Park JY, Yoo MJ, Kim MH: Comparison of surgical outcome between bursal and articular partial thickness rotator cuff tears. *Orthopedics* 26:387-390, 2003.

Authors compare the outcomes of patients with bursal (n = 13) versus articular (n = 24) partial-thickness rotator cuff tears treated with arthro-

scopic subacromial decompression and debridement (no repair). At 6-month follow-up, the pain score in the articular tear group decreased from 6.2 to 1.7, whereas in the bursal group scores dropped from 7.1 to 0.9. At this time, the bursal group also demonstrated statistically improved function with activities of daily living. However, at 2-year follow-up, differences between the two groups were not statistically significant.

Reed SC, Glossop N, Ogilvie-Harris DJ: Full thickness rotator cuff tears: a biomechanical comparison of suture versus bone anchor techniques. *Am J Sports Med* 24:46-48, 1996.

Authors perform a biomechanical study comparing suture versus bone anchor repairs of artificially produced rotator cuff tears on fresh-frozen human cadavers. Results demonstrate suture anchors being significantly stronger than suture-only repairs (mean values of strength to failure were 194 in the suture group and 261 in the anchor repair group). Anchor

insertion technique is also considered important to achieve optimal strength. Authors recommend the anchors be inserted into the edge of the subchondral bone, adjacent to the articular surface in a direction that produces approximately 90 degrees of pull to the anchor with the humerus at 30 degrees of abduction. Furthermore, the anchors should be countersunk below the bone surface.

Ruotolo C, Nottage WM: Surgical and nonsurgical management of rotator cuff tears. *Arthroscopy* 18:527-531, 2002.

Authors review the literature to evaluate outcomes of nonoperative and surgical management of rotator cuff tears. Authors conclude that surgical repair provides a higher rate of pain relief (85% vs. 50%) and return of strength than nonoperative treatment. In addition, the authors note that a chronic history of pain (>6-12 months) and large tears (>3 cm) have a poorer prognosis with nonoperative management.

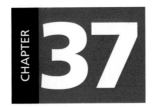

CHAPTER 37

Muscle Ruptures of the Shoulder

Introduction

- Although uncommon, muscle ruptures of the shoulder are associated with significant morbidity and disability.
- The incidence of these injuries is increasing with an aging athletic population with a greater frequency found in these groups.
- Etiology.
  - Trauma: typically low-energy eccentric contraction in middle-aged patient.
  - High association with anabolic steroid use.
  - Iatrogenic: rupture of repair following exposure for associated surgery.

Pectoralis Major

- Uncommon (probably underrecognized and underreported).
- Typically in weight lifters (bench press).
- Strong association with anabolic steroid use.
- No reported injuries in females.

Mechanism

- Excessive tension on a maximally eccentrically contracted muscle.
- Occurs during humerus extension at beginning of left (bench press).

Examination

- Hematoma, swelling, ecchymosis.
- Defect (axillary webbing).
  - Abduct to 90 degrees and flex to 45 degrees.
  - Compare with contralateral shoulder (Figure 37–1).
- Weak adduction and internal rotation.

Imaging

- Radiographs frequently negative.
- Magnetic resonance imaging (MRI) axial cuts can delineate anatomy and degree of tear (Figure 37–2).

Treatment

- Incomplete tear (more common).
  - Nonoperative includes rest, antiinflammatory medications, and physical therapy.
  - No bench press for 3 months.
- Complete tear.
  - Nonoperative associated with symptoms of cramping with heavy lifting and weakness (good results in 58% compared with 80% with repair).
  - Primary repair into a trough or with suture anchors (Figure 37–3).
    - Sternocostal head (deep origin with proximal insertion) (Figure 37–4).
      - Spirals 180 degrees.
      - More commonly injured than clavicular head (avulsion).
    - Clavicular head (superficial origin with distal insertion).
- Early repair has better outcome than late repair.

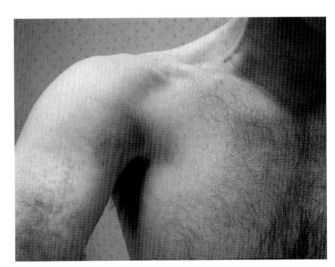

Figure 37–1:
Clinical photograph of a patient with a pectoralis major rupture. Note ecchymosis and loss of normal contour of the axilla ("webbing").

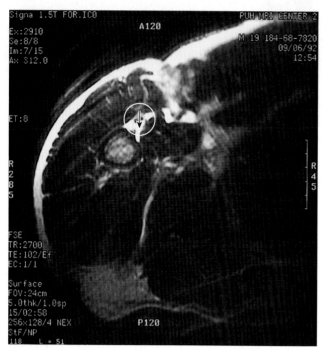

Figure 37–2:
Magnetic resonance imaging of pectoral muscle rupture. (From Miller MD, Howard RF, Plancher KD: *Surgical atlas of sports medicine.* Philadelphia, 2003, Saunders.)

Deltoid

- Unusual traumatic injury.
  - Most injuries are strains or partial tears with repetitive throwing (overuse) or from direct blow (acute trauma).
- Relatively common iatrogenic injury.
  - Following open rotator cuff repair.
  - Inadequate repair of deltoid back through drill holes in the acromion.

Examination

- Loss of normal contour.
- Weakness of abduction or flexion.
- Palpable defect.

Imaging

- Radiographs frequently negative.

Treatment

- Traumatic injury.
  - Incomplete: nonoperative with early range of motion and later strengthening.
  - Complete: open repair, arthroscopic repair also described.
- Iatrogenic injury.
  - Difficult (especially when noted late, which is often the case).

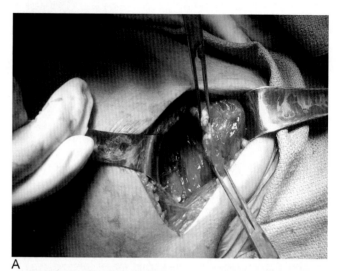

A

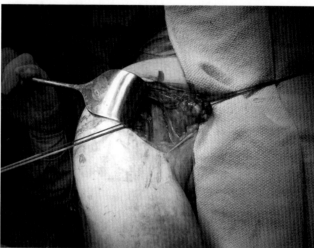

B

Figure 37–3:
Operative photographs of pectoralis major repair.
A, Deltopectoral exposure with retracted pectoralis tendon.
B, Suture anchors are placed near the tendon insertion.

- Deltoidplasty (mobilization and reattachment of the deltoid) should be considered, but it is often unsuccessful.

Latissimus Dorsi

- Humeral avulsions are rare.

Examination

- Local tenderness and pain with the shoulder in adduction and internal rotation.

Imaging

- Radiographs frequently negative.
- MRI helpful.

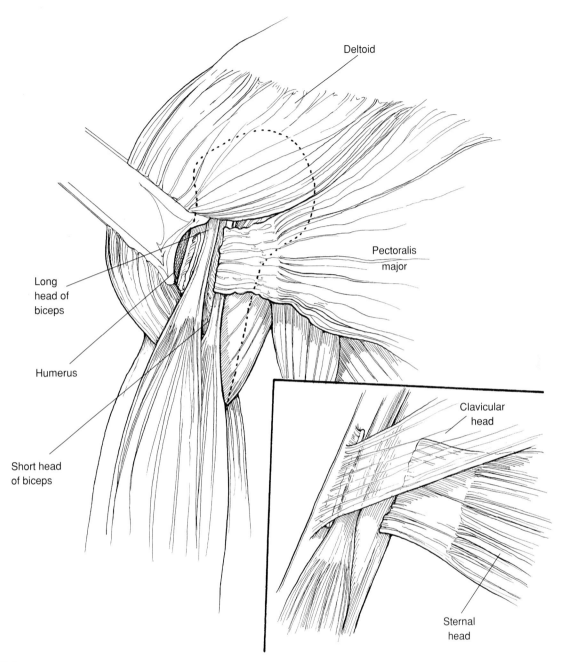

Figure 37–4:
Anatomy of a pectoralis major tear. (From Miller MD, Howard RF, Plancher KD: *Surgical atlas of sports medicine.* Philadelphia, 2003, Saunders.)

Treatment

- Typically conservative.
- Operative repair reserved for elite athletes.

Triceps

- Rare.

Mechanism

- Usually indirect during a fall on an outstretched hand (elderly patient).
- Eccentric stretch with weight lifting (associated with anabolic steroid use).

Examination

- Pain, swelling, weakness of elbow extension, palpable defect.

Imaging

- Radiographs—avulsion fracture commonly seen.
- Radial head fractures may occur simultaneously.
- MRI to clarify degree of injury and amount of retraction (operative planning).

Treatment

- Partial tear treated conservatively.
- Complete or near complete tear.
  - Primary repair.

Subscapularis

Mechanism

- Acute traumatic episode (violent external rotation or hyperextension).
- Following anterior glenohumeral dislocation (in patients older than age 30).
- Failure of repair following capsulotomy.

History

- Anterior shoulder pain.
- Pain with flexion.
- External rotation weakness.
- Popping with abduction (subluxating biceps tendon).

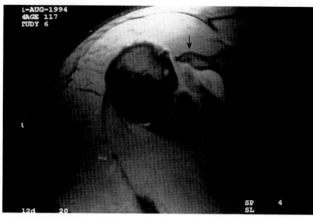

Figure 37–5:
Magnetic resonance imaging showing subscapularis tendon rupture.(From Miller MD, Howard RF, Plancher KD: *Surgical atlas of sports medicine.* Philadelphia, 2003, Saunders.)

Examination

- Increase in passive external rotation in adduction (compared with contralateral side).
- Positive lift-off test and belly-press test.

Imaging

- Radiographs can reveal an avulsion fracture on axillary.
- MRI—improved diagnostic accuracy (still commonly missed) (Figure 37–5).

Treatment

- Nonoperative: partial tear, low-demand asymptomatic patient without shoulder instability.
- Operative: complete tear, young patient, symptomatic subluxating biceps tendon.
  - May require Z-lengthening for chronic, retracted tears.
  - Complications.
    - Close proximity of axillary nerve and anterior humeral circumflex artery (Figure 37–6).
    - Repeat rupture.
    - Inadequate tissue for reconstruction (requires graft).

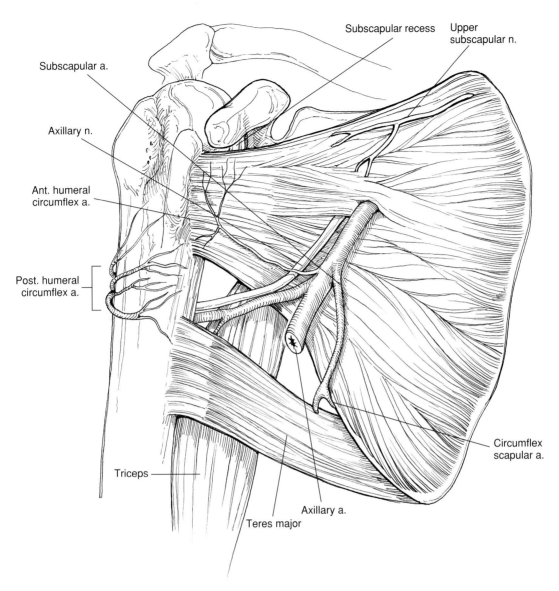

Figure 37–6:
Neurovascular anatomy surrounding subscapularis muscle insertion. (From Miller MD, Howard RF, Plancher KD: *Surgical atlas of sports medicine.* Philadelphia, 2003, Saunders.)

References

Aarimaa V, Rantanen J, Heikkila J, et al: Rupture of the pectoralis major muscle. *Am J Sports Med* 32:1256-1262, 2004.
> *The authors present a case series of 33 operatively treated pectoralis major ruptures and a meta-analysis of previously published cases. They concluded that early operative treatment is associated with better outcome than delayed treatment.*

Deutsch A, Altchek DW, Veltri DM, et al: Traumatic tears of the subscapularis tendon. Clinical diagnosis, MRI findings, and operative therapy. *Am J Sports Med* 25:13-22, 1997.
> *This reviews 14 cases of subscapularis tendon tear to determine the most predictive symptoms and physical examination findings associated with this condition. Surgical repair results in less pain and functional improvement.*

Henry JC, Scerpella TA: Acute traumatic tear of the latissimus dorsi tendon from its insertion. *Am J Sports Med* 28:577-579, 2000.
> *This case report demonstrated the utility of MRI and recommended acute repair in athletes. They cite studies that demonstrate measurable deficits in shoulder strength and function with loss of the latissimus dorsi muscle.*

Levy M, Goldberg I, Meir I: Fracture of the head of the radius with a tear or avulsion of the triceps tendon. *J Bone Joint Surg Br* 64:70-72, 1982.
> *These authors reported that radial head fractures are common in patients with triceps tendon injuries.*

Miller MD, Johnson DL, Fu FH: Rupture of the pectoralis major muscle in a collegiate football player. *Am J Sports Med* 21:475-477, 1993.

> *This is the first report of suture anchor use to repair ruptured pectoralis major tendons.*

Tarsney FF: Rupture and avulsion of the triceps. *Clin Orthop* 83:177-183, 1972.

> *Doubled the number of reports of triceps injuries in the literature at the time of publication. Reported the common finding of bony avulsion fragments on lateral radiographs.*

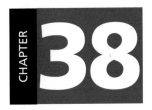

CHAPTER

Shoulder Loss of Motion

History, Physical Examination, and Imaging

- Adhesive capsulitis, also known as "frozen shoulder," denotes an idiopathic condition resulting in global loss of active and passive motion in the shoulder.
- Prevalence is estimated to be slightly greater than 2% of the population.
- Women comprise approximately 70% of patients.
- Twenty percent to thirty percent of patients will develop adhesive capsulitis in the contralateral shoulder.
- Several factors have been associated with adhesive capsulitis (Box 38–1).
- Pathology results from an intraarticular process defined by inflammation and fibrosis, which causes contracture of the capsule and a reduced intraarticular volume that produces a mechanical block to glenohumeral motion in all planes.
- Diabetics commonly have bilateral adhesive capsulitis and are usually unresponsive to most treatment.
- Progression of the condition can be described in three clinical and four arthroscopic stages (Box 38–2).
- Hannafin and Chiaia described four stages of adhesive capsulitis on the basis of history, physical examination, and arthroscopic findings (Box 38–3).
- Considered a self-limiting disease in many patients that takes 1 to 3 years for symptoms to completely resolve.

- Patients are aware of their limited shoulder motion, often associated with pain, which may limit their daily activities.
- Pain at rest and at night that is aggravated with extreme range of motion are common symptoms.
- Compensatory mechanisms, such as increased scapulothoracic motion, may result in additional symptoms (such as discomfort medial to the scapula).
- Examination should carefully document both active and passive range of motion.
- The large differential for shoulder stiffness must be considered and addressed during patient evaluation (Table 38–1).
- Associated conditions, such as rotator cuff disease, may produce greater loss in active motion.
- When measuring range of motion, it is critical that compensatory mechanisms be corrected for, such as a shoulder shrugging, trunk lean, and scapulothoracic motion.
  - Errors can be avoided by performing measurements in relation to the thorax rather than a vertical line drawn down to the floor.
  - Passive range of motion should be performed with the patient supine, which helps limit scapulothoracic movement, or by stabilizing the scapula with one hand.

Box 38–1	Factors Associated with Adhesive Capsulitis

Female gender
Diabetes
Thyroid disease
Autoimmune disease
Prolonged immobilization
Trauma
Older than 40 years
Myocardial infarction
Stroke

Box 38–2	Stages of Adhesive Capsulitis

Clinical

Stage I—Painful phase. Duration ranges from 2 to 9 months.
Stage II—Stiffening phase. Decrease in glenohumeral motion. Duration ranges from 4 to 12 months.
Stage III—Thawing phase. Gradual return of motion lasting months to years.

Arthroscopic

Stage 1—Patchy fibrinous synovitis
Stage 2—Capsular contraction, fibrinous adhesions, synovitis
Stage 3—Increased contraction, resolving synovitis
Stage 4—Severe contraction

Box 38–3 | Stages of Adhesive Capsulitis

Stage 1

Duration of symptoms: 0 to 3 months
    Pain with active and passive ROM
    Limitation of forward flexion, abduction, internal rotation, external rotation
    Examination with the patient under anesthesia: normal or minimal loss of ROM
    Arthroscopy: Diffuse glenohumeral synovitis, often most pronounced in the anterosuperior capsule
    Pathologic changes: Hypertrophic, hypervascular synovitis, rare inflammatory cell infiltrates, normal underlying capsule

State 2: "Freezing Stage"

Duration of symptoms: 3 to 9 months
    Chronic pain with active and passive ROM
    Significant limitation of forward flexion, abduction, internal rotation, external rotation
    Examination with the patient under anesthesia: ROM essentially identical to ROM when the patient is awake
    Anthroscopy: Diffuse, pedunculated synovitis (tight capsule with rubbery or dense feel on insertion of arthroscope)
    Pathologic changes: Hypertrophic, hypervascular synovitis with perivascular and subsynovial scar, fibroplasia, and scar formation in the underlying capsule

Stage 3: "Frozen Stage"

Duration of symptoms: 9 to 15 months
    Minimal pain except at end ROM
    Significant limitation of ROM with rigid "end feel"
    Examination with the patient under anesthesia: ROM identical to ROM when patient is awake
    Arthroscopy: No hypervascularity seen, remnants of fibrotic synovium can be seen. The capsule feels thick in insertion of the arthroscope, and there is a diminished capsular volume
    Pathologic changes: "Burned out" synovitis without significant hypertrophy or hypervascularity; underlying capsule shows dense scar formation

Stage 4: "Thawing Phase"

Duration of symptoms: 15 to 24 months
Minimal pain
Progressive improvement in ROM
Examination under anesthesia: data not available

ROM, Range of motion.
From Hannafin JA, Chiaia TA: *Clin Orthop Relat Res* 372:95–109, 2000.

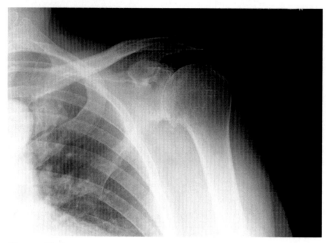

Figure 38–1:
Radiograph demonstrating osteoarthritis of the shoulder joint. Note the loss of the glenohumeral space.

provides a good assessment of rotator cuff tears, findings on arthrography have not demonstrated good correlation with motion loss. Magnetic resonance imaging (MRI) arthrography combines the benefits of both procedures and is excellent for evaluating associated pathology, such as a rotator cuff tear (Figure 38–2).

Types

- Adhesive capsulitis may be categorized into primary and secondary types.
- Primary (idiopathic) adhesive capsulitis is believed to result from a systemic disorder (inflammatory, immunologic, biochemical, endocrine), although a definite etiology is yet to be determined (Table 38–1).
- Idiopathic adhesive capsulitis normally results in global loss of motion.
- Secondary adhesive capsulitis is the result of a known intrinsic, extrinsic, or systemic disorder including posttraumatic and postoperative shoulder stiffness (Table 38–2).
- Secondary adhesive capsulitis can result in global loss of motion or reduced range of motion in specific planes depending on the underlying pathology and etiology.
  - Asymmetric loss of motion primarily results from scarring in the affected area, particularly along the interface between the proximal humerus and deltoid and conjoined tendon.
  - Contracture of the capsule and rotator cuff may also be present.
  - Particular patterns of limited motion can assist with planning rehabilitation protocols or operative management.
    - Reduced external rotation in adduction suggests contraction of the anterosuperior capsule and rotator interval.

- Evaluation of the cervical spine should be included in the examination.
- Standard radiographs are usually normal, particularly in idiopathic adhesive capsulitis. However, it provides radiologic evaluation of the glenohumeral joint and can help reveal arthritis, fractures, loose bodies, calcific tendinitis, abnormal bony morphology, dislocations, surgical hardware, and disuse osteoporosis (Figure 38–1).
- Arthrography has been recommended by some to confirm reduced intraarticular volume. Although it

Table 38–1: Proposed Pathogenic Mechanisms for Primary Frozen Shoulder

MECHANISM	DISORDER	PATHOLOGY	ETIOLOGY EXCLUDED BY
Autoimmume	Collagen-vascular disorders	Type IV reaction (to infarcted cuff tendon)	Absence of immune complexes and autoantibodies, no other affected joints
Inflammatory	Infectious arthritis	Viral, bacterial, or fungal infection	Absence of prodromal illness and systemic symptoms
Crystal arthropathy	CPPD disease and gout	Crystal deposition	Absence of recurrences, crystals, and inflammatory phases
Reactive arthropathy	Spondyloarthritides and ankylosing spondylitis	Seronegative arthritis	No systemic manifestations; normal joint fluid, no blood markers
Hemarthrosis	Hemoglobinopathies and trauma	Chemical irritation (hemosiderin)	No capsulitis or fibrositis with hemoglobinopathies
Paralytic	Suprascapular nerve palsy	Compression neuropathy	Absence of EMG or conduction abnormalities
Algodystrophy	Autonomic neuropathy	Neuropathic disturbance and hypervascularity	No sensory or vascular deficiency, stellate ganglion block not helpful
Degenerative	Rotator cuff tendon and degeneration/infarction	Microvascular infarction	Absence of tendon inflammation or infarction
Traumatic	Trauma and immobilization	Injury synovitis and tissue contracture	Brief shoulder stiffness after prolonged casting in the majority
Psychogenic	Hysteria and hypochondriasis	Depression, dependence, and chronic pain disorder	Similar MMPI between patients and controls
Fibrogenic	Cytokine induction of fibroplasia	Tissue contracture in response to cytokines, inflammatory cell products, and platelet-derived growth factor	No exclusion, current theory in text

CPPD, Calcium-pyrophosphate disease; EMG, electromyogram; MMPI, Minnesota Multiphasic Personality Inventory.
From *Instr Course Lect* 42:248, 1993.

- Limited external rotation in abduction is associated with contracture of the anteroinferior capsule.
- Decreased internal rotation in abduction or adduction and limited cross-chest adduction is suggestive of posterior capsular contraction.
- Extraarticular contractions must also be considered, such as in the rotator cuff muscles.

Treatment

- Controversy exists on optimal treatment, with several options available (Box 38–4).
- Treatment should be individualized according to the patient's need and stage of disease.
- A rehabilitation program is successful in the majority of cases of primary adhesive capsulitis and is recommended initially for the management of secondary adhesive capsulitis.
- Nonsteroidal antiinflammatory drugs (NSAIDs) and intraarticular steroid injections may benefit some patients during the inflammatory phase (early stages).
- Secondary adhesive capsulitis is often resistant to nonoperative management.
- Surgery is considered if no improvement is achieved after 6 months of conservative management.
- Severe limitation in motion postoperatively, such as after instability procedures, may indicate a poor glenohumeral articular joint relationship that can lead to advanced arthritic changes.
- Closed manipulation may be attempted in all conditions that do not involve extraarticular contracture.
- Contraindicated in patients with osteopenia, fractures, or previous surgical repair within the past 3 months because this may result in fracture, soft tissue damage, and nerve injury.
- Can be performed under general anesthesia, but interscalene blocks may provide greater control of postoperative pain and allow greater success in therapy. The regional block can be repeated following 2 postoperative days or continuously administered using an interscalene catheter.
- Manipulation is performed by stabilizing the scapula with one hand and using the other, placed just above the elbow, to rotate the arm in all planes with gradually increasing pressure until normal passive motion is restored.
- Arthroscopic release is a useful option in patients who have contraindications to or failed manipulation or would likely benefit from release before manipulation is performed.
  - Advantages of arthroscopy include the ability of detecting and correcting any coexisting pathology, examination of the results of manipulation (and making manipulation easier after release), precise and controlled release of structures and adhesions, and the ease in which it can be converted to an open approach.
  - Interscalene block is recommended to provide complete muscle paralysis and offer postoperative pain control.
  - A stiff shoulder with a reduced intraarticular volume can make the insertion of the arthroscope difficult and the area prone to articular injuries if insertion is applied with excessive force.

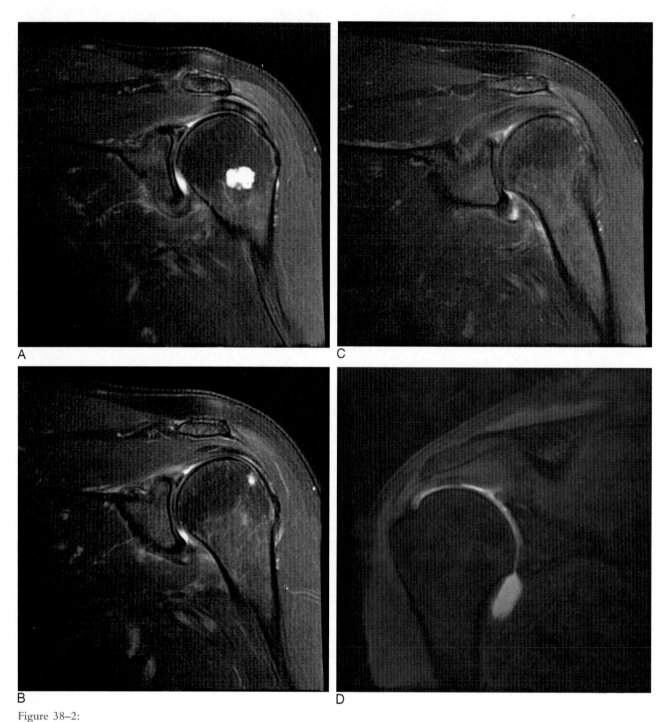

A

B

C

D

Figure 38–2:

A-C, Magnetic resonance imaging (MRI) arthrogram of a patient with adhesive capsulitis revealing a loss of the axillary pouch. **D-F,** MRI arthrogram of a normal patient for comparison. Note the difference in axillary pouch size compared with the patient with adhesive capsulitis.

(continued)

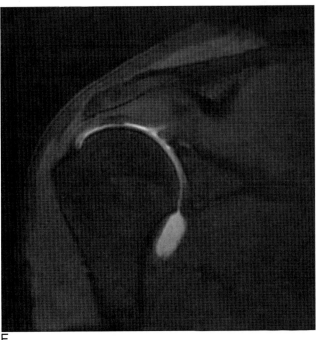

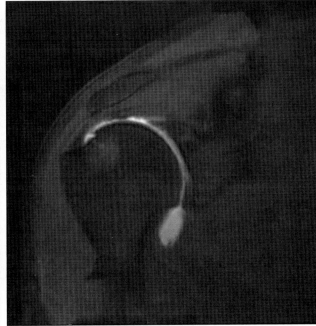

Figure 38–2, cont'd

- Damage of the articular surface can be reduced by using a slightly proximal posterior portal and entering the joint superiorly relative to the glenoid and over the humeral head, allowing the arthroscope to be inserted into the widest area of the joint (Figure 38–3).
- The joint should be examined for concomitant pathology and synovectomy performed if synovitis or synovial thickening is appreciated (usually present in early stages).
- Anterior release procedure is initiated by identifying the biceps tendon, marking the upper border of the rotator interval that is to be released, using electrocautery and shavers on surrounding scar tissue, and making sure to dissect down until the upper edge of the subscapularis tendon is visualized (rotator interval release). The release is taken all the way to the base of the coracoid (Figure 38–4A).
- Release of the rotator interval usually results in greater external rotation and inferolateral migration of the humeral head, which creates more space in the joint, facilitating arthroscopic instrumentation (Figure 38–4B).
- Manipulation is then performed in all planes. If only minimal improvement is achieved, release continues along the anteroinferior capsule while avoiding the axillary pouch.
- If internal rotation is still limited (> 40 degrees less in abduction than the contralateral arm) after the entire anterior capsule is released, a posterior capsule release is required.

- Posterior release is carried down from the biceps tendon origin to the posteroinferior rim of the glenoid.
- Open release is reserved for cases in which motion is still limited after arthroscopic treatment.
  - A deltopectoral incision is used and lysis of adhesions is performed across all the layers of dissection, making certain that all scarring between the deltoid and humerus is released (until free movement of the deltoid over the humeral head is achieved in all planes of motion). Dissection is assisted in this region with the arm abducted, allowing the deltoid to be lax, and using internal rotation to assist anterior to posterior release of subdeltoid adhesions.
  - Dissection is carried toward the subacromial space, the coracoacromial ligament is excised, and any surrounding adhesions removed, prior to releasing the rotator interval.
  - Manipulation is performed. If external rotation is still limited, the subscapularis muscle should be split and released from any adhesions. If limited external rotation persists, a lengthening Z-plasty of the subscapularis and capsule is recommended (Figure 38–5). If Z-plasty is performed, accurate documentation of range of motion limitations according to tendon tension is required to define a safe zone for early passive range of motion during rehabilitation.
  - Anterior and posterior capsules are released as needed.

Table 38–2: Differential Diagnoses of Shoulder Stiffness (Including Associated Diseases)

EXTRINSIC CAUSES		INTRINSIC CAUSES

Neurologic
Parkinson's disease
Autonomic dystrophy (RSD)
Intradural lesions
Neural compression
   Cervical disk disease
   Neurofibromata
Foraminal stenosis
Neuralgic amyotrophy
Hemiplegia
Head trauma

Muscular
Poliomyositis

Cardiovascular
Myocardial infarction
Thoracic outlet syndrome
Cerebral hemorrhage

Infectious
Chronic bronchitis
Pulmonary tuberculosis

Metabolic
Diabetes mellitus
Thyroid disease
Progressive systemic sclerosis (scleroderma)
Paget's disease

Neoplastic
Pancoast tumor
Lung carcinoma
Metastatic disease

Inflammatory
Rheumatologic disorders (see Box 38–3)
Polymyalgia rheumatica

Trauma
Surgery
   Axillary node dissection, sternotomy, thoracotomy
Fractures
   Cervical spine, ribs, elbow, hand, etc.

Medications
Isoniazid, phenobarbitone

Congenital
Klippel-Feil
Sprengel's deformity
Glenoid dysplasia
Atresia
Contractures
   Pectoralis major
   Axillary fold

Behavioral
Depression
Hysterical paralysis

Referred Pain
Diaphragmatic irritation
Gastrointestinal disorders
   Esophagitis
   Ulcers
   Cholecystitis

Bursitis
Subacromial
Calcific tendinitis
Snapping scapula

Biceps Tendon
Tenosynovitis
Partial or complete tears
SLAP lesions

Rotator Cuff
Impingement syndrome
Partial rotator cuff tears
Complete rotator cuff tears

Instability-Glenohumeral
Recurrent dislocation anterior and posterior
Chronic dislocation

Arthritides
Glenohumeral and acromio-clavicular
   Osteoarthritis
   Rheumatoid
   Psoriatic
   Infectious
   Neuropathic

Trauma
Fractures
   Glenoid
   Proximal humerus
Surgery
   Postoperative shoulder, breast, head, neck, chest

Miscellaneous
Avascular necrosis
Hemarthrosis
Osteochondromatosis
Suprascapular nerve palsy

SLAP, Superior labral anterior to posterior.
From Rockwood CA Jr, Matsen FA III, Wirth MA, Lippitt SB: *The shoulder*, 3rd ed. Philadelphia, 2004, Saunders.

Box 38–4	**Therapeutic Options for Adhesive Capsulitis**

Benign neglect
Home therapy
Supervised rehabilitation
Nonsteroidal antiinflammatory medications
Oral steroids
Intraarticular steroid injections
Therapeutic modalities
Distension arthrography
Closed manipulation
Open surgical release
Arthroscopic capsular release
Combination of above

Rehabilitation

- Rehabilitation protocols can be supervised, performed at home, or in a combination of the two.
- Range of motion and stretching exercises are the key elements in physical therapy.
- Therapeutic modalities assist in reducing pain and inflammation and relaxing muscles prior to exercises.
- Immediate postoperative rehabilitation can benefit from continuous use of an interscalene block and continuous passive motion.
- Aggressive stretching therapy in all planes can begin on the day following surgery, and the patient should be instructed on self-assisted stretching and a progressive

home program on discharge that can include supervised physical therapy.
- If Z-plasty is performed, stretching is restricted to only passive range of motion within the surgically documented "safe zone" for 4 weeks.
- Patients should be monitored for improvement, and necessary adjustments made to their rehabilitation depending on their individual needs and limitations.
- The strengthening phase of rehabilitation should not begin until the patient has regained pain-free global range of motion, which normally occurs at approximately 3 months.

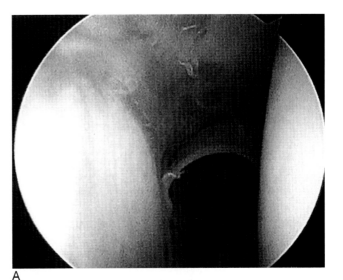

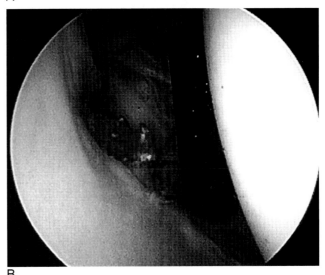

Figure 38–4:
A, Arthroscopic view of a patient with adhesive capsulitis. Note the severely contracted rotator interval, which is completely filled in with scar tissue. **B,** Arthroscopic view following release of the rotator interval from the base of the coracoid to the middle glenohumeral ligament.

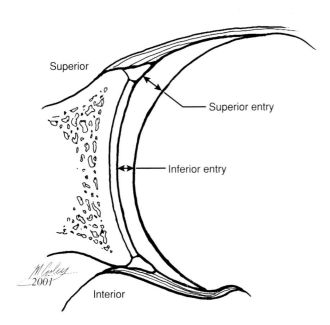

Figure 38–3:
Location of superior joint entry. (From Gartsman GM: *Shoulder arthroscopy.* Philadelphia, 2003, Saunders.)

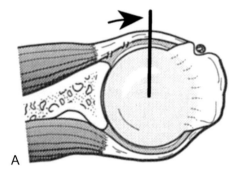

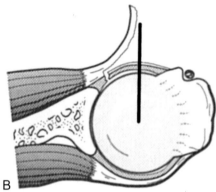

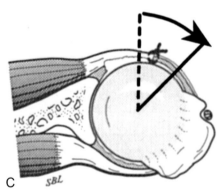

Figure 38–5:
Z-plasty lengthening of the subscapularis and capsule. A, The subscapularis tendon is exposed through a standard deltopectoral approach. **B,** The subscapularis tendon is detached off the lesser tuberosity and elevated off the anterior capsule. **C,** The anterior capsule is cut medial to its attachment on the lesser tuberosity, the arm is externally rotated, and the subscapularis is repaired to the lateral edge of the medial capsule, effectively lengthening the tendon. (From Matsen FA III, Lippitt SB, Sidles JA, Harryman DT II: *Practical evaluation of management of the shoulder.* Philadelphia, 1994, Saunders.)

Complications

- Chronic pain and stiffness.
- Instability.
- Reduced intraarticular volume enhances the risk for articular damage when forceful arthroscopic insertion is performed.

- Manipulation may produce fractures or tendon and ligament damage, especially in patients with contraindications.
- Extravasation of fluid with arthroscopic procedures.
- Axillary nerve is at risk during anterior capsule release.
- Division of the subscapularis tendon can occur if it is not adequately identified during arthroscopic procedures and is best avoided by converting to an open approach.
- If posterior release extends laterally past the glenoid rim, the superficial infraspinatus muscle at this region is at risk for injury, which would result in weak external rotation.
- Dissection medial to the base of the coracoid process places neurovascular structures at risk, including the musculocutaneous nerve.
- Interscalene blocks may be complicated by phrenic or laryngeal nerve block, pneumothorax, toxicity, brachial plexus injury, bronchospasm, and cardiac arrest.

References

Andersen NH, Sojbjerg JO, Johannsen HV, Sneppen O: Frozen shoulder: arthroscopy and manipulation under general anesthesia and early passive motion. *J Shoulder Elbow Surg* 7:218-222, 1998.
Authors study the effectiveness of arthroscopy and manipulation under anesthesia in 24 consecutive patients with refractory frozen shoulder (12 with primary and 12 with secondary adhesive capsulitis). Postoperative management included the use of a subacromial epidural catheter and supervised rehabilitation including the use of a continuous passive motion machine. After a 12-month follow-up, 75% of patients obtained normal or nearly full range of motion and 79% had minimal or no pain.

Arslan S, Celiker R: Comparison of the efficacy of local corticosteroid injection and physical therapy for the treatment of adhesive capsulitis. *Rheumatol Int* 21:20-23, 2001.
Authors compare the use of intraarticular injections (10 patients) to combined physiotherapy and nonsteroidal antiinflammatories (10 patients) in individuals affected with adhesive capsulitis. Evaluations were performed 2 and 12 weeks after treatment. Results demonstrated significant improvement in range of motion and pain in both groups. There were no significant differences between the two groups. The authors concluded that intraarticular injections and combined physiotherapy with nonsteroidal antiinflammatories were equally effective.

Griggs SM, Ahn A, Green A: Idiopathic adhesive capsulitis: A prospective functional outcome study of nonoperative treatment. *J Bone Joint Surg Am* 82:1398-1407, 2000.
Prospective study on 75 patients with idiopathic adhesive capsulitis treated with a specific four-direction shoulder-stretching exercise program including pendulum exercises and passive stretching exercises in forward elevation, external rotation, horizontal adduction, and internal rotation. Authors reported 90% subjective satisfaction among the patients with significant improvement in all ranges of motion. However, the authors note that approximately 40% of the patients still had abnormal shoulder function with measurable differences between the affected extremity and normal contralateral shoulder. Although this treatment appears to provide the majority of patients with satisfied results, the authors recommend that more aggressive and early treatment options be further studied to define optimal management of adhesive capsulitis.

Hannafin J, Chiaia T: Adhesive capsulitis: a treatment approach. *Clin Orthop Relat Res* 372:95-109, 2000.

Excellent review of the pathology, presentation, examination, diagnosis, staging, and treatment of adhesive capsulitis. The authors offer a four-stage classification system that is used to guide treatment. Stages are discussed individually with associated pathologic and clinical findings and optimal approaches to treatment.

Holloway GB, Schenk T, Williams GR, et al: Arthroscopic capsular release for the treatment of refractory postoperative or post-fracture shoulder stiffness. *J Bone Join Surg Am* 83:1682-1687, 2001.

Authors compare the outcomes of arthroscopic capsular release for postoperative stiffness, postfracture stiffness, and idiopathic adhesive capsulitis. Assessment of patients at a mean of 20 months after surgery revealed similar improvement in range of motion in all groups but significantly lower scores for pain, patient satisfaction, and functional activity among the postoperative stiffness group when compared with the patients with idiopathic or posttraumatic adhesive capsulitis.

Kivimaki J, Pohjolainen T: Manipulation under anesthesia for frozen shoulder with and without steroid injection. *Arch Phys Med Rehabil* 82:1188-1190, 2001.

Randomized trial study comparing the result of manipulation with and without steroid in 24 patients with adhesive capsulitis. Range of motion and shoulder symptoms were evaluated 1 day and 4 months following manipulation. Both groups demonstrated similar significant improvements in mobility and shoulder symptoms.

Long TR, Wass CT, Burkle CM: Perioperative interscalene blockade: an overview of its history and current clinical use. *J Clin Anesth* 14:546-556, 2002.

Anatomy, technique, anesthetic options, indications, results, and complications of interscalene blocks are reviewed.

Vad VB, Sakalkale D, Warren RF: The role of capsular distention in adhesive capsulitis. *Arch Phys Med Rehabil* 84:1290-1292, 2003.

Prospective study in 19 patients with Hannafin stage II adhesive capsulitis and 3 patients with Hannafin stage III using capsular distention with saline under fluoroscopy and a rehabilitation protocol. A minimum of 12 months after the procedure, evaluation demonstrated significant improvement in patients with stage II disease but only minimal improvement in patients with Hannafin stage III adhesive capsulitis.

Warner JJP: Frozen shoulder: diagnosis and management. *J Am Acad Orthop Surg* 5:130-140, 1997.

Author provides a comprehensive review of adhesive capsulitis including its epidemiology, anatomy, pathology, clinical and radiologic evaluation, and management. Nonoperative and surgical techniques including physical therapy, closed manipulation, and arthroscopic and open release are well described.

Warner JJP, Allen A, Marks PH, Wong P: Arthroscopic release for chronic refractory adhesive capsulitis of the shoulder. *J Bone Joint Surg Am* 78:1808-1816, 1996.

Authors report on their results of arthroscopic release in 23 patients with idiopathic adhesive capsulitis who failed nonoperative management including manipulation under anesthesia. Surgical technique is described and consists of careful portal placement, evaluation (and treatment) of concomitant pathology, anterior capsular release, and manipulation. Postoperatively, interscalene blocks or catheters were used for initial (inpatient) rehabilitation. At a mean of 39 months after surgery, all patients demonstrated significant improvement in range of motion, within a mean of 7 degrees of the normal contralateral shoulder. No complications were noted.

Yamaguchi K, Sethi N, Bauer GS: Postoperative pain control following arthroscopic release of adhesive capsulitis: a short-term retrospective review study of the use of an intra-articular pain catheter. *Arthroscopy* 18:359-365, 2002.

Retrospective study on the effectiveness of an intraarticular catheter for pain control following arthroscopic treatment of adhesive capsulitis. Authors comment that this technique allows arthroscopic-guided placement, long-lasting control of glenohumeral pain, and the ability to perform active range of motion (in contrast to the motor and sensory blockade produced by interscalene blocks).

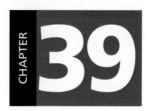

Nerve Entrapment at the Shoulder

Introduction

- Overhead athletes most commonly affected.
- Upper extremity nerve entrapments are often a result of ganglion cysts or traumatic injuries.
- Like all nerve entrapment syndromes, neurologic testing can help localize the location of the lesion.
- Examination should include muscle strength testing, sensory testing, and electromyographic studies.

Suprascapular Neuropathy

- Most frequently injured peripheral branch of the brachial plexus in athletes.
  - Especially in volleyball players (chronic traction injury) and throwing athletes.
- Mechanism.
  - Acute: traction injury, overzealous mobilization of retracted rotator cuff tears.
  - Chronic: overuse injury, ganglion, perilabral cyst associated with superior labral anterior to posterior tear, hypertrophied suprascapular ligament, scapular fracture callus.
  - Occurs at one of two locations, either at the anterior superior portion of the scapula as the nerve goes under the transverse scapular ligament or the spinoglenoid notch (Figure 39–1).
  - Suprascapular notch entrapment at the transverse scapular ligament affects both the supraspinatus and the infraspinatus because the nerve branch to the supraspinatus occurs immediately after the nerve traverses the scapular notch.
  - Spinoglenoid notch entrapment affects only the infraspinatus and not the supraspinatus because the entrapment occurs distal to the suprascapular nerve branch to the supraspinatus.
- Examination.
  - External rotation weakness in adduction and atrophy of the supraspinatus or the infraspinatus, or both (Figure 39–2).

- Nerve conduction velocities and electromyography may confirm the diagnosis (normal study does not rule out the diagnosis).
- Imaging.
  - Magnetic resonance imaging can sometimes be helpful if there is a cyst that is encroaching on these areas (Figure 39–3).
- Treatment.
  - Activity modification (overuse injury).
  - Alleviation of causative lesion (cyst decompression and labral repair).
  - Nerve or muscle transfer for irreparable injury.

Thoracic Outlet Syndrome

- Significant controversy surrounds the diagnosis and treatment of this entity.
- Typically involves compression of the brachial plexus and subclavian vessels as they pass between the scalene muscles and the first rib.
- Occurs more commonly in females than males.

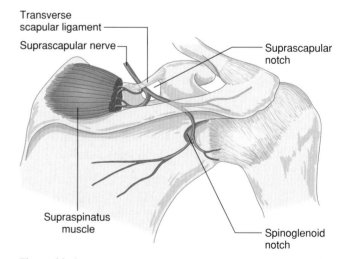

Figure 39–1:

Anatomy surrounding suprascapular nerve. (Redrawn from Moore TP, Hunter RE: *Oper Tech Sports Med* **4:9, 1996.)**

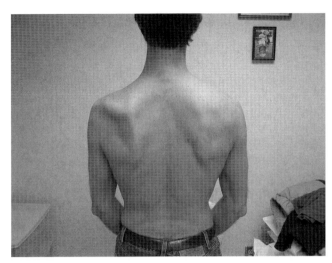

Figure 39–2:

Left shoulder infraspinatus muscle atrophy on clinical examination.

- History.
  - No pathognomic signs or symptoms.
  - Presentation dependent on specific structure compressed (94% to 97% with neurologic symptoms, vascular manifestations rare).
  - Most commonly intermittent pain and paresthesias usually in the ulnar nerve distribution.
  - Subjective weakness in 50% of patients.
  - No fixed deficits.
- Etiology includes the following:
  - Trauma with resultant fibrosis (reported in 20% to 86% of patients).
  - Cervical rib.
  - Clavicular fracture malunion or nonunion.
  - Aberrant origins of the scalenus muscles.
- Examination.
  - Adson test—loss of radial pulse or reproduction of symptoms during inspiration with head rotated to affected side.
  - Wright test—loss of radial pulse or reproduction of symptoms with ipsilateral arm extension, abduction, and external rotation during neck extension and rotation to contralateral shoulder (Figure 39–4).
  - Overhead stress test—reproduction of symptoms during repeated grasping of fists while positioned with the bilateral shoulders at 90 degrees of abduction and 90 degrees external rotation.
- Diagnosis.
  - Examination frequently inconclusive.
  - Nerve conduction velocities "across the thoracic outlet"—threshold of less than 60 m/second for surgery and comparison with contralateral side.
  - Typically a diagnosis of exclusion.
- Treatment.

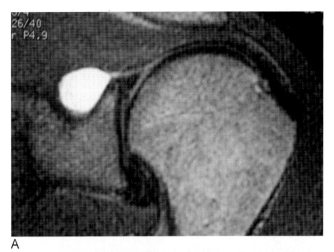

A

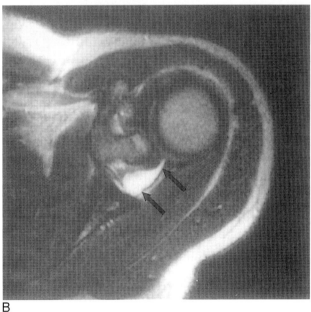

B

Figure 39–3:

A, Coronal magnetic resonance imaging (MRI) demonstrating suprascapular notch ganglion. **B,** Axial MRI demonstrating cyst and stalk arising from posterosuperior shoulder joint. (**A** from Miller MD, Cooper DE, Warner JJP: *Review of arthroscopy and sports medicine.* Philadelphia, 2002, Saunders; **B** from Moore TP, Hunter RE: *Oper Tech Sports Med* 4:10, 1996.)

- Nonoperative: postural training, muscle strengthening, nonsteroidal antiinflammatory drugs, biofeedback, ultrasound.
- Operative.
  - First rib resection.
  - Release of the scalene muscles.
  - Exploration of the supraclavicular fossa.
  - Claviculectomy.
  - Frequently associated with complications.
  - May require referral to thoracic or vascular surgeon.

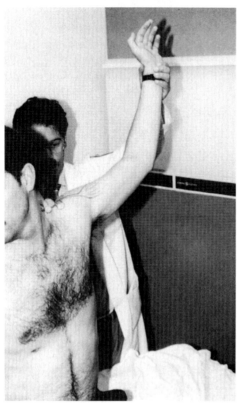

Figure 39–4:
The Wright test. (From Miller MD, Cooper DE, Warner JJP:
Review of arthroscopy and sports medicine. **Philadelphia, 2002,**
Saunders.)

Quadrilateral Space Syndrome

- Axillary nerve compression in the quadrilateral (quadrangular) space, which is bordered by both teres muscles (minor and major), the long head of the triceps, and the humerus.
- History.
  - Pain and paresthesias with the arm in the overhead position.
  - Can also occur in late cocking and acceleration phase of throwing.
- Imaging.
  - Angiogram may show a collusion of the circumflex scapular artery, which accompanies the axillary nerve through this space.
- Treatment.
  - Release of the quadrilateral space in refractory cases.

Long Thoracic Nerve

- Innervates the serratus anterior muscle, which retracts the scapula.
- Neuropathy causes medial winging of the scapula.
- Etiologies.
  - Compression (mass, crutch use).
  - Traction (swimmers).
  - Viral.
- History.
  - Scapulothoracic dyskinesis affecting shoulder function.
  - Weakness with overhead activities.
- Examination.
  - Unilateral medial winging of the scapula (push-up on wall).
- Treatment.
  - Typically observed for spontaneous resolution (up to 18 months).
  - Activity modification (swimmers).
  - Modified thoracolumbar brace with a scapular pad assists nerve regeneration by avoiding scapular winging and recurrent traction.
  - Recalcitrant cases with associated morbidity can be treated with pectoralis muscle transfer to inferior angle of the scapula.

References

Drez D Jr: Suprascapular neuropathy in the differential diagnosis of rotator cuff injuries. *Am J Sports Med* 4:43-45, 1976.

> *This landmark article recognized what was believed to be an unusual condition. The increased incidence of suprascapular neuropathy recently is likely related to a higher index of suspicion, largely because of articles such as this.*

Ferretti A, Declari A, Fontana M: Injury of the suprascapular nerve at the spinoglenoid notch. The natural history of infraspinatus atrophy in volleyball players. *Am J Sports Med* 26:759-763, 1998.

> *This article reported 38 volleyball players with suprascapular nerve entrapment. Athletes with no pain were treated conservatively. Athletes with pain were treated with surgical decompression. Most athletes were able to return to play without surgical intervention.*

Safran MR: Nerve injury about the shoulder in athletes, part 1. Suprascapular nerve and axillary nerve. *Am J Sports Med* 32:803-819, 2004.

Safran MR: Nerve injury about the shoulder in athletes, part 2. Long thoracic nerve, spinal accessory nerve, burners/stingers, thoracic outlet syndrome. *Am J Sports Med* 32:1063-1076, 2004.

> *These two articles offer a comprehensive overview of the current state of knowledge of nerve impingement about the shoulder.*

Vastamacki M, Goransson H: Suprascapular nerve entrapment. *Clin Orthop Relat Res* 297:135-143, 1993.

> *Largest study on suprascapular nerve entrapment. Open decompression was successful in most cases.*

CHAPTER 40

Upper Extremity Fractures

History, Physical Examination, and Imaging

- Fractures about the shoulder in young patients result from direct or high-energy trauma.
- Elderly patients with osteoporosis can incur fractures from simple falls.
- Associated injuries including other fractures and neurovascular damage are relatively common.
- Patients report a specific incident leading to their symptoms of pain, swelling, and limited ability to perform certain activities with their affected upper extremity.
- Inspection should document any bony deformities, swelling, bruising, and manner in which the patient holds or carries the affected arm.
- Puncture wounds at the site transform the injury into an open fracture.
- Physical examination will reveal tenderness along the injured site.
- It is critical to evaluate any possible nerve damage by testing sensation and motor function of all nerves that are distal to the site of injury.
- Possible vascular injury may present with pallor, prolonged capillary refill, or decreased/loss of pulses.
- Plain radiographic imaging is often sufficient to make the diagnosis.
- Computed tomography (CT) (and magnetic resonance imaging) can assist with further evaluation of occult or associated injuries or when planning for surgical treatment.

Types

Clavicle

- One of the most common bony injuries, constituting approximately 15% of all fractures.
- Can result from direct trauma or falls from an outstretched arm.
- Approximately 3% of patients have associated injuries.

- Classification according to site of injury was originally described by Neer (Box 40–1, Figures 40–1 to 40–5).
- Pain may limit the patient's ability to raise the arm.
- Patients often present with a deformity or "bump" at the injury site, with occasional tenting of the skin.
- Tenderness and crepitus are often present.
- The axillary, musculocutaneous, median, ulnar, and radial nerves should all be evaluated.
- CT imaging may be used to further evaluate uncommon medial injuries or complex acromioclavicular (AC) fractures.
- Group I and III fractures usually have satisfactory results when patients are placed in a sling for 6 weeks, with gentle shoulder exercises beginning after 2 weeks.
  - Open reduction and internal fixation (ORIF) is recommended with open fractures, neurovascular compromise, or severe tenting of the skin.
  - Shortening of 2 cm or greater has been associated with an increased risk of nonunion, persistent pain, and neurologic compromise, which have led some authors to recommend early surgical treatment.
  - Recalcitrant symptomatic cases and nonunions may necessitate ORIF (Figure 40–6).

Box 40–1 Classification of Clavicular Fractures

Group I (85%)—Middle third of clavicle
Group II (10%)—Lateral third of clavicle

- Type I—Between coracoclavicular and acromioclavicular ligaments. Minimal displacement
- Type II—(IIA) medial to both coracoclavicular ligaments, which remained attached (Figure 40–1) or (IIB) between the torn conoid and intact trapezoid ligaments (Figure 40–2)
- Type III—Intraarticular/acromioclavicular joint fractures (Figure 40–3)
- Type IV—Periosteal sleeve fracture with ligaments attached to the periosteum and proximal displacement (Figure 40–4)
- Type V—Comminuted fracture with ligaments attached to an inferior segment

Group III (5%)—Medial third of clavicle

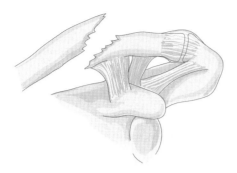

Figure 40–1:
Type IIA distal clavicular fracture. Conoid and trapezoid ligaments remain attached to distal segment while the proximal segment becomes displaced.

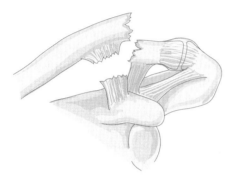

Figure 40–2:
Type IIB distal clavicular fracture. Conoid ligament is torn, allowing displacement of the proximal segment while the trapezoid ligament remains attached to the distal segment.

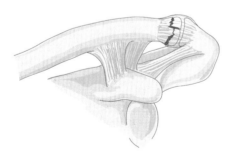

Figure 40–3:
Type III distal clavicular fracture involving the articular surface of the acromioclavicular joint.

- Segmental defects and shortening may require bone grafting (e.g., intercalary iliac crest grafting).
- Type I and minimally displaced types III to V lateral clavicular fractures usually do well with conservative management.

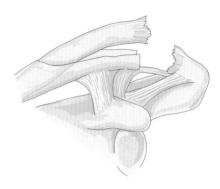

Figure 40–4:
Type IV distal clavicular fracture. Note that the coracoclavicular ligaments remained attached to either bone or periosteum as the proximal fractured fragment displaces through the superior periosteum.

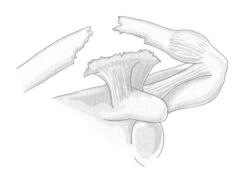

Figure 40–5:
Type V distal clavicle fracture. Comminuted fracture with acromioclavicular ligaments attached to inferior fracture segment.

- Significant displacement or AC stepoff may require surgical treatment.
- Type II lateral clavicular fractures are considered to be relatively unstable because of the unopposed pull by the sternocleidomastoid muscle on the medial fragment and the weight of the arm, and they have a higher rate of nonunion.
  - Classically treated surgically. However, recent studies have found conservative treatment to provide good results.
  - Fixation with a clavicular hook plate or intermedullary modified Hagie pins have resulted in good outcomes.
  - AC K-wires have been fraught with complications including nonunion and infection.

Scapula

- Comprises 3% to 5% of shoulder girdle injuries.
- Usually result from high-energy trauma including motor vehicle accidents and high falls.

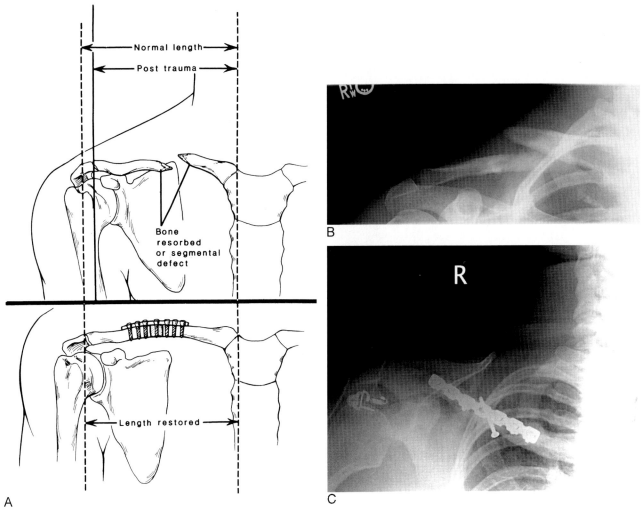

Figure 40–6:
Clavicle nonunion treated with open reduction and internal fixation (ORIF). **A,** Schematic of clavicular nonunion treated with open reduction, bone grafting, and internal fixation. **B,** Clavicle nonunion. **C,** Clavicle ORIF with iliac crest bonegraft (ICBG). (**A** from Craig EV: Fractures of the clavicle. In Rockwood CA Jr, Masten FA III, editors: *The shoulder*. Philadelphia, 1990, Saunders.)

As a result, associated injuries must be considered (Box 40–2).

- Frequently missed on initial examination because of the high rate (90%) of associated injuries and life-threatening status.
- Ninety percent of fractures are extraarticular, involving the neck, acromion, coracoid, body, or spine of the scapula.
- The bony Bankart lesion is the most common intraarticular fracture and is associated with shoulder instability, dislocations, and capsuloligamentous injury.
- High-energy intraarticular fractures usually result from extreme lateral forces that axially load the glenoid fossa.

- Radiographic visualization is occasionally difficult and may require CT evaluation, especially when intraarticular fractures are suspected (Figure 40–7).

Box 40–2	Injuries Associated with Scapular Fractures

Rib fractures (most common)
Pneumothorax
Pulmonary contusion
Head injury
Spinal cord injury
Brachial plexus injury

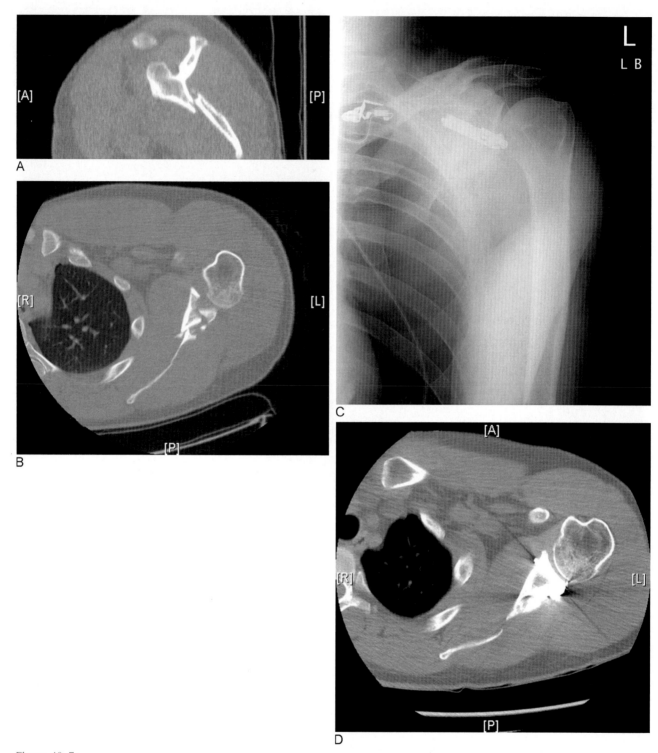

Figure 40–7:
Scapular body and intraarticular glenoid fracture. **A,** Displaced scapular body fracture on computed tomography (CT) scan.
B, Displaced, intraarticular glenoid fracture. **C,** Plain radiograph of glenoid fracture open reduction and internal fixation
(ORIF). **D,** CT scan of glenoid fracture ORIF.

- Arthroscopic visualization may be useful for subtle intraarticular glenoid fractures (Figure 40–8).
- Stryker notch view provides optimal visualization of the coracoid process.
- Most fractures are treated with immobilization (in sling and swathe) for a period of 6 weeks and early range of motion.
- ORIF (usually from a posterior approach) of a scapular neck fracture is indicated if there is greater than 1 cm of medial translation or greater than 40 degrees of angulation of the glenoid fossa (Box 40–3).
- Fractures of the coracoid process associated with nerve injury or complete AC injuries usually require surgical fixation.
- Surgical intervention of intraarticular fractures is indicated when there is involvement of one fourth of the anterior glenoid, one third of the posterior glenoid, or greater than 1 cm of displacement.
  - Fixation techniques use lag screws, 3.5-mm reconstruction plates, and bone grafting when necessary.

Proximal Humerus

- Makes up 4% to 5% of all fractures.
- The majority (85%) of fractures have only minimal displacement.
- Occurs most commonly in the older population affected with osteoporosis or in younger patients involved in high-energy trauma.
- The neck of the humerus has less density and mechanical strength than the rest of the shoulder bones and is at greatest risk for fracture.

- Nerve injury occurs in 30% of cases, and vascular damage to the axillary artery or its branches supplying the humeral head is less frequent.
  - Fractures of the neck risk damage to the ascending anterolateral branch of the anterior humeral circumflex, which supplies blood to the head of the humerus.
- The Neer classification is used to describe these fractures on the basis of displacement of 1 cm or 45-degree angulation of four parts as seen on plain films. The four parts include the (1) greater tuberosity, (2) lesser tuberosity, (3) humeral head, and (4) shaft (Figure 40–9).
- Examination often reveals significant swelling, discoloration, and tenderness about the proximal humerus and difficulty with active range of motion of the arm.
- The axillary, musculocutaneous, median, radial, and ulnar nerves and vascular integrity must also be evaluated.
- Shoulder trauma views are sufficient for diagnosis.
- Most nondisplaced or minimally displaced fractures can be managed conservatively with closed treatment, early passive motion at approximately 2 weeks, and advancement to active motion at 4 to 6 weeks.
- Fractures with significant displacement are usually considered for surgical treatment.
- Greater tuberosity fractures associated with anterior dislocations and lesser tuberosity fractures associated with posterior dislocation are usually minimally displaced after reduction and can be managed nonoperatively.
- Greater tuberosity fractures displaced greater than 5 to 10 mm may compromise function or have associated pathology of the rotator cuff muscles and are best treated with ORIF (usually through a deltoid-splitting approach) and rotator cuff repair if tears are present.
- Significant displacement of isolated lesser tuberosity fractures, which are rare, are treated by ORIF and rotator interval closure.
- Although infrequent, humeral neck fractures associated with glenohumeral dislocations should undergo ORIF prior to glenohumeral reduction to prevent further

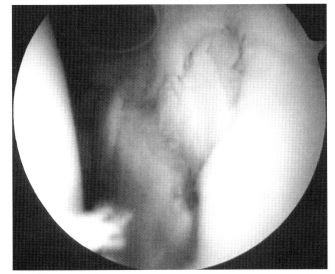

Figure 40–8:
Arthroscopic view of a displaced glenoid fracture that presented 1 month following injury.

Box 40–3	Indications for ORIF of Scapular Fractures

Scapular Neck

> 1 cm translation or
> 40 degrees of angulation of the glenoid fossa

Coracoid Process

Associated nerve injury or
Complete acromioclavicular injuries

Intraarticular Fractures

Involvement of one fourth of the anterior glenoid or
Involvement of one third of the posterior glenoid or
> 1 cm displacement

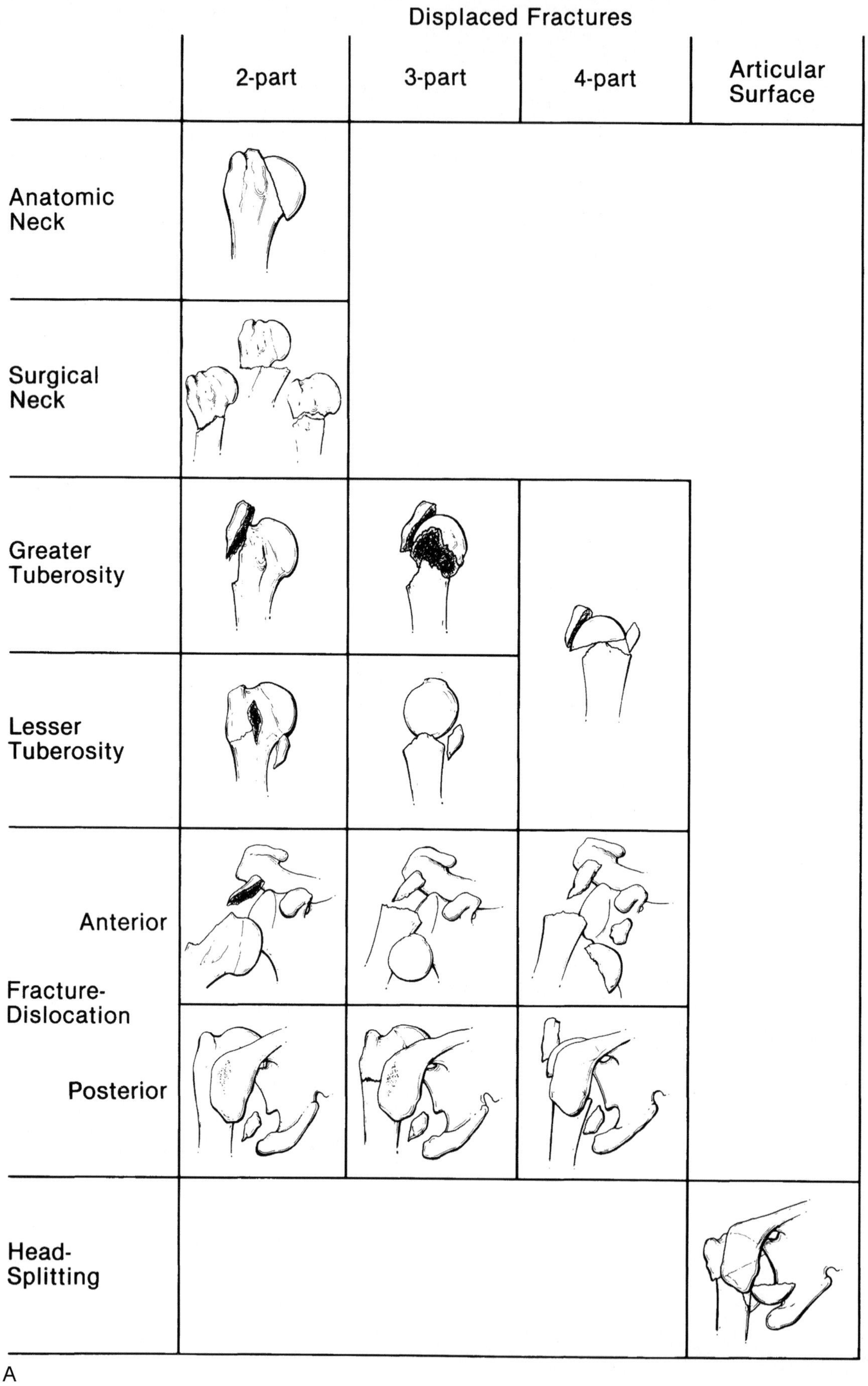

	Displaced Fractures			
	2-part	3-part	4-part	Articular Surface
Anatomic Neck	✎			
Surgical Neck	✎			
Greater Tuberosity	✎	✎		
Lesser Tuberosity	✎	✎	✎	
Fracture-Dislocation — Anterior	✎	✎	✎	
Fracture-Dislocation — Posterior	✎	✎	✎	
Head-Splitting				✎

A

Figure 40–9:

Proximal humerus fractures. **A,** Schematic of Neer's four-part classification of proximal humeral fractures.

(continued)

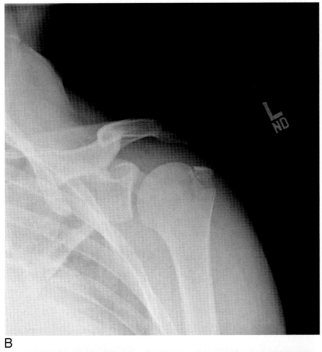

B

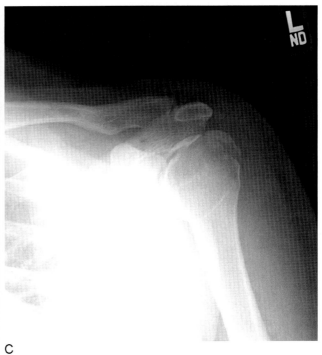

C

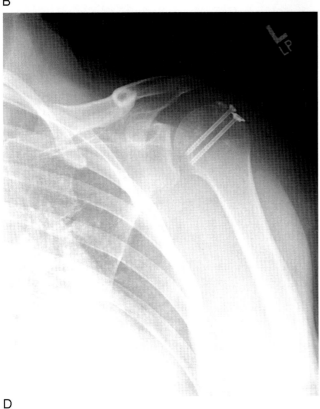

D

Figure 40–9, cont'd:
B and C, Plain radiographs of a greater tuberosity fracture. **D,** Radiograph of greater tuberosity fracture following open reduction and internal fixation. (**A** From Neer CS: *J Bone Joint Surg Am* 52:1077-1089, 1970.)

displacement and nerve injuries that may be seen with glenohumeral reduction attempts.
- Closed reduction of displaced two-part fractures can be attempted and supplemented with percutaneous pinning.
- ORIF of unstable two- and three-part fractures can involve intermedullary nails, tension banding, intraosseous sutures, or plate and screw fixation.

- Treatment of complex three- and four-part fractures is problematic and controversial. Generally, attempts at ORIF in younger patients and hemi or total arthroplasty in the elderly are advocated.
- Salvage arthroplasty can be a difficult but reasonable option when initial treatment fails.

Humeral Shaft

- Comprises 3% of all fractures.
- Approximately 18% of these fractures have an associated radial nerve injury resulting in either neurapraxia or axonotmesis.
- Tenderness, swelling, discoloration, and deformity at the site of injury are found during examination.
- Nerves distal to the fracture site include the median, radial, and ulnar nerves and must be tested during the examination.
- Patients with radial nerve injury often have difficulty or are unable to extend their wrist or fingers and have diminished sensation along the dorsum of the hand.

- Most of these fractures are successfully treated nonoperatively with a coaptation splint, hanging long arm cast, or functional braces.
- After 2 weeks in a coaptation splint, patients can then be fitted with a humeral fracture brace, which is worn until radiographic evidence of healing is noted, approximately at 6 to 8 weeks, and the patient continues with range-of-motion exercises of the shoulder, elbow, wrist, and hand.
- Malunion may occur and is allowable up to 3 cm of shortening, 20 degrees of anteroposterior angulation, or 30 degrees of varus or valgus angulation (Figure 40–10).

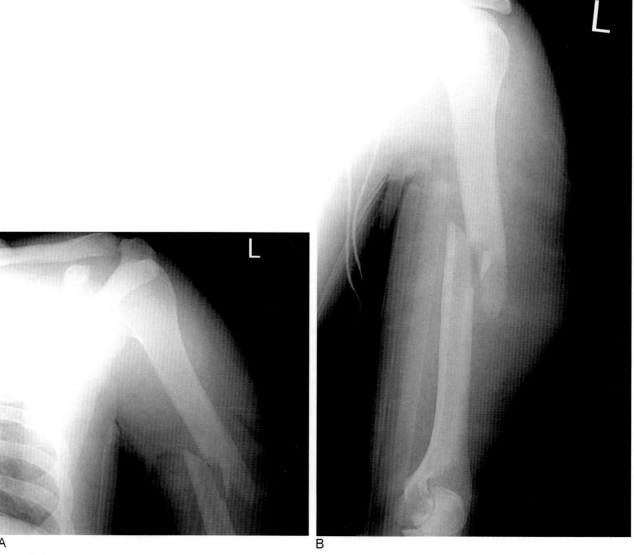

A

B

Figure 40–10:

A and B, Anteroposterior and lateral radiographs of a midshaft humerus fracture.

- Indications for surgical treatment include inability to maintain acceptable closed reduction, vascular or nerve injury, pathologic or segmental fractures, bilateral humeral fractures, polytrauma, and concomitant bone forearm fracture (Box 40–4).
- Intermedullary nails may be used within 3 cm proximal to the olecranon and up to 2 cm distal to the surgical neck (Figure 40–11).
- Open fixation is indicated in patients with small intermedullary canals, very proximal or distal fractures that cannot be corrected by intermedullary nailing, nonunions, and preexisting humeral deformity.
- Open fixation is usually performed using a 4.5-mm dynamic compression plate, ensuring five to six cortices proximal and distal to the fracture site (Figure 40–12).

Box 40–4	Indications for Surgical Management of Humeral Shaft Fractures

Inability to maintain acceptable closed reduction
Neurovascular injury
Pathologic fracture
Segmental fracture
Bilateral humeral fractures
Concomitant forearm fracture (floating elbow)
Polytrauma

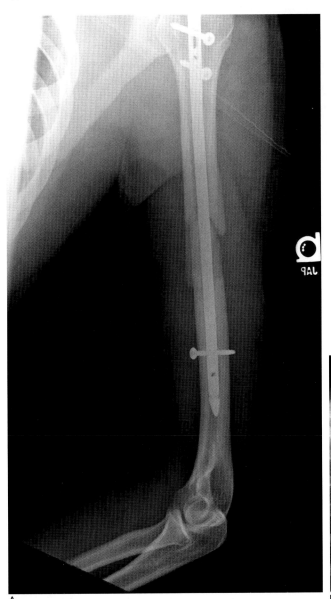

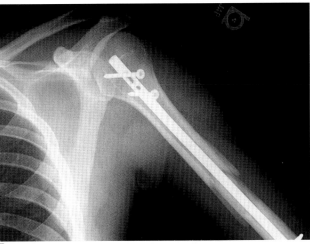

A   B

Figure 40–11:

A and B, Intramedullary nailing of a humerus fracture.

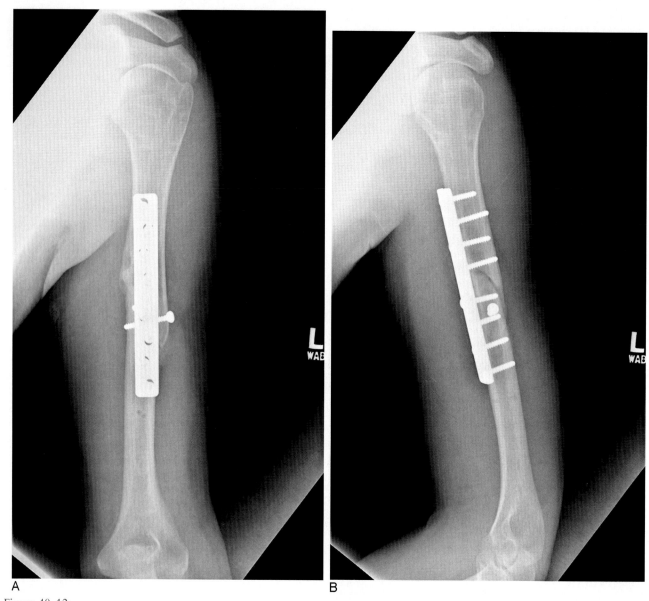

Figure 40–12:
A and **B,** Open reduction and internal fixation of humerus nonunion.

Rehabilitation

- Patients should be instructed to exercise the fingers, wrist, and elbow while in a splint to prevent stiffness.
- After the recommended period of immobilization, physical therapy is essential to regain motion and strength.

Complications

- Nonunion of all clavicular fractures approximates 1% to 4%, with 30% of nonunion reported in group II fractures.
- Malunion of clavicular fractures is common and can produce a cosmetic bony prominence, usually with no significant functional deficit.

- Neurovascular damage (after clavicular fractures) can be a delayed complication.
- Fractures and open surgical procedures that occur around the proximal area of the bicipital groove risk injury to the anterolateral branch of the anterior humeral circumflex, which is the main blood supply to the head of the humerus.
- Nonunion of humeral shaft fractures occurs in 7% of patients.
- Radial and other nerve injuries associated with fractures of the humerus should be closely observed. Full function normally returns within 6 months in 95% of cases.
- Flexion contractures of wrist and fingers can be avoided by placing the patient in a wrist splint and instructing him or her on appropriate stretching exercises.

References

Chapman JR, Henley MB, Agel J, Benca PJ: Randomized prospective study of humeral shaft fracture fixation: intramedullary nails versus plates. *J Orthop Trauma* 14:162-166, 2000.

Randomized prospective study comparing the use of locking antegrade intramedullary nails versus dynamic compression plates for the fixation of humeral shaft fractures in 84 patients. Outcomes demonstrated healed fractures at 16 weeks in 87% of the nail group and 93% of the plate group, with no statistical difference between the two groups. The authors noted that there was a significant association of shoulder pain and reduced shoulder range of motion in the group treated with intermedullary nails and reduced elbow range of motion in the patients managed with plate fixation. The authors comment that although most humeral shaft fractures can be managed nonoperatively, surgical correction, when indicated, can be performed with either of the previous techniques with reliable results.

Chen CY, Chao EK, Tu YK, et al: Closed management of percutaneous fixation of unstable proximal humerus fractures. *J Trauma* 45:1039-1045, 1998.

Prospective study evaluating the outcomes of closed reduction and percutaneous fixation (with K-pins and cannulated screws) in 19 patients with displaced two-part (n = 13) and three-part (n = 6) proximal humeral fractures. Technique is well described. Authors report 84% good to excellent results. Although considered technically demanding, this technique precludes extensive soft tissue dissection, minimizes surgical complications, and allows early rehabilitation.

Goss TP: The scapula: coracoid, acromial, and avulsion fractures. *Am J Orthop* 25:106-115, 1996.

Brief review of coracoid, acromial, and scapular avulsion fractures. Although most of these fractures can be successfully managed nonoperatively, the authors describe when surgical consideration is warranted.

Green A, Izzi J: Isolated fractures of the greater tuberosity of the proximal humerus. *J Shoulder Elbow Surg* 12:641-649, 2003.

Review article describing the anatomy, classification, presentation, evaluation, diagnosis, and management of isolated greater tuberosity fractures. The authors comment on the lack of well-defined diagnostic criteria, surgical indications, and substantial outcome studies. The authors report that displacement greater than 5 mm warrants consideration for surgical management.

Koch PP, Gross DFL, Gerber C: The results of functional (Sarmiento) bracing of humeral shaft fractures. *J Shoulder Elbow Surg* 11:143-150, 2002.

Authors report on outcomes of 67 humeral shaft fractures treated conservatively using functional bracing. Clinical healing was observed in 87% of cases, 95% of which had overall good to excellent results. The authors stress that nonoperative management remains the gold standard in light of new developing, less invasive surgical techniques.

Naranja RJ, Iannotti JP: Displaced three- and four-part proximal humerus fractures: evaluation and management. *J Am Acad Orthop Surg* 8:373-382, 2000.

Review article of the evaluation and management of three- and four-part proximal humerus fractures. A treatment algorithm is provided and described. Authors advise that valgus-impacted four-part fractures and displaced fractures in young patients with good bone stock should undergo ORIF. Older patients with poor bone stock appear to have better outcomes with early hemiarthroplasty. Surgical techniques are also reviewed.

Park MC, Murthi AM, Roth NS, et al: Two-part and three-part fractures of the proximal humerus treated with suture fixation. *J Orthop Trauma* 17:319-325, 2003.

Retrospective study evaluating the outcomes of two-part (n = 22) and three-part (n = 6) proximal humeral fractures in 27 patients treated with heavy nonabsorbable sutures. The authors stress the importance of incorporating the rotator cuff in the repair to provide further stability. The study demonstrated 78% excellent, 11% satisfactory, and 11% unsatisfactory results. The authors note these results are comparable with the more aggressive repairs implementing hardware while avoiding their inherent risks.

Der Tavitian J, Davison JNS, Dias JJ: Clavicular fracture non-union surgical outcome and complications. *Injury* 33:135-143, 2002.

Authors evaluate the outcomes and complications in patients who underwent surgical correction of clavicular fracture nonunions. Surgery was performed on 20 patients, 11 with midshaft, 8 with lateral third, and 1 with medial third fracture nonunions. Results demonstrated improved pain in 95% of patients, return of normal sleep in 94%, and resolution of deformity and neurologic symptoms in all patients. Literature review (from 24 publications comprising 301 patients) revealed 6% metal work, 15% soft tissue, and 2% scar complications, as well as an 8% rate of union failure. Authors note that midshaft fracture nonunions respond well to internal fixation with bone grafting, whereas fixation of lateral fracture nonunions are less predictable and difficult to perform.

Wentz S, Eberhardt C, Leonhard T: Reconstruction plate fixation with bone graft for mid-shaft clavicular non-union in semiprofessional athletes. *J Orthop Sci* 4:269-272, 1999.

Authors evaluate the outcomes of 19 atrophic and 3 hypertrophic midclavicular fracture nonunions surgically corrected with reconstruction plate fixation and bone grafting. Results demonstrated postoperative radiographic consolidation in all patients at an average of 14 weeks. Furthermore, pain, power, function, and range of motion all improved.

CHAPTER 41

Acromioclavicular, Sternoclavicular, and Clavicle Injuries

Introduction

- Both the acromioclavicular (AC) and the sternoclavicular joints are gliding joints with associated ligament support.
- The AC ligaments are contained within the AC joint capsule (superior component most significant).
- The coracoclavicular ligaments include the conoid and trapezoid ligaments.
- The AC ligaments are responsible for restricting anterior-posterior translation, and the coracoclavicular ligaments are responsible for restricting superior-inferior translation (Figure 41–1).

Acromioclavicular "Separations"

- AC joint injury is commonly referred to as a "shoulder separation" as compared with a "shoulder dislocation" (glenohumeral joint).
- Mechanism—direct trauma to anterosuperior aspect of acromion (driving shoulder into ground or another player).

Examination

- Clinical stepoff compared with contralateral side (comparison corrects for anatomic variation of joint except with bilateral injuries).
- Tenderness, excoriation, and ecchymosis at AC joint.
- Motion with manipulation of AC joint/shoulder.
- Restricted forward elevation and abduction secondary to pain.

Imaging

- Plain radiographs reveal degree of injury.
- Zanca view improves visualization of AC joint (30 degrees cephalad with less penetration).
- Views of bilateral joints for comparison (AC joint and coracoclavicular distance).
- Axillary lateral view for displacement in axial plane.

Classification

- Types I to VI (Figure 41–2).

- Determined by the ligaments disrupted and by the amount and direction of displacement of the distal clavicle (Box 41–1).
- Types I and II—cause injury to the AC joint but do not affect the coracoclavicular ligaments.
- Type III—injury to the coracoclavicular ligaments, but there is less than a 100% displacement comparison with the other side.
  - Coracoclavicular distances are measured and compared with the opposite side (Figure 41–3).
  - Hanging weights have been shown to not be necessary and only uncomfortable for the patient.
- Type IV—posterior displacement of the clavicle, sometimes into or through the trapezius.
  - Axillary views are necessary to make this diagnosis.
- Type V—superior displacement of the clavicle greater than 100% of the opposite side with buttonholing of the distal clavicle through the deltotrapezial fascia.
- Type VI—subcoracoid displacement of the distal clavicle.
  - Extremely rare.

Treatment

- Types I and II.
  - Nonoperative—taping, channeling of pads.
- Although controversial, treatment of types I to III is typically nonoperative.
  - Ice, rest, and nonsteroidal antiinflammatory drugs are typically the only treatment necessary.
  - A traditional sling may relieve pain in the initial period.
  - Pain usually resolves in as little as 2 weeks with types I and II but may last longer in type III AC separations.
  - Return to play may occur when the athlete has regained full and pain-free motion.
- Operative treatment is reserved for symptomatic chronic type III separations and type IV to VI separations.
- Primary repair is indicated early (Figure 41–4).
- Late reconstructions typically involve a Weaver-Dunn procedure, which is a transfer of the coracoacromial ligament into the end of the clavicle after a distal clavicle resection (Figure 41–5).

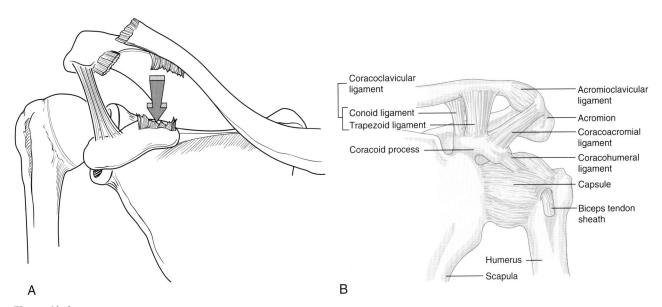

Figure 41–1:
A, The anatomy of the disrupted acromioclavicular (AC) joint. **B,** Anatomy of the AC ligamentous system. (**A** from Mazzocca AD, Sellards R, Garretson R, Romeo AA: Injuries to the acromioclavicular joint in adults and children. In Delee JC, Drez D Jr, Miller MD, editors: *Delee and Drez's Orthopaedic sports medicine: principles and practice,* 2nd ed. Philadelphia, 2003, WB Saunders; **B** redrawn from Klassen JF, Morrey BF, An K-N: *Oper Tech Sports Med* 5:62, 1997.)

Distal Clavicle Osteolysis

- This involves microtrauma to the distal clavicle.
- This occurs commonly in weightlifters.
- Radiographs may demonstrate cysts and osteopenia to the distal clavicle (Figure 41–6).

- Treatment involves restricting or modifying activities and arthroscopic or open distal clavicle resection.
  - Both techniques have equal efficacy in clinical studies.

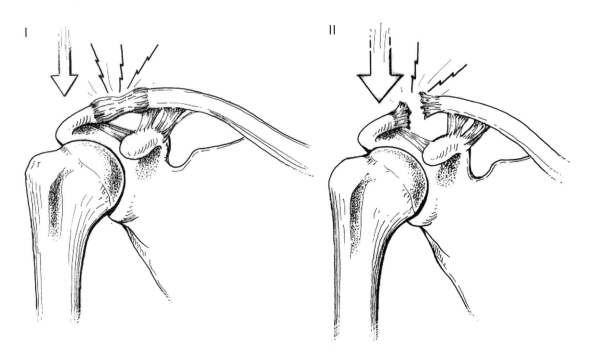

Figure 41–2:
Classification for acromioclavicular joint injuries types I to II.

(continued)

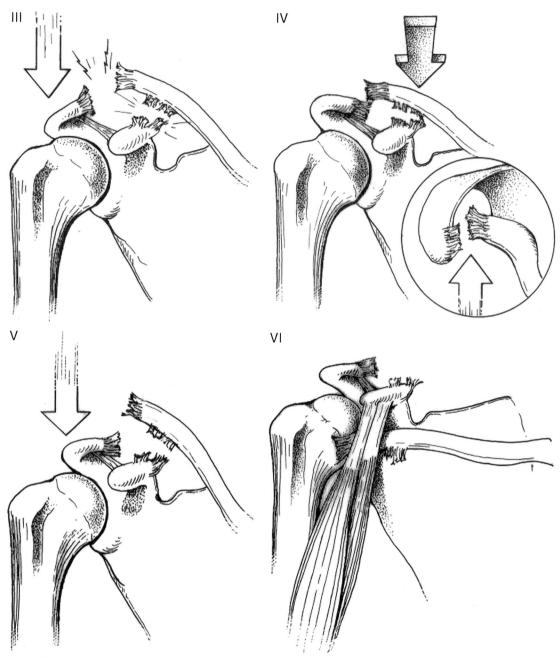

Figure 41–2, cont'd:

Classification for acromioclavicular joint injuries types III to VI. (From Ponce BA, Millett PJ, Warner JJP: *Oper Tech Sports Med* **12:36-37, 2004.)**

Acromioclavicular Arthritis

- This is commonly associated with impingement syndrome and rotator cuff disease.
- Physical examination is notable for painful cross-chest adduction and localized tenderness.
- Radiographs may show narrowing of the joint and osteophytes (Figure 41–7).
- Conservative treatment is typically considered initially.

Box 41–1	Classification of Acromioclavicular (AC) Separations

Type I Injury to the AC joint with intact ligaments
Type II Clavicle subluxed but not markedly elevated
Type III Clavicle elevated up to 100% of normal side
Type IV Clavicle elevated and posteriorly displaced
Type V Clavicle markedly elevated >100% of normal side
Type VI Clavicle completely dislocated and inferiorly displaced

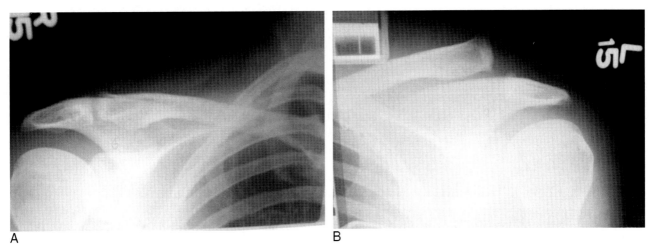

Figure 41–3:
Comparison radiographs demonstrate the amount of clavicle elevation. **A,** Normal right shoulder. **B,** Acromioclavicular separation of left shoulder.

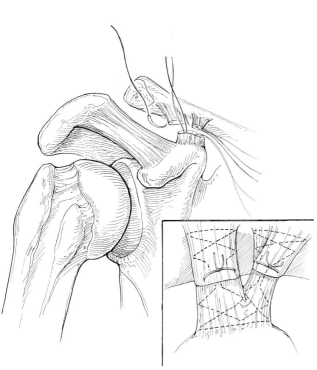

Figure 41–4:
Primary repair of acromioclavicular separation. (From Miller MD, Howard RF, Plancher KD: *Surgical atlas of sports medicine.* Philadelphia, 2003, WB Saunders.)

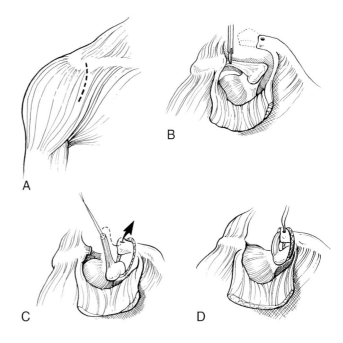

Figure 41–5:
Weaver-Dunn procedure. **A,** Skin incision. **B,** Distal clavicle resection. **C,** Mobilization of coracoacromial ligament and fixation of clavicle to the coracoid. **D,** Transfer of coracoacromial ligament to the clavicle. (From Miller MD, Cooper DE, Warner JJP: *Review of sports medicine and arthroscopy,* 2nd ed. Philadelphia, 2002, Saunders.)

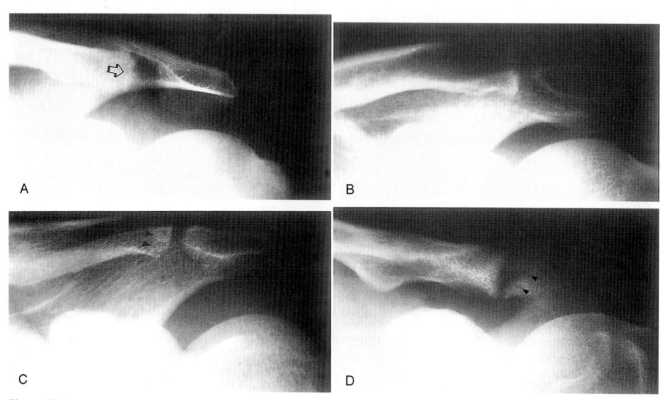

Figure 41–6:

The radiographic appearance of distal clavicle osteolysis. **A,** Widened acromioclavicular (AC) joint and loss of bone at distal clavicle. **B,** Bone loss and thinning of distal clavicle. **C,** Cystic changes of distal clavicle. **D,** Cystic changes and AC joint widening. (From Pitchford KR, Bernard RC: *Oper Tech Sports Med* 5:74, 1997.)

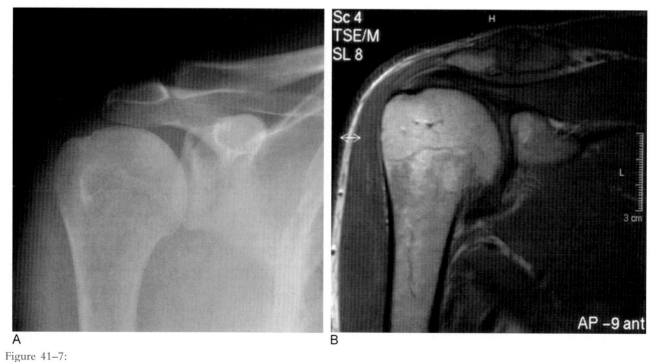

Figure 41–7:

The radiographic appearance of acromioclavicular joint arthritis. **A,** Plain radiography. **B,** MRI appearance. (From Nuber GW, Flannigan DC: Acromioclavicular joint pathology. In Miller MD, Cole BJ, editors: *Textbook of arthroscopy.* Philadelphia, 2004, Saunders.)

- AC injection with steroid/topical anesthetic may be helpful.
- Activity modification is generally recommended.
- Surgical options may be explored after conservative measures fail.
  - Distal clavicle excision is often done in conjunction with acromioplasty or rotator cuff surgery, or both.

Sternoclavicular Injuries

- These are typically more unusual than AC injuries and more difficult to treat.
- Although some radiographic views have been described to define the direction of displacement (serendipity view) (Figure 41–8), a computed tomography scan is most helpful (Figure 41–9).
- Acute anterior instability should be reduced if possible.

- Chronic anterior instability is typically treated nonoperatively.
- Posterior instability may benefit from closed reduction, particularly if it causes dysesthesia or vascular problems associated with great vessel compromise or occlusion.
- Physeal injuries can occur up to the 3rd decade in both AC and sternoclavicular injuries.
- Hardware should be avoided in both locations.

Clavicle Fractures

- Historically all clavicle fractures have been treated nonoperatively.
- Surgical indications for intramedullary fixation are evolving, particularly in significantly displaced fractures and chronic nonunions (Figure 41–10).

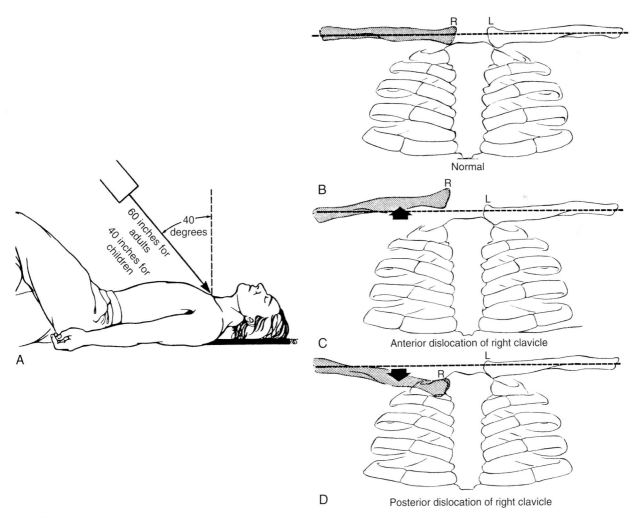

Figure 41–8:
Serendipity view. **A,** Patient positioning for serendipity view. **B,** Normal bony alignment of the sternoclavicular joint. **C,** Appearance of an anterior dislocation of the clavicle. **D,** Appearance of a posterior dislocation of the clavicle. (From Coupe KJ, Criswell AR, Tucker JJ: Fractures and dislocations of the shoulder girdle. In Brinker MR, editor: *Review of orthopaedic trauma.* Philadelphia, 2001, Saunders.)

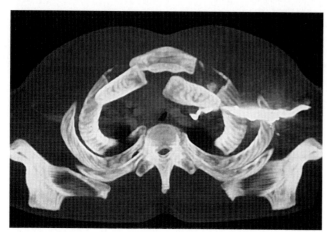

Figure 41–9:
Computed tomography of the sternoclavicular joint. (From Brinker MR, Miller MD: *Fundamentals of orthopaedics.* Philadelphia, 1999, Saunders.)

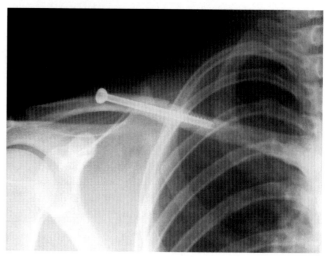

Figure 41–11:
Intermedullary fixation of a clavicle fracture.

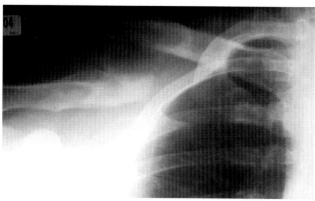

Figure 41–10:
Nonunion of the clavicle.

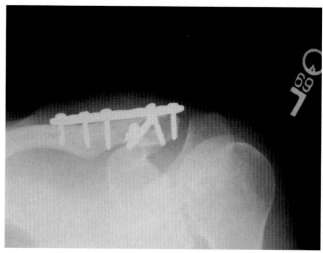

Figure 41–12:
Traditional plate and screw fixation of a clavicle fracture.

- Medial clavicle fractures with potential vascular compromise and distal clavicle fractures with significant displacement (more than 10 to 15 mm) should be considered for operative fixation.
- Treatment involves intramedullary devices or traditional plates and screws (Figures 41–11 and 41–12).

References

Bicos J, Nicholson GP: Treatment and results of sternoclavicular joint injuries. *Clin Sports Med* 22:359-370, 2003.
This is a review article of the most common current treatment strategies for sternoclavicular joint injury including diagnosis, initial management, conservative treatment options, and surgical treatment indications and options. Discussion also includes the most common complications of these treatment options and expected clinical results.

Chronopoulos E, Kim TK, Park HB, et al: Diagnostic value of physical tests for isolated chronic acromioclavicular lesions. *Am J Sports Med* 32:655-661, 2004.
This article serves as a review of some common physical examination points used in diagnosing AC pathology. The authors conclude that the cross-body adduction test is the most sensitive test for AC joint disease but does not have a high specificity associated with it.

Deshmukh AV, Wilson DR, Zilberfarb JL, Perlmutter GS: Stability of acromioclavicular joint reconstruction: biomechanical testing of various surgical techniques in a cadaveric model. *Am J Sports Med* 32:1492-1498, 2004.
This is a biomechanical study of the traditional Weaver-Dunn procedure and augmented Weaver-Dunn procedures. The authors are unable to advocate any one particular augmentation but do conclude that all augmentation procedures are biomechanically stronger forms of AC joint reconstruction.

Ernberg LA, Potter HG: Radiographic evaluation of the acromioclavicular and sternoclavicular joints. *Clin Sports Med* 22:255-275, 2003.
This is a review article discussing the most appropriate radiographic imaging studies for diagnosing and treating AC and sternoclavicular

joint injuries. *The authors provide indications for using plain radiograph, computerized tomography, and magnetic resonance imaging based on the suspected condition.*

Lemos MJ: The evaluation and treatment of the injured acromioclavicular joint in athletes. *Am J Sports Med* 26:137-144, 1998.
A review article discussing the history of management of AC separations, especially those that occur in athletes. The currently accepted classification system and the most appropriate treatment options for each type are discussed.

Nordqvist A, Petersson C, Redlund-Johnell I: The natural course of lateral clavicle fracture. (11-21) year follow-up of 110 cases. *Acta Orthop Scand* 64:87-91, 1993.
These authors followed a large group of patients with a lateral clavicle fracture and determined that more than 85% of the patients were asymptomatic at follow-up. The conclusion drawn by these authors is that lateral clavicle fractures heal well with only conservative management.

Renfree KJ, Wright TW: Anatomy and biomechanics of the acromioclavicular and sternoclavicular joints. *Clin Sports Med* 22:219-237, 2003.

This is a review article discussing the basic anatomy and biomechanics of the AC and sternoclavicular joints. The authors emphasize the importance in understanding the basic structure and function of the joint to properly treat injury.

Rudzki JR, Matava MJ, Paletta GA Jr: Complications of treatment of acromioclavicular and sternoclavicular joint injuries. *Clin Sports Med* 22:387-405, 2003.
This is a review article that discusses the most common complications of AC and sternoclavicular joint injury. Complications may come from the injury itself, conservative treatment, or surgical treatment. The authors provide information for rapid identification and management of these complications.

Salter EG, Nasca RJ, Shelley BS: Anatomical observations on the acromioclavicular joint and supporting ligaments. *Am J Sports Med* 15:199-206, 1987.
This is a cadaveric study that reviews the basics of AC joint anatomy including the intraarticular disc, the normal bony morphology, and the most common areas and types of ligament insertion at this joint. Understanding the anatomy has important implications in the management of AC joint disease.

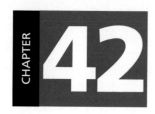

CHAPTER 42

Elbow Anatomy and Biomechanics

Introduction

- The elbow joint is a hinge-type (ginglymus) synovial joint formed by the humerus, radius, and ulna with three articulations and ligamentous support.
- It serves as a connection between the shoulder and hand, assisting placement of the hand in space.
- It allows the transfer of energy along the upper extremity kinetic chain, especially during overhead and throwing activities.
- The ulnohumeral joint is uniaxial in nature, with flexion and extension being its primary motion.
- The proximal radioulnar joint allows for forearm rotation.

Osteology

Distal Humerus

- The distal humeral shaft fans out to become the medial and lateral columns, which support the capitellum and trochlear "spool" in between (Figure 42–1). The columns, or condyles, are flanked by their respective epicondyles and are separated from each other by the coronoid fossa anteriorly and the olecranon fossa posteriorly.
- The very prominent medial epicondyle serves as an attachment site for the flexor-pronator muscles of the forearm and ulnar collateral ligament (Table 42–1).
- The lateral epicondyle is the attachment site for the extensor-supinator muscles of the forearm and the lateral collateral ligament complex (Table 42–2).

Ulna

- The larger proximal end of the ulna appears much like a pipe wrench with its jaws formed by the olecranon and coronoid process and its mouth by the trochlear notch (Figure 42–2).
- The proximal end clasps the distal humerus at the trochlea to form the ulnohumeral articulation, allowing movement in the flexion-extension plane.

- The lateral aspect of the coronoid process forms the greater sigmoid notch, which accepts part of the radial head to form the pivot-type radioulnar joint, allowing rotation of the distal radius about the distal ulna.
- Just distal to the radial notch is the supinator crest, which is the insertion site of the lateral ulnar collateral ligament proximally and the origin of the supinator muscle distally.

Radius

- The proximal disc-shaped head articulates with the ulna at the greater sigmoid notch of the ulna and its concave proximal surface receives the rounded capitellum to form the radiocapitellar articulation (Figure 42–2).
- The radius rotates about the ulna during pronation and supination and migrates approximately 1 to 2 mm proximally with pronation.
- A strong U-shaped annular ligament, attached to the anterior and posterior borders of the greater sigmoid notch, holds the head of the radius in position.

The Elbow Joint

- A hinge joint that allows extension between 0 and 5 degrees and flexion to 135 degrees or more (Figure 42–3).
- Flexion is limited by the anterior surfaces of the arm and forearm, tension of the posterior arm muscles, and the radial and ulnar collateral ligaments.
- Extension is mechanically blocked by the olecranon within its fossa and further limited by tension of the anterior arm muscles, elbow joint capsule, and the collateral ligaments.
- The elbow has approximately 3 to 5 degrees of varus, valgus, and rotational laxity throughout its range of motion.
- Pronation and supination occurring about the ulna and radius normally range from neutral to 90 degrees (Figure 42–3).
- Normal carrying angle is approximately 5 degrees in males and 10 degrees to 15 degrees in females (Figure 42–4).

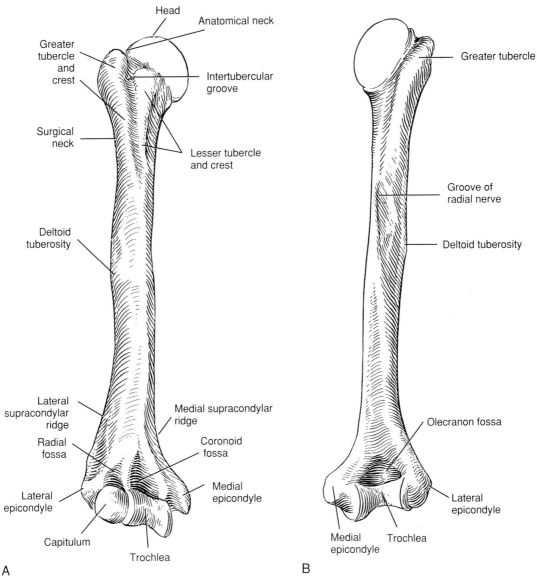

Figure 42–1:
Anterior (A) and posterior **(B)** views of the distal humerus. (From Jenkins DB, Hollinshead WH: *Hollinshead's functional anatomy of the limbs and back,* 8th ed. Philadelphia, 2002, Saunders.)

- The carrying angle is greatest when the elbow is extended and the forearm is supinated.
  - This allows the free movement of the arm without striking the hips during ambulation, especially when carrying heavy loads.
  - This angle is reduced with the forearm in pronation and flexion.
- Static stability of the joint is imposed by its bony architecture (most stable in extension), capsule, and strong surrounding ulnar and radial collateral ligaments (especially in flexion) (Figure 42–5, Table 42–3).
  - The bony articulations help resist valgus and varus stresses across the joint and are most stable with the elbow in extension.

- A relatively thin and weak fibrous capsule completely envelopes the joint and is well supported at its sides by the collateral ligaments.
  - It has a maximal volume of 15 to 30 ml at 80 degrees of flexion.
  - If hemarthrosis is present, the arm is held in flexion to reduce capsular distention and pain.
- The triangular-shaped ulnar collateral ligament with its apex attached to the base of the medial epicondyle is composed of a strong anterior band that attaches to the coronoid at the sublime tubercle and a weaker posterior band that connects to the medial edge of the olecranon. The primary stabilizer against valgus stress is the anterior band of the ulnar collateral ligament.

Table 42–1: Muscles of the Flexor Forearm

MUSCLE	ORIGIN	INSERTION	ACTION	INNERVATION
Superficial Muscles				
Flexor carpi radialis	Medial epicondyle of humerus (common flexor tendon)	Base of second metacarpal and possibly third metacarpal	Flexion and abduction (radial deviation) of hand	Median nerve
Flexor carpi ulnaris	Medial epicondyle of humerus (common flexor tendon); proximal two thirds of posterior surface of ulna	Pisiform bone	Flexion and adduction (ulnar deviation) of hand	Ulnar nerve
Palmaris longus	Medial epicondyle of humerus (common flexor tendon)	Palmar aponeurosis	Flexion of hand	Median nerve
Pronator teres	Medial epicondyle of humerus; coronoid process of ulna	Lateral surface of shaft of radius	Pronation of forearm (and hand)	Median nerve
Intermediate Muscle				
Flexor digitorum superficialis	Medial epicondyle of humerus (common flexor tendon); medial aspect of coronoid process of ulna; proximal half of radius distal to radial tuberosity	Middle phalanx of each of four fingers (medial four digits)	Flexion of middle phalanx of each of four fingers (medial four digits)	Median nerve
Deep Muscles				
Flexor digitorum profundus	Anterior and medial surfaces of proximal two thirds of ulna	Distal phalanx of each of four fingers (medial four digits)	Flexion of distal phalanx of each of four fingers (medial four digits)	Median and ulnar nerves
Flexor pollicis longus	Anterior surface of middle half of radius	Distal phalanx of thumb	Flexion of distal phalanx of thumb	Median nerve
Pronator quadratus	Distal fourth of ulna	Distal part of radius	Pronation of forearm (and hand)	Median nerve

From Jenkins DB, Hollinshead WH: *Hollinshead's functional anatomy of the limbs and back*, 8th ed. Philadelphia, 2002, Saunders.

- The lateral ulnar collateral complex (radial collateral ligament) is also triangular in shape and has a strong band that originates from the base of the lateral epicondyle, blends with the annular ligament of the radius, and inserts with the annular ligament at the posterior aspect of the greater sigmoid notch. The ulnar portion of this broad ligament also originates at the base of the lateral epicondyle and runs distally, posteriorly, and medially to insert on the ulna at the supinator crest (crista supinatorum). This portion is known as the lateral ulnar collateral ligament and is believed to be the primary constraint against posterolateral rotatory instability.
- Dynamic stability is provided by the various muscles that cross the joint.
- The coronoid and head of the radius lock into their respective fossae with full flexion of the joint and provide constraints to posterior translation of both forearm bones.
- There is less stability of the elbow joint in children because of the late fusion of the epiphyses around the joint. The proximal part of the olecranon fuses with the body of the ulna at 16 to 19 years of age, and the head of the radius fuses at 15 to 18 years of age.
- With overhead motion, the elbow experiences tensile forces along its medial aspect, compressive forces along its lateral aspect, and valgus extension forces along its posterior aspect (Figure 42–6).
- In overhead sports, valgus torque peaks during the late cocking and acceleration phases. The deceleration phase locks the olecranon within its fossa and can produce articular shear injuries.
- Pushups can produce compressive forces equal to 50% of a person's body weight across the joint and weightlifting may transmit forces up to three times body weight, reaching up to 3000 N of force across the radiohumeral and ulnohumeral joints.
- The radiocapitellar and ulnohumeral joints transmit 60% and 40% of axial loads, respectively, with the elbow in full extension.
- The small muscles about the elbow are unable to generate the proper amount of force required in sport activities depending on upper extremity limb strength and thus rely on the rest of the kinetic chain from the

Table 42–2:   Muscles of the Extensor Forearm

MUSCLE	ORIGIN	INSERTION	* ACTION	INNERVATION
Superficial Muscles				
Brachioradialis	Lateral supracondylar ridge of humerus; lateral intermuscular septum of arm	Lateral side of distal end of radius	Flexion of forearm	Radial nerve
Extensor carpi radialis brevis	Lateral epicondyle of humerus (common extensor tendon)	Base of third metacarpal	Extension of hand	Radial nerve
Extensor carpi radialis longus	Lateral supracondylar ridge and lateral epicondyle of humerus (common extensor tendon)	Base of second meta-carpal	Extension and abduction (radial deviation) of hand	Radial nerve
Extensor carpi ulnaris	Lateral epicondyle of humerus (common extensor tendon); proximal part of ulna	Base of fifth metacarpal	Extension and adduction (ulnar deviation) of hand	Radial nerve
Extensor digiti minimi	Lateral epicondyle of humerus (common extensor tendon)	Middle and distal phalanges of little finger	Extension and abduction of little finger	Radial nerve
Extensor digitorum	Lateral epicondyle of humerus; intermuscular septum; antebrachial fascia	Middle and distal phalanges of each of four fingers (medial four digits)	Extension of each of four fingers (medial four digits)	Radial nerve
Deep Muscles				
Abductor pollicis longus	Posterior surface of ulna and radius	Base of first metacarpal	Abduction and extension of thumb	Radial nerve
Extensor indicis	Posterior surface of ulna	Tendon of extensor digitorum; extensor expansion	Extension of index finger	Radial nerve
Extensor pollicis brevis	Posterior surface of radius	Proximal phalanx of thumb	Extension of proximal phalanx of thumb	Radial nerve
Extensor pollicis longus	Posterior surface of middle third of ulna	Distal phalanx of thumb	Extension of distal phalanx of thumb	Radial nerve
Supinator	Posterolateral surface of ulna below radial notch; lateral epicondyle; radial collateral and annular ligaments	Proximal shaft of radius	Supination of forearm (and hand)	Radial nerve

From Jenkins DB, Hollinshead WH: *Hollinshead's functional anatomy of the limbs and back*, 8th ed. Philadelphia, 2002, Saunders.

hips and trunks through the shoulder, elbow, hand, and wrist for optimal power.

Cubital Fossa

- A triangularly shaped soft tissue region anterior to the elbow joint with its base formed superiorly by an imaginary line connecting both humeral epicondyles and its lateral and medial sides outlined by the brachioradialis and pronator teres muscles, respectively.
- Its floor is composed of the brachialis and supinator muscles.
- Its roof is made up of deep fascia including the bicipital aponeurosis (lacertus fibrosis) and the overlying superficial fascia and skin.
- This fossa contains the biceps tendon, the brachial artery as it branches into its radial and ulnar arteries, the brachial veins, and portions of the median and radial nerves (Figure 42–7).

Muscles

- The brachialis is the main elbow flexor, and the triceps muscle is the main extensor.
- The biceps brachii is also a strong flexor of the elbow. In the flexed position, the biceps provides the majority of supination strength to the forearm.
- The triceps inserts onto the olecranon but also has a wide aponeurotic insertion via the anconeus.
- Medial triceps hypertrophy, most often seen in throwers and weightlifters, may cause ulnar nerve subluxation or neuritis. This can also lead to a "snapping" of the medial head of the triceps.
- The flexor-pronator group of muscles dynamically stabilizes the elbow against valgus stress, augmenting the restraint imparted by the ulnar collateral ligament.
- The extensor-supinator group provides dynamic stability against varus stress, enhancing the restraint afforded by the lateral ulnar collateral ligament complex.

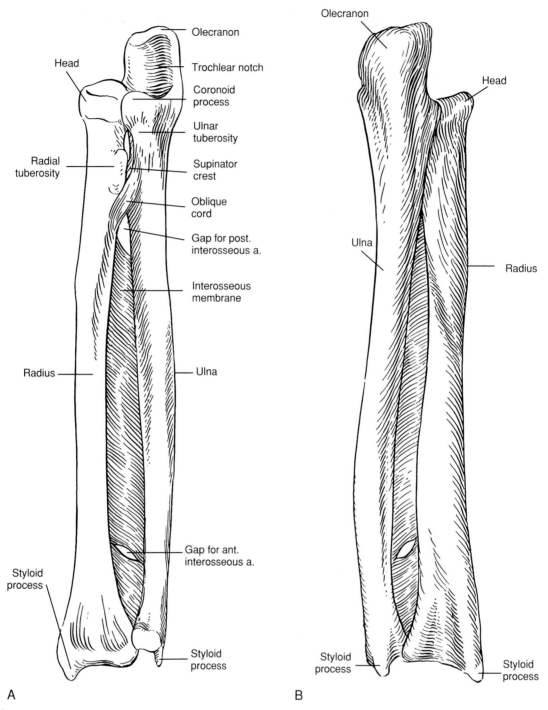

Figure 42–2:
Anterior (A) and posterior (B) views of the ulna and radius. (From Jenkins DB, Hollinshead WH: *Hollinshead's functional anatomy of the limbs and back,* 8th ed. Philadelphia, 2002, Saunders.)

Bursae

- The olecranon has a subcutaneous bursa, which resides superficially under the skin overlying the olecranon, and a subtendinous bursa, which lies between the triceps tendon and olecranon. (The subcutaneous bursa is more typically affected,

usually from falls, abrasions, or repetitive compression imposed on the posterior elbow against an unyielding surface.)
- The radioulnar bursa is located between the extensor digitorum, radiohumeral joint, and supinator muscle and can be irritated with repetitive wrist extension and is associated with lateral epicondylitis.

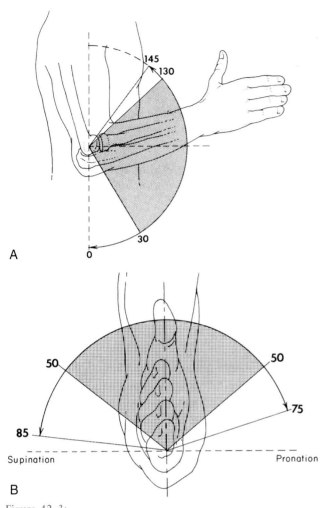

A

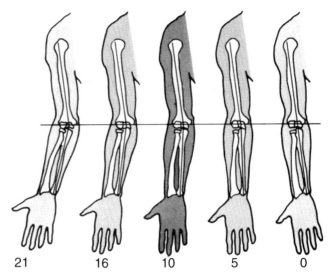

Figure 42–4:
Carrying angle. (From Lanz T, Wachsmuth W: *Praktische Anatomie*. ARM. Berlin, 1959, Springer.)

B

Figure 42–3:
A, Normal flexion and extension of the elbow. **B,** Normal pronation and supination. (From the Mayo Foundation. From Regan WD, Morrey BF: The physical examination of the elbow. In Morrey BF, editor: *The elbow and its disorders,* 2nd ed. Philadelphia, 1993, Saunders.)

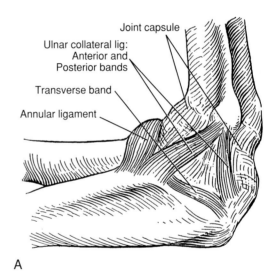

A

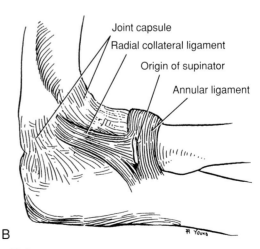

B

Figure 42–5:
Medial and lateral views of the ligaments about the elbow. **A,** Medial. **B,** Lateral. (From Jenkins DB, Hollinshead WH: *Hollinshead's functional anatomy of the limbs and back,* 8th ed. Philadelphia, 2002, Saunders.)

- The bicipitoradial bursa is interposed between the biceps tendon and anterior portion of the radial tuberosity.

Vessels

- The elbow joint receives its blood supply from articular arteries derived from the anastomosis around the elbow formed by branches of the brachial artery and recurrent branches of the ulnar and radial arteries (Figure 42–8).
- The brachial artery accompanies the median nerve as it passes the cubital fossa under the bicipital aponeurosis, medial to the biceps tendon, and then bifurcates to give off the radial and ulnar arteries.
- The profunda brachii artery is a large proximal branch of the brachial artery that accompanies the radial nerve in the spiral groove along the posterior humerus and gives

Table 42–3: Stabilizing Structure About the Elbow

Contribution to Resist Applied Varus Stress (3°)

	Extended	90°
LCL	14%	9%
Soft tissue, capsule	32%	13%
Osseous articulation	55%	75%

Contribution to Resist Joint Distraction (2.5 mm)

	Extended	90°
MCL	6%	78%
Soft tissue, LCL capsule	5%	10%
Osseous articulation	85%	9%

LCL, lateral collateral ligament; MCL, medial collateral ligament.
From Miller MD, Cooper DE, Warner JJP: *Review of sports medicine and arthroscopy,* Philadelphia, 2002, Saunders.

off anterior and posterior descending branches that help create part of the arterial anastomoses around the elbow.

Nerves

- The musculocutaneous, median, ulnar, and radial nerves are all terminal branches of the brachial plexus and provide innervation to muscles of the arm, forearm, and hand.

- The musculocutaneous nerve travels distally between the brachialis and biceps muscles and terminates as the lateral antebrachial cutaneous nerve at the lateral border of the biceps in the region of the cubital fossa and extends to supply sensation to the anterolateral forearm and volar radial aspect of thenar eminence (Figure 42–9).

- The median nerve, which originally travels lateral to the brachial artery, transitions to its medial side at the middle of the arm and accompanies it through the cubital fossa deep to the bicipital aponeurosis.

- After the radial nerve travels inferolaterally with the profunda brachii along the radial groove of the posterior humerus, it runs between the brachialis and brachioradialis muscles and passes anterior to the lateral epicondyle prior to dividing into its deep (motor) and superficial (sensory) branches (Figure 42–10).

- The ulnar nerve can be palpated as it travels posteriorly around the medial epicondyle and then through the cubital tunnel whose roof is formed by the cubital tunnel retinaculum and flexor carpi ulnaris aponeurosis and floor by the joint capsule and portions of the ulnar collateral ligament (Figure 42–11).

Text Continued on p. 362

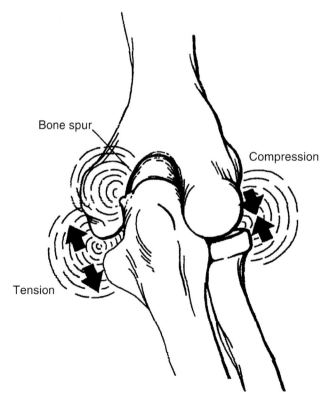

Figure 42–6:
Biomechanical forces within the elbow during throwing. (From Azar FM, Andrews JR, Wilk KE, Groh D: *Am J Sports Med* 28:22, **2002.)**

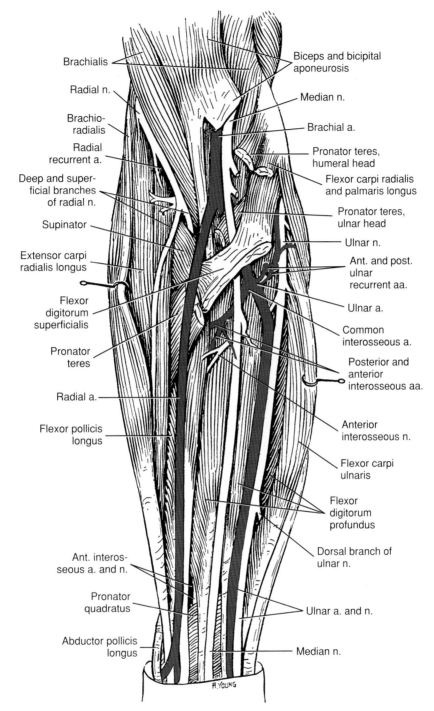

Brachialis

Radial n.

Brachio-radialis

Radial recurrent a.

Deep and super-ficial branches of radial n.

Supinator

Extensor carpi radialis longus

Flexor digitorum superficialis

Pronator teres

Radial a.

Flexor pollicis longus

Ant. interos-seous a. and n.

Pronator quadratus

Abductor pollicis longus

Biceps and bicipital aponeurosis

Median n.

Brachial a.

Pronator teres, humeral head

Flexor carpi radialis and palmaris longus

Pronator teres, ulnar head

Ulnar n.

Ant. and post. ulnar recurrent aa.

Ulnar a.

Common interosseous a.

Posterior and anterior interosseous aa.

Anterior interosseous n.

Flexor carpi ulnaris

Flexor digitorum profundus

Dorsal branch of ulnar n.

Ulnar a. and n.

Median n.

A. YOUNG

Figure 42–7:
Anterior view of the forearm and cubital fossa. (From Jenkins DB, Hollinshead WH: *Hollinshead's functional anatomy of the limbs and back,* 8th ed. Philadelphia, 2002, Saunders.)

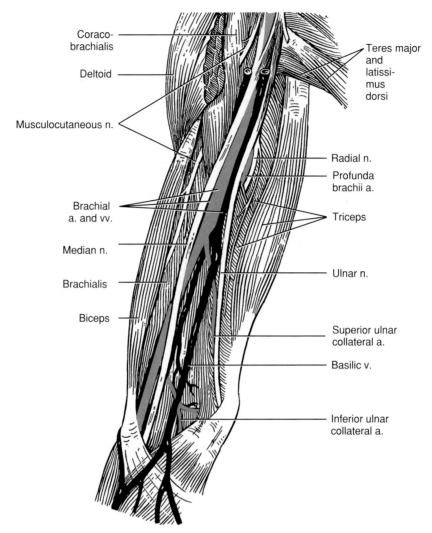

Figure 42–8:
Arteries about the elbow. (From Jenkins DB, Hollinshead WH: *Hollinshead's functional anatomy of the limbs and back,* 8th ed. Philadelphia, 2002, Saunders.)

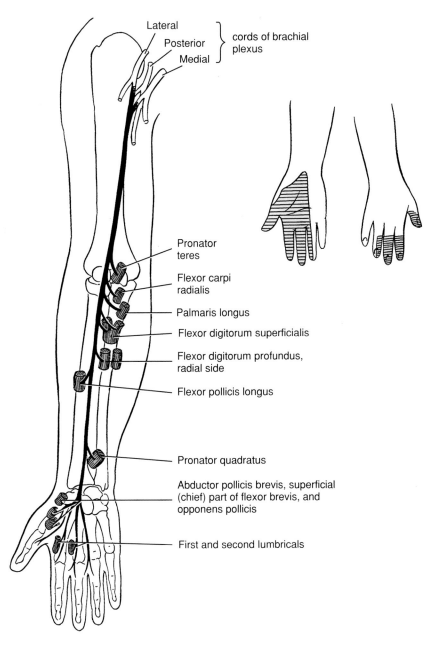

Figure 42–9:
Distribution of the median nerve. (From Jenkins DB, Hollinshead WH: *Hollinshead's functional anatomy of the limbs and back,* 8th ed. Philadelphia, 2002, Saunders.)

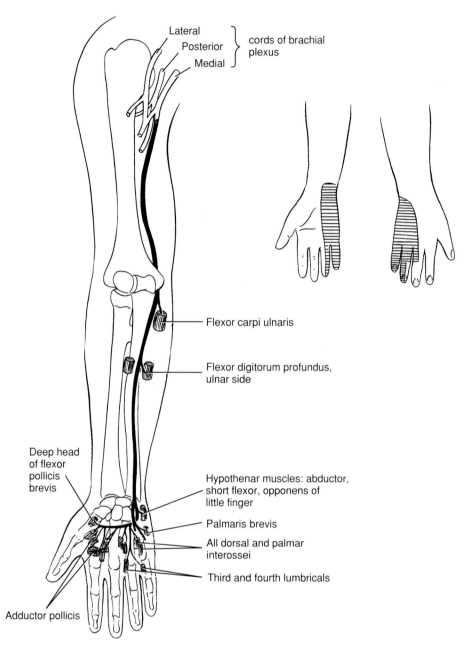

Figure 42–10:
Distribution of the ulnar nerve. (From Jenkins DB, Hollinshead WH: *Hollinshead's functional anatomy of the limbs and back,* 8th ed. Philadelphia, 2002, Saunders.)

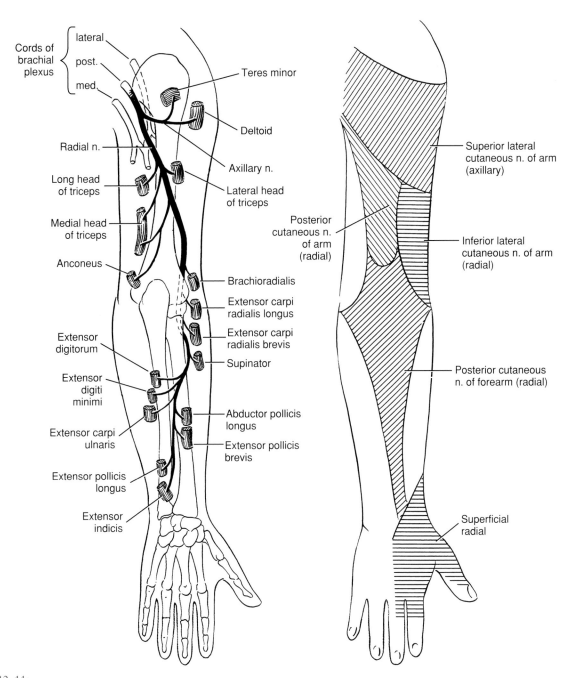

Figure 42–11:
Distribution of the radial nerve. (From Jenkins DB, Hollinshead WH: *Hollinshead's functional anatomy of the limbs and back,* 8th ed. Philadelphia, 2002, Saunders.)

References

Jenkins DB: *Hollinshead's functional anatomy of the limbs and back,* 6th ed. Philadelphia, 1991, Saunders.

 Orthopaedic anatomy textbook complete with figures and tables for study.

Miller MD: *Review of orthopaedics,* 3rd ed. Philadelphia, 2000, Saunders.

 Review text that concisely summarizes high yield topics for orthopaedics board examinations.

Morrey BF: *The elbow and its disorders,* 2nd ed. Philadelphia, 1993, Saunders.

 Definitive text describing pathologic conditions affecting the elbow and methods of treatment.

Elbow History, Physical Examination, and Imaging

History

- Age of the patient, hand dominance.
- Occupation, sports, activities.
- Acute versus chronic problem.
- Mechanism of injury.
- Environment in which the injury occurred.
- Pain: location, quality, severity, onset, timing, improving or exacerbating factors.
- Swelling or mass.
- Mechanical symptoms: stiffness, catching, locking.
- Neurologic symptoms: weakness, numbness, tingling.
- Medical comorbidities.
- Fractures or dislocations must be suspected in the acute setting.
- Elbow injuries are often overuse injuries and occur commonly in throwing athletes such as baseball pitchers who exert repetitive valgus stress to the elbow joint.
- History taking should include factors such as pitch count, innings pitched, accuracy, velocity, and phase of throwing that symptoms occur in for pitchers.

Physical Examination

- Inspection.
  - Skin.
  - Localized swelling.
  - Joint effusion.
  - Gross deformity.
  - Carrying angle.
    - Arm extended in anatomic position (palms forward).
    - Angle formed between upper arm and forearm.
    - Normal is 5 to 15 degrees of valgus.
    - Slightly increased (2 to 3 degrees) in females.
    - Less than 5 degrees: cubitus varus (gunstock deformity).
    - Greater than 15 degrees: cubitus valgus.
- Palpation.
- Bony prominences for tenderness or crepitus.
  - Medial epicondyle.
  - Medial supracondylar line of the humerus.
  - Olecranon.
  - Radial head.
  - Coronoid process.
  - Lateral epicondyle.
  - Lateral supracondylar line of the humerus.
- Soft tissues for generalized areas of tenderness, masses.
  - Medial.
    - Ulnar nerve.
    - Flexor-pronator mass.
    - Medial collateral ligament.
  - Posterior.
    - Olecranon bursa.
    - Triceps.
  - Lateral.
    - Mobile wad of three: brachioradialis, extensor carpi radialis longus (ECRL), extensor carpi radialis brevis (ECRB).
    - Lateral collateral ligament, annular ligament.
  - Anterior.
    - Antecubital fossa: biceps tendon, joint capsule.
- Range of motion (ROM).
  - Check both active and passive ROM.
  - Check for crepitus.
  - Elbow extension and flexion (normal 0 to 140 degrees).
    - Elbows must be held at the patient's side.
  - Forearm pronation and supination (normal 80 to 90 degrees each).
    - Elbows held at side, pencils in fist, rotate wrists.
  - Functional ROM is 30 to 130 degrees extension/flexion and 50 degrees of both pronation and supination.
  - Athletes require ROM closer to normal.
- Neurovascular.
  - Motor (screening examination).
    - Musculocutaneous.
      - Elbow flexion.
    - Radial.
      - Deep branch.
      - Elbow extension.
    - Posterior interosseous nerve (PIN).

363

- Wrist extension.
  - Median.
    - Anterior interosseous nerve (AIN).
    - "OK" sign.
  - Ulnar.
    - Finger abduction.
- Strength testing of elbow motion.
  - Graded 0 to 5.
  - Elbow flexors.
    - Primary: brachialis, biceps.
    - Secondary: brachioradialis, supinator.
  - Elbow extensors.
    - Primary: triceps.
    - Secondary: anconeus.
  - Pronators.
    - Primary: pronator teres, pronator quadratus.
    - Secondary: flexor carpi radialis.
  - Supinators.
    - Primary: biceps, supinator.
    - Secondary: brachioradialis.
- Sensation.
  - Dermatomal distribution.
    - C5 through T1.

- Peripheral nerve distribution.
  - Medial and lateral brachial cutaneous.
  - Medial and lateral antebrachial cutaneous.
  - Median, radial, ulnar (hand).
- Reflexes.
  - Biceps (C5).
  - Brachioradialis (C6).
  - Triceps (C7).
- Vascular.
  - Brachial, radial, ulnar pulses.
  - Color, temperature, capillary refill, skin or nail changes.
- Provocative testing.
  - Varus and valgus stress testing (Figure 43–1).
    - Performed at 0 and 30 degrees of elbow flexion.
      - Varus instability.
        - Integrity of lateral collateral ligament.
        - Humerus fully internally rotated.
        - Outward force applied to forearm.
      - Valgus instability.
        - Integrity of medial collateral ligament.
        - Humerus fully externally rotated.
        - Outward force applied to forearm.

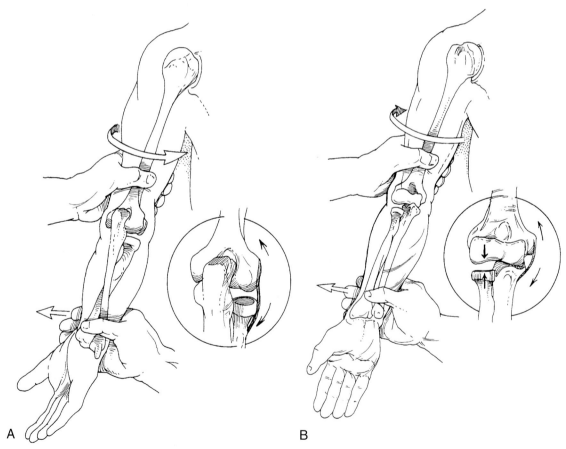

A   B

Figure 43–1:

Varus (A) and valgus (B) instability testing of the elbow. (From Morrey BF: *The elbow and its disorders,* 2nd ed. Philadelphia, 1994, Saunders.)

- ○ Must be compared with the contralateral side.
- ○ 3- to 4-mm difference can indicate instability.
- Pivot-shift test (Figure 43–2).
  - ○ Used to evaluate for posterolateral elbow instability.
  - ○ With patient supine, supinate forearm, extend elbow, and exert simultaneous axial compression and valgus stress.
  - ○ Apprehension signifies true instability.
- Lateral epicondylitis.
  - ○ Pain at the origin of the ECRB.
  - ○ Pain increased with resisted wrist extension with elbow extended and forearm pronated.
- Medial epicondylitis.
  - ○ Pain at the origin of the flexor-pronator mass.
  - ○ Pain increased with resisted wrist flexion with forearm supinated.
- Cubital tunnel syndrome.
  - ○ Compressive neuropathy of the ulnar nerve.
  - ○ Pain, numbness, tingling in medial forearm, 4th and 5th digits.
  - ○ Tinel's sign: symptoms elicited with tapping on the nerve behind the medial epicondyle.
  - ○ Compression over the cubital tunnel is the most sensitive test.
  - ○ Sustained hyperflexion of elbow may elicit symptoms.
- Examination of the upper extremity must also include examination of the cervical spine, shoulder, hand, and wrist.

Imaging

- Plain radiographs.
- Anteroposterior view (forearm supinated).
  - ○ Good visualization of the medial and lateral epicondyles, radiocapitellar articular surface.
  - ○ Measurement of the carrying angle.
- Lateral view (90 degrees of flexion, forearm neutral).
  - ○ Good visualization of the distal humerus, elbow joint, coronoid, olecranon.
  - ○ True lateral view of the joint shows three concentric arcs.
  - ○ Posterior fat pad sign indicates joint effusion.
- Oblique views.
  - ○ Medial oblique improves visualization of the trochlea, olecranon, and coronoid.
  - ○ Lateral oblique improves visualization of the radiocapitellar joint, medial epicondyle.
- Radial head view (Figure 43–3).
  - ○ 45-degree caudal tilt lateral.

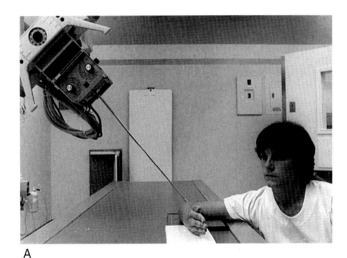

A

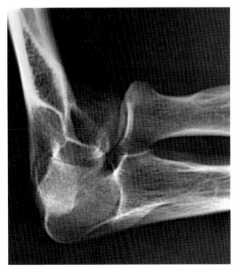

B

Figure 43–3:
Radial head view. **A**, Patient positioning. **B**, Radiographic appearance. (Morrey BF: *The elbow and its disorders*, 3rd ed. Philadelphia, 2000, Saunders.)

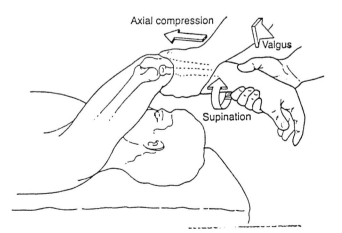

Figure 43–2:
Lateral pivot shift test of the elbow for posterolateral rotatory instability. (From Miller MD, editor: *Review of orthopaedics*, 4th ed. Philadelphia, 2004, Saunders.)

- Axial views.
  - Evaluation of the epicondyles, olecranon fossa, and ulnar sulcus.
- Stress radiographs.
  - Done in 45 to 90 degrees of flexion with fluoroscopic guidance.
  - Varus or valgus stress applied, compared with neutral views.
  - Opening greater than 2 mm demonstrates ligamentous injury.
- Computed tomography scan.
  - Great for bony detail.
  - Intraarticular or complex fracture patterns.
- Arthrogram.
  - Capsular tearing.
  - Intraarticular loose bodies.
- Magnetic resonance imaging.
  - Great for soft tissue detail.
  - Osteochondritis dissecans.
  - Biceps tendon injury.

- Ligamentous injury.
- Neurovascular structures.
- Tumors.

References

Green DP: *Green's operative hand surgery,* 4th ed. New York, 1999, Churchill Livingstone.
  Classic two volume reference text describing pathologic conditions of the upper extremity.

Morrey BF: *The elbow and its disorders,* 2nd ed. Philadelphia, 1993, Saunders.
  Definitive textbook describing pathologic conditions affecting the elbow and methods of treatment.

Topper SM: Hand and microsurgery. In Miller MD, editor: *Review of orthopaedics,* 3rd ed. Philadelphia, 2000, Saunders.
  Review text that concisely summarizes high yield topics for orthopaedics board examinations.

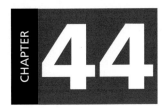

Elbow Arthroscopy

Introduction

- Elbow arthroscopy is a technically demanding procedure secondary to the limited joint space and close proximity of neurovascular structures.
- Thorough study of elbow anatomy has led to the development of relatively safe techniques.

Indications

- Diagnostic.
- Loose bodies.
- Articular cartilage pathology.
- Osteochondritis dissecans.
- Debridement of osteophytes.
- Lysis of adhesions.
- Arthrofibrosis.
- Rheumatoid arthritis—synovectomy.
- Few intraarticular fractures.
- Radial head fracture and resection.
- Septic arthritis.
- Pigmented villonodular synovitis.
- Degenerative joint disease (mild to moderate).
- Synovial chondromatosis.

Contraindications

- Extensive arthrofibrosis.
- Severe ankylosis.
- Severe degenerative joint disease.
- Previous elbow surgery that distorts anatomy (ulnar nerve transposition).
- Capsular contraction.
- Complex regional pain syndrome.

Surgical Technique

- A 4-mm 30-degree arthroscope is typically used.
- The radial head, epicondyles, olecranon, and median and ulnar nerves should be marked with a surgical marker.

Positioning

- The patient may be placed in a supine, lateral decubitus, or prone position.
  - Supine position.
    - Advantages: facilitates use of regional block anesthesia, safe conversion from regional to general anesthesia, superior airway maintenance, standard and familiar anatomic references.
    - Disadvantages: limited and difficult posterior compartment access, timely setup, arm instability requiring additional equipment or personnel support, costly suspension device, limited manipulation of the elbow.
  - Prone position.
    - Advantages: simple setup, arm stability (additional support not required), easy manipulation of the elbow, improved posterior access, gravity allows neurovascular structures to fall away from surgical site, may convert to open procedure.
    - Disadvantages: unfamiliar anatomic orientation, uncomfortable position for regional anesthesia, conversion from regional to general anesthesia is difficult and requires redraping, respiratory compromise in patients at risk, ventilation is difficult, setup and procedure may not be possible in patients with reduced shoulder mobility (e.g., patients with glenohumeral arthritis or adhesive capsulitis).
  - Lateral decubitus position.
    - Combines advantages of supine and prone positions.

Portals

- Nine established utility portals have been described (Figure 44–1). The most commonly used portals include the direct lateral, anterolateral, anteromedial, straight posterior, and posterolateral portals.
- Direct lateral portal.
  - Lies in the middle of the triangle formed by the lateral epicondyle, olecranon process, and radial head. This portal is established first and allows for joint distention.

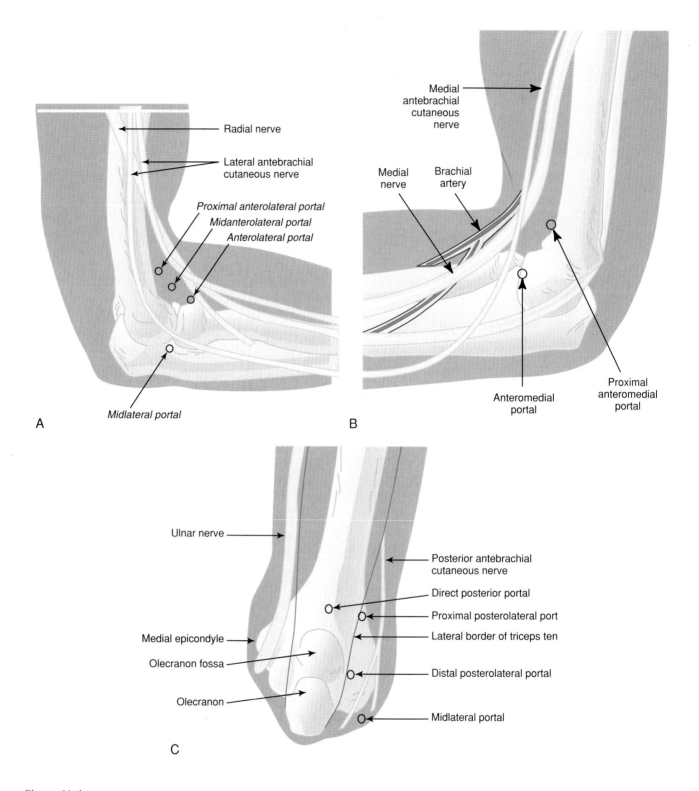

Figure 44–1:
Arthroscopic portals. **A,** Lateral portals. **B,** Medial portals. **C,** Posterior portals.(From Miller MD, Cole BJ, editors: *Textbook of arthroscopy*. Philadelphia, 2004, Saunders.)

It also provides excellent visualization of the posterior chamber.

- Anterolateral portal.
  - Established 3 cm distal and 1 cm anterior to the lateral epicondyle. This portal traverses the extensor carpi radialis brevis muscle and lies beneath the radial nerve.
- Anteromedial portal.
  - Entry site is 2 cm distal and 2 cm anterior to the medial epicondyle. May be established under direct visualization using an 18-gauge needle or by use of Wissinger rod technique. This portal traverses the pronator teres and flexor digitorum superficialis tendons passing posteriorly to the median nerve and brachial artery. This portal allows great visualization of the anterior and lateral compartments.
- Straight posterior portal.
  - Lies 3 cm proximal to the olecranon tip and passed through the triceps tendon.
- Posterolateral portal.
  - Placed 3 cm proximal to the olecranon tip and lateral to the triceps tendon.
- Posterior portals are great working portals for procedures within the posterior compartment.
- Neurovascular structures are at risk with portal placement as described in Figure 44–1.
  - Cadaveric studies have evaluated the proximity of neurovascular structures to portal entry sites.
  - Distention of the joint and elbow position during portal placement displaces structures away from portal entry sites and minimizes the risk of inadvertent neurovascular injury.
  - Severely arthritic joints may have diminished volume space and therefore an increased risk of neurovascular injury.

Rehabilitation

- Postsurgical rehabilitation can follow a four-phase program and is tailored according to the surgery performed and the patient's needs.
  - Phase I begins immediately after surgery concentrating on regaining full elbow flexion and controlling pain and inflammation.
  - Phase II begins after pain and inflammation have subsided and consists of strengthening and range-of-motion exercises.
  - Phase III starts after the patient has pain free full range of motion and emphasizes progressive strengthening exercises and returning the extremity to normal activity.
  - Phase IV works on gradually returning the patient to unrestricted activity and sport-specific needs.

Complications

- Neurovascular injuries are of greatest concern during elbow arthroscopy and can range from transient neuropraxia to complete disruption of nerves and vessels.
  - Superficial cutaneous nerves are at risk with portal placement.
  - The radial nerve is at greatest risk in proximity to the anterolateral portal.
  - The median nerve and brachial artery are at greatest risk with anteromedial portal placement.
  - Use of the posteromedial portal is not recommended because it risks injury to the posterior antebrachial cutaneous, ulnar, and median nerves and the brachial artery.
  - Injury to neurovascular structures may be avoided by limiting incisions to the skin only and using a hemostat to perform blunt dissection down to the capsule, preferably in a direction parallel to underlying nerves. Establishing portals under direct visualization is also advised when possible.
- Articular cartilage injury.
- Fluid extravasation, which can lead to compartment syndrome.
- Synovial-cutaneous fistula, most commonly seen at the anterolateral portal site.
- Arthrofibrosis.

References

Andrews JR, Baumgarten TE: Arthroscopic anatomy of the elbow. *Orthop Clin North Am* 26:671-677, 1995.
  Discussion of arthroscopic portals and anatomy.

Hsu, JC, Yamaguchi, K: Elbow: anaesthesia, patient positioning, portal placement, normal arthroscopic anatomy, and diagnostic arthroscopy. In Miller MD, editor: *Textbook of arthroscopy.* Philadelphia, 2004, Elsevier.
  Arthroscopy text that describes the arthroscopic techniques for the elbow and other joints. Color plates serve as an arthroscopic atlas.

Kelley EW, Morrey BF, O'Driscoll SW: Complications of elbow arthroscopy. *J Bone Joint Surg Am* 83:25-34, 2001.
  Retrospective review describing the complications from elbow arthroscopy.

Miller MD, Cole BJ: *Textbook of arthroscopy.* Philadelphia, 2004, Saunders.
  Arthroscopy text that describes the arthroscopic techniques for the elbow and other joints. Color plates serve as an arthroscopic atlas.

Morrey BF: Arthroscopy of the elbow. In Morrey BF, editor: *The elbow and its disorders.* Philadelphia, 1985, Saunders.
  Definitive textbook describing pathologic conditions affecting the elbow and methods of treatment.

O'Driscoll SW, Morrey BF: Arthroscopy of the elbow: diagnostic and therapeutic benefits and hazards. *J Bone Joint Surg Am* 74:84-94, 1992.
  Review of the Mayo experience with elbow arthroscopy.

Phillips BB: Arthroscopy of the upper extremity. In Canale ST, editor: *Campbell's operative orthopaedics,* 10th ed. Philadelphia, 2003, Mosby.
  Classic five-volume orthopaedics reference.

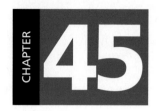

Elbow Instability

- Relative stability of the elbow joint is conferred by conforming bony articular surfaces and capsuloligamentous restraints and surrounding muscles.

Medial Collateral Ligament Injury

- The medial collateral ligament plays a key role as the primary soft tissue stabilizer of the elbow in both valgus and distraction stress. The radial head is a secondary stabilizer to valgus stress.
- The medial ligamentous complex is made up of three well-defined portions.
  - Anterior oblique—primary medial stabilizer, inserts on the sublime tubercle of the ulna.
  - Posterior oblique.
  - Transverse oblique.
- Mechanism of injury typically involves repetitive trauma secondary to excessive valgus stress in a throwing athlete. Maximal valgus forces are generated during the late cocking and acceleration phases of throwing.
- Examination findings include localized medial tenderness and laxity to valgus stress.
  - Valgus stress should be applied with the elbow at 30 degrees of flexion in both the supinated and pronated positions.
- Valgus instability may lead to development of arthrosis of the posteromedial tip of the olecranon and the radiocapitellar joint. Ulnar neuropathy may result from traction injury or impingement from osteophytes.
- Routine x-ray examination includes anteroposterior, lateral, and two oblique projections. Chronic cases may demonstrate degenerative changes of the olecranon or radiocapitellar joint. Gravity stress radiographs demonstrate medial joint space widening in approximately half of cases. Magnetic resonance imaging (MRI) with arthrogram may demonstrate incompetence of the ligament and extravasation of fluid around the humerus or ulna without extracapsular leakage (T sign).
- Initial treatment includes rest, bracing, and therapy.

- Surgery is indicated for competitive throwing athletes with acute complete ruptures and patients with chronic instability who have failed conservative treatment.
  - The anterior oblique band of the ligament is reconstructed with tendon graft (usually palmaris or plantaris) secured through drill holes in the ulna and medial epicondyle.
  - The ulnar nerve may be transposed anteriorly for symptomatic ulnar nerve involvement.
  - Rehabilitation is regimented, and athletes are allowed to return to a supervised throwing program after 4 months. Return to competitive play takes 1 year.

Lateral Collateral Ligament Injury

- The lateral ligamentous complex of the elbow extends from the lateral epicondyle and inserts on the annular ligament. The main lateral stabilizer of the elbow, the lateral ulnar collateral ligament, is a separate band that inserts on the supinator crest of the ulna.
- The lateral collateral ligament plays a secondary role in varus stability.
- Injury is often a sequela of traumatic elbow dislocation or subluxation. Injury less commonly results from varus stress.
- Symptoms may include sensation of popping or clicking or locking. Patients characteristically complain of symptoms of instability when using their arms to push themselves up from a seated position.
- Posterolateral rotatory instability may be demonstrated by the lateral pivot shift test.
  - Subluxation of the radiocapitellar joint is detected as a prominence as a valgus stress and axial load is applied with the forearm supinated and the elbow held at 30 degrees of flexion.
  - This test is most easily done with the patient supine and the shoulder abducted and fully externally rotated. As the elbow is progressively flexed, the subluxed radial head reduces and a clunk may be detected.

- Posterolateral rotatory instability may also be detected by supinating the forearm with the elbow held at 30 degrees of flexion while stabilizing the medial epicondyle. The examiner looks for the olecranon to "roll off" the distal humerus with supination of the forearm.
- Stress radiographs may demonstrate joint subluxation. MRI may show ligament degeneration.
- Operative treatment includes reconstruction of the lateral ulnar collateral ligament with tendon graft and capsular imbrication.

Elbow Dislocation

- Simple dislocation involves disruption of the capsuloligamentous structures. Most commonly posterolateral in direction (80%).
- Bony injuries are common and may include fractures of the radial head and neck, coronoid, capitellum, epicondyles, and olecranon.
- Reduction maneuver includes traction, correction of displacement, and elbow flexion.
  - Neurovascular status must be assessed both before and after reduction. A nerve deficit that appears following reduction requires exploration.
  - Postreduction stability should be assessed.
- Most simple dislocations of the elbow are stable and can be managed nonsurgically. Fracture-dislocations in which the fracture does not compromise stability may be treated nonsurgically.
  - Nonoperative management includes a 3- to 5-day period of immobilization, followed by early range of motion.

- Surgical algorithm for unstable cases involves reconstruction of the articular elements, particularly the ulnohumeral joint.
  - At least 50% of the coronoid must be present for stability.
  - Fifty percent of the olecranon is required to maintain stability.
  - The radial head is a secondary stabilizer of the elbow, in that it becomes the primary stabilizer to valgus instability if medial collateral ligament is torn or attenuated.
- If instability persists despite fracture fixation (or in simple dislocations with instability), repair or reconstruction of the lateral collateral ligament complex and common extensor tendon should be performed. Further soft tissue reconstruction including repair of the medial collateral ligament and common flexor-pronator origin is performed if necessary.
- A hinged external fixator may be added if necessary.
- Complications include stiffness, instability, heterotopic ossification, and myositis ossificans.

References

O'Driscoll SW, Bell DF, Morrey BF: Posterolateral rotatory instability of the elbow. *J Bone Joint Surg Am* 73:440-446, 1991.
  This is a landmark article describing posterolateral rotatory instability of the elbow. O'Driscoll and colleagues describe the condition and their early experience with operative repair.

Yadao MA, Savoie FH III, Field LD: Posterolateral rotatory instability of the elbow. *Instruct Course Lect* 53:607-614, 2004.
  Review of posterolateral instability of the elbow and surgical technique for ligament reconstruction.

CHAPTER 46

Tendon Injuries about the Elbow

Introduction

- Tendon ruptures usually occur from an activity that places a muscle under excessive load. This usually occurs during an eccentric contraction. Direct blows and lacerations may also cause tendon injury.
- Ruptures usually occur at musculotendinous or tendo-osseous junction. These are typically watershed areas of blood supply.
- Commonly affects the dominant arm of middle-aged males. Competitive athletes of all ages may be affected, especially those routinely lifting heavy weights as a part of their training regimen.
- Degenerative changes secondary to repetitive microtrauma may predispose to tendon rupture. A number of systemic conditions (rheumatoid arthritis, renal failure) may weaken tendons. Anabolic steroids and corticosteroid injections predispose to tendon rupture as well.

Distal Biceps Tendon Ruptures

- Only 3% to 5% of biceps tendon ruptures occur distally.
- Distal ruptures typically cause greater weakness than proximal biceps tears.

History

- Patients typically present with pain, swelling, and ecchymosis to the antecubital fossa.
- In cases of acute rupture, patients may report hearing or feeling a "pop" at the time of injury.
- Patients may also complain of weakness with elbow flexion and supination.

Examination

- A defect may be palpable within the tendon substance.
- Proximal migration of the muscle belly occurs with contraction.
- This may not occur if a complete tear is maintained distally by the lacertus fibrosis.
- Weakness with resisted supination and elbow flexion relative to the opposite arm.
- Partial ruptures may present with less dramatic weakness and are more difficult to diagnose.

Imaging

- Standard radiographs should be evaluated for bony avulsion or fracture.
- Magnetic resonance imaging (MRI) shows tendon rupture and is helpful for differentiation between partial and complete tears. MRI may also be used to assess degree of tendon retraction.

Treatment

- Partial tendon rupture may be treated with splinting in flexion and subsequent rehabilitation. Some authors recommend treating more extensive partial tears by excising the remaining tendon and then performing an anatomic repair.
- Acute complete ruptures are treated with repair of the tendon to the radial tuberosity.
- A double-incision technique as described by Boyd and Anderson is commonly used (Figure 46–1).
  - An anterior incision is used to locate the retracted tendon, which is passed down to its anatomic insertion site on the radial tuberosity.
  - A muscle-splitting posterolateral approach is used to expose the radial tuberosity and anatomically reattach the ruptured tendon.
- Anterior approaches with and without the use of suture anchors have also been described.
- Chronic complete ruptures with retraction may be repaired using a fascia lata or semitendinosus graft.

Distal Triceps Rupture

- Distal avulsion or rupture of the triceps tendon is rare.
- Typically a small piece of bone from the tip of the olecranon is avulsed with the tendon.
- Congenital or metabolic bone disorders such as Marfan's syndrome, osteogenesis imperfecta, or hypothyroidism

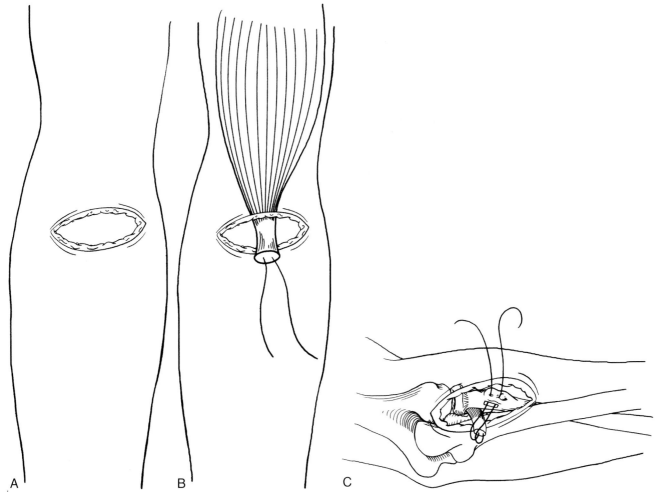

Figure 46–1:
Technique of Boyd and Anderson for reinserting biceps tendon into radial tuberosity. **A,** Skin incision. **B,** Retrieving tendon. **C,** Burrhole in radial tuberosity with passage of sutures. (Modified from Canale ST, editor: *Campbell's operative orthopaedics,* 10th ed. Philadelphia, 2003, Saunders.)

may exist and produce a weak insertion site. Injury may also be associated with olecranon bursitis.

History and Examination

- Pain, swelling, and ecchymosis to the distal posterior arm are common.
- Weakness of elbow extension is detected on physical examination.

Imaging

- Radiographs may demonstrate bony avulsions (Figure 46–2).
- MRI is helpful to confirm the diagnosis and assess degree of retraction.

Treatment

- Triceps avulsions are surgically reattached to the insertion site using transosseous tunnels and suture (Figure 46–3). Fracture fragments of less than 50% of the olecranon are excised.

- Turndown flaps and fascial grafts may be used in chronic cases with retraction.

Rehabilitation of Tendon Injuries

- Range-of-motion exercises typically begin no earlier than 3 weeks after surgical repair.
- The repaired muscle should not begin active exercises for 6 to 9 weeks.
- Powerful activity of the affected muscle should be avoided for 4 to 6 months.

Complications

- Neurovascular injury during surgical repair.
- Loss of motion (slight loss of supination is common after biceps repair).
- Heterotopic ossification—especially with two-incision biceps repairs.

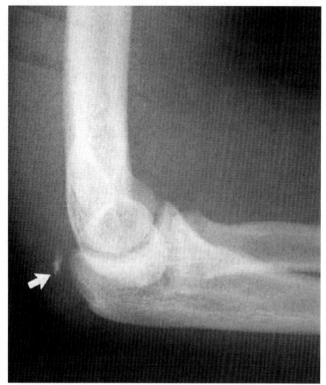

Figure 46–2:
Triceps tendon rupture with small avulsion fragment of ole-cranon. (From DeLee JC, Drez D Jr, Miller MD, editors: *DeLee and Drez's orthopaedic sports medicine, principles and practice,* 2nd ed. Philadelphia, 2003, Saunders.)

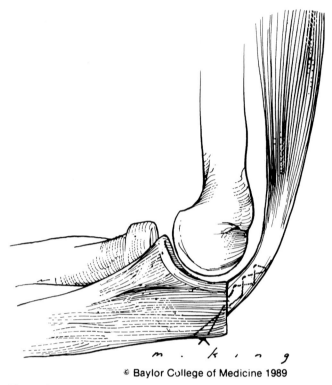

© Baylor College of Medicine 1989

Figure 46–3:
Triceps tendon reinsertion approximating the joint surface after olecranon fracture excision. (From DeLee JC, Drez D Jr, Miller MD, editors: *DeLee and Drez's orthopaedic sports medicine, principles and practice,* 2nd ed. Philadelphia, 2003, Saunders.)

- Radioulnar synostosis.
- Reduced strength, particularly if diagnosis and repair is delayed.
- Repair failure.

References

Azar FM: Traumatic disorders. In Canale ST, editor: *Campbells operative orthopaedics,* 10th ed. Philadelphia, 2003, Mosby.
Classic five volume orthopaedics reference.

Bennett JB, Mehlhoff TL: Soft tissue injury and fractures. In *DeLee and Drez's orthopaedic sports medicine, principles and practice,* 2nd ed. Philadelphia, 2003, Saunders.
Reference text covering all aspects of sports medicine.

Bernstein AD, Breslow MJ, Jarawi LM: Distal biceps tendon ruptures: a historical perspective and current concepts. *Am J Orthop* 30:193-200, 2001.
Excellent review of diagnosis and treatment for injuries to the distal biceps tendon.

Boyd HB, Anderson LD: A method for reinsertion of the distal biceps brachii tendon. *J Bone Joint Surg Am* 43:1041-1046, 1961.
Boyd describes his method for anatomic reinsertion of the biceps tendon and early results.

Sollender JL, Rayan GM, Barden GA: Triceps tendon rupture in weight lifters. *J Shoulder Elbow Surg* 7:151-153, 1998.
Sollender and colleagues present four weightlifters with triceps tendon raptures, two of whom had received local steroid injections for pain in the triceps. All four patients had taken oral anabolic steroids before injury.

Stannard JP, Bucknell AL: Rupture of the triceps tendon associated with steroid injections. *Am J Sports Med* 21:482-485, 1993.
Local steroid injections and a history of anabolic steroid abuse are implicated in a case report of a patient with rupture of the triceps tendon.

Strauch RJ, Michelson H, Rosenwasser MP: Repair of rupture of the distal tendon of the biceps brachii: review of the literature and report of three cases treated with a single anterior incision and suture anchors. *Am J Orthop* 2:151-156, 1997.
Strauch and colleagues describe their technique and results with biceps repair using a single incision and suture anchors.

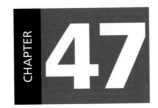
Nerve Entrapment

Introduction

- Repetitive activities requisite to certain sports predispose athletes to entrapment neuropathies of the upper extremity. For instance, throwing a baseball or serving a tennis ball places considerable valgus load at the elbow, which may predispose to cubital tunnel syndrome.
- Pathophysiology of axonal injury involves interference with the intraneural circulation. Persistent ischemia leads to fibrosis and irreversible injury, underscoring the importance of early diagnosis and treatment.
- Nerve compression leading to a disruption of flow of nutrients and waste products along the course of an axon lowers the threshold for compression at another site, the so-called *double crush phenomenon*. Outcome of surgical decompression may be suboptimal unless all sites of compression are addressed.

Pronator Syndrome

- The median nerve may be compressed around the elbow at four anatomic sites.
  - Between a supracondylar process and the ligament of Struthers.
  - Beneath the edge of the bicipital aponeurosis (lacertus fibrosis).
  - Between the ulnar and humeral heads of the pronator teres.
  - Deep to the aponeurotic arch of the flexor digitorum superficialis.
- Patients complain of pain in the volar proximal forearm exacerbated by repetitive, strenuous activity. Patients may also complain of paresthesias in radial three and one-half digits.
- Motor weakness is unusual.
- Provocative tests include exacerbation of symptoms with resisted forearm pronation or extreme elbow flexion. Phalen's and Tinel's test at the wrist are negative.
- Electromyography (EMG)/nerve conduction studies (NCS) are typically unreliable for diagnosis.

- Nerve exploration and decompression should address all possible sites of compression.

Anterior Interosseus Nerve Syndrome

- Isolated anterior interosseus nerve (AIN) palsy manifests as weakness in the AIN innervated muscles, leading to a characteristic pinch deformity due to weakness of the flexor pollicis longus (FPL) and flexor digitorum profundus (FDP) to index (inability to make the "OK" sign).

Carpal Tunnel Syndrome

- Compression of the median nerve in the carpal tunnel is most commonly caused by flexor tenosynovitis, although a multitude of other conditions may also play a role. Sports activities involving repetitive flexion or grasping activities are frequently encountered.
- The carpal tunnel is bounded superiorly by the transverse carpal ligament, which extends from the pisiform and hamate ulnarly to the scaphoid and trapezium radially. The carpal tunnel contains the median nerve and the tendons of the flexor digitorum superficialis, flexor digitorum profundus, and flexor pollicis longus.
- The palmar cutaneous branch of the median nerve branches from the median nerve proximal to the wrist and passes superficial to the transverse carpal ligament. This supplies sensation to the radial aspect of the palm and therefore remains uninvolved in carpal tunnel syndrome. The motor branch to the thenar muscles typically branches distal to the transverse carpal ligament (extraligamentous, recurrent pattern of branching); however, anatomic variants are common.
- Symptoms include numbness or tingling in the radial three and one-half digits and hand clumsiness or weakness.
- Sensory testing should include two-point discrimination (normal < 5 mm) or vibratory threshold. Motor testing may demonstrate weakness of the thenar muscles. Pressure

over the carpal canal (Durkin's compression test) is the best test and will provoke symptoms. Percussion of the median nerve over the carpal tunnel may cause paresthesias into median nerve distribution (positive Tinel's test). Persistent wrist flexion may also exacerbate symptoms (positive Phalen's test).

- EMG/NCS are helpful to confirm the diagnosis.
- Steroid injection benefits patients with mild, intermittent symptoms most; it may serve a diagnostic purpose as well.
- Carpal tunnel release may be done open or endoscopically. The most common cause of persistent symptoms following endoscopic decompression is incomplete release of the transverse carpal ligament.

Radial Tunnel Syndrome

- Sites of radial nerve entrapment include the following:
  - Fibrous bands at the level of the radial head.
  - Engorged leash of recurrent radial vessels (Leash of Henry).
  - Tendinous margin of the extensor carpi radialis brevis.
  - As the posterior interosseus nerve enters the supinator muscle (arcade of Frohse, *most common site of entrapment*).
- Patients complain of pain distal to the extensor origin along the radial tunnel. There is no motor or sensory dysfunction. Must be considered in the differential diagnosis of lateral epicondylitis.
- Findings include tenderness to palpation along the radial tunnel. Pain may also be reproduced by resisted middle finger extension and resisted forearm supination with elbow extended.
- EMG/NCS are usually not helpful.
- Surgical decompression should be considered after exhaustive nonoperative measures.

Posterior Interosseus Nerve Syndrome

- Pain as in radial tunnel syndrome *plus* weakness in posterior interosseus nerve (PIN) innervated muscles (extensor carpi radialis brevis, supinator, extensor carpi ulnaris, extensor digitorum communis, abductor pollicis longus, extensor pollicis longus and brevis).
- Same anatomic sites of compression as with radial tunnel syndrome.
- EMG/NCS are useful.
- Decompression offers more favorable results than radial tunnel syndrome.

Superficial Radial Nerve Compression Syndrome

- Also called Wartenberg's syndrome, a compressive neuropathy of the sensory branch of the radial nerve in the distal forearm may be caused by external compression, trauma, or a scissor-like action between the tendons of the extensor carpi radialis longus and brachioradialis as the forearm is pronated.
- Steroid injection is diagnostic and therapeutic.
- Surgical decompression is warranted in refractory cases.

Cubital Tunnel Syndrome

- Sites of ulnar nerve compression around the elbow include the following.
  - The arcade of Struthers—a fascial arcade through which the ulnar nerve passes in the arm.
  - The medial intermuscular septum in the arm.
  - Subluxing medial head of the triceps.
  - Beneath the cubital tunnel retinaculum (Osbourne's ligament), possibly exacerbated in some patients who may have an anconeus epitrochlearis (a vestigial muscle extending from the medial epicondyle to the medial olecranon).
  - The flexor carpi ulnaris aponeurosis.
- Ulnar nerve subluxation over the medial epicondyle, seen in 15% of the population, may predispose to neuritis of the ulnar nerve. Repetitive valgus stress to the elbow, commonly seen in pitchers and tennis players, may also lead to irritation of the ulnar nerve.
- Symptoms include pain at the medial elbow and paresthesias in the ulnar one and one-half fingers. Weakness of the ulnar nerve innervated muscles of the hand may manifest as diminished dexterity or as weakness in grip or pinch strength. Atrophy of the hand intrinsics is seen late.
- Provocative maneuvers include pressure over the ulnar nerve to both assess sensitivity and provoke symptoms, percussion along the course of the nerve (Tinel's sign), and full elbow flexion with the wrist extended. Wartenberg's test assesses the strength of the adductor pollicis; weak grasp between the extended thumb and index finger is a positive test. Decreased sensation along the dorso-ulnar aspect of the hand or weakness of the FDP of the ring and small fingers localizes the compression proximally and not within Guyon's canal.
- Radiographs of the elbow should be obtained in patients with a history of trauma or diminished elbow motion looking for bony impingement of the nerve within the cubital tunnel.
- EMG/NCS may confirm nerve compression at the level of the elbow.

- Early symptoms may resolve with bracing to prevent extremes of elbow flexion. Surgical intervention includes simple decompression, subcutaneous or submuscular anterior transposition, and medial epicondylectomy. Branches of the medial brachial and medial antebrachial cutaneous nerves should be identified and preserved.

Ulnar Tunnel Syndrome

- Entrapment of the ulnar nerve as it passes through the ulnar tunnel (Guyon's canal) at the wrist may lead pure motor, pure sensory, or mixed symptoms. The ulnar nerve bifurcates to form a deep motor and superficial sensory branch within the canal.
- The ulnar nerve travels with the ulnar artery through Guyon's canal. The transverse carpal ligament forms the floor of the canal, and the volar carpal ligament forms the roof. The ulnar border is formed by the hook of the hamate and the radial border by the pisiform.
- Compressive etiologies include ganglia, hook of hamate fractures, and thrombosis or aneurysm of the ulnar artery (hypothenar hammer syndrome).
- Patients may complain of wrist pain with radiation into the small and ring fingers. Intrinsic weakness and atrophy occur late.
- Fractures of the hook of the hamate (common in baseball players) may be detected on carpal tunnel views of the wrist or computed tomography scan. Ganglia may be detected on magnetic resonance imaging. Allen's test and Doppler studies may be useful to evaluate the ulnar artery.
- EMG/NCS is useful to localize the level of the lesion.

- Operative decompression is performed in cases that fail conservative management. Concomitant carpal and cubital tunnel syndrome may be addressed surgically with carpal tunnel release, which increases the volume within Guyon's canal as well.

Thoracic Outlet Syndrome

- Entrapment neuropathy of the lower trunk of the brachial plexus between the anterior and middle scalene muscles and the first rib or a cervical rib.
- Presents with numbness and tingling along the ulnar border of the hand and hand weakness. Medial arm and forearm paresthesias may also be present (compression is proximal to the origin of the medial brachial and antebrachial cutaneous nerves).
- Treatment involves decompression ± first rib or cervical rib resection.

References

Green DP, Hotchkiss RN, Pederson WC, editors: *Green's operative hand surgery,* vol 1 and 2, 4th ed. New York, 1999, Churchill Livingstone.
Classic two-volume reference text describing pathologic conditions of the upper extremity.

Miller MD: *Review of orthopaedics,* 3rd ed. Philadelphia, 2000, Saunders.
Review text that concisely summarizes high yield topics orthopaedics board examinations.

Morrey BF: *The elbow and its disorders,* 2nd ed. Philadelphia, 1993, Saunders.
Definitive textbook describing pathologic conditions affecting the elbow and methods of treatment.

CHAPTER 48

Elbow Overuse Injuries

- Overuse injury is a nonspecific term that may be applied to a spectrum of conditions affecting the upper extremity. Please note that other chapters within this section provide coverage of such topics as well.

Lateral Epicondylitis

- Also referred to as "tennis elbow," this condition is a common cause of lateral elbow pain among athletes and nonathletes. Mechanism of injury typically involves repetitive elbow extension and supination, which is common in racquet sports.
- The extensor carpi radialis brevis tendon is most commonly affected just distal to its origin on the lateral epicondyle; tendons of the extensor carpi radialis longus and extensor digitorum communis may be affected as well. Pathophysiology involves microtears within the tendon substance, leading to subsequent tendon degeneration and angiofibroblastic hyperplasia. This condition is thus more aptly termed "tendinosis."
- Patients report pain and tenderness of the lateral elbow that is exacerbated with activities involving wrist dorsiflexion and supination.
- Pain and tenderness slightly distal to the lateral epicondyle is elicited on examination and is pronounced with resisted wrist dorsiflexion with the elbow fully extended. Diminished grip strength with the elbow in an extended versus flexed position may also be observed; serial measurements may be used to quantify response to treatment.
- Radiographs may demonstrate calcifications within the extensor tendon substance, suggesting chronic degeneration; radiographs are also helpful to rule out lateral compartment pathology. Magnetic resonance imaging (MRI) shows abnormal signal within the tendon substance but is rarely necessary for diagnosis.
- Most patients respond favorably to nonoperative treatment, which is divided into three phases.
  - Phase I begins when acute symptoms are present. Includes rest, ice massage, nonsteroidal antiinflammatory drugs formal therapy (stretches,

trigger point massage), modalities (ultrasound, iontophoresis), counterforce bracing, and therapeutic steroid injection (Figure 48–1).
  - Phase II begins when acute phase and severe pain is gone. Continue stretching and modalities, add gentle conditioning program, and gradually return to work/sport activities.
  - Phase III begins when almost all pain is gone: continue to increase strengthening and flexibility, full return to competitive sports, equipment and ergonomics modification.
    - Recommended racquet modifications include a more flexible frame, lighter weight, larger head, larger grip, looser string tension, and use of a two-handed backstroke.
- Surgery is reserved for patients with refractory symptoms of at least 6 months' duration. Most commonly this involves debridement of abnormal appearing tendon and repair of the tendon back to the lateral epicondyle, which has been decorticated to a bleeding cancellous surface. Arthroscopic debridement is gaining popularity. Anconeus muscle transfer is also described for recurrent cases.
- Failure to address concomitant radial tunnel syndrome may lead to incomplete relief of symptoms (see Chapter 47).

Medial Epicondylitis

- Also referred to as "golfer's elbow," medial epicondylitis is much less common than lateral epicondylitis. Activities producing a valgus force at the elbow may lead to degeneration at the origin of the flexor-pronator tendon complex at the medial epicondyle (medial conjoint tendon); the flexor carpi radialis and pronator teres are usually affected.
- Patients complain of medial elbow pain and tenderness.
- Physical examination elicits pain at a point just distal to the medial epicondyle that is exacerbated with resisted wrist flexion and forearm pronation.
- Treatment is basically the same as for lateral epicondylitis.

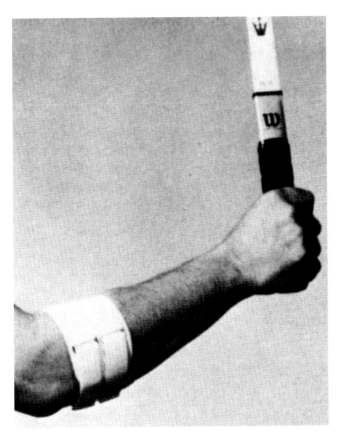

Figure 48–1:
Lateral elbow counterforce brace. (From Morrey BF: *The elbow and its disorders.* **Philadelphia, 1985, Saunders.)**

- Concomitant cubital tunnel syndrome and valgus instability are common and should also be addressed (see Chapters 45 and 47).

Triceps Tendinitis

- Tendinitis of the triceps occurs secondary to repetitive elbow extension.
- Posterior elbow pain and tenderness is exacerbated with elbow extension.
- Conservative treatment is largely successful (three-phase rehabilitation protocol outlined previously).
  - Partial tendon rupture should be considered in refractory cases.
- Olecranon spurs often seen—these are calcifications of tendon insertion and can lead to bursal symptoms. The degeneration of the tendon insertion is primary pathology.

Osteochondritis Dissecans of the Capitellum

- Repetitive compression to the radiocapitellar joint may lead to osteochondral injury. Athletes participating in throwing and racquet sports and gymnastics are commonly affected.
- Osteochondritis dissecans (OCD) is believed to result from ischemia to subchondral bone, secondary to infarction or trauma, which leads to subsequent changes in the overlying cartilage. OCD of the capitellum usually affects teenagers and young adults.
  - Diffuse osteochondrosis of the capitellum seen in children is called Panner's disease and may represent a similar disease process.
- Patients typically present with activity-related lateral elbow pain. Mechanical symptoms including popping, catching, and locking may be present.
- Radiographs and MRI are usually diagnostic and help to guide treatment.
- Skeletally immature patients are typically treated nonoperatively with rest and avoidance of aggravating activity. Elbow arthroscopy is advocated for skeletally mature patients or younger patients with pronounced mechanical symptoms. Size and stability of the lesion guides treatment. Drilling of the defect to stimulate healing may be done for larger lesions that are stable, whereas debridement and abrasion chondroplasty versus microfracture is favored for smaller, unstable lesions.

Valgus Extension Overload/Posteromedial Impingement

- Repetitive valgus stress in throwing athletes may lead to chondromalacia of the tip of the olecranon and posteromedial trochlea followed by formation of osteophytes between the olecranon and trochlea. This may lead to posteromedial impingement, which predominantly limits elbow extension and results in pain with throwing.
- Radiographs and MRI are helpful for diagnosis and to rule out stress fracture of the olecranon.
- Chronic cases refractory to rest and rehabilitation may be treated with arthroscopic debridement of chondromalacia and posteromedial osteophytes (Figure 48–2).

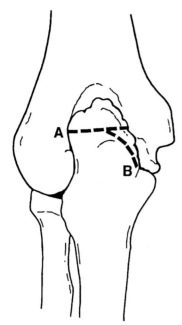

Figure 48–2:
Resection of posteromedial osteophytes. (From Canale ST, editor: *Campbell's operative orthopaedics,* 10th ed. Philadelphia, 2003, Saunders.)

References

Almekinders LC: Tendinitis and other chronic tendinopathies. *J Am Acad Orthop Surg* 6:157-164, 1998.
Discussion of the etiology of tendon problems and the efficacy of available treatments.

Chen FS, Rokito AS, Jobe FW: Medial elbow problems in the overhead-throwing athlete. *J Am Acad Orthop Surg* 9:99-113, 2001.
Valgus instability, valgus extension overload, posteromedial impingement, medial epicondylitis, and ulnar neuropathy are presented.

Ciccotti MG: Epicondylitis in the athlete. *Instruct Course Lect* 48:375-81, 1999.
Epicondylitis can be caused by sports-related activities and may be confused with other pathologic entities affecting the elbow. Nonsurgical treatment is usually successful, but surgical treatment is often successful in resistant cases.

Kobayashi K, Burton KJ, Rodner C, et al: Lateral compression injuries in the pediatric elbow: Panner's disease and osteochondritis dissecans of the capitellum. *J Am Acad Orthop Surg* 12:246-254, 2004.
Lateral compression injuries of the elbow in preadolescent and adolescent patients include Panner's disease and OCD. Panner's disease and OCD likely represent a continuum of disordered endochondral ossification.

Morrey BF, Regan WD: Tendinopathies about the elbow. In Delee JC, Drez D Jr, Miller MD, editors: *Delee and Drez's orthopaedic sports medicine,* 2nd ed. Philadelphia, 2003, Saunders.
Reference text covering all aspects of sports medicine.

Petrie RS, Bradley JP: Osteochondritis dissecans of the humeral capitellum. In Delee JC, Drez D Jr, Miller MD, editors: *Delee and Drez's orthopaedic sports medicine,* 2nd ed. Philadelphia, 2003, Saunders.
Reference text covering all aspects of sports medicine.

Phillips BB: Arthroscopy of the upper extremity. In Canale ST, editor: *Campbell's operative orthopaedics,* 10th ed. Philadelphia, 2003, Mosby.
Classic five-volume orthopaedics reference.

CHAPTER 49

Elbow Loss of Motion

- Functional range of elbow motion.
  - Extension-flexion: 30 to 130 degrees.
  - Pronation-supination: 50 degrees each (100 degrees total).
- Deficits in pronation or supination may result from radiocapitellar or proximal radioulnar joint pathology or pathology in the forearm or wrist. Stiffness in flexion or extension usually results from ulnohumeral joint pathology.

Etiology

- Causes of elbow stiffness may be classified as intrinsic or extrinsic (Box 49–1).
- Intrinsic block to elbow motion commonly results from posttraumatic arthritis and osteoarthritis. Posteromedial olecranon osteophytes commonly cause flexion contracture in throwing athletes.
- Extrinsic etiologies include contractures of the joint capsule or surrounding muscles (brachialis, biceps, or triceps muscles). Hemarthrosis following minor trauma may lead to guarding and the development of soft tissue contracture.

Examination

- Assess the integrity of soft tissues surrounding the elbow.
- Passive and active range of motion should be recorded.
- Neurovascular assessment.

Imaging

- Anteroposterior, lateral, and oblique radiographs of the elbow.
- Forearm and wrist radiographs should be obtained for rotational deficits.
- Computed tomography may be helpful in cases of severe deformity or heterotopic ossification.
- Magnetic resonance imaging may be useful in cases with instability.

Treatment

- Institution of early motion following elbow injury is key for prevention.
- Nonoperative treatment includes physical therapy, followed by splinting.
- Surgical algorithm for refractory cases takes into account the cause of stiffness, degree of articular degeneration, and functional demands of the patient. Arthroscopy is a valuable tool for debridement and assessment of articular damage. Surgery should only be considered in patients who are willing to comply with regimented postoperative rehabilitation.
  - Soft tissue releases (arthroscopic or open) are favored in cases with little or no degenerative changes and may be performed after the inflammatory phase of soft tissue healing is over (3 to 6 months postinjury).
  - Limited bony debridement is beneficial in patients with moderate articular degenerative changes. Outerbridge-

---

Box 49–1	Causes of Elbow Stiffness by Location of Pathology

Extrinsic
   Skin, subcutaneous tissue
   Capsule (posterior/anterior)
   Collateral ligament contracture
   Myostatic contracture (posterior/anterior)
   Heterotopic ossification
Intrinsic
   Articular deformity
   Articular adhesions
   Impinging osteophytes
      Olecranon
      Coronoid
   Fibrosis that impinges on:
      Olecranon fossa
      Coronoid fossa
   Loose bodies
Mixed

Strauch RJ, Rosenwasser MP: From Bruno RJ, Lee ML, *J Am Acad Orthop Surgeons* 10:106–116, 2002.

Kashiwagi ulnohumeral arthroplasty is reserved for patients with severe spurring as etiology for limited motion.

- Younger patients with full-thickness loss of articular cartilage are candidates for interposition arthroplasty (distraction fascial arthroplasty) or arthrodesis. Total elbow arthroplasty is reserved for older, low-demand patients with stiffness who have severe degeneration of the ulnohumeral joint.

- Heterotopic ossification should not be excised until the bone appears mature (trabeculae). Extensive debridement may destabilize the elbow. Often, removal of the heterotopic ossification (HO) requires excision of the collateral ligaments. In these cases, ligament reconstruction with placement of a hinged fixator has shown good results. HO may be minimized or prevented with the use of bisphosphonates (inhibit mineralization of osteoid) or indomethacin (inhibits prostaglandin formation). Perioperative radiation may also prevent recurrence; a single dose of 800 or 1000 cGy divided over five doses should begin within 48 hours postoperatively.

References

Bruno RJ, Lee ML, Strauch RJ, Rosenwasser MP: Posttraumatic elbow stiffness: evaluation and management. *J Am Acad Orthop Surg* 10:106-116, 2002.

The extent of degenerative changes guides treatment for this condition. Soft tissue releases, debridement arthroplasty, resurfacing arthroplasty, and total elbow arthroplasty are presented.

Gates HS III, Sullivan FL, Ubaniak JR: Anterior capsulotomy and continuous passive motion in the treatment of post traumatic flexion contracture of the elbow: a prospective study. *J Bone Joint Surg Am* 74:1229-1234, 1992.

Anterior capsulotomy is an effective treatment of posttraumatic flexion contracture of the elbow. Although the postoperative use of continuous passive motion did not significantly improve mean active extension, it did improve active flexion and the total arc of motion.

Hastings H II, Graham TJ: The classification and treatment of heterotopic ossification about the elbow and forearm. *Hand Clin* 10:417-437, 1994.

Review of the risk factors, pathophysiology, pathoanatomy, and the potential role for reconstructive procedures.

Kashiwagi D: Osteoarthritis of the elbow joint: intraarticular changes and the special operative procedure, Outerbridge-Kashiwagi method. In Kashiwagi D, editor: *Elbow joint.* Amsterdam, 1985, Elsevier Science Publishers.

The technique for ulnohumeral arthoplasty is presented within this comprehensive text of pathologic conditions affecting the elbow.

Kim SJ, Kim HK, Lee JW: Arthroscopy for limitation of motion of the elbow. *Arthroscopy* 11:680-683, 1995.

Twenty-five patients with limitation of motion of the elbow joint caused by the intraarticular pathologies were treated with arthroscopic procedures. The total range of motion improved by 24 degrees, and 23 patients were satisfied with their results.

Mansat P, Morrey BF: Semiconstrained total elbow arthroplasty for ankylosed and stiff elbows. *J Bone Joint Surg Am* 82:1260-1268, 2000.

A semiconstrained total elbow arthroplasty was performed in 13 patients with a preoperative range of elbow motion of 30 degrees or less. Complications including reoperation were frequent, but the outcome was successful in the majority of patients.

McAuliffe JA, Wolfson AH: Early excision of heterotopic ossification about the elbow followed by radiation therapy. *J Bone Joint Surg Am* 79:749-755, 1997.

Excision of heterotopic ossification about the elbow was performed 3 to 10 months after the initial injury and followed by radiation therapy to prevent recurrence in eight patients. On the basis of this experience, it seems that the generally recommended 12- to 18-month delay between injury and excision, to allow for maturation of heterotopic bone and thus to lessen the likelihood of recurrence, may be eliminated.

Morrey BF: Distraction arthroplasty: clinical applications. *Clin Orthop* 293:46-54, 1993.

The concept of a hinged-joint distraction device appears to have broad clinical application in those circumstances in which both joint motion and joint stability are simultaneous treatment goals.

Weiss AP, Sachar K: Soft tissue contractures about the elbow. *Hand Clin* 10:439-451, 1994.

Motion-directed therapy often improves or eliminates elbow contracture if it is recognized early in treatment. Progressive soft tissue contracture, with or without the concomitant development of heterotopic ossification, is best treated by surgical release. This article discusses the operative technique and the results of treatment.

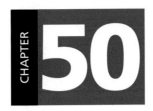

CHAPTER 50

Wrist and Hand Anatomy and Biomechanics

Kinematics

- Wrist motion involves three degrees of freedom: flexion/extension, radial/ulnar deviation, and pronation/supination.
- The radiocarpal joint contributes $\frac{2}{3}$ of wrist extension and $\frac{1}{3}$ of wrist flexion. The midcarpal joint contributes $\frac{1}{3}$ of wrist extension and $\frac{2}{3}$ of wrist flexion.
- Maximal grip strength is achieved with 35 to 40 degrees of extension and slight ulnar deviation.
- In an ulnar neutral wrist, 80% of compressive load is borne across the radiocarpal articulation and 20% across the ulnocarpal articulation.

Carpal Bones

- The carpal bones are divided into a proximal row (scaphoid, lunate, triquetrum, and pisiform) and distal row (trapezium, trapezoid, capitate, and hamate) (Figure 50–1).
- Ossification begins with the capitate at 1 year of age and progresses in a counterclockwise direction (Box 50–1).
- The scaphoid and trapezium form the lateral wall of the carpal tunnel and the triquetrum and hamate the medial wall. The median nerve lies radial to the tendons of the flexor digitorum profundus and superficialis; the flexor pollicis longus tendon lies radial to the nerve (Figure 50–2).
- The scaphoid is the most commonly fractured carpal bone. Branches of the radial artery supply the scaphoid in a retrograde fashion, the most important of which enter distally at the dorsal ridge; fractures of the proximal third of the scaphoid are prone to develop avascular necrosis of the proximal fragment.
- The pisiform is a sesamoid bone within the tendon of the flexor carpi ulnaris.
- The hamate has a prominent volar process, the hook of the hamate, which is commonly injured with a direct blow in golfers, tennis players, and baseball players.
  - A carpal tunnel radiographic view may show pisiform or hook of hamate fracture.

- Often, a computed tomography scan is necessary to define these injuries and should be obtained when clinical suspicion is high.

Metacarpals

- The five metacarpal bones are numbered from lateral to medial.
- The metacarpal heads have dorsal tubercles that serve as attachment sites for the collateral ligaments.
- Each metacarpal has an epiphysis in the head, except for the first metacarpal, which has an epiphysis in its base.
- The metacarpal shaft serves as the origin of the interossei muscles, and the metacarpal bases serve as points for tendon insertion (Box 50–2).
- The deep transverse metacarpal ligament stabilizes the heads of the second to fifth metacarpals.

Phalanges

- The digits are properly referred to as the thumb, index, long, ring, and small finger.
- The digits are composed of a proximal, middle, and distal phalanx, except for the thumb, which has only a proximal and distal phalanx.
- The epiphysis of each bone is in its base.

Radiocarpal/Ulnocarpal Joint

- The wrist joint is enveloped with a thin fibrous capsule that attaches proximally to the distal radius and ulna and distally to the first row of carpal bones. Stability is imparted to the joint by multiple surrounding ligaments (Box 50–3).
- The radius has facets for articulation with the scaphoid and lunate; the ulna articulates with the triquetrum through the triangular fibrocartilage complex.
- The triangular fibrocartilage complex (TFCC) stabilizes the distal radioulnar joint and is a load-bearing structure between the carpus and the ulna (Figure 50–3).

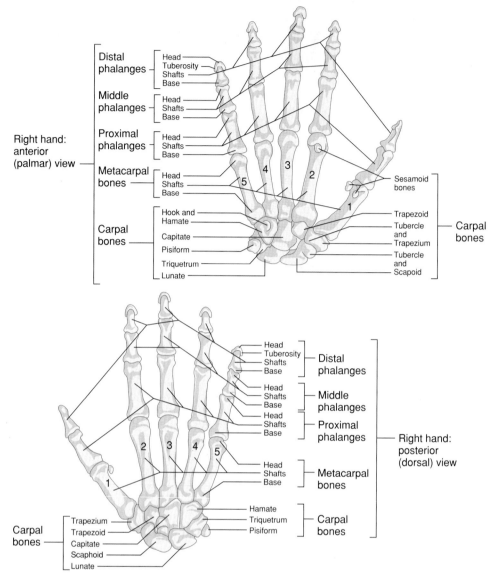

Figure 50–1:
Wrist and hand osteology. (Modified from Thompson JC: *Netter's concise atlas of orthopaedic anatomy*. Teterboro, NJ, 2002, Multimedia USA.)

- The TFCC is composed of the articular disc (triangular fibrocartilage proper), volar ulnocarpal ligaments, meniscal homologue, ulnar collateral ligament, dorsal and palmar radioulnar ligaments, and the floor of the extensor carpi ulnaris sheath.
- Similar to the menisci of the knee, the TFCC consists of a peripheral vascular zone and central avascular zone. Peripheral tears have the ability to heal, whereas central tears do not.
- Innervation of the joint derives from the anterior interosseous branch of the median nerve, the posterior interosseous branch of the radial nerve, and the dorsal and deep branches of the ulnar nerve.

Box 50–1	Carpal Bone Ossification

Capitate: 1 year
Hamate: 1 to 2 years
Triquetrum: 3 years
Lunate: 4 to 5 years
Scaphoid: 5 years
Trapezium: 5 to 6 years
Trapezoid: 5 to 7 years
Pisiform: 9 to 12 years

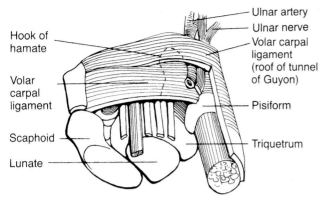

Figure 50–2:
Anatomy of the carpal tunnel. (From DeLee JC, Drez D Jr: *Orthopaedic sports medicine: principles and practice.* Philadelphia, 1994, Saunders.)

Box 50–3	Ligamentous Structures about the Wrist Joint

Volar radiocarpal ligaments
   Radioscaphocapitate ligament
   Radioscapholunate ligament
   Radiolunotriquetral ligament
Dorsal radiocarpal ligament
Dorsal Intercarpal ligament
Radial collateral ligament
Ulnar collateral ligament
Triangular fibrocartilage complex

Midcarpal and Intercarpal Joints

- The midcarpal joint is an ellipsoid joint through which ⅓ of wrist extension and ⅔ of wrist flexion occurs.
- Carpal bones within a row are stabilized by intrinsic ligaments. Ligament disruption may lead to instability.
  - Scapholunate ligament—disruption may lead to dorsal intercalated segment instability.
  - Lunotriquetral ligament—disruption may lead to volar intercalated segment instability.

Carpometacarpal Joints

- The thumb carpometacarpal joint is created between the trapezium and base of the first metacarpal. It is a saddle-type joint and a common site for arthritis.
- Motion of the carpometacarpal joints includes flexion, extension, adduction, and abduction, with the thumb having the greatest range of motion and the ability to be opposed to the other digits.

Metacarpophalangeal Joints

- Ellipsoid type joints between the heads of the metacarpals and bases of the proximal phalanges allow

Box 50–2	Tendon Insertions at the Metacarpal Bases

First metacarpal—abductor pollicis longus
Second metacarpal—extensor carpi radialis longus (dorsal), flexor carpi radialis (volar)
Third metacarpal—extensor carpi radialis brevis (dorsal), flexor carpi radialis (volar)
Fifth metacarpal—extensor carpi ulnaris (dorsal) and flexor carpi ulnaris (volar)

flexion, extension, adduction, abduction, and circumduction.
- Each joint is enclosed by a capsule strengthened by radial and ulnar collateral ligaments and a volar plate.
  - Collateral ligaments are tight in flexion and lax in extension.
  - The thumb ulnar collateral ligament is important to stabilize pinch, and injury to this structure is referred to as *gamekeeper's thumb.*

Interphalangeal Joints

- Uniaxial hinge joint permitting only flexion and extension.
- Collateral ligaments are tight in extension and lax in flexion.
- Dorsal (Cleland's) and volar (Grayson's) digital cutaneous ligaments stabilize the neurovascular bundles with finger motion.

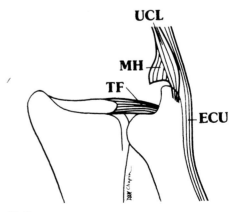

Figure 50–3:
The triangular fibrocartilage complex. ECU, Extensor carpi ulnris; MH, meniscal homologue; TF, triangular fibrocartilage; UCL, ulnar collateral ligament. (From Weissman BN, Sledge CB: *Orthopedic radiology.* Philadelphia, 1986, Saunders.)

Muscles

- The extensor retinaculum, a transverse fibrous band extending from the distal radius laterally to the styloid process of the ulna medially, overlies the extensor tendons crossing the wrist. Six extensor compartments are present (Figure 50–4).
- Distinct pathologic conditions are associated with each extensor compartment (Box 50–4).
- The anatomic snuffbox is bounded radially by the tendons of the abductor pollicis longus and extensor pollicis brevis and ulnarly by the extensor pollicis longus; the scaphoid and trapezium form the floor. The deep branch of the radial artery may be palpated within the snuffbox.

Box 50–4	**Extensor Compartments at the Wrist**

Abductor pollicis longus and extensor pollicis brevis—de Quervain's tenosynovitis
Extensor carpi radialis longus and brevis—intersection syndrome
Extensor pollicis longus—drummers wrist and rupture following distal radius fractures (more common with nondisplaced fractures
Extensor digitorum and extensor indicis—extensor tenosynovitis
Extensor digiti minimi—Vaughn Jackson syndrome (ischemic rupture in rheumatoids)
Extensor carpi ulnaris—tendinitis or subluxation of the tendon may occur

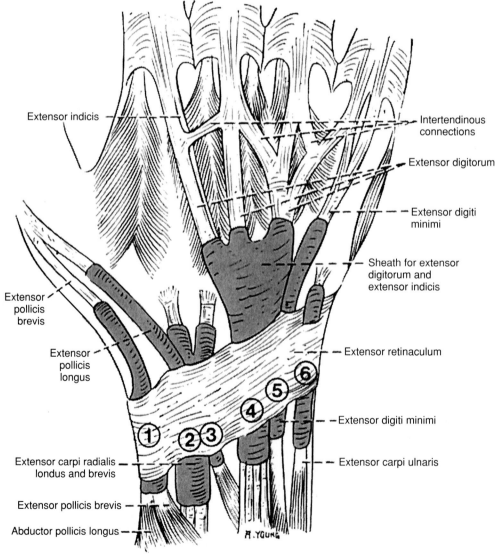

Figure 50–4:

Extensor compartments of the wrist. (From Jenkins DB: *Hollinshead's functional anatomy of the limbs and back,* 6th ed. Philadelphia, 1991, Saunders.)

- Metacarpophalangeal (MCP) and interphalangeal joint flexion and extension are achieved through the complex integrated action of the flexor tendons and intrinsic apparatus (Figure 50–5).
- The flexor digitorum superficialis tendon inserts at the dorsolateral aspect of the shaft of the middle phalanx and produces proximal interphalangeal flexion (PIP); the flexor digitorum profundus tendon inserts at the volar base of the distal phalanx producing distal interphalangeal flexion.

- Dorsal interossei muscles (abductors of the fingers) and volar interossei (adductors) also contribute to MCP flexion and PIP extension.
- Lumbricals originate on the flexor digitorum profundus tendons and insert on the radial lateral band of the extensor mechanisms; the lumbricals flex the MCP and extend the PIP joints.
- The thenar and hypothenar groups both include opponens, abductor, and flexor muscles.
- The thenar group also contains the adductor pollicis, which is critical for pinch strength.

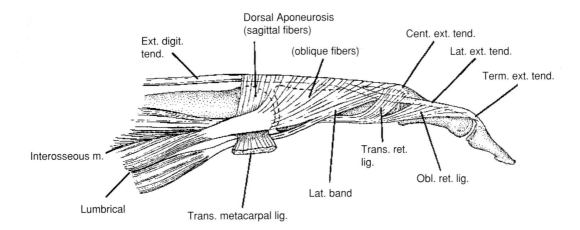

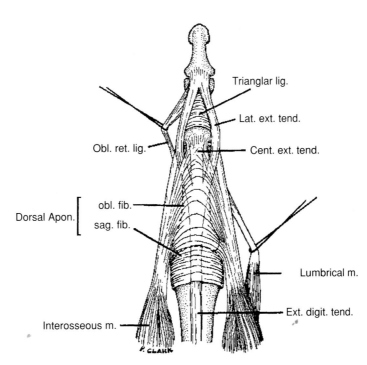

Figure 50–5:
Extensor apparatus of the digit. (From Miller MD: *Review of orthopaedics,* 4th ed. Philadelphia, 2004, Saunders. Modified from Bora FW: *The pediatric upper extremity.* Philadelphia, 1986, Saunders.)

Flexor Tendon Sheath

- Protects and nourishes the flexor tendons and maintains the flexor tendons in position throughout wrist and hand motion, preventing bowstringing.
- Includes five annular pulleys and three intervening cruciate pulleys in the fingers and two annular pulleys and one cruciate pulley in the thumb (Figure 50–6).
  - The A2 and A4 pulleys derive from bone at the proximal and middle phalanx, respectively, and are the most important in preventing bowstringing.

Vasculature

- The hand is supplied by the radial and ulnar arteries, which anastomose to form the deep and superficial palmar arches.
  - The deep palmar arch lies proximal to the superficial arch.
  - The ulnar artery is the major contributor to the superficial arch; radial artery is the major contributor to the deep arch.
  - Branches from the deep arch primarily supply the thumb and radial index finger; branches from the superficial arch primarily supply the other fingers.
  - In the digit, digital arteries lie dorsal to the digital nerves.

Ulnar Nerve

- Proximal to the wrist, gives off palmar and dorsal cutaneous branches that supply sensation to the ulnar aspect of the hand.
- The ulnar nerves passes through Guyon's canal at the wrist, formed by the pisiform (ulnar border), hook of the hamate (radial border), transverse carpal ligament (floor), and volar carpal ligament (roof). The nerve lies ulnar to the artery within the tunnel and divides into a superficial and deep branch.

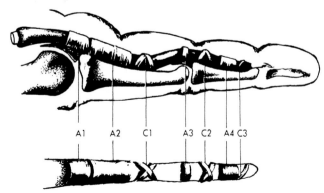

Figure 50–6:
Flexor pulleys. (From Tubiana R: *The hand.* **Philadelphia, 1985, Saunders.)**

- The ulnar nerve supplies sensory innervation to the ulnar one and one-half digits. Ulnar innervated muscles in the hand include the hypothenar muscles, medial two lumbricals, the interossei, the adductor pollicis, and the deep head of the flexor pollicis brevis.

Median Nerve

- The palmar cutaneous nerve branches from the median nerve approximately 5 cm proximal to the wrist crease and pass superficial to the carpal tunnel to supply sensation to the thenar eminence.
- The median nerve enters the wrist within the carpal tunnel, which is a frequent site of compression.
  - The motor branch of the median nerve most commonly branches just beyond the ligament with a recurrent pathway to supply the thenar muscles; however, other anatomic patterns are common.
- Median nerve innervated muscles in the hand include the radial two lumbricals, the opponens pollicis, abductor pollicis brevis, and the superficial head of the flexor pollicis brevis. Sensory innervation to the volar surfaces and dorsal tips of the radial three and one-half digits is provided by the median nerve.

Radial Nerve

- The superficial branch of the radial nerve supplies sensation to the lateral dorsum of the hand.

References

Agur AMR, Lee MJ: *Grant's atlas of anatomy,* 10th ed. Philadelphia, 1999, Lippincott, Williams and Wilkins.
Comprehensive anatomy textbook with detailed illustrations.

Hoppenfeld S, deBoer P: *Surgical exposures in orthopaedics,* 3rd ed. Philadelphia, 2003, Lippincott, Williams and Wilkins.
Comprehensive textbook of surgical exposures, complete with stepwise dissection instructions and full-scale drawings.

Jebson JL, Kasdan ML, editors: *Hand secrets,* 2nd ed. Philadelphia, 2002, Hanley and Belfus.
Review book written in question-and-answer format.

Miller MD, Gomez BA: Anatomy. In Miller MD, editor: *Review of orthopaedics,* 3rd ed. Philadelphia, 2000, Saunders.
Review textbook bridging multiple orthopaedic topics, well-suited for examination preparation.

Thompson JC: Chapter 4 (forearm anatomy) and Chapter 5 (hand anatomy). In Thompson JC, editor: *Netter's concise atlas of orthopaedic anatomy.* Teterboro, NJ, 2002, Multimedia USA.
Condensed version of illustrations pertinent to orthopaedic study.

Topper SM: Hand and microsurgery. In Miller MD, editor: *Review of orthopaedics,* 3rd ed. Philadelphia, 2000, Saunders.
Review textbook bridging multiple orthopaedic topics, well-suited for examination preparation.

CHAPTER 51

Wrist and Hand History, Physical Examination, and Imaging

History

- Age of the patient, hand dominance.
- Occupation, sports, activities.
- Acute versus chronic.
- Mechanism of injury.
- Environment in which the injury occurred.
- Pain: location, quality, severity, onset, timing, improving or exacerbating factors.
- Swelling or mass.
- Mechanical symptoms = stiffness, catching, locking.
- Neurologic symptoms = weakness, numbness, tingling.
- Medical comorbidities.

Physical Examination

Inspection

- Skin.
  - Color, temperature, moisture, scars, lesions.
  - Palmar skin much thicker, fixed by fascia.
- Nails.
  - Color, shape.
  - Paronychia or eponychia.
- Attitude or posture.
  - At rest, the metacarpophalangeal (MCP), proximal interphalangeal (PIP), and distal interphalangeal (DIP) joints are slightly flexed and the fingers cascade.
- Gross deformity.
  - Ulnar drift of fingers.
  - Swan neck: PIP hyperextended, DIP flexed (Figure 51–1).
  - Boutonniere: PIP flexed, DIP hyperextended (Figure 51–2).
  - Mallet finger: DIP flexed.
  - Trigger finger.
  - Rotational or angular deformities.
- Localized swelling.
  - Heberden's nodes at the DIP joint.
  - Bouchard's nodes at the PIP joint.
- Joint effusion.
- Muscle atrophy.
  - Thenar or hypothenar muscles.
  - Intrinsics.

Palpation

- Bony prominences for tenderness or crepitus.
  - Radial and ulnar styloids.
  - Radiocarpal joint.
  - Lister's tubercle.
  - Anatomic snuffbox (scaphoid).
    - Outlined by extensor pollicis longus (EPL), abductor pollicis longus (APL), extensor pollicis brevis (EPB).
  - Carpal bones.
  - Metacarpals.
  - Phalanges.
- Soft tissues for generalized areas of tenderness, masses.
  - Flexor tendons/sheaths.
  - Extensor tendon compartments (6).
    - 1=APL, EPB.
    - 2=extensor carpi radialis longus (ECRL), extensor carpi radialis brevis (ECRB).
    - 3=EPL.

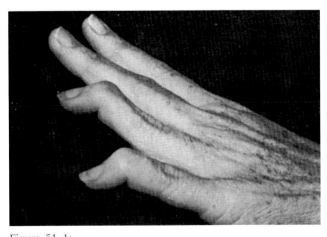

Figure 51–1:

Swan neck deformity. (From Green DP, Hotchkiss RN, Pederson WC, editors: *Green's operative hand surgery,* **4th ed. New York, 1999, Churchill Livingstone.)**

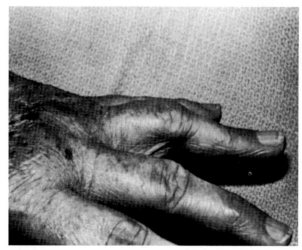

Figure 51–2:
Boutonniere deformity. (From Green DP, Hotchkiss RN, Pederson WC, editors: *Green's operative hand surgery,* **4th ed. New York, 1999, Churchill Livingstone.)**

- 4=extensor digitorum communis (EDC), extensor indicis proprius (EIP).
- 5=extensor digiti minimi (EDM).
- 6=extensor carpi ulnaris (ECU).
- Carpal tunnel.
- Scapholunate area.
- Thenar and hypothenar eminences.
- Palm for nodules.
- Distal fingertips.

Range of Motion

- Wrist.
  - Flexion (normal 80 degrees).
  - Extension (normal 75 degrees).
  - Radial deviation (normal 15 to 20 degrees).
  - Ulnar deviation (normal 30 to 40 degrees).
- Finger.
  - MCP.
    - Extension/flexion (normal 0 to 90 degrees).
    - Abduction/adduction (normal 0 to 20 degrees).
  - PIP.
    - Extension/flexion (normal 0 to 110 degrees).
  - DIP.
    - Extension/flexion (normal 10 to 80 degrees).
- Thumb.
  - Carpo-metacarpal (CMC).
    - Palmar abduction/adduction (normal 70 degrees).
  - MCP.
    - Extension/flexion (normal 0 to 50 degrees).
  - Interphalangeal (IP).
    - Extension/flexion (normal 10 to 90 degrees).
  - Opposition.
    - Thumb to small finger.

Neurovascular

- Motor (screening examination).
  - Posterior interosseous nerve (PIN).
    - Wrist and finger extension.
    - Thumb abduction and extension.
  - Anterior interosseous nerve (AIN).
    - "OK" sign: thumb IP flexion, index PIP flexion.
  - Motor recurrent branch (median nerve).
    - Thumb opposition.
  - Ulnar nerve.
    - Finger abduction/adduction.
- Strength.
  - Graded 0 to 5.
  - Wrist flexion.
    - Flexor carpi radialis.
    - Flexor carpi ulnaris.
    - Palmaris longus.
  - Wrist extension.
    - Extensor carpi radialis longus.
    - Extensor carpi radialis brevis.
    - Extensor carpi ulnaris.
  - Pronation.
    - Pronator quadratus.
  - Finger PIP flexion.
    - Flexor digitorum superficialis.
  - Finger DIP flexion.
    - Flexor digitorum profundus.
  - Finger extension.
    - Extensor indicis proprius (index finger).
    - Extensor digitorum communis.
    - Extensor digiti minimi (small finger).
  - Finger abduction.
    - Dorsal interossei (4).
    - Abductor digiti minimi.
  - Finger adduction.
    - Volar interossei (3).
  - Finger MCP flexion and PIP extension.
    - Lumbricals.
  - Thumb IP flexion.
    - Flexor pollicis longus.
  - Thumb MCP flexion.
    - Flexor pollicis brevis.
  - Thumb extension.
    - Extensor pollicis longus.
    - Extensor pollicis brevis.
    - Abductor pollicis longus.
  - Thumb abduction.
    - Abductor pollicis longus.
    - Abductor pollicis brevis.
  - Thumb adduction.
    - Adductor pollicis.
  - Thumb opposition.
    - Opponens pollicis.
  - Small finger opposition.

- ○ Opponens digiti minimi.
- Sensation.
  - Dermatomal distributions.
    - ○ C6 = Thumb, index.
    - ○ C7 = Long.
    - ○ C8 = Ring, small.
  - Peripheral nerve distributions.
    - ○ Superficial sensory (radial).
    - ○ Palmar cutaneous (median).
    - ○ Dorsal sensory (ulnar).
  - Two-point discrimination.
    - ○ Dynamic and static.
    - ○ Normal is 6 mm or less.
    - ○ May increase with age.
- Reflexes.
  - Hoffmann's sign.
    - ○ Flick long finger distal phalanx.
    - ○ Positive (pathologic) when thumb or index DIP spontaneously flexes.
- Vascular.
  - Radial and ulnar pulses.
  - Color, temperature, capillary refill.
  - Doppler arches, digital pulses.
  - Allen test for radial and ulnar artery patency.

Provocative Testing

- Carpal tunnel syndrome.
  - Pain, numbness, and tingling of thumb, index, long, and radial half of the ring finger.
  - Compression over the carpal tunnel is the most sensitive test.
  - Tinel's sign.
  - Phalen test.
  - Weak thenar musculature.
- Kanavel's signs (purulent tenosynovitis).
  - Flexed posture.
  - Tenderness of flexor sheath.
  - Fusiform swelling.
  - Pain on passive extension.
- Froment's sign.
  - Patient holds paper between thumb and index.
  - Examiner attempts to pull paper away.
  - Flexion of thumb PIP indicates adductor weakness, possible ulnar nerve palsy.
- Finkelstein's test.
  - Pain with ulnar deviation and thumb in palm.
  - First extensor compartment tenosynovitis.
- CMC grind.
  - Rotation and axial compression of thumb CMC joint.
  - Pain indicates arthritis at CMC and/or MCP joint.
- Flexor digitorum profundus (FDP) injury.
  - Inability to flex DIP with PIP stabilized in extension.
- Flexor digitorum superficialis (FDS) injury.
  - Inability to flex PIP with MCP stabilized in extension.
- Valgus thumb instability.
  - Apply valgus stress with thumb MCP stabilized.

- Laxity may indicate ulnar collateral ligament strain: skier's (acute) or gamekeeper's (chronic) thumb.

Imaging

- Plain radiographs.
  - Posteroanterior (PA), lateral, and oblique views (wrist, hand, or single digit).
  - Three smooth arcs of carpus on PA view.
    - ○ Ulnar variance.
    - ○ Scapholunate angle (normal 30 to 60 degrees) on lateral view.
    - ○ Spilled tea cup sign: lunate dislocation on lateral view (Figure 51–3).
  - Radial and ulnar deviation views.
  - Clenched fist anteroposterior (AP) view.
    - ○ Scapholunate interval widening.
  - Scaphoid (navicular) view.
  - Brewerton view.
    - ○ AP with metacarpals inclined 65 degrees.
    - ○ Good visualization of the metacarpal head and neck region.
  - Carpal tunnel view.
    - ○ Volar trapezium, pisiform, and hook of the hamate fractures.
- Stress views.
  - Gamekeeper's thumb.
- Ultrasound.
  - Differentiation between cystic and solid mass.
- Bone scan.
  - Septic arthritis.
  - Occult fracture.
  - Reflex sympathetic dystrophy.
- Computed tomography scan.
  - Distal radio-ulnar joint (DRUJ) injuries.
  - Carpal fractures, especially hook of the hamate (Figure 51–4).
  - Bony detail of tumors.

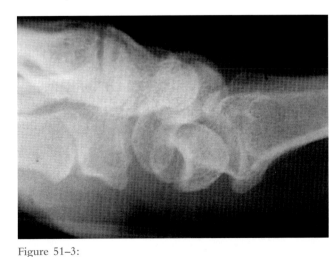

Figure 51–3:
Lunate dislocation. (From Lichtman DM, Alexander AH: *The wrist and its disorders,* **2nd ed. Philadelphia, 1998, Saunders.)**

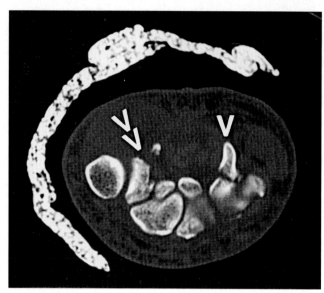

Figure 51–4:
Hamate and trapezium fractures. (From Lichtman DM, Alexander AH: *The wrist and its disorders,* 2nd ed. Philadelphia, 1998, Saunders.)

- Magnetic resonance imaging.
  - Infections, synovitis.
  - Scaphoid fracture or avascular necrosis (AVN).
  - Kienbock's disease (AVN of the lunate).
  - Triangular fibrocartilage complex injury.
  - Soft tissue masses.

References

Green DP, Hotchkiss RN, Pederson WC, editors: *Green's operative hand surgery,* 4th ed. New York, 1999, Churchill Livingstone.
  Comprehensive hand surgery textbook.

Lichtman DM, Alexander AH: *The wrist and its disorders,* 2nd ed. Philadelphia, 1998, Saunders.
  Comprehensive textbook focused on the normal wrist and its various pathologies.

Topper SM: Hand and microsurgery. In Miller MD, editor: *Review of orthopaedics,* 3rd ed. Philadelphia, 2000, Saunders.
  Review textbook bridging multiple orthopaedic topics and well-suited for examination preparation.

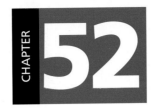

Wrist Arthroscopy

Introduction

- Wrist arthroscopy is often used when history, physical examination, and imaging have failed to produce an adequate diagnosis and treatment plan.
- Can be used both diagnostically and therapeutically for several wrist conditions.
- Advantages over open approaches are similar to other arthroscopic procedures and include direct visualization of the articular surfaces and stability of the intrinsic ligaments, less surgical dissection, less postoperative pain, faster recovery, and earlier return to work and activities of daily living.
- With the development of smaller, effective equipment and standardized techniques, wrist arthroscopy is becoming as common as arthroscopy of the knee and shoulder.

Indications

- Diagnostic.
  - Chronic wrist pain, unresponsive to conservative treatment.
- Intercarpal ligament tears.
- Extrinsic radiocarpal wrist ligament tears.
- Triangular fibrocartilage complex (TFCC) injuries.
  - Traumatic or degenerative.
- Internal fixation of intraarticular distal radius and scaphoid fractures.
- Carpal instability.
- Articular cartilage or osteochondral injuries.
- Dorsal ganglion excision.
- Contracture release.
- Bony excision procedures (proximal row carpectomy, radial styloidectomy, excision of distal ulna, partial resection/wafer procedures).
- Loose bodies.
- Synovectomy or synovial biopsy.
- Joint lavage for infection.
- The indications for wrist arthroscopy are still evolving.

Surgical Technique

- Supine position with the affected hand in a traction device (Figure 52–1).
- Traction towers have the additional advantage of being able to place the wrist in various degrees of flexion or radial/ulnar deviation, allowing a greater amount of visualization and access during arthroscopic procedures.
- A 2- to 3-mm scope with an angle of 25 to 30 degrees is most commonly used.
- A 1.5- to 2-mm scope may be more appropriate for the distal radioulnar joint in a small wrist.
- Fluid distention.
  - Most commonly by a gravity-flow system.
  - Other systems: hand pump, mechanical pump, pressure sensing.
- Available equipment should include a joint probe, grasping and basket forceps, power shaver and burr, suction basket, and occasionally small arthroscopic knives.
- Diagnostic arthroscopy should proceed in a systematic fashion.
- Debridement and therapeutic procedures should address underlying pathology and correspond to the patient's symptoms.

Portals

- Because of the greater concentration of neurovascular structures on the volar aspect of the wrist, the dorsal aspect of the wrist is principally used for arthroscopic portal entry.
- Five radiocarpal, four midcarpal, and two distal radioulnar portals are available for wrist arthroscopy (Figure 52–2).
- Radiocarpal portals (5).
  - Defined in accordance with their relationship to the dorsal compartments.
  - The 3-4 portal is the principal and initial portal site.
    - Lies approximately 1 cm distal to Lister's tubercle, between the extensor digitorum communis and extensor pollicis longus tendons.

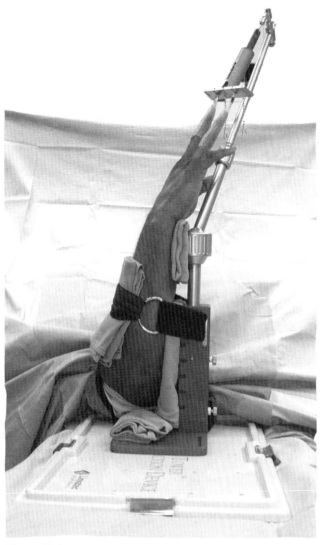

Figure 52–1:

Traction tower. (From Miller MD, Cole BJ: *Textbook of arthroscopy*. Philadelphia, 2004, Saunders.)

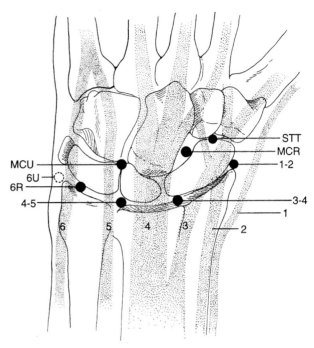

Figure 52–2:

Arthroscopic wrist portals. (From Miller MD, Osborne JR, Warner JJP, Fu FH: *MRI-arthroscopy correlative atlas*. Philadelphia, 1997, Saunders.)

- ○ Established using an 18-gauge needle placed between the extensor digitorum communis and extensor pollicis longus tendons at an angle corresponding to the volar and radial tilt.
- ○ The joint is then distended with 5 to 10 ml of fluid and the arthroscope introduced through a skin incision created with a No. 11 scalpel blade.
- ○ Provides good visualization of the volar radioscapholunate ligament, other radial ligaments, and the TFCC.
- • The 4-5 portal assists with instrument insertion.
  - ○ Located between the extensor digitorum communis and extensor digiti minimi tendons, approximately 1 cm ulnar to the 3-4 portal.

- ○ Provides visualization of the ulnar side of the radiocarpal joint, ulnocarpal ligaments, and the TFCC.
- • The 6R portal can be used for inflow, outflow, instrumentation, and visualization.
  - ○ Located radial to the extensor carpi ulnaris.
  - ○ Provides good visualization of the TFCC, ulnolunate, ulnotriquetral, scapholunate, and interosseous lunotriquetral ligaments.
- • The 6U portal is sometimes used for joint distention and outflow.
  - ○ Located ulnar to the extensor carpi ulnaris but is not commonly used because of the risk to the nearby dorsal ulnar sensory nerve.
- • The 1-2 portal is ideally suited for radial styloidectomy.
  - ○ Located distal to the radial styloid between the extensor carpi radialis longus and extensor pollicis brevis tendon.
  - ○ Provides visualization similar to the 3-4 portal.
  - ○ Not frequently used because of the proximity of the superficial sensory radial nerve and the radial artery as it passes through the anatomic snuffbox.
- • Midcarpal portals (4).
- • Should be used routinely in wrist arthroscopy procedures.
- • Essential in evaluating carpal (scapholunate and lunotriquetral) instability.

- Arthroscopic probes usually cannot enter between normal carpal joints.
- The midcarpal radial and ulnar portals are the most frequently used and the best for evaluating carpal mobility.
- The midcarpal radial portal.
  - Located 1 cm distal to the 3-4 radiocarpal portal, in line with the radial border of the third metacarpal, between the extensor carpi radialis brevis and extensor digitorum communis tendons.
  - Allows visualization of the midcarpal space, scapholunate, scaphocapitate, and scaphotrapezoid articulations.
- The midcarpal ulnar portal.
  - Located 1 cm distal to the 4-5 radiocarpal portal, in line with the shaft of the fourth metacarpal, between the extensor digitorum communis and extensor digitorum minimi tendons.
  - Provides good visualization of the lunotriquetral, lunocapitate, and triquetrohamate articulations.
- The scaphotrapezial-trapezoid portal.
  - Located between the extensor carpi radialis longus and extensor carpi radialis brevis tendons.
  - Best located with traction on the thumb and index finger.
  - Allows evaluation of the distal aspect of the scaphoid and its articulations with the trapezoid and trapezium.
- The triquetrohamate portal.
  - Located ulnar to the extensor carpi ulnaris, just proximal to the ulnar base of the fifth metacarpal and is occasionally used as an inflow or outflow portal.
- Distal radioulnar portals (2).
  - Used to examine the distal radioulnar joint when necessary and not accessible by general wrist arthroscopy.
  - The two portals used are located proximal and distal to the ulnar head and allow visualization of the proximal and distal radio-ulnar joint (DRUJ), respectively.
  - The distal portal lies just proximal to the TFCC and can evaluate its undersurface.

Complications

- Simple diagnostic and debridement procedures have minimal risk.
- Damage to neurovascular, ligament and tendon structures.

- Risks during portal placement can be reduced by using blunt dissection down to the wrist joint.
- The 6U radiocarpal portal is noted for its increased risk of injury to the dorsal ulnar sensory nerve.
- The 1-2 radiocarpal portal risks injury to the superficial sensory radial nerve and the radial artery.
- The distal and proximal distal radioulnar portals risk injury to the TFCC and the posterior interosseous nerve, respectively.
- Reflex sympathetic dystrophy.
- Tendon irritation/iatrogenic rupture.
- Chondral injuries.

Postoperative Care

- Sterile dressing, splint.
- Splint removed at first postoperative visit.
- Evaluate wounds, range of motion.
- Hand therapy not routinely required.
- Full recovery from most diagnostic procedures by 6 weeks.

References

Green DP, Hotchkiss RN, Pederson WC (eds): *Green's operative hand surgery,* 4th ed. New York, 1999, Churchill Livingstone.
 Comprehensive hand surgery textbook.

Koman LA, Poehling GC, Toby EB, et al: Chronic wrist pain: indications for wrist arthroscopy. *Arthroscopy* 6:116-119, 1990.
 A review of 54 consecutive arthroscopies of the radiocarpal and midcarpal joints in 53 patients with chronic wrist pain. The authors recommended arthroscopy for patients with the diagnosis of wrist pain of longer than 3 months' duration. Common indications include defects of the triangular fibrocartilage and lesions of the articular cartilage including loose bodies, which are easily detectable and treatable with wrist arthroscopy.

Miller MD: Sports medicine. In Miller MD, editor: *Review of orthopaedics,* 3rd ed. Philadelphia, 2000, Saunders.
 Review textbook bridging multiple orthopaedic topics, well-suited for examination preparation.

Miller MD, Cole BJ: *Textbook of arthroscopy.* Philadelphia, 2004, Saunders.
 Comprehensive textbook detailing arthroscopic techniques for all the major joints.

Poehling GG, Siegel DB, Koman LA, et al: Arthroscopy of the wrist and elbow. In DeLee JC, Drez D Jr, editors: *Orthopaedic sports medicine.* Philadelphia, 1993, Saunders.
 Comprehensive textbook of the principles and the practice of sports medicine.

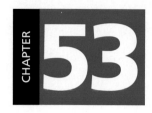

Carpal Instability

Classification (Figure 53–1)

Carpal Instability Dissociative (CID)

- Involves disruption of an intercarpal ligament within a carpal row. Can be dorsal intercalated segment instability (DISI) or volar intercalated segment instability (VISI).
- DISI: may result from disruption of the scapholunate ligament or unstable scaphoid fractures.
  - Examination: dorsoradial point tenderness, grip weakness, limited motion.
    - Positive Watson's test: radial deviation of the wrist while stabilizing the tuberosity of the scaphoid with volar pressure induces dorsal subluxation of the proximal pole of the scaphoid.
  - Imaging.
    - Anteroposterior (AP) view: scapholunate (SL) interval increased greater than 3 mm (Terry Thomas' sign, accentuated on closed fist view AP); scaphoid foreshortening—cortical ring sign (Figure 53–2).
    - Lateral: lunate dorsally flexed, scaphoid palmarly flexed. Scapholunate angle greater than 70 degrees (Figure 53–3). Increased radiolunate and capitolunate angles.
    - Magnetic resonance imaging: disruption of SL ligament.
  - Scapholunate advanced collapse (SLAC) is a typical pattern of arthritis that results from long-standing scapholunate dissociation (Figure 53–4). Degenerative arthritis begins between the tip of the radial styloid and the scaphoid, later to involve the entire radioscaphoid joint. This progresses to the lunocapitate joint and then the rest of the carpus. The radiolunate joint is usually spared.
  - Surgical algorithm for scapholunate dissociation takes into account the acuity of presentation, reducibility of the deformity, and degree of arthrosis. Acute cases are treated effectively with SL ligament repair ± capsulodesis, whereas either a proximal row carpectomy (PRC) or any of a variety of selective fusions may be done for chronic cases with arthrosis. The treatment of unstable scaphoid fractures and malunions is determined by the degree of scaphoid nonunion advanced collapse (SNAC) changes in the carpus.
- VISI: results from disruption of the lunotriquetral ligament.
  - Examination: ulnar-sided pain/tenderness, painful click or clunk with ulnar deviation and supination.
    - Positive ballottement test: palmar and dorsal displacement of the triquetrum while stabilizing the scaphoid reproduces characteristic pain.
  - Imaging.
    - AP—may see disruption of proximal arc.
    - Lateral—acutely one usually sees nothing. Over time the lunate palmarly flexes (Figure 53–3). Capitolunate angle less than 30 degrees or normal.
    - Treatment options include multiple pin fixation (early), LT fusion (chronically), ulnar shortening osteotomy.

		Midcarpal Instability	
Dissociative CID	SL Tear (DISI)	Lunate	LT Tear (VISI)
		Radiocarpal Instability	
		Non-dissociative CIND	

Figure 53–1:

Wrist instability diagram. Carpal instability dissociative (CID) results from intercarpal ligament rupture or carpal fracture. Scapholunate dissociation results in dorsal intercalated segmental instability (DISI), and lunotriquetral dissociation results in volar intercalated segmental instability (VISI). Carpal instability nondissociation (CIND) typically results from extrinsic carpal ligament rupture and may be either radiocarpal or midcarpal. (From Howard RF: Hand and microsurgery. In Miller MD, editor: *Review of orthopaedics,* 4th ed. Philadelphia, 2004, Saunders.)

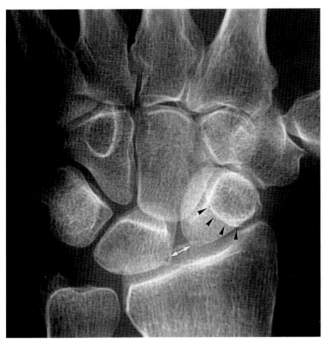

Figure 53–2:
Posteroanterior wrist film shows increased scapholunate interval and foreshortened scaphoid with cortical ring sign indicative of dorsal intercalated segmental instability. (From Garcia-Elias M: Carpal instabilities and dislocations. In Green DP, Hotchkiss RN, Pederson WC, editors: *Green's operative hand surgery,* 4th ed. New York, 1999, Churchill Livingstone.)

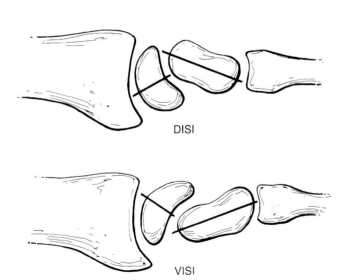

Figure 53–3:
Patterns of carpal instability as seen on lateral radiographs. Dorsal intercalated segment instability (DISI) is present when the lunate lies volar to the capitate but is flexed dorsally. Volar intercalated segmental instability (VISI) is present when the lunate lies dorsal to the capitate and is flexed volarly. (From McCue FC, Bruce JF: The wrist. In DeLee JC, Drez D Jr, editors: *Orthopaedic sports medicine: principles and practice.* Philadelphia, 1994, Saunders.)

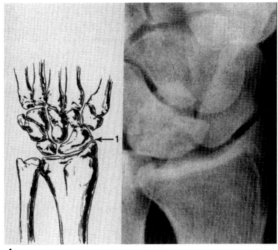

A

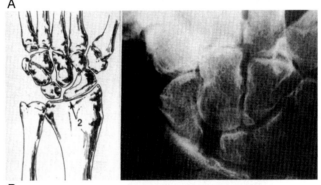

B

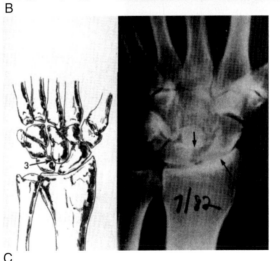

C

Figure 53–4:
Stages of scapholunate advanced collapse (SLAC). Pattern of arthrosis seen with chronic scapholunate dissociation. **A**, Stage I. **B**, Stage II. **C**, Stage III. (From Watson HK, Ballet FL: *J Hand Surg Am* 9:358-365, 1984.)

Carpal Instability Nondissociative (CIND)

- Instability between the radius and proximal carpal row, between carpal rows, or both.
- May result from laxity or disruption of radiocarpal or midcarpal ligaments. "Adaptive" midcarpal instability can

result from conditions leading to malalignment (malunited distal radius fracture).

- Examination: laxity, clunking sensation as lunate suddenly dorsiflexes as one goes from radial to ulnar deviation. Slight palmar pressure with the examiner's thumb on the capitate as the wrist is deviated from radial to ulnar accentuates the clunk.
- Imaging: cineradiography may demonstrate the "clunk" with radial or ulnar deviation.
- Treatment includes activity modification/splinting and selective fusion. Open repair and pinning is recommended for ulnar translocation. Various ligament reconstructions have been described for midcarpal instability; however, midcarpal fusion appears most reliable.

Carpal Instability Combined (CIC)

- Combines features of both CID and CIND.
- Perilunate instability.
  - Typically occurs following extreme wrist extension.
  - Mayfield described the typical sequence of carpal destabilization (Figure 53–5). The arc of injury progresses counterclockwise in four stages and may

include ligament disruption (lesser arc pattern) or carpal bone fracture (greater arc).
  - SL dissociation or scaphoid fracture.
  - Lunocapitate (midcarpal joint) dissociation.
  - Lunotriquetral (LT) disruption or triquetrum fracture.
  - Lunate dislocation (usually volar).
- Early open reduction, ligament repair, and pinning are recommended. Greater arc injuries require open reduction and internal fixation.

Carpal Instability Longitudinal (CIL)

- Traumatic disruption of the proximal and distal rows and intermetacarpal bases.
- May be axial radial, axial ulnar, or combined.
- Treatment includes reduction and pinning, prolonged casting.

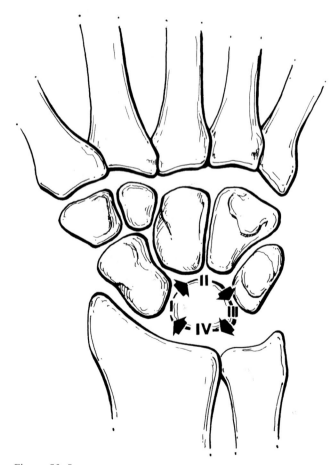

Figure 53–5:
Four stages of perilunate injury. (From McCue FC, Bruce JF: The wrist. In DeLee JC, Drez D Jr, editors: *Orthopaedic sports medicine: principles and practice.* **Philadelphia, 1994, Saunders.)**

References

Bednar JM, Osterman AL: Carpal instability: evaluation and treatment. *J Am Acad Orthop Surg* 1:10-17, 1993.
Instability patterns and treatment algorithm are presented.

Garcia-Elias M: Carpal instabilities and dislocations. In Green DP, Hotchkiss RN, Pederson WC, editors: *Green's operative hand surgery,* 4th ed. Philadelphia, 1999, Churchill Livingstone.

Howard RF: Hand and microsurgery. In Miller MD, editor: *Review of orthopaedics,* 4th ed. Philadelphia, 2004, Saunders.
Review textbook bridging multiple orthopaedic topics, and well-suited for examination preparation.

Kozin SH: Perilunate injuries: diagnosis and treatment. *J Am Acad Orthop Surg* 6:114-120, 1998.
Review of diagnosis and injury patterns of perilunate injuries. Treatment modalities are reviewed.

McCue FC, Bruce JF, Koman JD: The wrist in the adult. In DeLee JC, Drez D Jr, Miller MD editors: *DeLee and Drez's orthopaedic sports medicine,* 2nd ed. Philadelphia, 2003, Saunders.
Comprehensive textbook of the principles and the practice of sports medicine.

Shin AY, Battaglia MJ, Bishop AT: Lunotriquetral instability: diagnosis and treatment. *J Am Acad Orthop Surg* 8:170-179, 2000.
Review of lunotriquetral instability and methods of treatment.

Topper SM: Hand and microsurgery. In Miller MD, editor: *Review of orthopaedics,* 3rd ed. Philadelphia, 2000, Saunders.
Review textbook bridging multiple orthopaedic topics, well-suited for examination preparation.

Topper SM, Wood MB, Cooney WP: Athletic injuries of the wrist. In Cooney WP, Linschied RL, Dobyns JH, editors: *The wrist: diagnosis and operative treatment.* St Louis, 1998, Mosby.
Textbook focused on the diagnosis and treatment of wrist disorders.

Walsh JJ, Berger RA, Cooney WP: Current status of scapholunate interosseus ligament injuries. *J Am Acad Orthop Surg* 10:32-42, 2002.
Review of methods used to treat these injuries.

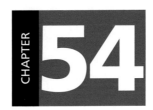

Ulnar-Sided Wrist Pain

Introduction

- Ulnar-sided wrist pain represents a wide spectrum of conditions that are often difficult to diagnose on history and physical examination alone.
- There are both intraarticular and extraarticular causes, and the workup should proceed in a systematic fashion to evaluate for all possible etiologies.
- Pain may arise acutely or progressively from trauma, repetitive microtrauma, tendon and anatomic abnormalities, neuropathy, or degenerative disease.
- A limited differential diagnosis includes fractures, triangular fibrocartilage complex (TFCC) injury, ulnar impaction syndrome, extensor carpi ulnaris tendonopathy, lunotriquetral ligament injury, pisotriquetral arthritis, ganglion cysts, and ulnar neuropathy.
- It is the physician's responsibility to sort out various contributing factors and proceed with an appropriate workup to arrive at a diagnosis.
- Advanced knowledge of wrist anatomy can guide the physical examination and narrow the differential diagnosis, but advanced imaging and/or wrist arthroscopy are often required to confirm the diagnosis.

History, Physical Examination, and Imaging

- Note the patient's age, sex, hand dominance, occupation, and activities.
- History taking should address prior surgery; recent or remote trauma; and the onset, duration, frequency, intensity, and quality of the pain.
- A complete physical examination as described in Chapter 51 should be performed and augmented with provocative maneuvers and special tests specific to the conditions being considered.
- Comparison with the unaffected extremity is an integral part of the examination.

- Initial radiographic evaluation should include a standard three-view (anteroposterior [AP], lateral, and oblique) series of the wrist.
- Evaluate for evidence of fracture, dislocation, arthritis, ulnar variance, and any other abnormalities.
- A computed tomography scan is recommended when further evaluation of the bony anatomy is required.
- Magnetic resonance imaging (MRI) and ultrasound can both be used to further assess the soft tissue structures about the wrist.
- Arthrography is a very sensitive test for evaluating the integrity of the TFCC, but in general, MRI provides more information and has largely replaced arthrography.
- Diagnostic arthroscopy is more frequently used in undiagnosed cases, providing the advantage of a dynamic evaluation and the ability to concurrently perform therapeutic procedures.
- Electromyography and nerve conduction studies are considered for symptoms of ulnar neuropathy.

Triangular Fibrocartilage Complex Injury

- The anatomy of the TFCC is shown in Figure 54–1.
- A very common cause of ulnar-sided wrist pain.
- Etiologies include acute compression injuries or repetitive microtrauma from activities involving frequent pronation and supination of the wrist.
- Degenerative tears are often associated with ulnar impaction syndrome.
- Patients often present with pain at the ulnocarpal joint that may be associated with popping or clicking.
- Tenderness is usually appreciated slightly palmar to the extensor carpi ulnaris.
- Pain can often be reproduced on physical examination by applying an axial load to an ulnarly deviated wrist and ranging it through supination and pronation.
- Lester described a "press test," in which the patient is asked to lift himself or herself out of a chair while bearing weight on the extended wrists; he considered the test to be 100% sensitive.

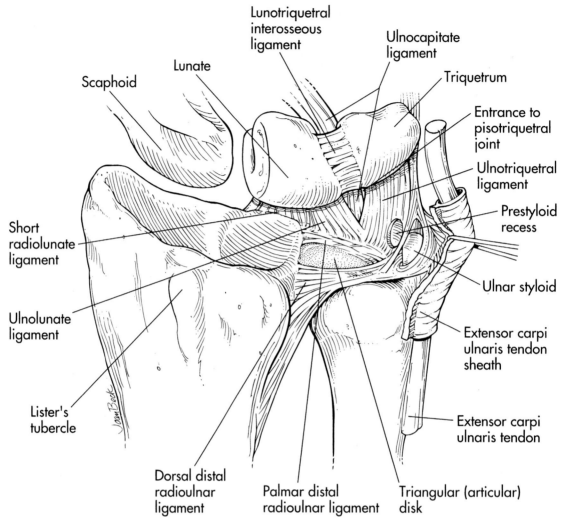

Figure 54–1:
Anatomy of the triangular fibrocartilage complex. (From Cooney WP, Linscheid RL, Dobyns JH: *The wrist: diagnosis and operative treatment.* St Louis, 1998, Mosby.)

- Standard AP radiographs for evaluating ulnar variance should be performed with the shoulder abducted 90 degrees, the elbow flexed 90 degrees, and the hand flat on the cassette, placing the distal radioulnar joint in neutral forearm rotation.
- A three-compartment arthrography, with injections of radiopaque dye into the carpal, midcarpal, and distal radioulnar joints, is positive when dye leaks from one compartment to another. This also allows localization of the tear from the leaking site.
- Arthroscopy is gradually replacing arthrography as the diagnostic test of choice, which not only provides direct visualization but also offers the option of therapeutic repair.
- Diagnostic arthroscopy can be supplemented with fluoroscopy to assess instability within the joints.

- Palmer and Werner devised a classification system that separates traumatic and degenerative TFCC tears and assists in determining treatment (Table 54–1).
- When not associated with instability, subluxations, or displaced fractures, TFCC tears are initially managed with immobilization, nonsteroidal antiinflammatory drugs (NSAIDs), and avoidance of aggravating activities.
- Failure of conservative management after 6 months is an indication for arthroscopic or open repair.
- Treatment is aimed at restoring normal anatomy and function.
- Failure to correct an associated ulnar positive variance that has led to an ulnar abutment syndrome will usually result in failure of TFCC repairs, secondary to inadequate decompression of the ulnocarpal joint.

Table 54–1:   Classification of Injuries of the TFCC

CLASS	DESCRIPTION	TREATMENT
Traumatic Lesions (Type 1)		
1A	Horizontal tear adjacent to sigmoid notch*	Debridement
1B	Avulsion from ulna ± ulnar styloid fracture	Suture repair
1C	Avulsion from carpus; exposes pisiform	Debridement
1D	Avulsion from sigmoid notch	Debridement
Degenerative Lesions (Type 2)		
2A	Thinning of TFCC without perforation†	
2B	Thinning of disc with chondromalacia	
2C	Perforation of disc with chondromalacia	
2D	Perforation of disc, chondromalacia, partial tear of lunotriquetral ligament	
2E	Perforation of disc, chondromalacia, complete tear of lunotriquetral ligament, ulnocarpal degenerative joint disease	

TFCC, Triangular fibrocartilage complex.
*Most common.
†Treatment for degenerative lesions includes debridement of loose degenerated discs, intraarticular resection of the ulnar head, and debridement of lunotriquetral ligament tears with percutaneous pinning of the lunotriquetral joint based on the pathology present.
From Miller MD, Cooper DE, Warner JJP, et al: *Review of sports medicine and arthroscopy.* Philadelphia, 2002, WB Saunders.

- In acute tears, operative management generally consists of debriding central tears and repairing peripheral tears, which have a rich vascular supply similar to meniscal tears in the knee.
- Debridement is carried out until there are no loose edges and a smooth rim of TFCC is created.
- The dorsal and palmar radioulnar ligaments must be preserved.
- Because class 2 lesions are associated with ulnar variation and impaction, surgical treatment focuses on decompression of the ulnocarpal joint (typically ulnar shortening).
- Tightening of the ulnocarpal ligaments makes this an ideal procedure in cases in which lunotriquetral instability exists.
- Open wafer (class 2A-C) or arthroscopic wafer (class 2C) are alternative options.
- Limited ulnar head resection or a Suave-Kapandji procedure are recommended for class 2E lesions (the Suave-Kapandji procedure involves arthrodesis of the distal radioulnar joint (DRUJ) and creation of a pseudoarthrosis at the ulnar neck).
- Distal ulnar resection for cases with ulnar positive variance is believed to have less morbidity than ulnar osteotomy procedures.
- After debridement and/or ulnar shortening, the extremity should be removed from traction and axial load is applied to the wrist in ulnar deviation while repeatedly ranging it through pronation and supination.
- If popping or clicking is noted, further debridement or further ulnar shortening may be required.

Ulnocarpal Impaction Syndrome

- Often found in conjunction with TFCC tears as explained previously.
- May be associated with posttraumatic or idiopathic premature closure of the radial epiphysis (as seen in a Madelung deformity).
- Patients present with ulnar-sided pain that is exacerbated when the wrist is axially loaded in ulnar deviation.
- Ulnar variance is measured as described previously.
- Excessive styloid length can be described as an ulnar styloid process index greater than 0.22, which is calculated by subtracting the ulnar variance from the ulnar styloid length and dividing by the width of the ulnar head.
- "Stylocarpal impaction" is sometimes observed in patients with long ulnar styloids with impaction between the styloid and triquetrum.
- Radiographic evaluation may reveal cystic or sclerotic changes along the lunate or ulnar head.
- Initial treatment involves activity modifications, NSAIDs, and occasionally steroid injections.
- Surgical options include epiphyseal arrest in children or ulnar shortening after growth plate closure.
- The wafer osteotomy described by Feldon and colleagues involves resection of 2 to 4 mm of cartilage and bone underlying the TFCC.
- Posttraumatic arthritis responds to ulnar head resection as described by Darrach, arthrodesis and ulnar pseudoarthrosis as described by Sauve-Kapandji, or a hemi-resection-interposition arthroplasty as described by Bowers.

Extensor Carpi Ulnaris Tendinitis/Subluxation

- Usually results from repetitive forceful pronation and supination activities as seen in tennis players that put extreme topspin on the tennis ball.
- Patients present with pain, swelling, and occasionally "snapping" along the extensor carpi ulnaris (ECU) that can be reproduced or exacerbated with active ulnar deviation in supination.
- Tendon subluxation and reduction may be appreciated with supination and pronation, respectively.
- Repetitive microtrauma can result in tendon irritation and lead to tearing or stretching of the ECU sheath and subsequent subluxation with a popping sensation reported by the patient.
- It is important to distinguish this condition from TFCC pathology.
- A local anesthetic/steroid injection into the ECU sheath can be diagnostic/therapeutic.

- Initial management consists of immobilization in a long arm cast with the forearm in pronation and the wrist in slight dorsiflexion for up to 6 weeks.
- NSAIDs can assist with controlling the initial inflammatory phase.
- Debridement of the sheath is recommended in cases of chronic tendinitis that have failed conservative management.
- Chronic instability of the ECU is treated with reconstruction of the fibro-osseous tunnel using a flap of the extensor retinaculum.

Lunotriquetral Ligament Injury

- Uncommon and often difficult to diagnose.
- Patients typically present with mild to moderate ulnar-sided wrist pain that can be exacerbated with translation of the triquetrum onto the lunate.
- Arthrography is only positive with complete ligament disruption.
- MRI may demonstrate the lesion, but often arthroscopy is required to make the definitive diagnosis.
- Mild cases can be treated with a splint for 2 weeks, followed by reevaluation.
- Partial tears typically respond to a period of immobilization that allows ligament healing and resolution of symptoms related to inflammation.
- Chronic cases or severe acute cases can lead to carpal instability and collapse and should be surgically repaired.
- Surgical options include lunotriquetral reduction and pinning or arthrodesis for more advanced chronic cases.

Pisotriquetral Arthritis

- Usually the result of a posttraumatic degenerative process, often from a remote fall onto the ulnar side of an extended wrist.
- Examination often reveals tenderness at the pisotriquetral joint with or without crepitus on pisotriquetral grind maneuver.
- Treatment is usually conservative with splinting, NSAIDs, and occasionally steroid injections.
- Surgical excision of the pisiform is considered in recalcitrant cases.

Ganglion Cyst

- Mucin-filled cyst that accounts for 50% to 70% of soft tissue tumors of the hand.
- Most commonly arise from a nearby joint capsule or tendon sheath.
- May be dorsal or volar but most arise dorsally from the scapholunate ligament (Figure 54–2).

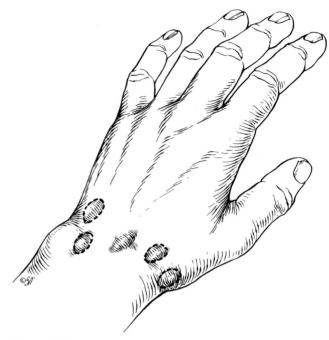

Figure 54–2:
Dorsal wrist ganglion locations. (From Green DP, Hotchkiss RN, Pederson WC, editors: *Green's operative hand surgery,* **4th ed. New York, 1999, Churchill Livingstone.)**

- The main body of the cyst may be located elsewhere from its origin, separated by a pedicle.
- Patients may present with symptoms of pain, weakness, or cosmetic concerns.
- Some ganglions may be occult and only evident with marked wrist flexion or extension.
- Some may become large and affect wrist motion or cause nerve impingement.
- Aspiration is associated with a 15% to 20% recurrence rate.
- Recurrence can be decreased to less than 10% by surgical excision that can be performed either open or arthroscopically.
- Failure to excise the origin (stalk) of the cyst increases the risk of recurrence.
- Excision may result in transient stiffness, scarring and decreased range of motion.

Ulnar Neuropathy

- Discussed in Chapter 47.

References

Green DP, Hotchkiss RN, Pederson WC (eds): *Green's operative hand surgery,* 4th ed. New York, 1999, Churchill Livingstone.
   Comprehensive hand surgery textbook.

Lichtman DM, Alexander AH: *The wrist and its disorders,* 2nd ed. Philadelphia, 1997, Saunders.

Comprehensive textbook focused on the normal wrist and its various pathologies.

Palmer AK: Triangular fibrocartilage complex lesions: a classification. *J Hand Surg Am* 14:594–606, 1989.

Drawing on 10 years of clinical experience, a classification system for degenerative and traumatic injuries to the TFCC lesions is presented. This classification is based on the clinical examination, routine x-ray films, wrist arthrograms, wrist arthroscopy, and wrist arthrotomy.

Topper SM: Hand and microsurgery. In Miller MD, editor: *Review of orthopaedics,* 3rd ed. Philadelphia, 2000, Saunders.

Review textbook bridging multiple orthopaedic topics, well-suited for examination preparation.

Topper SM, Wood MB, Ruby LK: Ulnar styloid impaction syndrome. *J Hand Surg Am* 22:699–704, 1997.

A case series of eight patients with an excessively long ulnar styloid that was affecting the triquetrum, causing pain secondary to chondromalacia and synovitis. All patients were treated by open partial ulnar styloidectomy and evaluated clinically and radiographically at an average of 34 months. All had reduction in pain and all but one returned to previous employment without restrictions.

CHAPTER 55

Wrist and Hand Overuse Injuries

De Quervain's Disease

- Overuse of the wrist and hand may lead to stenosing tenosynovitis of the first dorsal compartment at the wrist (abductor pollicis longus and extensor pollicis brevis). Racket sport athletes and golfers are prone to develop de Quervain's.
- Symptoms include dorsoradial wrist pain and swelling. Crepitus over the tendons may be detected with thumb motion.
  - Positive Finkelstein's test—ulnar deviation of the wrist with the thumb in the palm reproduces symptoms.
- Nonoperative treatment includes avoidance of aggravating activities, splinting of the thumb and wrist, nonsteroidal antiinflammatory drugs (NSAIDs), and local steroid injection.
- Surgical release of the first dorsal compartment should be considered in cases that fail nonoperative treatment.
  - Recurrent symptoms following release are usually secondary to incomplete decompression. Anatomic variations of the first dorsal compartment may include multiple tendon slips of the abductor pollicis longus (APL) and separate subcompartments. The superficial radial nerve and radial artery should be protected.

Intersection Syndrome

- Forceful, repetitive wrist motion may lead to tenosynovitis of the second dorsal compartment (extensor carpi radialis longus and brevis). This condition is commonly diagnosed in rowers ("oarsman's wrist") and golfers.
- Athletes may complain of pain and characteristic **crepitance** ("squeakers") in the radial distal forearm. Pain and swelling are localized more proximal in the forearm than de Quervain's at the location where the tendons of the first dorsal compartment cross over the second dorsal compartment.
- Nonoperative treatment includes splinting, NSAIDs, and local steroid injection.

- Surgical decompression of the second dorsal compartment with excision of the inflamed synovium or bursa between the two compartments is recommended for cases that fail conservative modalities for 3 months.

Extensor Pollicis Longus Tenosynovitis

- Symptoms of extensor pollicis longus tenosynovitis include dorsoradial wrist pain aggravated by thumb motion. The point of maximal tenderness may be located just distal to Lister's tubercle.
- Nonoperative modalities are usually successful; however, chronic tenosynovitis may lead to tendon rupture.

Extensor Carpi Ulnaris Tendinitis/Subluxation

- The extensor carpi ulnaris is secured tightly against the ulnar groove. Translation of the tendon with wrist rotation is resisted by the extensor sheath. Trauma to the extensor retinaculum (hypersupination or ulnar deviation injury) or tenosynovitis of the tendon may allow the tendon to slide out of its groove. These conditions are common in racket sport athletes.
- Patients with tendinitis present with pain along the dorso-ulnar border of the wrist and forearm exacerbated with resisted wrist extension. Subluxation presents with a painful snapping sensation with supination and ulnar deviation. It may be possible to displace the tendon from its groove manually.
- Tendinitis typically resolves to conservative treatment, including rest, NSAIDs, splinting, and injection.
- Subluxation that presents acutely may be treated with immobilization in a long arm cast with the forearm in pronation. Chronic and refractory cases are treated by surgical reconstruction of the ulnar septum of the sixth dorsal compartment with a strip of extensor retinaculum.

Flexor Carpi Radialis and Flexor Carpi Ulnaris Tendinitis

- Athletes who engage in forceful, repetitive wrist flexion may develop inflammation of the wrist flexor tendons.
- Symptoms include volar radial/ulnar wrist and forearm pain. Symptoms are elicited with resisted wrist flexion and radial/ulnar deviation.
- Nonoperative treatment includes rest, splinting, NSAIDs, and steroid injection.
- Surgical release of the flexor carpi radialis yields good results but is rarely necessary.

Acute Calcific Tendinitis of the Flexor Carpi Ulnaris

- Acute onset of excruciating pain in the volar ulnar wrist with no history of trauma may represent acute calcific tendinitis.
- Radiographs may show fluffy soft tissue calcification.
- May be misdiagnosed as cellulitis.
- Typically responds well to immobilization, ice, NSAIDs, and injection.

Trigger Finger

- Stenosing tenosynovitis of the digital flexor tendon sheath typically occurs beneath the A1 pulley. Athletes may participate in sports with repetitive and prolonged gripping and grasping. Pathophysiology involves fibrous metaplasia of the A1 pulley.
- Symptoms include pain, triggering, and episodes of locking. Tenderness is easily localized on physical examination.
- Nonoperative treatment includes antiinflammatory medications and local steroid injection. A maximum of three steroid injections should be given.
- Open or percutaneous release of the A1 pulley is usually curative.
  - Recurrent triggering following release may be secondary to a bulbous enlargement of the flexor tendon and may require reduction flexor tenoplasty. The radial digital nerve of the thumb is at risk with release of the thumb A1 pulley.

Reference

Wolfe S: Tenosynovitis. In Green DP, Hotchkiss RN, Pederson WC, editors: *Green's operative hand surgery,* 4th ed. Philadelphia, 1999, Churchill Livingstone.
   Comprehensive hand surgery textbook.

Finger Injuries

Introduction

- Frequent use of the hands in sports, occupations, daily activities, and hobbies subjects them to a high risk of injury.
- Multiple anatomic structures of the hands and fingers are at risk.
- A thorough history and physical examination combined with the appropriate plain radiographs usually reveals the diagnosis.
- Failure to make the proper diagnosis and treat accordingly can result in limited hand function and lead to permanent disability.
- Closed injuries of the hand are often missed on the initial evaluation.
- Early diagnosis and treatment results in the most successful outcomes.
- A comprehensive review of all finger injuries is beyond the scope of this book, but this chapter includes many commonly encountered conditions.

History, Physical Examination, and Imaging

- Patients usually present with a traumatic incident that produces limited finger function.
- Injuries can be either open or closed and occasionally produce a gross deformity.
- The time of injury and environment in which the injury occurred are important considerations.
- Mechanism of injury, particular disability, and aggravating motions should be noted.
- If the injury involves penetration of the skin, a tetanus booster may be required.
- The physical examination should be performed systematically and include assessment of the skin, muscles, tendons, ligaments, joints, nerves, and vascular supply of the hand and fingers.
- Plain radiographs of the hand or affected finger(s) should include posteroanterior, lateral, and oblique views.
- Occasionally, careful exploration of a wound is required at the initial evaluation.

Jersey Finger

- Avulsion of the flexor digitorum profundus (FDP) at its insertion on the volar surface of the distal phalanx.
- Commonly occurs in football players or other athletes from grabbing an opponent's jersey and forcing a flexed distal interphalangeal (DIP) joint into extension.
- Results in loss of active DIP joint flexion.
- The ring finger is affected most frequently.
- Early diagnosis is critical to prevent permanent disability caused by extensive fibrosis, scarring, and contracture.
- Physical examination often reveals a swollen, tender finger along the volar surface of the DIP joint and the inability to actively flex the distal phalanx with the proximal interphalangeal (PIP) joint stabilized in extension.
- PIP joint and metacarpophalangeal (MCP) joint flexion is preserved because of the intact flexor digitorum superficialis (FDS) tendon and lumbrical muscles.
- Plain radiographs may demonstrate a bony avulsion at the insertion site on the volar base of the distal phalanx.
- The FDP tendon may be retracted and difficult to retrieve.
- The retracted tendon end may be appreciated on radiographs if a bony fragment is present or may only be seen on magnetic resonance imaging.
- A classification system derived by Leddy and Packer is based on the final location of the retracted tendon and helps to guide treatment (Table 56–1).
- A fourth type was later added by Smith.
- Early repair is recommended, although some believe it can be postponed up to 3 months in some injuries.
- Type I injuries are dysvascular and require surgical management within 7 to 10 days to provide optimal results.
- Repair can be performed using a pullout suture over a button.
- Repair may require a separate incision to retrieve a retracted tendon and should ensure that the tendon is passed under the annular pulleys to prevent bowstringing.

Table 56–1: Leddy Classification of Profundus Avulsions

TYPE	TENDON RETRACTION LEVEL	REPAIR	INTERVAL/TREATMENT
I	Palm	(Dysvascular)	7-10 days
II (most common)	PIPJ (held by vinculum longus)		3 mo
III	A4 pulley (held by bony avulsion fragment)	ORIF fragment	
IIIa	Type III but profundus also avulses off fracture fragment	Treatment based on level of tendon retraction	

ORIF, Open reduction and internal fixation; PIPJ, proximal interphalangeal joint.
From Miller MD, editor: *Review of orthopaedics*, 4th ed. Philadelphia, 2004, Saunders.

- Tethering of the repaired tendon to an adjacent tendon creates an active flexion lag of the adjacent digit because they share a common muscle belly.
- Delayed repairs are complicated by extensive scarring and are best managed by simple observation, tendon grafting, or DIP arthrodesis.
- Tendon repairs are the weakest between postoperative days 6 and 12.
- Postoperative care involves dynamic splinting and rehabilitation including passive flexion and active extension exercises (Kleinert's protocol).

Flexor Tendon Injury

- Flexor tendons may be partially or fully avulsed or lacerated.
- The FDS may be injured in isolation or in conjunction with the FDP tendon.
- FDS tendon rupture is indicated by lack of PIP joint flexion with all unaffected fingers held in full extension by the examiner.
- The small finger FDS test is unreliable up to 30% of the time.
- Patients with partial injuries may demonstrate full range of motion but often have weak and painful resisted motion.
- Complete ruptures of both the FDS and FDP will result in loss of PIP and DIP flexion.
- Flexor tendon injuries are classified by zone (Figure 56–1).
  - Zone 1: fingertip to the FDS insertion on the middle phalanx.
  - Zone 2: FDS insertion to the distal palmar crease ("no man's land").
  - Zone 3: distal palmar crease to the distal aspect of the transverse carpal ligament.
  - Zone 4: carpal tunnel.
  - Zone 5: wrist crease to the musculotendinous junction.
- Ruptured flexor tendons (>60% of the cross-sectional area) should be repaired acutely to restore normal function.
- Delayed repair is associated with increased adhesion formation.
- Recommended repair technique includes the use of a core suture augmented with a running epitendinous suture.

- The strength of repair is directly proportional to the number of core suture strands crossing the repair site.
- Epitendinous sutures add strength and may reduce the incidence of adhesion formation.
- Following repair, the hand is immobilized in a dorsal splint with the wrist in 30 degrees of flexion, the MCP joints in 60 degrees of flexion, and the PIP and DIP joints in full extension.
- Rehabilitation consists of early motion with gradual progression from passive to active-assisted to active range-of-motion protocols, based on the quality of repair, patient compliance, and reliability of the therapist.

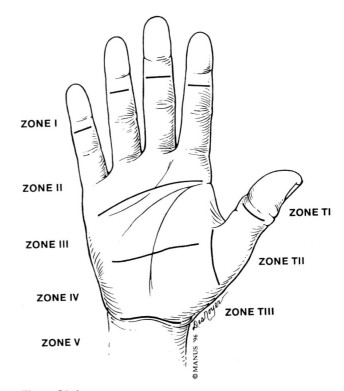

Figure 56–1:
Zones of tendon injury. (From Green DP, Hotchkiss RN, Pederson WC, editors: *Green's operative hand surgery*, 4th ed. New York, 1999, Churchill Livingstone.)

Mallet Finger

- Also referred to as "drop finger" or "baseball finger," this injury results when the terminal extensor tendon is avulsed from its insertion on the dorsal surface of the distal phalanx.
- The mechanism of injury is forceful flexion of an extended finger at the DIP joint.
- Can occur from attempting to catch a baseball or being struck by a volleyball.
- May also result from a laceration or an avulsion fracture of the distal phalanx.
- Some patients will not seek early evaluation if the injury produces little pain and the deformity does not interfere with daily activities.
- A chronic untreated mallet finger may gradually produce a disabling swan neck deformity.
- Initial presentation may reveal ecchymosis, swelling, and tenderness over the dorsal DIP joint, but occasionally these signs will be completely absent.
- All patients will demonstrate some degree of extensor lag at the DIP joint.
- Plain radiographs may demonstrate a bony avulsion or volar subluxation of the distal phalanx.
- Most cases can be managed nonoperatively with strict splint immobilization of the DIP joint for 6 to 8 weeks, followed by nighttime splinting for another 4 to 6 weeks.
- The PIP joint should not be immobilized to avoid unnecessary joint stiffness.
- Most bony mallet injuries can also be treated nonoperatively with closed reduction and splint immobilization for 6 to 8 weeks.
- Bony mallet injuries involving more than 50% of the articular surface, those producing volar subluxation of the distal phalanx, or those associated with significant malrotation may require open reduction and internal fixation (ORIF).

Extensor Mechanism Rupture (Central Slip Injury)

- Avulsion of the central slip from its insertion at the dorsal base of the middle phalanx usually occurs either from forced flexion of an extended PIP joint or may be secondary to a volar PIP joint dislocation in the acute setting.
- PIP joint dislocation will produce an obvious deformity, but the joint is often relocated prior to presentation and should be noted in the patient's history.
- May occur insidiously in patients with rheumatoid arthritis.
- Physical examination often reveals tenderness and ecchymosis over the dorsal aspect of the PIP joint in an acute injury.

- Many patients are still capable of extending the PIP joint through the intact lateral bands, but weakness of extension is often appreciated.
- The lateral bands subluxate volarly and act as PIP joint flexors.
- The intrinsic muscle forces on the DIP joint are increased, resulting in compensatory hyperextension.
- The resulting position of PIP flexion and DIP hyperextension is called a *boutonniere deformity*.
- This deformity may take up to 3 weeks to become apparent after a traumatic injury.
- Treatment of traumatic ruptures involves splinting the PIP joint in extension, with the DIP and MCP joints free, for 6 to 8 weeks.
- The DIP joint should be actively stretched in flexion to prevent contracture.
- Acute surgical repairs are indicated in irreducible avulsion fractures and open injuries that require irrigation and debridement.
- A tendon graft or local extensor mechanism flap may be required to attain adequate length.
- Treatment of chronic injuries must address the resulting boutonniere deformity.
- Repairs should only be performed after full passive range of motion of the joints is restored.
- Severe chronic deformities may require arthroplasty or fusion.

Sagittal Band Rupture (Extensor Tendon)

- Most commonly results from forceful flexion or extension injuries that cause the extensor tendon to subluxate or dislocate and tear the sagittal band.
- May also result from lacerations.
- Commonly seen in boxing and martial arts.
- The long finger is the most commonly affected.
- Patients often present with pain and loss of active extension at the MCP joint and may complain of a popping sensation as the tendon glides over the dorsum of the joint with range of motion.
- Acute injuries can be managed with an extension splint for 4 to 6 weeks.
- Delayed diagnosis may require surgical repair with centralization and stabilization of the extensor tendon.

Collateral Ligament Injuries of the PIP and MCP Joints

- A jammed finger usually results in damage to the collateral ligament of the PIP joint.
- Damage to the MCP joint collateral ligament is seen more often among athletes and usually involves the radial collateral ligament.

- Radial collateral ligament tears are more common than ulnar collateral ligament tears.
- Physical examination reveals tenderness along the side of the joint and is exacerbated when stress is applied to the affected side.
- PIP joint collateral ligament injuries respond well to 3 to 6 weeks of buddy taping.
- MCP joint injuries are splinted with the MCP joint in 50 degrees of flexion.
- Surgical repair of a complete tear of the index PIP radial collateral ligament is controversial, although repair of the index MCP radial collateral ligament is generally accepted.

Ulnar Collateral Ligament Injury of the Thumb MP Joint

- Also referred to as a skier's thumb (acute) or gamekeeper's thumb (chronic).
- Originally described in Scottish gamekeepers who suffered attritional wear of the ulnar collateral ligament from repeatedly twisting the head and neck of hares.
- Now commonly associated with skiers who forcefully abduct their thumbs from holding onto their ski poles during a fall.
- Partial or complete tears result from forceful valgus stress (abduction or radial deviation) of the thumb MCP joint.
- Avulsions of the ligament most frequently occur from its distal attachment on the proximal phalanx.
- Patients often present with pain, swelling, and occasionally gross radial deviation of the thumb MCP joint.
- Physical examination reveals tenderness at the ulnar aspect of the MCP joint and instability with valgus stress (must be compared with the contralateral thumb).
- Valgus stress testing must be performed with the MCP joint fully flexed and then fully extended.
- In the fully flexed position, radial deviation of the thumb greater than 35 degrees implies complete ulnar collateral ligament avulsion.
- In the fully extended position, any degree of instability is secondary to ligament avulsion.
- Plain radiographs should be obtained to rule out an avulsion fracture.
- Stress radiographs can further assess the severity of the injury.
- Partial ruptures are treated with a thumb spica cast for 4 to 6 weeks, followed by physical therapy to restore range of motion and strength.
- Complete ruptures may be associated with an interposition of the adductor pollicis aponeurosis between the torn ends (Stener's lesion), which may prevent healing (Figure 56–2).

- Surgical indications include displaced avulsion fractures, complete tears, and joint subluxation.
- Surgery consists of ORIF of any displaced bony fragments, removal of the Stener's lesion, and reattachment of the ligament to the proximal phalanx with a suture anchor.
- Chronic cases require abductor tendon advancement, ligament reconstruction, or tendon graft, because primary repair is usually not possible.
- Postoperatively, patients are treated with a thumb spica cast followed by rehabilitation.

Radial Collateral Ligament Injury of the Thumb MCP Joint

- This rare injury results from forceful varus stress (adduction or ulnar deviation) applied to the thumb MCP joint.
- Not as incapacitating as ulnar collateral ligament injuries.
- The thumb often remains functional, even with complete disruption of the ligament.
- Most partial and complete tears respond to splint immobilization.

Dorsal PIP Dislocation (Volar Plate Injury)

- The most common articular injury in the hand.
- More common than volar PIP dislocations.

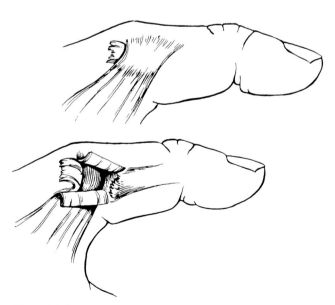

Figure 56–2:
Stener's lesion. (From Green DP, Strickland JW: The hand. In DeLee JC, Drez D Jr, editors: *Orthopaedic sports medicine: principles and practice.* **Philadelphia, 1994, Saunders.)**

- Produces avulsion of the volar plate and is classified into three types.
- Type I involves hyperextension of the joint and volar plate avulsion.
  - This injury is successfully treated by reduction and buddy taping for 2 weeks.
- Type II is characterized by complete dorsal dislocation with volar plate avulsion and bilateral collateral ligament disruption.
  - These are best managed by reduction and extension block splinting in 20 to 30 degrees of flexion for 3 to 6 weeks.
- Type III injury is considered a fracture-dislocation with comminution of the joint.
  - Stable fracture-dislocations (involving < 30% of the articular surface) can initially be managed conservatively with reduction and extension block splinting, followed by gradual straightening over a period of 4 to 6 weeks.
  - Unstable fracture-dislocations (>30% of the articular surface) and irreducible dislocations require traction, ORIF, or volar plate arthroplasty.
  - Injuries with extensive comminution may require arthroplasty or arthrodesis.
- The key to all treatment is restoration of articular congruity.

Volar PIP Dislocation

- Not as common as dorsal PIP dislocations.
- Mechanism of injury usually involves an axial load on a flexed PIP joint.
- Severe dislocation advances the distal condyles of the proximal phalanx through the extensor mechanism and ruptures the central slip.
- In rotational injuries, the proximal phalanx may disrupt a lateral band and cause it to subluxate.
- Injuries that appear stable and have an intact central slip can be treated by buddy taping and protected rehabilitation.
- Injuries that disrupt the central slip are managed with closed reduction and splinting of the PIP joint in extension.
- Dislocations involving interposition of the lateral band are best reduced by flexing the MCP and PIP joints and applying longitudinal traction to pull the condyles back under the middle phalanx.
- Open reduction is required if the dislocation is irreducible by closed means.
- Unstable associated fractures may require pinning and/or open surgical repair.

Metacarpophalangeal Joint Dislocation

- Less common than PIP joint dislocations.
- Dorsal dislocations occur from forceful hyperextension and are much more common than volar dislocations.

- Reduction of dorsal dislocations should be performed by hyperextending the proximal phalanx while applying a volarly directed force with the wrist and interphalangeal joints in flexion (relaxing the flexor tendons).
- Following closed reduction, a short period of buddy taping is often sufficient to restore full finger function.
- Reduction may be blocked by interposition of the volar plate within the joint and a buttonhole effect produced by trapping of the metacarpal head between the flexor tendons and lumbricals.
- Clinical evaluation of these injuries reveals puckering of the skin, intraarticular sesamoids, and parallelism of the proximal phalanx and metacarpal on radiographs.
- In irreducible fractures requiring open means, a dorsal approach carries less risk of injury to the digital arteries and nerves.
- Postoperatively, the finger is placed in an extension block splint for 1 week followed by progressive range of motion.
- Closed reduction of volar dislocations involves hyperflexion of the MP joint and a dorsally directed pressure on the proximal phalanx.
- Open reduction is required if closed reduction is not possible.

Thumb Dislocations

- Simple dislocations of the thumb can be managed by closed reduction and thumb spica cast immobilization for approximately 3 weeks.
- Similar to PIP dislocations, irreducible thumb dislocations usually suggest interposition of the volar plate and require open reduction.

Metacarpal Fractures

- Metacarpal fractures are common injuries in adults.
- Fractures can occur at the base, shaft, neck, or head of the metacarpal.
- The most common is a fracture of the fifth metacarpal neck, termed a *boxer's fracture*.
- Boxer's fractures occur from striking an object on the ulnar aspect of a closed fist.
- Physical examination must focus on the degree of malrotation, best appreciated by having the patient slowly make a fist and observing for overlap of the fingers.
- Each finger should point toward the scaphoid tubercle.
- Must compare with the contralateral hand.
- Malrotation is the least tolerated deformity in metacarpal fractures.
- Radiographic evaluation must describe any displacement, angulation, rotation, and shortening.
- The second and third metacarpals are inherently more rigid and tolerate less angulation than the more mobile fourth and fifth metacarpals.

- Second and third metacarpal shaft fractures can tolerate 10 degrees of angulation, whereas the fourth and fifth can tolerate 20 and 30 degrees, respectively.
- Metacarpal neck fractures of the index and long fingers can tolerate 15 degrees of angulation, whereas neck fractures of the ring and small fingers can tolerate 30 and 50 degrees, respectively.
- Fractures of the metacarpal head are rare.
- Minimally displaced fractures that fall within the above limits of angulation and are not malrotated can be successfully managed in splint or cast immobilization for 3 to 4 weeks.
- Immobilization in the intrinsic plus position is recommended—MCP in 80 to 90 degrees of flexion and the PIP and DIP joints in full extension.
- Significantly displaced, malangulated, or malrotated fractures can be treated with percutaneous pinning or open reduction internal fixation (ORIF).
- Percutaneous pinning can be achieved by intramedullary fixation or through fixation to an adjacent bone with pins removed at 4 weeks.
- Some comminuted fracture patterns may respond better to traction and external fixation.
- The most common complications of metacarpal fractures include loss of knuckle prominence, joint stiffness, and posttraumatic arthritis.

Thumb Metacarpal Base Fractures

- Second most common metacarpal fracture and the most common fracture of the thumb.
- Most frequently seen in the dominant hand of males younger than 30 years.
- The mechanism of injury is an axial force applied to a partially flexed thumb.
- Fractures may be extraarticular or intraarticular (Figure 56–3).
- Transverse extraarticular fractures without significant displacement can be managed by closed reduction and immobilization in a thumb spica cast for 4 to 6 weeks.
- Oblique and significantly displaced extraarticular fractures are best treated with closed reduction and percutaneous pinning.
- Bennett's fracture is an intraarticular fracture-subluxation of the metacarpal base with proximal, dorsal, and radial subluxation caused by the abductor pollicis longus.
- Treatment depends on the degree of articular involvement, with closed reduction and immobilization acceptable for fractures involving less than 20% of the articular surface and ORIF recommended for those involving greater than 30%.

- Rolando's fracture is a T- or Y-shaped intraarticular fracture with comminution.
- Treatment depends on the degree of comminution, with percutaneous pinning, external fixation, or ORIF with or without bone grafting appropriate in different patterns of injury.

Phalangeal Fractures

- Divided into intraarticular and extraarticular base, diaphyseal, neck, and condylar fractures of the distal, middle, or proximal phalanges.
- The distal phalanx is the most commonly fractured bone in the hand and usually involves the thumb or long finger.
- Tuft fractures of the distal phalanx are often associated with nailbed injuries.
- Stable, minimally displaced fractures can be treated with immobilization in casts, splints, or buddy taping for approximately 3 weeks.
- Unstable, significantly displaced fractures can be managed by closed reduction and percutaneous pinning.
- ORIF is usually reserved for irreducible, unstable, or incongruent articular surface fractures.
- Significantly comminuted fractures may require traction.

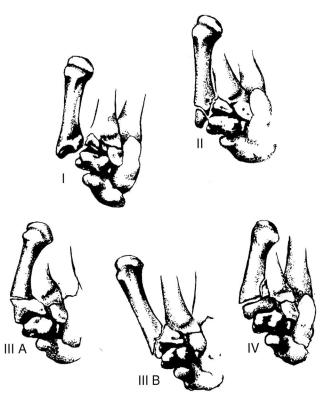

Figure 56–3:
Classification of first metacarpal base fractures. (From Green DP, O'Brien ET: *South Med J* 65:807, 1972.)

- Intraarticular fractures have a high incidence of arthritis and a poorer prognosis in general.
- Range-of-motion exercises should be implemented early to avoid joint stiffness.

References

Buchler U, McCollam SM, Oppikofer C: Comminuted fractures of the basilar joint of the thumb: combined treatment by external fixation, limited internal fixation and bone grafting. *J Hand Surg* 16A:556-560, 1991.

A case series of 13 patients receiving combined treatment reviewed retrospectively at an average follow-up of 35 months. The majority had a good subjective result and the overall union rate was 100%, although focal articular irregularities were commonly seen radiographically and strength and range of motion were decreased as compared with the contralateral thumb.

Green DP, Hotchkiss RN, Pederson WC, editors: *Green's operative hand surgery*, 4th ed. New York, 1999, Churchill Livingstone.

Comprehensive hand surgery textbook.

Jebson PGL, Engber WD, Lange RH: Dislocations and fracture-dislocations of the carpometacarpal joints. *Orthop Rev* 23:19-28, 1994.

This article reviews the pertinent anatomy, mechanism of injury, evaluation, and treatment of patients with carpometacarpal joint injuries.

Kozin SH, Bishop AT: Gamekeeper's thumb: early diagnosis and treatment. *Orthop Rev* 23:797-804, 1994.

A comprehensive review article describing the diagnosis and treatment of gamekeeper's thumb.

Leddy JP, Packer JW: Avulsion of the profundus tendon insertion in athletes. *J Hand Surg* 2:66-69, 1977.

A review of 36 avulsions of the flexor profundus tendon insertion in athletes seen during a 5-year period, giving a classification scheme and treatment recommendations.

Lichtman DM, Alexander AH: *The wrist and its disorders,* 2nd ed. Philadelphia, 1997, WB Saunders.

Comprehensive textbook focused on the normal wrist and its various pathologies.

Lister GD, Kleinert HE, Kutz JE, et al: Primary flexor tendon repair followed by immediate controlled mobilization. *J Hand Surg* 2:441-451, 1977.

A study of the results of immediate repair and controlled mobilization in 156 severed flexor tendons in 68 patients occurring over an 18-month period.

Smith JH: Avulsion of a profundus tendon with simultaneous intra-articular fracture of the distal phalanx [case report]. *J Hand Surg* 6A:600-601, 1981.

Case report where a fourth type of profundus tendon avulsion was classified.

Stener B: Displacement of the ruptured ulnar collateral ligament of the metacarpophalangeal joint of the thumb: a clinical and anatomical study. *J Bone Joint Surg Br* 44:869-879, 1962.

The classic article describing the Stener lesion in gamekeeper's thumbs.

Topper SM: Hand and microsurgery. In Miller MD, editor: *Review of orthopaedics,* 3rd ed. Philadelphia, 2000, WB Saunders.

Review textbook bridging multiple orthopaedic topics, well-suited for examination preparation.

Wehbe MA, Schneider LH: Mallet fractures. *J Bone Joint Surg Am* 66:658-669, 1984.

A review of 160 mallet fingers followed for an average of more than 3 years in which the authors reported no advantage of surgical intervention over conservative treatment in obtaining a good result.

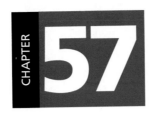

CHAPTER 57

Concussion in Sport

Introduction

- Concussion is a common yet serious injury in the athletic population.
- There is not a universal definition agreed on by everyone.
- Committee on Head Injury Nomenclature of the Congress of Neurological Surgeons defines it as "a clinical syndrome characterized by immediate and transient posttraumatic impairment of neural function, such as alteration of consciousness, disturbance of vision, equilibrium, etc., due to brainstem involvement."
- A more general definition is any trauma-induced alteration in mental status that *may or may not* include loss of consciousness (LOC).
- Note that LOC is not a requirement to have sustained a concussion.
- Boxing, football, ice hockey, and soccer are the most common sports associated with an increased risk of head injury.
- Remember, many athletes feel a pressure to return to play quickly and therefore may not be forthcoming regarding injuries or symptoms related to a head injury.
- Long-term deficits in the form of postconcussional syndrome (see later) have been described after a single event; however, if identified and properly managed, most concussive injuries result in a good prognosis with minimal deleterious effects.

Pathophysiology

- Pathophysiology is not well understood. Several mechanisms have been proposed. Likely a combination of all of them.
- Mechanical: in animal models, acceleration and deceleration forces on the brain have been demonstrated to cause axonal damage (axotomy) from shear-strain.
- Coup injury—a forceful blow to a resting, mobile head typically producing a brain injury deep to the point of cranial impact.

- Contrecoup injury—a moving head colliding against an immobile object typically producing maximal brain injury opposite the site of cranial impact.
- Vascular: loss of autoregulation of the brain's blood supply leading to vascular engorgement, increased intracranial pressure, and in severe cases (second impact syndrome) brain herniation (Figure 57–1).
- Metabolic: high energy demands within brain after a concussive injury combined with a decrease in cerebral blood flow result in the alterations in mental status.

History and Physical Examination

- Variable presentation is not uncommon.
- In some instances, the athletes may be obviously down and injured on the field.
- Other times, they will report to you on the sidelines complaining of a "ding" or saying that they have had their "bell rung."
- Therefore a high index of suspicion and a careful serial neurologic examination is necessary.
- Signs and symptoms of concussion must be addressed (Box 57–1).
- Headache is most commonly reported symptom and may be seen in up to 70% of athletes who sustain a concussion.
- Headaches may have a variable presentation and can be described as pressure, throbbing, or pulsatile. The complaints can be generalized, localized, bilateral, or unilateral.
- The athlete's general appearance and behavior can provide some clues as to the presence of a concussion.
  - Dazed look.
  - Unequal pupils.
  - Slurred speech.
  - Restlessness.
  - Vomiting.
  - Abnormally aggressive or emotional behavior.
- Evaluation of peripheral sensation and strength.
- Cranial nerve evaluation is essential (Table 57–1).

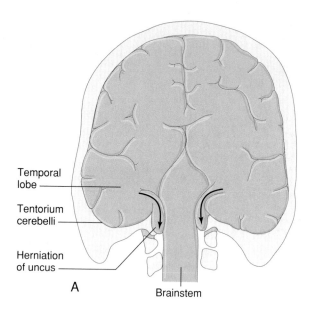

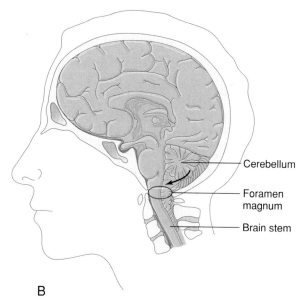

Figure 57–1:
Second impact syndrome. A, Anteroposterior view of cerebral swelling and resulting downward force causing herniation. **B,** Lateral view. (Redrawn from Cantu RC: Clin Sports Med 17:37-44, 1998.)

- Examination of cognition should focus on attention, concentration, speed of mental processes, and memory (Table 57–2).
- The Standardized Assessment of Concussion (SAC) test is a guide to help test all aspects of mental function that may be affected by concussion (Box 57–2).
- Orientation to person, place, and time should be noted.
- Attention.
  - Months of the year backward.
  - Repeating a series of numbers forward and backward.
  - Counting backward from 100 by 3s or 7s.

- Memory.
  - Retrograde amnesia may be present.
  - Questions to test memory should include recall of the play being run at the time of the injury, score of the game, outcomes of recent games, and even current news events.
  - Ask the athlete to repeat a list of objects immediately and at 5 minutes.
- Coordination.
  - Romberg or modified Romberg.
  - Finger to nose.
  - Finger to finger.
  - Tandem gait.

Imaging

- Because concussions are a metabolic process rather than structural injury, traditional imaging techniques, such as computed tomography (CT) and magnetic resonance imaging (MRI), may initially be normal.
- CT and MRI, however, are still valuable techniques for identifying associated injuries such as cerebral bleeds and skull fractures.

Classification/Grading

- No universally accepted classification or grading system.

Box 57–1	**Signs and Symptoms of Concussion**

Signs Observed by Staff

Appears to be dazed or stunned
Is confused about assignment
Forgets plays
Is unsure of game, score, or opponent
Moves clumsily
Answers questions slowly
Loses consciousness
Shows behavior or personality change
Forgets events prior to play (retrograde)
Forgets events after hit (posttraumatic)

Symptoms Reported by Athlete

Headache
Nausea
Balance problems or dizziness
Double or fuzzy/blurry vision
Sensitivity to light or noise
Feeling sluggish or slowed down
Feeling "foggy" or groggy
Concentration or memory problems
Change in sleep pattern (appears later)
Feeling fatigued

From Lovell M, Collins M, Bradley J: Return to play following sports-related concussion. *Clin Sports Med* 23: 421-441, 2004.

Table 57–1:   Cranial Nerves

CRANIAL NERVE	NAME	TEST
I	Olfactory N.	Smell a familiar odor
II	Optic N.	Visual acuity and peripheral vision
III	Oculomotor N.	Pupillary response
IV	Trochlear N.	Eye tracking
V	Trigeminal N.	Facial sensation and motor function
VI	Abducens N.	Lateral eye movements
VII	Facial N.	Facial expression and taste
VIII	Auditory N.	Hearing
IX	Glossopharyngeal N.	Swallow and "ah"
X	Vagus N.	Gag reflex
XI	Spinal accessory N.	Shoulder shrugging
XII	Hypoglossal N.	Tongue motion and strength

- Classification is typically based on presence of duration of LOC or confusion and evidence of posttraumatic amnesia (PTA).
- Some concussion classifications place greater emphasis on the duration of confusion and PTA, whereas others place more emphasis on LOC regardless of the amnestic period (Table 57–3).

Table 57–2:   Head Injury Evaluation

ABCs Evaluate and maintain an airway!

LOC: Evaluate level of consciousness before moving. Clear C-spine.

Vital signs: increased intercranial pressure→increased BP and decreased pulse.

Orientation: person, place, and time.

Memory: before and after injury. What happened? Score? What did they do before game?

Balance: Romberg test—stand with feet together and eyes closed. Maintain balance for 20 sec.

Cranial nerves:

Smell
Visual acuity
Pupil reflex
Lateral eye movement
Sensation to face
Eye movement
Facial expression
Hearing
Swallow
HR normal
Shrug shoulders
Stick out tongue

Strength, coordination, and sensation

SAC: Test initially and periodically after the injury to evaluate for any decline in mental function.

Exertional testing: All testing should be repeated after exertion before athlete is cleared to return to play.

The athlete should not return to play if there is any loss of consciousness, disorientation, or symptom. *Remember, headache is a symptom!*

ABC, Airway, breathing, circulation; BP, blood pressure; HR, heart rate; LOC, level of consciousness; SAC, Standardized Assessment of Concussion.

Box 57–2   Standardized Assessment of Concussion

Orientation (1 point each)

Month
Date
Day of week
Year
Time (within 1 hour)
Orientation score: 5

Immediate Memory (1 Point for Each Correct, Total over Three Trials)

	Trial 1	Trial 2	Trial 3
Word 1			
Word 2			
Word 3			
Word 4			
Word 5			

Immediate memory score: 15

Concentration

Reverse digits (1 point each for each string length)

Go to next string length if correct on first trial. Stop if incorrect on both trials.

3-8-2	5-1-8
2-7-9-3	2-1-6-8
5-1-8-6-9	9-4-1-7-5
6-9-7-3-5-1	4-2-8-9-3-7

Months of the year in reverse order (1 point for entire sequence correct)

Dec-Nov-Oct-Sep-Aug-Jul-Jun-May-Apr-Mar-Feb-Jan
Concentration score: 5

Delayed recall (approximately 5 minutes after immediate memory; 1 point each)

Word 1
Word 2
Word 3
Word 4
Word 5
Delayed recall score: 5

Summary of Total Scores

Orientation: 5
Immediate memory: 15
Concentration: 5
Delayed recall: 5
Total score: 30

The following may be performed between the immediate memory and delayed recall portions of this assessment when appropriate:

Neurologic Screening

Pupils
Recollection of the injury
Strength
Sensation
Coordination

(continued)

Box 57–2	Standardized Assessment of Concussion—cont'd

Exertional Maneuvers

1 40-yard sprint
5 sit-ups
5 push-ups
3 knee bends

From Asthagiri AR, Dumont AS, Sheehan JM: *Clin Sports Med* 22:559-576, 2003.

Initial Management

- Always suspect a neck injury in an athlete with a concussion.
- The airway, breathing, and circulation (ABCs) should be the first priority if the athlete is unconscious in the field.
- The cervical spine should be immobilized in the unconscious athlete until it can be cleared clinically or radiographically, or both.
- Initial treatment.
  - Remove player from the game.
  - Perform a careful neurologic examination.
  - Observe him or her on the bench.
  - Repeat serial examinations as needed.
- Remember that exertional testing is an important component to the evaluation.

Return to Play

- The decision to allow an athlete to return to play after an injury is a difficult one.

- Currently no set algorithm exists, and the decision should be individualized to each athlete, the circumstances surrounding the injury, and serial neurologic examinations.
- The following noted in Table 57–4 are recommendations.
- An athlete who is symptomatic from a head injury must not participate in contact or collision sports until all cerebral symptoms have subsided for a period of 7 days prior to return to play!

Postconcussional Syndrome

- Symptoms consist of headache, especially with exertion, labyrinthine disturbance, fatigue, irritability, and impaired memory and concentration.
- True incidence is unknown.
- Typically correlates well with the duration of posttraumatic amnesia.
- Again, return to competition must be deferred until all symptoms have abated and diagnostic studies are normal.
- Consideration for advanced imaging with CT may be necessary in cases in which symptoms persist or are severe.

Second Impact Syndrome

- Second impact syndrome (SIS) is defined as rapid brain swelling and herniation following a second head injury.
- Well-described syndrome that can result in rapid death.
- Typically, the athlete is still symptomatic from the first injury and returns to play before completely clearing his or her sensorium.

Table 57–3: Recent Concussion Grading Scales

GUIDELINE	GRADE 1	GRADE 2	GRADE 3
Cantu	1. No loss of consciousness 2. Posttraumatic amnesia lasts < 30 min	1. Loss of consciousness lasts > 5 min OR 2. Posttraumatic amnesia lasts > 30 min	1. Loss of consciousness lasts > 5 min OR 2. Posttraumatic amnesia lasts > 24 hr
Colorado	1. Confusion without amnesia 2. No loss of consciousness	1. Confusion with amnesia 2. No loss of consciousness	1. Loss of consciousness (of any duration)
American Academy of Neurology	1. Transient confusion 2. No loss of consciousness 3. Concussion symptoms, mental status changes resolve in < 5 min	1. Transient confusion 2. No loss of consciousness 3. Concussion symptoms, mental status change lasts > 15 min	1. Loss of consciousness (brief or prolonged)
Cantu	1. No loss of consciousness OR 2. Posttraumatic amnesia, signs/symptoms last > 30 min	1. Loss of consciousness lasts < 1 min OR 2. Posttraumatic amnesia lasts > 30 min but < 24 hr	1. Loss of consciousness lasts > 1 min OR 2. Posttraumatic amnesia lasts > 24 hr OR 3. Postconcussion signs or symptoms last > 7 days

From Lovell M, Collins M, Bradley J: *Clin Sports Med* 23:421-441, 2004.

Table 57–4: Concussion Management

CLASSIFICATION	GRADE	SIGNS/SYMPTOMS	1ST CONCUSSION	2ND CONCUSSION	3RD CONCUSSION
Colorado Medical Society	I	(+) Confusion (−) Amnesia (−) LOC	Return to play if symptoms resolve within 20 min	Terminate contest; return to play if without symptoms for 1 wk	Terminate contest; return to play if without symptoms for 3 mo
	II	(+) Confusion (+) Amnesia (−) LOC	Terminate contest; return to play if without symptoms for 1 wk	Terminate contest; return to play if without symptoms for 1 wk	Terminate season; return to play if without symptoms next season
	III	(+) LOC	Terminate contest; hospital evaluation; return to play in 1 mo after 2 consecutive wk without symptoms	Terminate season; return to play if without symptoms next season	Terminate season; strongly discourage return to contact or collision sports
Cantu grading system	I	(+) Amnesia <30-min duration (−) LOC	Return to play if asymptomatic for 1 wk*	Return to play in 2 wk after 1 wk without symptoms	Terminate season; return to play next season if asymptomatic
	II	(+) LOC < 5-min duration OR (+) Amnesia >30 min but <24-hr duration	Return to play if asymptomatic for 2 wk*	Return to play in 1 mo (consider season) after 1 wk without symptoms	Terminate season; return to play next season if asymptomatic
	III	(+) LOC >5-min duration OR (+) Amnesia >24-hr duration	Return to play in 1 mo after 1 wk without symptoms*	Terminate season; return to play next season if asymptomatic	Consider no further contact sports
American Academy of Neurology	I	(+) Confusion is transient (−) LOC * Symptoms <15-min duration	May return to play if symptoms clear within 15 min	Terminate contest; may return to play if without symptoms on exertion for 1 wk	
	II	(+) Confusion is transient (−) LOC * Symptoms >15-min duration	Terminate contest; may return to play if without symptoms on exertion for 1 wk	Terminate contest; may return to play if without symptoms on exertion for 2 wk; terminate season with any CT/MRI scan abnormalities	
	III	(+) LOC	Terminate contest; hospital evaluation if LOC persists or neurolog abnormality; if LOC brief, return to play in 1 wk if no symptoms on exertion; if LOC prolonged (>1 min), return in 2 wk if no symptoms on exertion	Terminate contest; return to play after 1 mo without symptoms*	

LOC, Loss of consciousness.
*CT or MRI scans if signs or symptoms persist.
Data from Bailes JE, Cantu RC: Head injuries in athletes. *Neurosurgery* 48:26–46, 2001.
From Asthagiri AR, Dumont AS, Sheehan JM: *Clin Sports Med* 22:559–576, 2003.

- Often the second injury is a relatively minor head injury that occurs shortly after previous head injury.
- Note that SIS can occur without LOC after either of the injuries.

The author reviews the current understanding and describes the pathophysiology, incidence, and management of the SIS. SIS is a potentially fatal diagnosis, and removal from competition and play is imperative until all cerebral symptoms have subsided for at least 1 week.

References

Cantu RC: Second-impact syndrome. *Clin Sports Med* 17:37–44, 1998.

Cantu RC: Post-traumatic retrograde and antegrade amnesia. Pathophysiology and implications in grading and safe return to play. *J Athletic Training* 36:244–248, 2001.

This review article stresses the importance of retrograde and antegrade posttraumatic amnesia as in the neurologic assessment and as predictive outcome values in the head-injured athlete.

Collins MW, Field M, Lovell MR, et al: Relationship between post-concussion headache and neuropsychological test performance in high school athletes. *Am J Sports Med* 31:168-173, 2003.

Headache is a common symptom after concussion. Cognitive testing on high school athletes who report headache after head injury has demonstrated some degree of deficit on tests of reaction time and memory. This suggests that any degree of headache after head injury is significant.

Lovell MR, Collins MW, Iverson GL, et al: Grade 1 or "ding" concussions in high school athletes. *Am J Sports Med* 32:47-54, 2004.

In a prospective study of 43 high school athletes, these authors demonstrate an adverse effect to memory and cognition at 36 hours after a grade 1 head injury. This raises concern regarding some current recommendations in the management of the grade 1 concussion that suggest

athletes may return to play after only 15 minutes of being asymptomatic after the initial event.

McCrea M, Guskiewicz KM, Marshall SW, et al: Acute effects and recovery time following concussion in collegiate football players: the NCAA concussion study. *JAMA* 290:2556-2563, 2003.

An increasing number of head injuries in collegiate football is causing more attention to be focused on predicting length of recovery and therefore return to play. Length to symptom resolution is variable, and many factors are involved, making it difficult to sort out exactly what factors have the most influence on symptom resolution.

Proctor MR, Cantu RC: Head and neck injuries in young athletes. *Clin Sports Med* 19:693-715, 2000.

Mild to moderate concussions have become recognized as an epidemic in sports and can have an impact on the scholastic performance of the young athlete. This article reviews the epidemiology of head and neck injuries and presents the basic pathophysiology and criteria for return to play of the young athlete after suffering head and neck injuries.

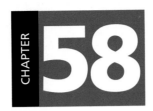
Basic Anatomy of the Spinal Column

Introduction

- The spinal column is composed of 7 cervical, 12 thoracic, and 5 lumbar vertebrae (not including 5 immovable sacral and 1 coccygeal) (Figure 58–1).
- On the basis of the three-column concept (excluding atlas and axis) proposed by Dennis, the spinal segments are composed of the following columns (Figure 58–2).
  - Anterior column: anterior longitudinal ligament (ALL), the anterior half of the vertebral body, and the intervertebral disc (IVD).
  - Middle column: posterior longitudinal ligament (PLL), the posterior half of vertebral body, and the IVD.
  - Posterior column: neural arch, posterolateral facet complexes, laminae, spinous process, ligamentum flavum, and the interspinous and supraspinous ligaments.
- All bony elements surrounding the canal vary in cortical and cancellous osseous composition and angled trajectories, width, and/or length.
- Various kinematic dynamics are associated with the normal cervical, thoracic, and lumbar spine (Table 58–1).
- In the normal, human spine, sagittal balance is represented by a vertical plum line that stems from the odontoid process, crosses the C7 vertebra and the T12-L1 region, and intersects with the posterior aspect of the sacrum.
- Alteration in the distribution of biomechanical forces to the spine may alter the morphology and alignment of the spinal column, resulting in neurologic compromise.

Cervical Spine

- The high cervical region, composed of the atlas (C1) and axis (C2), are co-components of the craniovertebral junction.
- The lower cervical spine (C3-C7) is known as the subaxial spine and is distinct from the high cervical vertebrae by the presence of uncovertebral joints and the morphology of the vertebral bodies.

- The lateral masses of the cervical spine are thinnest at C6 and C7 and are composed of the superior and inferior articular processes.
- The spinal canal adopts a triangular configuration with a varied sagittal diameter, but approximately 17 to 18 mm from C3 to C6 and 15 mm at C7, ±5 mm, respectively.
- The anterior column of the cervical spine transmits 36% of the applied load, whereas each pair of the facets transmits 32% of the total load.

Thoracic Spine

- The thoracic spinal column is composed of 12 vertebrae, is mechanically stiffer, has greater kyphosis,

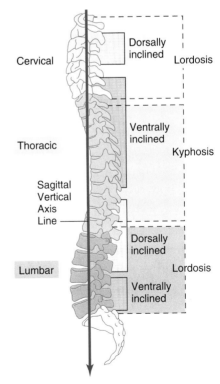

Figure 58–1:
Balance of sagittal contour.

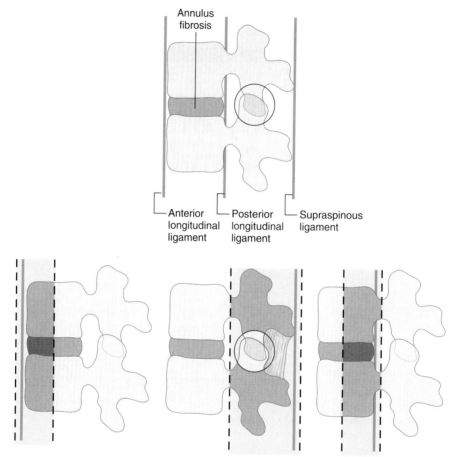

Figure 58–2:
Three-column classification of spinal instability.

and is less mobile due to rib attachments than the cervical spine.
- The thoracic vertebral bodies are heart shaped and the spinal canal is circular.
- The thoracic spinal canal is smaller in diameter than the cervical and lumbar regions.
- The anteroposterior spinal column is designed to accommodate greater amounts of translation, whereas the lower aspect is constructed to combat amounts of rotational forces.

- Various ligamentous structures are noted to account for the articular processes of the ribs.

Lumbar Spine

- The lumbar spine is composed of five kidney-shaped vertebrae.
- The lumbar spinal canal exhibits a triangular morphology.
- The pedicles vary in height but increase in width and medial inclination from L1 to L5.

Table 58–1: Kinematics of the Normal, Adult Spinal Column			
REGION	**FLEXION/EXTENSION**	**LATERAL BENDING**	**ROTATION**
Occipitoatlantal joint	30-40 degrees	8 degrees	4 degrees
Atlantoaxial joint	10 degrees	0 degrees	45-50 degrees
Lower cervical spine	50-60 degrees	60 degrees (>½ rotation in lower region)	60 degrees
Thoracic spine	75 degrees (flexion > extension: flexion greater caudally: lower segments > higher segments)	75 degrees (lower segments > higher segments)	70 degrees (higher segments > lower segments)
Lumbar spine	85 degrees (flexion > extension)	30 degrees	10 degrees (diminishes near lumbosacral junction)

- Less motion is located at L5-S1 due to the iliolumbar ligament and transition zone to the sacral body.

Spinal Nerves and Cord

- The spinal cord continues from the medulla, exiting at the foramen magnum and terminating at the level of T12-L1 or L2-L3 at the conus medullaris and extends caudally as the cauda equina.
- The spinal cord has transverse enlargements at the cervical and lumbar levels.
- Three meninges cover the spinal cord: the dura mater, arachnoid, and pia mater, which are continuations from the brain.
- The spinal cord is divided between the white (nerve fibers and glia) and gray (cell bodies of efferent and interneurons) matter.
- Gray matter consists of anterior and posterior horns, which are responsible for motor and sensory function, respectively (Figure 58–3).
- The white matter is divided into anterior, posterior, and lateral columns.
- Sensation of pressure, proprioception, tactile discrimination, and vibration are represented by the ascending tracts of the posterior column.
- Pain, temperature, and light touch sensations cross the opposite side and travel to the thalamus by the lateral spinothalamic tract of the lateral column.
- The spinal cord also includes the descending motor lateral corticospinal tract. Crude touch is representative of the ascending sensory tract, whereas the descending anterior corticospinal tract is responsible for motor function.
- The spinal column consists of 31 pairs of spinal nerves (8 cervical, 12 thoracic, 5 lumbar, 5 sacral, 1 coccygeal).
- The spinal nerve is composed of ventral/dorsal roots (sensory and motor functions) with ventral/dorsal rami.
- Rami are composed of preganglionic (white) and postganglionic (gray) fibers.
- The outer region of the IVD is innervated by the sinuvertebral nerve, and the posterior muscles and facets are innervated by the dorsal ramus.
- Dermatome and myotome classifications are established to represent various innervations and functions of the spinal nerves.
- The anterior spinal artery (ASA) provides 60% to 70% of the cord's vascular supply. The spinal cord's vascular supply is also provided by two brainstem-originating medullary feeders and additional medullary feeders from ascending cervical and vertebral arteries. The central gray matter is minimally supplied by the two posterior spinal arteries.
- As a diagnostic standard, a canal anteroposterior diameter less than 13 mm has been established as congenital stenosis.
- At the level of C1, the spinal cord occupies one half of the spinal canal, and at the C5 to C7 level the cord expands and occupies three fourths of the vertebral foramen. The canal diameter is even more diminished in the thoracic spine, allowing less free space for the spinal cord.

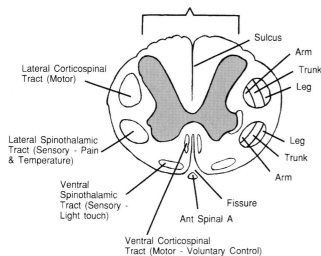

POSTERIOR FUNICULI
[Dorsal Columns]
(Sensory - Deep touch, Prop, Vib)

Sulcus
Arm
Trunk
Leg

Lateral Corticospinal Tract (Motor)

Lateral Spinothalamic Tract (Sensory - Pain & Temperature)

Leg
Trunk
Arm

Ventral Spinothalamic Tract (Sensory - Light touch)

Fissure
Ant Spinal A

Ventral Corticospinal Tract (Motor - Voluntary Control)

Figure 58–3:
Cross-section of the spinal cord. Prop, Proprioception; Vib, vibratory sense. (From Shuler FD: Anatomy. In Miller MD, editor: *Review of orthopaedics*, 4th ed. Philadelphia, 2004, Saunders.)

References

An HS, Gordin R, Renner K: Anatomic considerations for plate-screw fixation of the cervical spine. *Spine* 16(suppl):S548-S51, 1991.
> *This study provides insight regarding the varied dimensions of the pedicles throughout the cervical spine. Moreover, the study addresses and suggests optimal screw-pedicle trajectories to obtain optimal screw-plate fixation with decrease risk of complications.*

An HS, Riley LH: *An atlas of surgery of the spine.* Philadelphia, 1998, Lippincott Williams & Wilkins.
> *This atlas provides exceptional and copious illustrations of the anatomy of the spinal column. Furthermore, the textbook elaborately addresses the numerous avenues for operative intervention of various spine conditions in an informative, anatomically guided fashion.*

Burrows EH: The sagittal diameter of the spinal canal in cervical spondylosis. *Clin Radiol* 14(77):77-86; 1963.
> *This study suggested parameters regarding the diameter of the sagittal, cervical, spinal canal and the effects on it by spondylosis.*

Crossman AR, Neary D: *Neuroanatomy.* London, 2000, Churchill Livingstone.
> *This work provides a very comprehensive review of the neuroanatomy of the human body, with copious color-coded illustrations and discussion entailing, among others, the spinal cord and its functions.*

Denis F: The three column spine and its significance in the classification of acute thoracolumbar spinal injuries. *Spine* 8:817-831, 1983.
Key study providing three-column concept of spinal instability in thoracolumbar spinal injuries, which are also apropos to the cervical spine.

Dickman CA, Spetzler RF, Sonntag VKH: *Surgery of the craniovertebral junction.* New York, 1998, Thieme Medical Publishers.
This textbook provides a comprehensive evaluation of the anatomy, function, various disorders, diagnostic techniques and criteria, and operative management options as pertaining to the craniovertebral junction.

Edgar M, Ghadially J: Innervation of the lumbar spine. *Clin Orthop* 11:35-41, 1976.
The study reports that the sinuvertebral nerves are pain generators in the spine.

Knightly JJ: Anatomy and biomechanics of the lumbar spine. In Batjer HH, Loftus CM, editors: *Textbook of neurological surgery principles and practice.* Philadelphia, 2002, Lippincott Williams & Wilkins.
An informative book chapter addressing the anatomy and biomechanics of the lumbar spine. In particular, the chapter provides informative data regarding the lumbar facet joint alignment and function.

Lee CK, Rauschning W, Glenn W: Lateral lumbar spinal canal stenosis: classification, pathologic anatomy and surgical decompression. *Spine* 13:313-320, 1980.
This study describes the course of the exiting nerve root in the lumbar spine and proposes three distinct zones: the entrance, mid, and exit zones.

Panjabi MM, Takata K, Goel V, et al: Thoracic human vertebrae. Quantitative three-dimensional anatomy. *Spine* 16:888-901, 1991.
This study provides a quantitative three-dimensional analyses of the thoracic vertebrae. The study elaborates on the thoracic vertebra's transition zones and various dimensions of thoracic anatomic structures and their relationship to each other. As such, the study's findings provide valuable information to more precisely guide the clinical and surgical management of the patient.

Parke WW, Gammell K, Rothman R: Arterial vascularization of the cauda equina. *J Bone Joint Surg Am* 63:53-62, 1981.
The study refers to the clinical importance of the vascularity associated with the spine's neural structures.

Rydevik BL, Brown MD, Lundborg G: Pathoanatomy and pathophysiology of nerve root compression. *Spine* 9:7-15, 1984.
This study further provided evidence of the pathoanatomy and pathophysiology of nerve root compression and expanded the understanding of the etiology of nerve root symptoms.

Rydevik BL, Holm S, Brown MD, et al: Nutrition of spinal nerve roots: the role of diffusion for the CSF. *Trans Orthop Res Soc* 9:276, 1984.
This study reported that spinal fluid accounts for 58% of the nutrition of the spinal nerve.

Watanabe R, Parke WW: Vascular and neural pathology of lumbosacral spinal stenosis. *J Neurosurg* 64:64-70, 1986.
This study noted that the formation of arachnoiditis and scarring surrounding the nerve roots and impedance of spinal fluid at the level of stenosis may obstruct nutrition to the neural elements.

White AA, Panjabi M: *Clinical biomechanics of the spine,* 2nd ed. Philadelphia, 1990, Lippincott Williams & Wilkins.
This second edition builds on the seminal work provided by White and Panjabi in the first edition of this text and continues to fuse principles of orthopaedics with biomechanics to address the clinical aspects and anatomic underpinnings of spinal biomechanics.

Wolff J: *Das Gesetz der Transformation der Knochen.* Berlin, 1892, Hirschwald.
This seminal work presents Wolff's laws of bone remodeling. The principles of these fundamental laws provide the basis explaining the relationship between applied forces and bone response.

Zindrick MR, Wiltse LL, Doornik A, et al: Analysis of the morphometric characteristics of the thoracic and lumbar pedicles. *Spine* 2:160-166, 1987.
A quantitative analyses of the morphology of the thoracic and lumbar pedicles. The study made claims regarding the width, height, and inclination of the pedicles in relation to the vertebral body.

CHAPTER 59

Cervical Spine Injuries

Introduction

- Cervical spine injuries in sports are uncommon but can produce significant disability.
- They most commonly occur in sports resulting in excessive axial loads applied to the head that transmit forces through the cervical spine.
- Normally, the cervical spine dissipates much of the forces experienced through the paravertebral muscles, intervertebral discs, and normal lordosis of the spine.
- The neck is at greatest risk when the lordotic curve is straightened, at approximately 30 degrees of flexion, because of its diminished ability to disperse axial load forces.
- Protective equipment may not prevent cervical injuries. Preventing activities that apply axial load to the cervical spine, such as in "spearing" (which is banned), is a far more effective means of prevention.
- These injuries can often be divided into upper cervical injuries (occiput, atlas, axis), lower cervical injuries (C3-C7), neurapraxia ("stingers" and "burners") (Figure 59–1), and transient quadriplegia.
- Approximately 50% of cervical spine movement occurs at the upper cervical spine.

History, Physical Examination, and Imaging

- If present at the time of injury, the cervical spine should be stabilized and appropriate advanced trauma life support (ATLS) protocol followed, which initially includes the assessment of the airway, breathing, and circulation.
- Helmets (and shoulder pads) generally should not be removed prior to arrival at a medical facility unless the airway is compromised or inaccessible, the helmet is unable to control the head, or the face mask cannot be removed.
- Spinal injury must be presumed in all unconscious patients or those who complain of neck pain or neurologic symptoms.

- A detailed history from the patient and witnesses should be documented including the cause of injury and subsequent medical status of the patient.
- Location, duration, radiation of pain, and other neurologic symptoms should be noted.
- Bilateral extremity paresthesias and weakness suggest a spinal cord injury rather than a nerve root lesion or neurapraxia.
- Neurologic assessment should be performed on the field and repeated on arrival at a medical facility.
- The cervical spine examination should make note of tenderness, range of motion (if cleared from the cervical collar), and neurologic evaluation in accordance with spinal levels by assessing sensation, muscle strength, and appropriate reflexes of both upper and lower extremities (Figure 59–2).

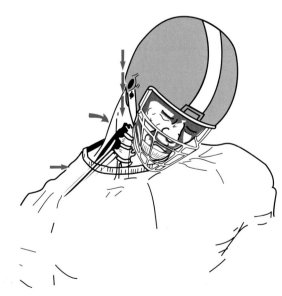

Figure 59–1:
"Stingers" or "burners." (From Warren WL, Bailes JE: *Clin Sports Med* 17:99-110, 1998.)

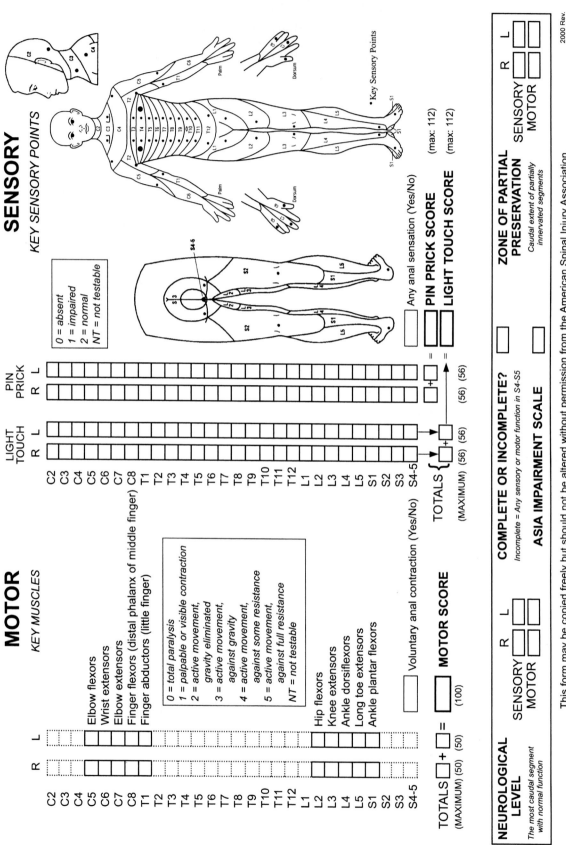

Figure 59–2:

American Spine Injury Association standard neurologic classification of spinal cord injury. (American Spinal Injury Association: *International standards for neurological and functional classification of spinal cord injury.* Chicago, 2002, American Spinal Injury Association.)

- Initial radiographic evaluation must include all seven cervical vertebrae and the C7-T1 disc space.
- Lateral radiographs should be evaluated for any prevertebral soft tissue swelling, fractures, instability, and malalignment.
- Soft tissue swelling on lateral radiographs suggests underlying cervical spine injury if the retropharyngeal enlargement is greater than 7 mm at C2 and greater than 22 mm at C4-C5.
- Anteroposterior cervical radiographs can help assess spinous process alignment.
- Odontoid views demonstrate the lateral masses of C1 and C2, and the odontoid should be assessed for fractures, instability, or abnormal alignment.
- Oblique views provide visualization of the intervertebral foramen, pedicles, and facet joints.
- When all of the previously mentioned radiographs are within normal limits, flexion/extension views or magnetic resonance imaging (MRI) can be ordered to evaluate cervical ligamentous injury.
- Flexion/extension cervical views are suggestive of instability if there is translation greater than 3.5 mm and angulation greater than 11 degrees.
- Computed tomography (CT) is ideal in delineating fracture patterns and demonstrating detailed bony anatomy.
- MRI is the imaging modality of choice when soft tissue evaluation is desired.

Types

Spinal Cord Injuries

- Spinal cord injuries are usually due to compression or contusion rather than transections.
- These injuries cannot be defined until spinal shock has resolved, identified by the return of the bulbocavernosus reflex.
- Any presence of motor or sensory function below the affected level, such as sacral sparing, indicates an incomplete cord injury.
- Complete cord injuries are characterized by loss of function below a specific level.

- American Spine Injury Association impairment scale further classifies cord injury (Table 59-1).
- Central cord syndrome is the most common cord injury and usually presents with greater motor and sensory loss in the upper extremities than lower extremities.
- Anterior cord syndrome is the second most common cord injury and has the worst prognosis. Classic presentation includes motor loss below the affected level (lower extremities > upper extremities) with sparing of posterior column function (proprioception, deep pressure sensation, and vibration).
- Brown-Sequard syndrome has the best prognosis of all the cord injuries and is characterized by ipsilateral motor and proprioception loss and contralateral pain and temperature loss.
- Posterior cord syndrome is a very rare injury and results in the loss of proprioception, vibration, and sensation to deep pressure with preserved motor function.
- Initial treatment should include stabilization of the cervical spine with a hard cervical collar and control of neurogenic shock with fluids and vasopressors if present.
- Patients who present within 8 hours of injury should be administered methylprednisolone (30 mg/kg bolus followed by infusion at 5.4 mg/kg/hr) for 24 hours if started within 3 hours of injury or 48 hours if started later.

Upper Cervical Injuries

Occipital Condyle Fractures

- These are rare fractures and are associated with other spinal fractures in one third of cases.
- Cranial nerve palsies may be present on examination (especially CN IX, X, XI, and XII).
- CT imaging may help assess and classify the type of fracture: nondisplaced impaction fractures (type I); basilar skull fracture extending into the foramen magnum (type II); and avulsion of the alar ligament from rotational or lateral bending (type III).
- Types I and II fractures can be managed with a hard cervical collar for 2 to 3 months.

Table 59-1:	American Spine Injury Association (ASIA) Impairment Scale (Frankel Scale)
GRADE	**DESCRIPTION**
A—Complete	No motor or sensory function is preserved in the sacral segments S4-S5
B—Incomplete	Sensory but not motor function is preserved below the neurologic level and includes the sacral segments S4-S5
C—Incomplete	Motor function is preserved below the neurologic level, and more than half of key muscles below the neurologic level have a muscle grade < 3
D—Incomplete	Motor function is preserved below the neurologic level, and at least half of key muscles below the neurologic level have a muscle grade of 3 or more
E—Normal	Motor and sensory function are normal

From American Spinal Injury Association: *International standards for neurological and functional classification of spinal cord injury.* Chicago, 2002, American Spinal Injury Association.

- Type III fractures are considered unstable and are best managed with halo immobilization or surgically by occipitocervical fusion.

Atlanto-Occipital Dislocation

- Atlanto-occipital dislocations, resulting from hyperextension, translation, rotation, and distraction, can cause severe neurologic injury and even death.
- Several radiographic measurements have been described to detect atlanto-occipital dislocation (Figure 59–3).
- Classification is based on direction of displacement. Longitudinal distraction without dislocation (type I), anterior displacement of the occiput (type II) is the most common; and posterior displacement of the occiput (type III).

Atlas Fracture

- Results from axial loading and correlates with the head position during injury.
  - Axial load with the head in extension results in posterior arch fractures.
  - Axial load with the head in flexion results in anterior arch fractures.
  - A four-part burst pattern is commonly known as a Jefferson fracture.
- Fifty percent of these fractures are associated with other cervical spine fractures.
- Isolated atlas fractures are not usually associated with neurologic injury in light of the large spinal cord space at this level.

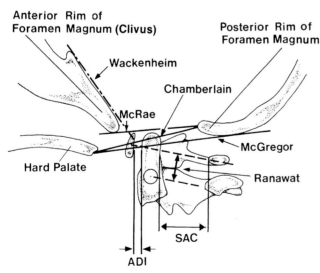

Figure 59–3:
Craniocervical radiographic criteria to evaluate normal alignment. ADI, Atlantodens interval; SAC, space available for the cord. (From Lauerman WC, McCall BR: In Miller MD, editor: *Review of orthopaedics,* 4th ed. Philadelphia, 2004, Saunders.)

- Fracture stability is dependent on the integrity of the transverse atlantal ligament.
- Indications of instability and disruption of the transverse ligament are noted by an atlanto-dens interval greater than 4 mm on lateral plain radiographs, lateral mass spreading greater than 6.9 mm on anteroposterior open-mouth plain radiographs, and bony avulsion or tear of the transverse atlantal ligament as seen on CT and MRI, respectively.
- Isolated stable C1 fractures can be treated in a hard cervical collar.
- Unstable C1 fractures can initially be treated with a halo vest.
- Malunion, nonunion, or persistent instability requires C1 C2 fusion.

Atlantoaxial Rotatory Subluxation

- Traumatically results from flexion, extension, and rotational forces.
- The patient usually complains of suboccipital pain and decreased rotation on examination.
- The head may be tilted to the subluxated joint side and rotated in the opposite direction.
- Imaging will reveal asymmetric positioning of the odontoid in relation to the lateral masses of the atlas.
- Classification is based on the degree of translation of the atlas to the axis.
- Initial treatment consists of skeletal traction for reduction and halo immobilization.
- Chronic atlantoaxial instability is treated with C1-C2 arthrodesis.

Odontoid Fracture

- Typically from flexion, although extension and rotational may be causative factors.
- One fourth of cases are associated with a neurologic deficit.
- Classification is divided into three types.
  - Type I—fracture of the distal tip; stable if less than 2 mm displacement.
  - Type II—fracture at the base of the dens; most common type.
  - Type III—fracture extending into the body of the axis.
- Stable type I fractures are treated with a rigid cervical collar for 2 to 3 months and followed up with flexion/extension cervical views.
- Type II fractures, with less than 6 mm of displacement, can be managed with halo immobilization for 2 to 3 months.
- Surgical intervention may be considered in type II cases with displacement greater than 6 mm, angulation greater than 10 degrees, nonunion, persistent instability, or inability to maintain reduction.

- Type III fractures are best treated with closed reduction and halo immobilization.

Axis Isthmus Fracture (Hangman's Fracture)

- Results from hyperextension, axial load, and rebound flexion.
- Neurologic injury is uncommon with bilateral C2 isthmus fractures; however, associated subaxial cervical injuries may produce neurologic deficits.
- Classification is based on amount of displacement.
  - Type I—vertical fracture with less than 3 mm of displacement and no angulation.
  - Type II—fractures with more than 3 mm of anterolisthesis and angulation.
  - Type IIa—angulation and no anterior translation, suggesting disruption of the posterior longitudinal ligament and intervening disc.
  - Type III—vertical fracture with significant anterolisthesis.
- Type I fractures can be treated with a rigid orthosis for 2 to 3 months.
- Type II fractures are treated with traction reduction and halo immobilization.
- Traction should not be applied to type IIa fractures because of ligamentous injury.
- Type III fractures have the highest risk of producing neurologic deficits; therefore, treatment often involves open reduction with stabilization.

Lower Cervical Injuries

Compression-Flexion and Compressive-Extension Fractures

- Compression-flexion (CF) injuries account for 20% of lower cervical fractures and are characterized by anterior vertebral compression with posterior element distraction.
- Stable CF injuries may be treated with a rigid cervical collar for 2 to 3 months.
- Unstable CF injuries without posterior ligament disruption may be managed with halo immobilization.
- CF injuries with posterior ligament disruption or neurologic involvement, or both, require anterior decompression, fusion, and instrumentation.
- Compression-extension (CE) injuries are characterized by failure of the posterior ligament that progresses from posterior arch fractures (stage I and II) through increasing degrees of anterolisthesis of the superior vertebral body to the anterior vertebral body (stages III to V).
- Stable CE injuries (stages I and II) can usually be managed with a hard collar, whereas unstable injuries (stages III to V) may require reduction and fusion.
- Vertical compression fractures make up 15% of lower cervical fractures and most often involve the C5-C6 level.

- Minimal fracture deformity can be treated in a rigid cervical collar.
- Significant fractures without much displacement can be managed with halo immobilization.
- Fractures with significant displacement or neurologic injury necessitate anterior decompression and fusion.

Distraction Injuries

- Distraction-flexion (DF) injuries account for 10% of lower cervical fractures.
- These injuries are commonly managed by reduction and skeletal traction.
- If instability is present, cervical fusion should be considered.
- MRI should be performed prior to surgery to determine the presence of a herniated disc, which would require discectomy.
- Distraction-extension (DE) injuries, which comprise 20% of lower cervical fractures, result from tensile failure in extension.
- Brace treatment is difficult in DE injuries and may require either halo immobilization or reduction and fusion.

Lateral Flexion Injuries

- Account for 20% of lower cervical injuries. Stage I injuries result in an ipsilateral fracture, whereas stage II injuries are composed of contralateral ligamentous or bony failure and vertebral displacement.
- Stable stage I injuries can be managed by external immobilization for 2 to 3 months.
- Unstable stage I and stage II injuries may necessitate reduction and surgical stabilization.

Neurapraxia ("Stingers" and "Burners")

- Reports incidence between 49% and 65% in collegiate football players.
- Results from traction or compression of the brachial plexus or nerve roots and is the most common athletic cervical neurologic injury.
- Activities causing extremely forceful lateral neck flexion can compress the nerves of the ipsilateral side or stretch the brachial plexus of the opposite side.
- Compression may result from poorly fitting equipment such as shoulder pads.
- Patients complain of unilateral radiating pain, burning, paresthesias, and occasionally weakness of the upper extremity.
- The C5, C6, and C7 myotomes are the most often affected.
- Bilateral symptoms or lower extremity symptoms suggest spinal cord injury.
- Symptoms usually resolve within seconds or minutes but can last hours or days.
- Physical examination may reveal pain and weakness of the affected upper extremity.

- Treatment is most often conservative.
- Radiographs and MRI may be considered to rule out fractures or disc herniation.
- If symptoms resolve, and the patient demonstrates pain-free full range of cervical motion and an intact neurologic examination, the patient may safely return to play.
- Persistent symptoms may require further evaluation, and the patient should be restricted from play until full recovery is achieved.

Cervical Sprains and Strains

- Strains describe injuries to the muscle-tendon unit.
- Sprains are defined as ligamentous injuries and have potential for cervical instability.
- Patients present with pain, tenderness, and limited range of motion.
- Radiographs may demonstrate straightening of the lordotic cervical spine.
- Initially, cervical sprains are treated with collar immobilization and analgesics.
- If initial radiographs were normal, flexion/extension views should be performed when symptoms have resolved to evaluate for any persistent instability.
- MRI should be considered in patients with persistent symptoms.

Cervical Disc Herniation

- Patients may present with radicular symptoms and neck pain.
- Physical examination should attempt to determine the level affected by neurologic examination.
- Radiographs should rule out any fractures, degenerative disease, or other bony pathology.
- MRI may demonstrate the presence and severity of disc herniation.
- Initial management is conservative.
- Persistent neurologic symptoms are an indication for surgical decompression.

Transient Quadriplegia

- Occurs in approximately 7 per 10,000 collegiate football players.
- Commonly associated with an axial load injury with hyperextension or hyperflexion.
- A pincer-like mechanism of injury in which the cord is compressed between cervical segments and the posterior ligamentum flavum within a decreased spinal canal diameter.
- The patient experiences a temporary loss of motor or sensory function, or both, usually lasting minutes but sometimes persisting for days.
- Complaints of bilateral burning dysesthesias, paresthesias, loss of sensation in the extremities, and weakness ranging from mild decrease in strength to complete paralysis.

- Torg and colleagues demonstrated that several of these cases were associated with spinal stenosis. The Torg ratio, measured by dividing the sagittal canal diameter by the width of the vertebral body, indicates stenosis when values are less than 0.8 (Figure 59–4). This ratio has a poor positive predictive value and should not be considered for screening athletes.
- Klippel-Feil syndrome, intervertebral disc disease, and congenital or acquired stenosis are predisposing factors to spinal cord injury.
- If all studies are normal and symptoms have completely resolved, the patient may return to play; however, several authorities believe that patients with any of the previously mentioned predisposing factors should be prohibited form participating in contact sports.

Spear Tackler's Spine

- Subset of football players with a radiographic evidence of developmental stenosis, loss of the normal lordotic curve, and posttraumatic changes that predisposed them to spinal cord injury and is a contraindication to participation in collision and contact sports.
- These changes develop from poor tackling techniques (spearing—in which axial load is applied to a straightened cervical spine, such as when the neck is flexed at 30 degrees) or other similar activities.

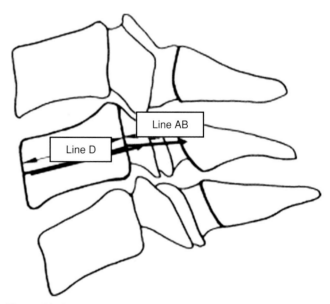

Figure 59–4:
Torg ratio.
(From Weinberg J, Rokito S, Silber JS: *Clin Sports Med* 22:493-500, 2003.)

Rehabilitation and Return to Play

- Proper rehabilitation is essential to recover range of motion, posture, and strength (Box 59–1).
- Paracervical and paraspinal strengthening exercises should be emphasized to increase the neck's ability to withstand contact forces.
- The strengthening regimen should begin with isometric exercises, advanced slowly with increasing concentric resistive exercises, and end by implementing eccentric strengthening exercises once painless full range of motion is achieved.
- Patients must be instructed on proper playing techniques to avoid further potential injury.
- There is no single, generalized criterion to follow when deciding whether to return an athlete to play.
- Patients should be prohibited from returning to play until neurologic symptoms and neck pain have resolved and they have returned to their preinjury strength and function.
- Congenital abnormalities, such as odontoid agenesis, odontoid hypoplasia, os odontoid, type I Klippel-Feil (fusion of the cervical and upper thoracic vertebra with synostosis), and atlanto-occipital fusion are absolute contraindications to contact sports.
- Other absolute contraindications include atlantoaxial instability, C1-C2 fusion, and irrecoverable spinal cord injuries.

Box 59–1 | **Return to Play**

No Contraindications

- Fewer than three episodes of a prior burner/stinger lasting < 24 hours, with full range of cervical motion without any evidence of a neurologic deficit
- One episode of transient quadriparesis/quadriplegia with full range of cervical motion, no evidence of a residual neurologic deficit, and no evidence of a herniated disc or instability

Relative Contraindications

- Prolonged symptomatic burner/stinger or transient quadriparesis lasting > 24 hours
- Three or more previous episodes of either a stinger/burner or two episodes of transient quadriparesis/quadriplegia; the patient must have full cervical range of motion and strength without neck discomfort

Absolute Contraindications

- More than two previous episodes of transient quadriparesis/quadriplegia
- Clinical history, physical examination findings, or imaging confirmation of cervical myelopathy/melomalacia
- Continued cervical neck discomfort, decreased range of motion, or any evidence of a neurologic deficit from baseline after any cervical spine injury

From Vaccaro AR, Watkins B, Albetr TJ, et al: *Orthopedics* 24:699–703, 2001.

References

Allen BL, Ferguson RL, Lehman TR, O'Brien RP: A mechanistic classification of closed, indirect fractures and dislocations of the lower cervical spine. *Spine* 7:1-27, 1982.
> *The article proposed a spine injury analysis on the basis of mechanistic principles based on neck position or applied forces, or both, at the time of injury. The article proposes categories of phylogenies of injury that are further stratified into stages of injury severity.*

Anderson LD, D'Alonzo RT: Fractures of the odontoid process of the axis. *J Bone Joint Surg Am* 56:1663-1674, 1974.
> *Study suggests a classification of occipital condyle fractures.*

Bracken M: Steroids for acute spinal cord injury. *Cochrane Database Syst Rev* 3: CD001046, 2002.
> *This study is a systematic review based on evidence-based principles assessing randomized-controlled trials (RCTs) addressing the therapeutic efficacy of steroid use in acute spinal cord injury. The study concluded that methylprednisolone steroid therapy has shown efficacy when administered within 8 hours of injury. The study also addressed benefits of extended dose maintenance and the need for further RCT studies.*

Bucholz RW, Burkhead WZ: The pathologic anatomy of fatal atlanto-occipital dislocations. *J Bone Joint Surg Am* 61:248-250, 1979.
> *This study underlined the high incidence of atlanto-occipital dislocations and traumatic spondylolisthesis of the axis in fatal multiple trauma patients.*

Clarke CR: *The cervical spine,* 2nd ed. Philadelphia, 2004, Lippincott Williams & Wilkins.
> *The most recent, comprehensive, multiauthored textbook addressing issues related specifically to the cervical spine. The textbook provides a very comprehensive section on high and low cervical spine injuries, entailing epidemiology, classification, diagnostic methods, and treatment options.*

Denis F: The three column spine and its significance in the classification of acute thoracolumbar spinal injuries. *Spine* 8:817-831, 1983.
> *Key study providing three-column concept of spinal instability in thoracolumbar spinal injuries, which are also apropos to the cervical spine.*

Fielding JW, Hawkins RJ: Atlanto-axial rotatory fixation. *J Bone Joint Surg Am* 59:37-44, 1977.
> *The authors proposed a four-part classification of atlantoaxial rotatory fixation.*

Hurley R: *The cervical spine surgery atlas.* Philadelphia, 2003, Lippincott Williams & Wilkins.
> *This atlas provides numerous illustrations regarding cervical spine anatomy and numerous operative techniques in addressing various cervical spine disorders.*

Levine AM, Edwards CC: The management of traumatic spondylolisthesis of the axis. *J Bone Joint Surg Am* 67:217-226, 1985.
> *This article proposed a modification to Effendi's three-part classification system of traumatic spondylolisthesis of the axis.*

Powers B, Miller MD, Kramer RS, et al: Traumatic anterior atlanto-occipital dislocation. *Neurosurgery* 4:12-17, 1979.
> *Suggestion of radiographic criterion, known as the Power's ratio, used for measurement of atlanto-occipital joint injuries.*

Simpson MJ, Sutton D, Rizzolo SJ, Cotler JM: Traumatic injuries of the adult lower cervical spine. In An HS, Simpson MJ, editors: *Surgery of the cervical spine.* Baltimore, 1994, Williams & Wilkins.

This book chapter provides a very comprehensive description and treatment of various lower cervical spine injuries in the adult patient. The chapter incorporates various diagrams, illustrations, and images to underline various principles regarding cervical spine injuries.

Smith GW, Robinson RA: The treatment of certain cervical spine disorders by the anterior removal of the intervertebral disc and interbody fusion. *J Bone Joint Surg Am* 40:607-624, 1958.

Seminal report of anterior cervical discectomy and interbody spine surgery technique to address cervical spine disorders.

Vaccaro AR, Cotler JM: Traumatic injuries of the adult upper cervical spine. In An HS, Simpson MJ, editors: *Surgery of the cervical spine.* Baltimore, 1994, Williams & Wilkins.

This book chapter provides a comprehensive description and treatment of various upper cervical spine injuries in the adult patient. The chapter incorporates various diagrams, illustrations, and images to underline various principles regarding cervical spine injuries.

Wackenheim A: *Roentgen diagnosis of the craniovertebral region.* Berlin, 1974, Springer-Verlag.

Seminal textbook underlining various radiographic parameters of normal and abnormal pathology at the craniovertebral junction.

White AA, Panjabi M: *Clinical biomechanics of the spine,* 2nd ed. Philadelphia, 1990, Lippincott Williams & Wilkins.

This second edition builds on the seminal work provided by White and Panjabi in the first edition of this text and continues to fuse principles of orthopaedics with biomechanics to address the clinical aspects of spinal biomechanics. The text provides, among many topics, solid foundations and concepts regarding cervical spine injuries.

CHAPTER 60

Disc Disease

Introduction

- Disc disease is more common with age.
- Disc disease can result in the following.
  - Disc degeneration.
    - Disc metabolism may alter with age or due to systemic or local factors, biomechanical effects, immune factors, and genetic disposition.
  - Intervertebral disc (IVD) prolapse.
    - Displacement of the nucleus can result in compression of the spinal cord or its nerve roots. This typically affects the lower nerve root of the affected segment.
  - Spondylosis.
    - Interbody height decreases, osteophytes may form, instability may develop, segmental or overall deformity may arise, and disc bulging may occur.
- Compression of the affected nerve root will result in dysfunction of that root, causing pain, numbness, and weakness of the muscles innervated by that nerve root and loss of reflexes controlled by that nerve root.
- Treatment options vary with the degree of disc disease, type and duration of symptoms, associated spinal comorbidities, and spine location.
- Mainstay of treatment entails conservative management (medications, physical therapy, modalities), epidural steroid injections, surgical decompression, and in selected cases disc arthroplasty.

Intervertebral Disc

- The IVD is a complex structure that mainly assumes the role as the shock absorber of the spinal column.
- Composed of an inner region (nucleus pulposus) and an outer region (annulus fibrosus) (Figure 60–1).
- Contributes 20% to 30% of the spinal column height.
- Bordered anteriorly by the anterior longitudinal ligament, posteriorly by the posterior longitudinal ligament (PLL), and superiorly and inferiorly by the cartilaginous endplates.

- Cartilaginous endplates are composed of hyaline cartilage and are vascularly supplied by the cortical matrix of the vertebra.
- Underlining cortical and cancellous bone of the adjacent vertebral body varies.
- Type I and type II collagens predominantly comprise the annulus and nucleus, respectively (Table 60–1).
- Covalent collagen cross-links further contribute to the tensile strength of the IVD.
- Collagen fibers represent 20% of the nucleus pulposus and 70% of the outer annulus.
  - With disc degeneration, collagen cross-linking decreases in the annulus and collagen synthesis increases in the nucleus.
- The matrix of the nucleus consists of large amounts of proteoglycans (consisting of a centralized hyaluronan filament and linked glycosaminoglycans) that contribute to the compressive strength of the disc.
  - Small-typed proteoglycans, consisting of biglycan, decorin, lumican, and fibromodulin, are responsible for the organization of collagen and fibril formation.

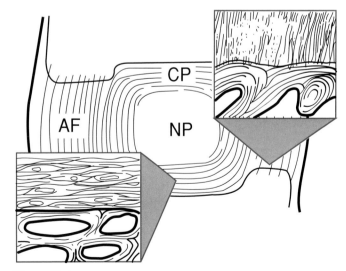

Figure 60–1:
Schematic representation of orientation of fibers in disc and endplate. AF, Annulus fibrosus; CP, cartilaginous endplate; NP, nucleus pulposus.

Table 60–1:	Collagen Composition of Intervertebral Disc	
	COLLAGEN TYPE	**% OF TOTAL COLLAGEN**
Annulus Fibrosus	I	80 outer 0 Inner
	II	0 outer 80 Inner
	III	Possible traces
	V	3
	VI	10
	IX	1-2
	XI	1
Nucleus Fibrosus	II	75-80
	VI	15-20
	IX	1-2
	XI	3

From Eyre DR, Benya P, Buckwalter J, et al: The Intervertebral disc. Part B: basic sciences perspectives. In Frymoyer JW, Gordon SL, editors: *New perspectives on low back pain.* Park Ridge, IL, 1989, American Academy of Orthopaedic Surgeons.

- Large-type proteoglycans (large amounts of keratin and chondroitin sulfate) mainly entail aggrecan, which is primarily responsible for water retention and, in large part, to the disc's compressive strength.
- Proteoglycan synthetic activity is maximum in the inner annulus; however, this activity is one third lower in adults in comparison with young individuals.
- In the aging process, chondroitin and keratin sulfate ratios decrease and the ability for proteoglycans to bind with hyaluronan filaments decreases, thus increasing the risk of disc degeneration.
- The nucleus (85% water content) is more hydrated than the annulus (78% water content).
- Regarding the annulus, the inner region is composed of more fibrocartilaginous tissue, whereas the outer region is composed more of collagen fibrils and a neurovascular supply.
  - Nutrition is diffused through the endplates; however, with age, blood supply to the endplates and outer annulus decrease.
  - Nicotine use decreases blood supply and nutrition to the disc.
- Various biomechanical processes encompass the disc and its degeneration. Furthermore, applied force is not uniform throughout the disc and is also dependent on body position.
- Motion is greater at the IVDs, and compressive and tensile forces are distributed throughout the spinal column.
- Normal cervical and lumbar spines exhibit a lordotic curvature, and the thoracic spine a kyphotic morphology, mainly attributed to the configuration of the IVDs and applied stresses attributed to bipedalism.
- The height of the IVDs is greater at the anterior aspect of the interspace, which may account for the natural cervical lordotic alignment.

- Loss of lordosis or kyphosis is attributed to dehydration of the IVDs, which mainly occurs anteriorly, largely accredited to posterior resistance due to uncovertebral joint and articular facet stability.
- Such manifestations may contribute to altered or ensuing biomechanical forces throughout the spine, resulting in initial reactive hyperostosis of the adjacent vertebral rims and development of a spondylotic bar with possible coupling of posterior disc protrusion.
- Posterior disc herniation either contained by the PLL or extruded material and/or foraminal stenosis may contribute to impingement of the exiting nerve root and could produce radiculopathic symptoms.
  - Due to such altered biomechanics attributed to disc herniation, osteophytes and facet joint degeneration can also ensue and may lead to ligamentum flavum buckling and potential contribution to stenosis of the neural elements.
  - Interbody height loss, due to disc degeneration, may also lead to facet joint overriding and the development of spondylolisthesis.
- Hypermobility at the adjacent levels may further induce hypertrophy at the respective motion segment and threaten encroachment on the spinal cord and nerve roots.
- Manifestation of pain is attributed to compression or stretching of the sinuvertebral nerve and altered integrity or distortion of the apophyseal facet joints, ligamentous elements, and spinal column musculature.

Cervical Disc Disease

- Can affect any of the eight cervical roots and the terminal branches of the brachial plexus.
- Unusual in young athletes but can occur in conjunction with trauma.
- Individuals may develop axial neck pain (with or without referred pain), cervical radiculopathy, and/or myelopathy.
- Examination should be tailored to address the following:
  - Dermatomal pain distribution and type of pain.
  - Neurologic findings (reflex changes, numbness, paresthesias, and/or weakness).
  - Neck range of motion to evaluate underlying pathology and symptom exacerbation.
  - Presence of myelopathic signs and symptoms include the following:
    - Clumsy hands.
    - Motor and sensory weakness/dysfunction.
    - Gait abnormalities.
    - Spasticity (clonus, hyperreflexia, Babinski's sign).
    - Sphincter dysfunction.
    - Positive Lhermitte's sign.
    - Positive Hoffman's sign.
- Plain radiographs are helpful but usually poor indicators in individuals older than 40 years.

- Myelography is beneficial to determine acute disc herniation and spondylosis but difficult to evaluate intradural lesion and its extent and differentiation between soft and hard disc protrusions.
- Computed tomography (CT) is advantageous to determine extent of cord compression and stenosis and differentiate bony from soft tissue compression.
- Magnetic resonance imaging (MRI) is advantageous to determine associated spinal cord lesions and extent of cervical disc disease.
- Operative management is pursued if conservative treatment fails in axial or radicular pain, progression of nerve or cord pathology, and the presence of myelopathic symptoms.
  - Surgical treatment may consist of anterior or posterior approaches or a combination of both.
  - Operative treatment is dependent on the type, extent, and location of the lesion; degree of cervical contour; and, at times, surgeon's experience.

Thoracic Disc Disease

- Thoracic involvement is uncommon.
- The majority of patients are asymptomatic.
- Can affect any of the 12 thoracic nerve roots but typically the lower roots.
- Presentation is typically vague, with nonspecific radiating chest and upper back pain.
- MRI is the most helpful study but requires a high index of suspicion to request this study.
- The thoracic spinal canal is small; thus, the risk of myelopathic symptoms to develop is high.
- A thorough differential diagnosis is essential to rule out intraabdominal, intrathoracic, or retroperitoneal pathology; neurologic or metabolic disorders; and the presence of spinal infections, neoplasm, traumatic fractures, spinal deformity, congenital manifestations, autoimmune disease, and referred cervical or shoulder pain.
- Conservative treatment focuses on bracing, antiinflammatories, therapy, and modalities.
- Operative intervention is indicated for myelopathy with or without radiculopathy, for persistent radiculopathy that is nonresponsive to conservative treatment for at least 6 months, or for progressive symptoms and decreased quality of life.

Lumbar Disc Disease

- Can affect any of the lumbar levels.
- More common than any other spinal region.
- In the lumbar spine, the nucleus is located more posteriorly in comparison with the thoracic spine and is also characterized by a high water content that diminishes with age (Figure 60–2).

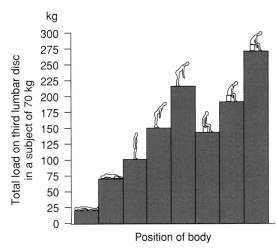

Figure 60–2:
Lumbar disc pressure. (Redrawn from Hackley DR, Wiesel SW: *Clin Sports Med* 12:465-485, 1993.)

- Disc herniation usually causes impingement of traversing nerve roots and associated neurologic findings (Table 60–2).
- In the elderly, spinal stenosis and spondylolisthesis with or without stenosis may also develop.
- Physical examination entails a careful bone and soft tissue palpation, range of motion, spinal balance and patient behavior evaluation, and motor-sensory function (Figure 60–3).
- In addition, the neurologic examination can include provocative tests such as the following:

Table 60–2:	Clinical Features of Herniated Lumbar Discs

L3–4 Disc; L4 Nerve Root

Pain	Lower back, hip, posterolateral thigh, across patella, anteromedial aspect of leg
Numbness	Anteromedial thigh and knee
Weakness	Knee extension
Atrophy	Quadriceps
Reflexes	Knee jerk diminished

L4–5 Disc; L5 Nerve Root

Pain	Sacroiliac region, hip, posterolateral thigh, anterolateral leg
Numbness	Lateral leg, first webspace
Weakness	Dorsiflexion of great toe and foot
Atrophy	Minimal anterior calf
Reflexes	None or absent posterior tibial tendon reflex

L5–S1 Disc; S1 Nerve Root

Pain	Sacroiliac region, hip, posterolateral thigh/leg
Numbness	Back of calf; lateral heel, foot, and toe
Weakness	Plantarflexion of foot and great toe
Atrophy	Gastrocnemius and soleus
Reflexes	Ankle jerk diminished or absent

From Boden SD, Wiesel SW, Laws ER, et al: *The aging spine*. Philadelphia, 1991, WB Saunders.

- Straight, contralateral, and reverse straight leg raising tests.
- Lasegue's maneuver (foot dorsiflexion can exacerbate pain of straight leg raising).
- Bowstring's sign.
- Waddell's sign (inappropriate findings consistent with malingering).
- Careful search for cauda equina syndrome should be elicited on history and examination.
- Various risk factors have been noted that contribute to low back pain and sciatica (Table 60–3).

- Differential diagnosis is relatively similar in scope as for the thoracic spine.
- Plain radiographic films usually appear normal with respect to the presence of disc herniation; however, such imaging is advantageous for evaluation for the presence of spinal alignment, interbody height, infection, spondylosis, and spondylolisthesis.
- CT and myelogram are helpful in determining presence of a herniated disc and stenosis, but false-positive rates are high.
- Bone scan and discography are poor indicators for lumbar disc disease and associated manifestations.

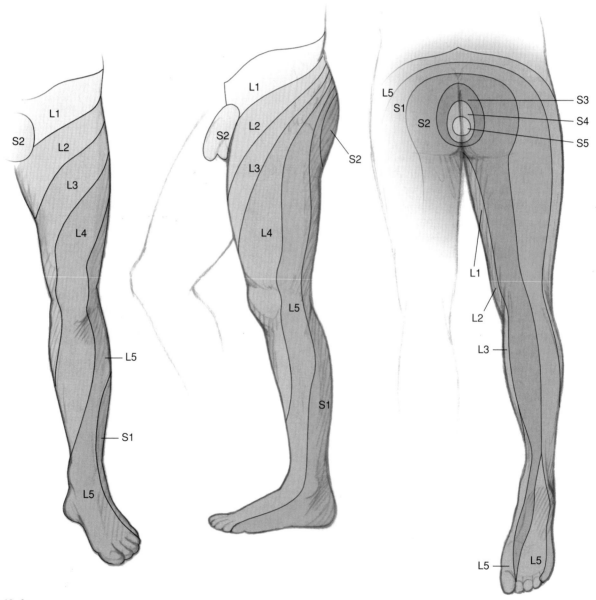

Figure 60–3:
Lumbosacral dermatomes. (From Albert TJ, Singh K: Low back pain and sciatica. In Fitzgerald RH, Kaufer H, Malkani AL, editors: *Orthopaedics*. St Louis, 2002, Mosby.)

Table 60–3:	Risk Factors for Low Back Pain and Sciatica	
OCCUPATIONAL	**INDIVIDUAL**
Heavy physical work	1. Age and sex
Static work postures	2. Posture
Frequent bending and twisting	3. Anthropometry
Lifting, pushing, and pulling	4. Muscle strength
Repetitive	5. Physical fitness
Vibrations	6. Spine mobility
	7. Smoking (?)

From Albert TJ, Singh K: Low back pain and sciatica. In Fitzgerald RH, Kaufer H, Malkani AL editors: *Orthopaedics.* St Louis, 2002, Mosby.

- MRI is ideal to determine extent of disc disease and degree of stenosis.
- Conservative treatment is the mainstay of initial treatment and includes activity modification, antiinflammatories, physical therapy, modalities, and injections.
- Depending on the specific diagnosis and pathology, injections can include facet blocks, selective nerve root injections, and epidural steroid injections.
- Operative intervention is indicated for cauda equina syndrome, persistent neurologic signs and symptoms that are nonresponsive to conservative treatment for at least 6 weeks, or for progressive symptoms and decreased quality of life.

References

An HS: *Principles and techniques of spine surgery.* Philadelphia, 1998, Lippincott Williams & Wilkins.

This textbook provides a thorough discussion with regard to many spine-related conditions and their respective diagnostic and management options. Furthermore, this text provides numerous illustrations and figures that aid in the understanding of each topic at hand.

An HS, Riley LH: *An atlas of surgery of the spine.* Philadelphia, 1998, Lippincott Williams & Wilkins.

This atlas provides exceptional and copious illustrations that address the numerous avenues for operative intervention of disc-related pathology. In addition, this text provides thorough discussion regarding the indications and contraindications associated with each spine procedure.

Battie MC, Videman T, Gibbons LE, et al: 1995 Volvo Award in clinical sciences. Determinants of lumbar disc degeneration: a study relating lifetime exposures and magnetic resonance imaging findings in identical twins. *Spine* 20:2601-2612, 1995.

The study stressed the importance of various environmental and familial factors that could contribute to disc degeneration.

Battie MC, Videman T, Gill K, et al: 1991 Volvo Award in clinical sciences. Smoking and lumbar intervertebral disc degeneration: an MRI study of identical twins. *Spine* 16:1015-1021, 1991.

This study reported a strong association that smoking increases the risk of IVD degeneration.

Brain WR, Northfield D, Wilkinson M: The neurological manifestations of cervical spondylosis. *Brain* 75:187-225, 1952.

This work represents possibly the earliest account distinguishing cervical spondylotic myelopathy as a distinct entity.

Brown CW, Deffer PAJ, Akmakjian J, et al: The natural history of thoracic disc herniation. *Spine Suppl* 17:S97-S102, 1992.

This work provides a thorough review of the natural history of thoracic disc herniation.

Buckwalter JA: The fine structure of human intervertebral disc. In White AAI, Gordon SL, editors: *Symposium on idiopathic low back pain.* St Louis, 1982, Mosby.

This book chapter is an informative resource that illustrates the fine anatomic composition of the IVD. In addition, this work further stresses the importance of the various IVD factors that contribute to its tensile and compressive strength.

Clarke CR. *The cervical spine,* 2nd ed. Philadelphia, 2004, Lippincott Williams & Wilkins.

The most recent, comprehensive, multiauthored textbook addressing issues related specifically to the cervical spine. The textbook provides a comprehensive section on cervical disc disease, entailing epidemiology, classification, diagnostic methods, and treatment options.

Clarke E, Robinson PK: Cervical myelopathy: a complication of cervical spondylosis. *Brain* 79:483-510, 1956.

This work provided one of the earliest descriptions of the various effects associated with cervical spondylotic myelopathy.

Fardon DF, Milette PC: Nomenclature and classification of lumbar disc pathology. Recommendations of the Combined Task Forces of the North American Spine Society, American Society of Spine Radiology, and American Society of Neuroradiology. *Spine* 26:E93 E113, 2001.

This review is a solid resource in providing a thorough and up-to-date description of the nomenclature and classification of lumbar disc pathology. The work provides various educational schematics, illustrations, and discussion on the various stages of lumbar disc-related pathology.

Fessler RG, Sturgill M: Review: complications of surgery for thoracic disc disease. *Surg Neurol* 49:609-618, 1998.

This review article addresses advantages and disadvantages associated with various thoracic operative procedures to address thoracic disc-related pathology.

Gower W, Pedrini V: Age related variations in protein-polysaccharides from human nucleus pulposus, annulus fibrosus and costal cartilage. *J Bone Joint Surg Am* 51:1154-1162, 1969.

This study demonstrated that IVD dehydration is related to age. In addition, this work also noted the altered ability of the disc to accommodate forces as a result of dehydration.

Johnstone-Bayliss MT: The large proteoglycans of the human intervertebral disc: changes in their biosynthesis and structure with age, topography, and pathology. *Spine* 20:674-684, 1995.

The study addresses the role and composition of large proteoglycans as pertaining to the human IVD. The authors further delineate the biochemical processes and other factors associated with these proteoglycans and their function with respect to age, topography, and pathology in human disc metabolism.

Mixter WJ, Barr JS: Rupture of the intervertebral disc with involvement of the spinal canal. *N Engl J Med* 211:210-215, 1934.
> *Seminal work describing the presence of symptoms related to a herniated disc. This work further described one of the earliest accounts of operative management of a herniated disc.*

Nachemson A: The load on lumbar disks in different positions of the body. *Clin Orthop* 45:107-122, 1966.
> *This study stressed that the IVD is subjected to varying degrees of force, dependent on body position.*

Naylor A: The biophysical and biochemical aspects of intervertebral disc herniations and degeneration. *Ann R Coll Engl* 31:32-35, 1962.
> *This study explains the various forces acting on the IVD and their role in disc tear, degeneration, and prolapse.*

Smith GW, Robinson RA: The treatment of certain cervical spine disorders by the anterior removal of the intervertebral disc and interbody fusion. *J Bone Joint Surg Am* 40:607-624, 1958.
> *Seminal report of anterior cervical discectomy and interbody spine surgery technique to address cervical spine disorders.*

Urban JP, McMullin JF: Swelling pressure of the lumbar intervertebral discs: influence of age, spinal level, composition, and degeneration. *Spine* 13:179-187, 1988.
> *This study highlights the various factors that are at play in the altered composition of the IVD, primarily pertaining to the association of diminished disc water content with age.*

Waddell G, McCulloch JA, Kummel E, Venner RM: Nonorganic physical signs in low-back pain. *Spine* 5:117-125, 1980.
> *In the evaluation of low back pain, this study denoted various physical signs that are nonorganic in nature and could suggest malingering.*

Williams RW: Microlumbar discectomy: a conservative surgical approach to the virgin herniated lumbar disc. *Spine* 3:175-182, 1978.
> *This work was instrumental in ushering in a new era of surgical disc management via microdiscectomy.*

Dealing with Low Back Pain

Introduction

- Low back pain (LBP) is one of the top five reasons for physician visits.
- After upper respiratory infections, LBP is the second leading cause for work absenteeism.
- LBP most commonly results from low back strains or sprains.
- Reports indicate a 60% to 85% lifetime prevalence of LBP in the general population.
- Only 14% of cases last 2 or more weeks, whereas 80% to 90% resolve within 6 weeks.
- Risk factors for LBP are numerous.
  - Increasing age.
  - Smoking.
  - Heavy lifting activities.
  - Psychological distress.
  - Severe scoliosis.
  - Drug abuse.
  - Previous history of LBP.
- Prevalence of specific injuries varies among sports, reflecting primary activities that correspond to certain mechanisms of injury.

History

- Algorithm (Figure 61–1).
- Identify if symptoms predominantly involve the back or leg to help differentiate axial back pain from radicular pain.
- The evaluating physician should document the location, quality, duration, onset, radiation, and alleviating and aggravating factors.
- Elicit for an eventful mechanism of injury to help distinguish between traumatic or atraumatic causes.
- An athlete's sport, position, repetitive motions during play, and training regimen help define potential traumatic or overuse injuries.
- Previous back injuries and back pain should be reviewed, along with their prescribed therapies and outcomes.

- Review of symptoms should include "red flag" questions (Table 61–1). When present, they are suggestive of malignancy or infection and should be evaluated further. In these cases, plain radiographs and advanced imaging studies, combined with appropriate blood work, should be considered.
- Bowel and bladder dysfunction (incontinence or retention) with saddle anesthesia may indicate a possible cauda equina syndrome and must be recognized as an emergency.
- LBP may be secondary to referred pain (e.g., peptic ulcer disease, aortic aneurysm, pelvic inflammatory disease, cholecystitis, nephrolithiasis, pancreatitis, retroperitoneal abscess).
- Psychosocial factors that may contribute to the patient's symptoms should be documented, especially in cases in which the symptoms are inconsistent with the history, examination, and imaging studies.

Physical Examination

- Only about 1% of patients present with associated neurologic signs.
- Inspection should include noting any evidence of scoliosis, kyphosis, and cutaneous lesions overlying the spine (e.g., psoriasis, café au lait spots—neurofibromatosis, vesicles—herpes zoster, pilonidal cysts, hair patch—spina bifida, needle marks—intravenous drug abuse).
- Gait patterns should be observed for waddling, splinting or antalgic gait, and difficulty with toe or heel walking.
- Palpation of the paraspinous muscles may be notable for tenderness found with sprains and strains.
- Normally direct percussion of the spinous processes should not elicit pain.
- Range-of-motion testing may demonstrate stiffness or exacerbation of pain with certain movements.
- Pain with extension that is relieved with flexion is more consistent with neural compression and posterior element pathology (spinal stenosis, spondylolysis, spondylolisthesis, facet arthrosis, etc.).

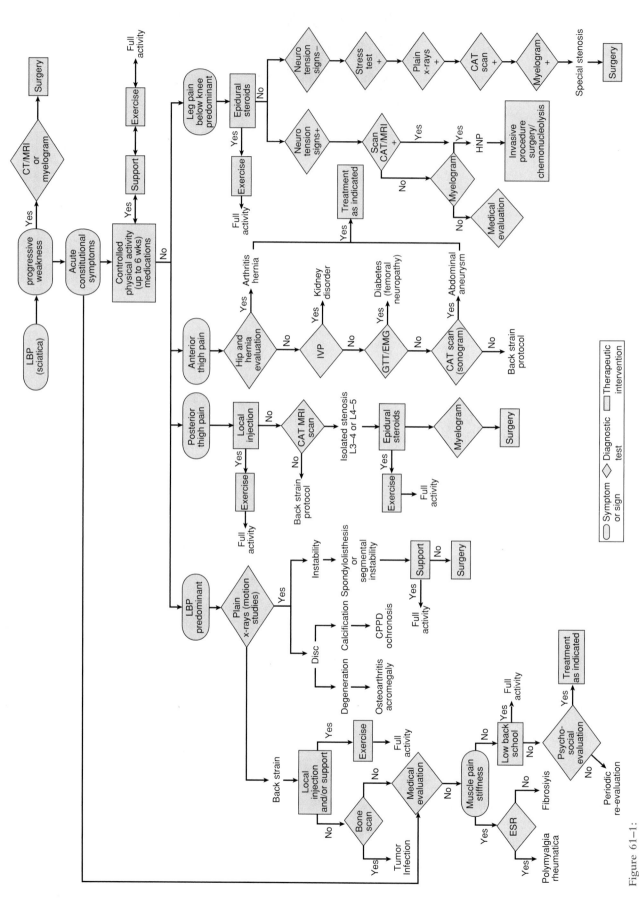

Figure 61–1:

Algorithm for the differential diagnosis of low back pain. CAT/CT, Computed tomography; CPPD, calcium pyrophosphate dihydrate disease; EMG, electromyography; ESR, erythrocyte sedimentation rate; GTT, glucose tolerance test; IVP, intravenous pyelogram; LBP, low back pain; MRI, magnetic resonance imaging. (Redrawn from Wiesel SW, Delahay JN, Connell MC, editors: *Essentials of orthopaedic surgery*. Philadelphia, 1993, Saunders.)

Table 61–1: "Red Flag" Symptoms

Fever
Chills
Night pain
Night sweats
Weight loss

- Pain with flexion that is relieved with extension is more consistent with disc pathology (symptomatic degenerative disc and herniated disc).
- Strength, sensation, and reflexes should be conducted, paying attention to specific nerve root levels (Table 61–2).
- An examination of the abdomen, the pelvis, and rectum may be necessary to check for masses or other pathology that may produce referred pain to the low back.
- The Waddell test can be performed by lightly pinching the skin of the lower back and indicates psychogenic pain if the patient complains of extreme distress. Additional Waddell tests should be performed to help distinguish nonorganic etiology.

Imaging

- In the absence of trauma, significant neurologic symptoms, or red flag signs, imaging studies are not indicated until patients have failed a 6-week trial of conservative treatment.
- "Abnormal" findings on imaging studies can occur in asymptomatic patients and should be carefully correlated with the patient's symptoms and examination findings.
- Initial imaging studies should begin with plain anteroposterior and lateral radiographs.
- Oblique lumbar views can help identify a pars defect as a break in the neck of the Scottie dog (Figure 61–2).
- Dynamic flexion and extension views may help identify evidence of instability and the presence of a spondylolisthesis.
- When advanced imaging is necessary, magnetic resonance imaging (MRI) is the modality of choice and can provide details about the disc, show evidence of neurologic compression, and identify the presence of neoplasms and/or infections.

- Computed tomography (CT) imaging, with or without myelography, is recommended in patients unable to undergo MRI, with question of neural compression secondary to bony anomalies or with fractures requiring further detail.
- A bone scan can serve as a screening tool in children and adolescent patients with back pain.
- Although controversial, selective discography can help confirm symptomatic disc changes seen on MRI but is unreliable in patients with psychogenic or symptomatic multilevel pathology.
- Discography should be performed at the level of interest and one or two normal control levels.
- Anesthetic injections may be used diagnostically or therapeutically.

Differential Diagnosis

- The differential for back pain can be divided into degenerative, traumatic, infectious, neoplastic, endocrine/metabolic, congenital, and miscellaneous disorders (Table 61–3).
- Ninety-eight percent of LBP is caused by mechanical factors such as degenerative disease, spinal stenosis, spondylolisthesis, herniated disc, and musculoskeletal strains.
- Young and adolescent athletes should be considered separately from the adult population because it has been reported that LBP in young athletes results from spondylolysis in 47% of cases and hyperlordosis in 25% of cases compared with the 48% of discogenic etiologies in adults.

Herniated Disc

- Most commonly seen in participants of collision sports or weightlifting in young and middle-aged adults.
- An acute onset of symptoms may result from a traumatic event.
- The patient may report greatest relief when lying supine, when intradiscal pressure is lowest, and increased pain when sitting in a flexed position.
- A Valsalva maneuver (e.g., straining, coughing, sneezing) may also exacerbate pain found in lumbar radiculopathy.

Table 61–2: Findings in Lumbar Disc Disease

LEVEL	NERVE ROOT	SENSORY LOSS	MOTOR LOSS	REFLEX LOSS
L1–L3	L2, L3	Anterior thigh	Hip flexors	None
L3–L4	L4	Medial calf	Quadriceps, tibialis anterior	Knee jerk
L4–L5	L5	Lateral calf, dorsal foot	EDL, EHL	None
L5–S1	S1	Posterior calf, plantar foot	Gastrocnemius/soleus	Ankle jerk
S2–S4	S2, S3, S4	Perianal	Bowel/bladder	Cremasteric

EDL, Extensor digitorum longus; EHL, extensor hallicus longus.
From Lauerman WC, McCall BR: Spine. In Miller MD, *Review of orthopaedics*, 4th ed. Philadelphia, 2004, Saunders.

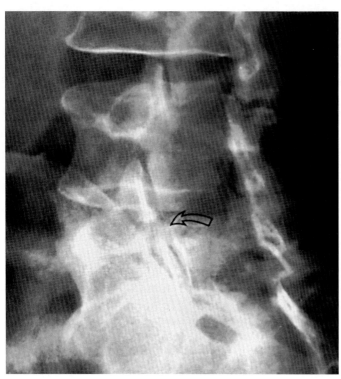

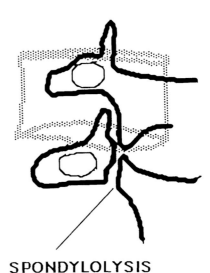

SPONDYLOLYSIS

Figure 61–2:
Radiographic evidence of a spondylolysis. (From Helms CA: *Fundamentals of skeletal radiology.* Philadelphia, 1989, Saunders.)

- The patients may demonstrate an abnormal gait, decreased range of motion, and paraspinous tenderness secondary to muscle spasm.
- In severe, chronic cases, muscle atrophy can occur.
- Herniated discs most frequently occur at L4-L5 followed by the L5-S1 disc.

- The herniation is typically posterolateral where the posterior longitudinal ligament is the weakest.
- Central herniations can present as back symptoms and, if large enough, can result in compression of the cauda equina.
- Symptoms and neurologic findings are often specific to the nerve level involved (Table 61–2).

Table 61–3: Differential Diagnosis of Disorders in the L-Spine

EVALUATION	BACK STRAIN	HNP	SPINAL STENOSIS	SPONDYLOLISTHESIS/ INSTABILITY	TUMOR	SPONDYLO- ARTHROPATHY	METABOLIC	INFECTION
Predominant pain (leg versus back)	Back	Leg	Leg	Back	Back	Back	Back	Back
Constitutional symptoms				+	+		+	
Tension sign		+						
Neurologic examination		+	+ After stress					
Plain x-ray studies			+	+	±	+	+	±
Lateral motion x-ray studies				+				
CT scan		+	+		+			+
Myelogram		+	+					
Bone scan					+	+	+	+
ESR					+	+		+
Ca/P/alk phos					+			

Ca/P/alk phos, Calcium alkaline phosphatase; CT, computed tomography; ESR, erythrocyte sedimentation rate; HNP, herniated nucleus pulposus.
From Weinstein, JN, Wiesel SW: *The lumbar spine.* Philadelphia, 1990, WB Saunders.

- Straight leg test performed between 30 and 70 degrees is sensitive for L4-L5 and L5-S1 disc herniations but not very specific.
- A positive femoral nerve tension sign is suggestive of L2-L3 or L3-L4 disc pathology.
- Contralateral straight leg raise is considered the most specific test for disc herniation but lacks sensitivity.
- Although plain radiographs are often ordered during initial evaluation, MRI is considered the imaging study of choice when disc herniation is suspected, especially in acute cases with neurologic symptoms.

Spondylolysis

- Spondylolysis represents a defect in the pars interarticularis and is the most common cause of LBP in young and adolescent athletes.
- Common in athletes who perform repetitive hyperextension activities of the back (e.g., gymnasts, football linemen, and dancers), resulting in stress-type fractures.
- Hereditary risk factors have been associated with several cases.
- May lead to spondylolisthesis.
- Symptoms often include LBP that is exacerbated with hyperextension and relieved when these activities are avoided.
- Physical examination usually demonstrates reproducible pain with provocative hyperextension and may reveal tight hamstrings.
- Lateral and oblique plain radiographic views demonstrate the majority of cases with the so-called Scottie dog lesion that shows a defect at the neck of the "dog" (Figure 61–2).
- CT scan and bone scan may help provide additional information.
- Single-photon emission computed tomography (SPECT) has been shown to be the most sensitive method for detecting this injury.

Spondylolisthesis

- Spondylolisthesis refers to the anterior slippage of one vertebra on another.
- The L4-L5 and L5-S1 vertebrae are the usual levels involved.
- This condition may remain asymptomatic until an acute injury occurs.
- Five types (Figure 61–3) and five grades of slippage (Figure 61–4).
- The isthmic type is most common.
- A heart-shaped buttock may be appreciated with the vertical position of the sacrum.
- The patient presents with LBP and may demonstrate a waddle gait, hamstring tightness, and postural abnormalities on examination.

- In some cases, neural compression can lead to radicular symptoms.
- Radiographs demonstrate the lesion and grade of spondylolisthesis.
- CT scan or bone scan can assist in making the diagnosis.

Lumbar Degenerative Disease/Spondylosis

- Spondylosis, degeneration of the lumbar spine, is a naturally occurring process.
- With age, the intervertebral disc desiccates and the amount of fibrous tissue increases, while the surrounding ligaments thicken and osteophytes form, producing a stiffer spine.
- Disc degeneration progresses through stages. Initially there are annular tears and ligament stretching, followed by further tearing and laxity, and it finally ends with loss of disc height.
- A hereditary predisposition and trauma may produce accelerated changes in some individuals.
- By age 79, nearly 100% of the population demonstrates some degree of lumbar spondylosis.
- However, radiographic evidence of spondylosis correlates poorly with clinical symptoms, making it difficult to attribute back pain to localized degenerative disease.
- Similarly, MRI findings must be carefully correlated with clinical findings.
- The presence of a "high-intensity zone" on MRI is characterized by a high intensity signal in the posterior annulus on T2-weighted images and has been correlated with an annular disruption, but its association with symptomatic discs is controversial.
- MRI may also reveal a decreased signal within the disc space (dark disc) on T2-weighted images, which may represent disc degeneration or simply dehydration.
- Although controversial, if surgical intervention is being considered, discography can be used to correlate MRI findings with clinical symptoms.

Apophyseal Ring Fractures

- The ring apophysis circumscribes the cartilaginous growth plate during adolescence and usually ossifies at 12 years of age.
- Originally separated from the vertebral body by hyaline cartilage, the ring apophysis fuses with the body between 14 and 21 years of age, signifying the end of longitudinal growth of the spine.
- Fractures of the ring apophysis are unique to the adolescent population, often resulting in avulsions that displace posteriorly into the canal attached to the intervertebral disc.
- Injury commonly results from either trauma or repetitive hyperflexion stresses.

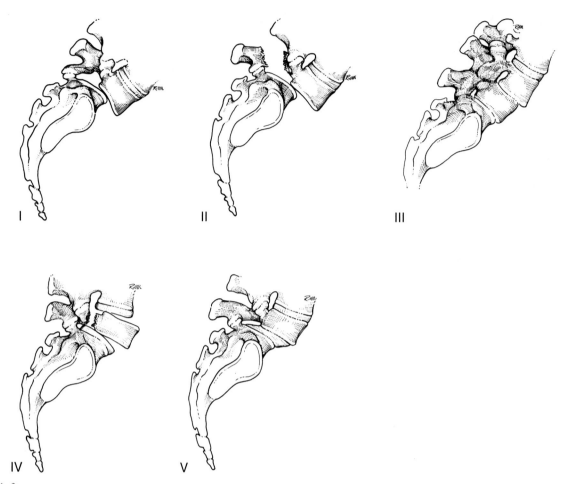

Figure 61–3:
Five types of spondylolisthesis. **I,** Type I dysplastic. **II,** Isthmic. **III,** Degenerative. **IV,** Traumatic. **V,** Pathologic. (From Freeman BL III: Scoliosis and kyphosis. In Canale ST, editor: *Campbell's operative orthopaedics,* 10th ed. Philadelphia, 2003, Mosby.)

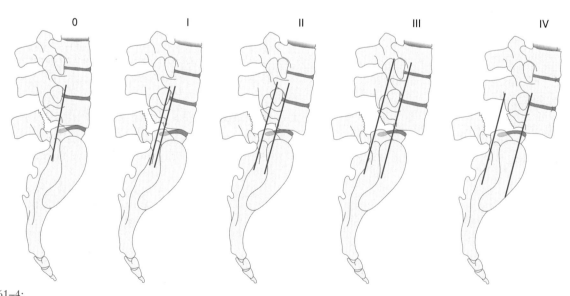

Figure 61–4:
Grading system for spondylolisthesis. (Redrawn from Borenstein DG, Wiesel SW: *Low back pain: Medical diagnosis and comprehensive management.* Philadelphia, 1989, Saunders.)

- Signs and symptoms are similar to those found with herniated discs and often lack neurologic complaints.
- Straight leg raise and contralateral straight leg raise test may be positive.
- Radiographs may demonstrate avulsion off the vertebral body and are best appreciated on lateral views.
- CT imaging may better define and diagnose these injuries.

Vertebral Osteomyelitis and Discitis

- Difficult to differentiate between discitis and osteomyelitis because they are a continuum of the same disease process.
- Typically seen in younger patients, diabetics, and those who are immunosuppressed.
- Most commonly attributed to a bacterial infection (predominantly *Staphylococcus aureus*) that results from hematogenous seeding.
- Back pain is the most common presenting symptom.
- Constitutional symptoms, fever, and systemic signs and symptoms are uncommon.
- Unless systemically ill, white blood cell count is typically normal.
- Erythrocyte sedimentation rate (ESR), complete blood count, C-reactive protein, and blood cultures must be included in the laboratory evaluation.
- ESR has been reported to be elevated in 90% of cases and blood cultures positive in 50% of cases.
- Radiographs are usually normal in the acute phase but may demonstrate erosions and sclerosis of the endplate and diminished disc space in advanced cases.
- When plain radiographs are normal, MRI is ideal for accurate diagnosis.

Initial Treatment Options

- Symptoms of acute LBP are usually self-limiting.
- Initial management should consist of antiinflammatories, activity modifications (removal from competition and practice), patient education, and reassurance.
- Symptomatic relief may be provided through the use of heat, ice, massage therapy, ultrasound, traction, and transcutaneous electrical nerve stimulation.
- Bed rest is not advised for greater than 48 hours because prolonged bed rest has been found to be detrimental to recovery.
- Use of immobilization in generalized LBP is controversial and should be used when specific etiologies are being treated (e.g., spondylolysis with increased uptake on bone scan).
- Patients with radicular symptoms that persist may be tried on a short-term regimen of low-dose oral steroids, epidural steroid injections, or selective nerve root injections.

- Opiates and muscle relaxants should be used judiciously but can be considered for severe breakthrough pain and spasm in the acute phase; however, they should not be used for chronic LBP (greater than 6 weeks).

Specific Interventions

- Patients with herniated discs who have significant weakness or pain, despite extensive nonoperative treatment with correlating findings on imaging studies, are candidates for surgical intervention.
- Persistent symptomatic spondylolytic defects may require open reduction, internal fixation, and bone grafting.
- Grades 1 and 2 spondylolisthesis can be treated nonoperatively and followed closely. Athletes and the family should be told that progression would require removal from competition and possibly surgical intervention.
- Patients with spondylolisthesis with intractable symptoms, progression, or slippage greater than 50% may require surgical intervention with posterolateral fusion. Decompression and nerve root exploration is controversial but should be performed in patients with radicular symptoms.
- Reduction of spondylolisthesis is also controversial; however, it is typically reserved for patients with unacceptable deformity or severe kyphosis.
- Symptomatic degenerative disease unresponsive to conservative management with positive discography and MRI findings may be considered for spinal fusion.
- Apophyseal ring fractures often respond to nonoperative management and bracing, but may require excision of the bony fragment and disc material if neurologic deficits and pain continue.
- Whenever possible, discitis and osteomyelitis are managed nonoperatively initially with parenteral antibiotics followed by oral antibiotics. If possible, tissue biopsy for culture and sensitivity should be obtained prior to beginning antibiotic therapy. The use of immobilization should be individualized.

Rehabilitation

- Proper rehabilitation is essential in relieving symptoms and preventing reinjury.
- Traditional teaching focuses on flexion exercises for patients with posterior element pathology, whereas those with disc disease should focus on extension exercises.
- Regardless of the pathology, most rehabilitation programs should focus, to some degree, on components of lumbar stabilization, abdominal strengthening, and aerobic conditioning.

• Stretching and strengthening exercises of the abdomen, back, and hip should be included in the regimen, with restrictions in accordance with the underlying pathology.

References

An HS, Vaccaro AR, Dolinskas CA, et al: Differentiation between spinal tumors and infections with magnetic resonance imaging. *Spine* 16:S334-S338, 1991.

This study reports on the MRI findings pertaining to infections of the spinal column. This study also distinguishes such findings from those of spinal tumors. This study further brings attention to the fact that spinal infections often occur in the anterior vertebral column, may involve disc spaces, and could highly exhibit contiguous vertebral involvement.

Bell GR, Rothman RH: The conservative treatment of sciatica. *Spine* 9:54-56, 1984.

This work recommends the utilization of 2-week bed rest with gradual mobilization and the use of aspirin for the treatment of acute sciatica. Furthermore, the work stresses the importance of a standardized program of patient education, including home exercises, proper body mechanics, and pain control, and the adherence to at least a 3-month conservative therapy regimen before surgical avenues are recommended.

Boden SD, Davis DO, Dina TS, et al: Abnormal magnetic-resonance scans of the lumbar spine in asymptomatic subjects. A prospective investigation. *J Bone Joint Surg Am* 72:403-408, 1990.

This study highlighted the importance that radiographic findings must be properly correlated with clinical signs and symptoms. In the study's evaluation of asymptomatic individuals with LBP, MRI noted the occurrence of disc herniations and spinal stenosis that were not associated with symptoms.

Collier BD, Johnson RP, Carrera GF, et al: Painful spondylolysis or spondylolisthesis studied by radiography and single-photon emission computed tomography. *Radiology* 154:207-211, 1985.

This study noted the efficacy of SPECT in comparison with planar bone scintigraphy in the detection and localization of pars defects in LBP individuals with spondylolysis or spondylolisthesis. In non-LBP individuals with spondylolysis or spondylolisthesis, the posterior neural arch was normal on SPECT imaging.

Deyo RA, Diehl AK, Rosenthal M: How many days of bed rest for acute low back pain? A randomized clinical trial. *N Engl J Med* 315:1064-1070, 1986.

This randomized clinical trial noted that appropriateness to recommend 2 days of bed rest in individuals with acute LBP rather than longer periods of bed rest. The results suggested that with 2 days of bed rest, no perceivable difference in clinical outcome is noted in comparison with longer periods of rest and, as such, could lead to reduction in absenteeism from work and its associated economic implications.

Deyo RA, Tsui-Wu YJ: Descriptive epidemiology of low-back pain and its related medical care in the United States. *Spine* 12:264-268, 1987.

This epidemiologic study noted the variations in prevalence in LBP as pertaining to age, sex, race, region, and educational status. The study also noted that general practitioners are initially sought for medical care in the event of symptoms arising pertaining to LBP. This study suggested a scheme to address various nonbiologic factors pertaining to LBP.

Fredrickson BE, Baker D, McHolick WJ, et al: The natural history of spondylolysis and spondylolisthesis. *J Bone Joint Surg Am* 66:699-707, 1984.

This radiographic study suggested a hereditary predisposition as pertaining to the presence of a spondylolytic defect and a strong association with spina bifida occulta. The study further noted that the presence of a slip in adolescence was unlikely to progress after adolescence.

Frymoyer JW, Pope MH, Clements JH, et al: Risk factors in low-back pain. An epidemiological survey. *J Bone Joint Surg Am* 65:213-218, 1983.

This epidemiologic study presents a thorough discussion and evaluation of various risk factors contributing to LBP.

Kirkaldy-Willis WH, Wedge JH, Yong-Hing K, Reilly J: Pathology and pathogenesis of lumbar spondylosis and stenosis. *Spine* 3:319-328, 1978.

This study provided a fundamental understanding of the pathology and pathogenesis of lumbar spondylosis and stenosis.

Kostuik JP, Harrington I, Alexander D, et al: Cauda equina syndrome and lumbar disc herniation. *J Bone Joint Surg Am* 68:386-391, 1986.

This study suggested two classifications (modes) of patients presenting with cauda equina syndrome secondary to a centralized disc herniation. The study noted the association of bladder dysfunction in such patients and stressed the importance of timing for surgery.

Shen FH, Samartzis D, Andersson GBJ: Nonoperative management of acute and chronic low back pain. *J Am Acad Orthop Surg* (in press).

This review provides a thorough discussion of the epidemiologic factors, pathophysiology, clinical manifestations, diagnosis, and management in individuals with acute or chronic LBP.

Waddell G, Main CJ, Morris EW, et al: Chronic low-back pain, psychologic distress, and illness behavior. *Spine* 9:209-213, 1984.

This study reported on various methods to assess distress and psychological behavior in individuals with chronic LBP.

Waddell G, McCulloch JA, Kummel E, Venner RM: Nonorganic physical signs in low-back pain. *Spine* 5:117-125, 1980.

In the evaluation of LBP, this study denoted various physical signs that are nonorganic in nature that could suggest malingering.

Weber H: Lumbar disc herniation. A controlled, prospective study with ten years of observation. *Spine* 8:131-140, 1983.

The study evaluated the clinical outcome of patients treated operatively and nonoperatively for lumbar disc herniations on the basis of symptoms and signs.

Wiesel SW, Cuckler JM, Deluca F, et al: Acute low-back pain. An objective analysis of conservative therapy. *Spine* 5:324-330, 1980.

This study noted the importance of bed rest in the management of individuals with acute back pain. The authors reported that proper bed rest can decrease time lost from work and that the use of analgesic medication with bed rest can lead to decreased pain, but not necessarily hasten return to work.

Wiltse LL, Winter RB: Terminology and measurement of spondylolisthesis. *J Bone Joint Surg Am* 65:768-772, 1983.

This work presents a thorough discussion and evaluation of the pathology and biomechanics of spondylolisthesis. Moreover, the work presents and clarifies a classification scheme as pertaining to spondylolisthesis.

CHAPTER 62

Spondylolysis/Spondylolisthesis

Introduction

- Spondylolysis is described as a defect of the pars interarticularis without any slip of one vertebra on another.
- The pars defect may be unilateral or bilateral and generally occurs at the L4-L5 or L5-S1 level.
- Spondylolisthesis occurs when there is anterior or posterior displacement of one vertebra over another (with or without pars defect) and is graded on the basis of percent of displacement (Figure 62–1).
  - Grade I: 0% to 25%.
  - Grade II: 25% to 50%.
  - Grade III: 50% to 75%.
  - Grade IV: 75% to 100%.
  - Grade V (spondyloptosis): >100%.
- Usual mechanism is repetitive hyperextension of the lumber spine.
- Risk factors that have been identified for progression include the following (Table 62–1):
  - Remaining growth potential.
  - Radiographic characteristics of bony anatomy.
- Spondylolisthesis may occur in linebackers, weightlifters, and wrestlers, but 40% to 60% of such cases in athletes manifest in gymnasts.
- Cause is usually thought to be a stress fracture, but other possible causes include congenital dysplasia, facet degeneration, or traumatic fracture.

Classification

- Spondylolisthesis has been documented in no other species other than the human race.
  - Attributed to bipedalism and lordotic lumbar spine.
- Wiltse/Newman/MacNab classification is most widely accepted (Table 62–2); however, other helpful classifications exist (Table 62–3).
  - Dysplastic.
    - Genetic disposition.
    - Congenital defect of inferior L5 facet or superior S1 fact without pars defect or elongation.
      - Symptomatic and progressive.
      - Compression of cauda equina may develop with slips greater than 25 to 30 degrees.
  - Isthmic.
    - Most common.
    - Defect of pars interarticularis.
    - Fracture can be lytic fatigue or secondary to trauma.
  - Degenerative.
    - Most common at L4-L5 level.
      - Attributed to checkrein effects of the iliolumbar ligament at L5-S1 level, which minimizes motion.
    - Mainly occurs in sixth decade of life and predominantly in females.
    - Associated with disc disease, spondylosis, and/or stenosis.
    - Slip does not exceed 30 degrees and rotation has a unilateral preference.
  - Traumatic.
  - Pathologic.
    - Associated with certain congenital syndromes and disease.

Diagnosis

- Spondylolysis and spondylolisthesis can be asymptomatic and found incidentally.
- Rule out other causes of low back pain in children! Differential diagnosis includes the following:
  - Discitis.
  - Osteoid osteoma.
  - Tumor.
  - Herniated disc.
  - Rheumatoid spondylitis.
  - Muscle strain/sprain.
- Positive single leg hyperextension.
- Negative straight leg raise.
- Restricted forward flexion of the hips and back, tight hamstrings, flat buttock (due to vertical sacrum), anterior protrusion of the pelvis, and pelvic waddling gait.
- Anteroposterior (AP) and lateral radiographs.

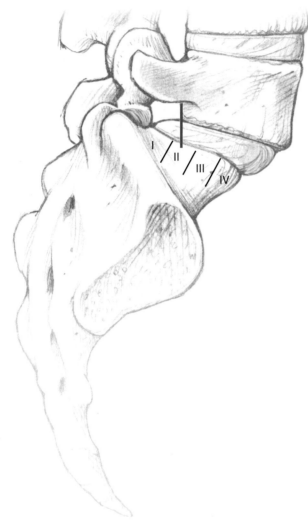

Figure 62–1:
Meyerding's classification for degree of slip. (From Jenis LG, An HS: Lumbar spondylolisthesis. In Fitzgerald RH Jr, Kaufer H, Malkani AL, editors: *Orthopedics*. St Louis, 2002, Mosby.)

Table 62–1:	Risk Factors for Progression of Spondylolisthesis

Clinical Risk Factors
Growth years (9 to 15 years of age)
Girls > boys
Episodes of back pain
Postural deformity or gait abnormality caused by hamstring spasm
Roentgenographic Risk Factors
Dysplastic (type I) spondylolisthesis
Dome-shaped, vertical sacrum
Trapezoid-shaped L5 vertebral body
≥50% slip (grades III and IV)
Increasing slip angle
Instability or excessive motion on flexion-extension views

Freeman BL III: Scoliosis and kyphosis. In Canale ST, editor: *Campbell's operative orthopaedics* 9th ed. St Louis, 1998, Mosby.

Table 62–2:	Wiltse Classification of Spondylolisthesis
CLASS	**DESCRIPTION**
I: Congenital	Congenital anomaly of the lumbosacral junction
II: Isthmic	Stress fracture or healed intact but elongated pars interarticularis
III: Degenerative	Secondary to intersegmental instability
IV: Traumatic	Acute fractures in area other than pars interarticularis
V: Pathologic	Due to intrinsic bone disease leading to fracture and slippage

Jenis LG, An HS: Lumbar spondylolisthesis. In Fitzgerald RH Jr, Kaufer H, Malkani AL, editors: *Orthopedics*. St Louis, 2002, Mosby.

- Flexion and extension views help identify possible instability in spondylolisthesis.
- Plain radiographs consider oblique views to help identify lesion.
- Variety of radiographic measurements help to characterize and describe the deformity (Figures 62–2 and 62–3).
- In early cases, plain radiographs may be negative but often a stress reaction may begin to become apparent after 3 to 6 weeks of symptoms.
- Bone scan—only helpful in an acute situation.
- Single-photon emission computed tomography—most sensitive test.
- Computed tomography (CT) scan is helpful to assess healing.
- CT myelogram is helpful for characterizing bony anatomy and isolating location of neural compression.
- Magnetic resonance imaging is generally not helpful unless you are attempting to rule out other conditions such as disc herniation; however, such imaging can help delineate degree of stenosis and neural accommodation.

Spondylolysis

- Nonoperative treatment.
  - Few are symptomatic. If identified incidentally, then observation is indicated.

Table 62–3:	Marchetti and Bartolozzi Classification of Spondylolisthesis

I. Developmental
  High dysplastic
  Low dysplastic
II. Acquired
  Traumatic
    Acute fracture
    Stress fracture
  Postsurgery
  Pathological
  Degenerative

Jenis LG, An HS: Lumbar spondylolisthesis. In Fitzgerald RH Jr, Kaufer H, Malkani AL, editors: *Orthopedics*. St Louis, 2002, Mosby.

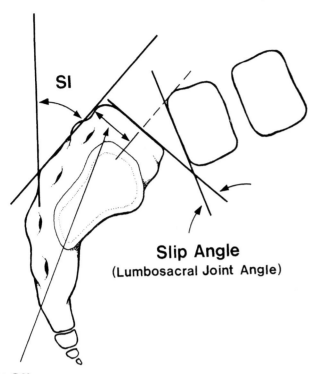

% Slip

Figure 62–2:
Measurement of slip angle in spondylolisthesis. SI, Sacral inclination. (From Lauerman WC, McCall BR: Spine. In Miller MD: *Review of orthopaedics,* **4th ed. Philadelphia, 2004, Saunders.)**

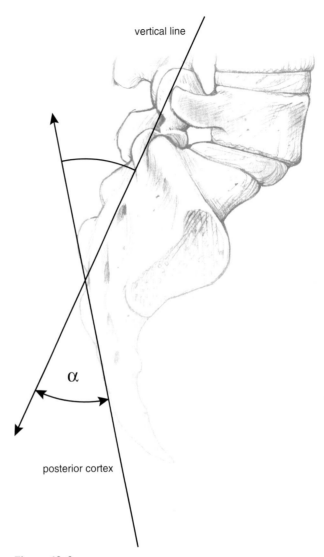

Figure 62–3:
Measurement of sacral inclination in spondylolisthesis. (From Jenis LG, An HS: Lumbar spondylolisthesis. In Fitzgerald RH Jr, Kaufer H, Malkani AL, editors: *Orthopedics.* **St Louis, 2002, Mosby.)**

- The mainstay of treatment for symptomatic spondylolysis is rest or activity modification, or both.
- After initial inflammatory phase may initiate back and abdominal strengthening and hamstring stretching.
- Bracing may be helpful and is done with a lumbosacral orthosis that places the lumbar spine in slight flexion.
- Bracing may have a role especially in cases of positive bone scan.
- There is uncertainty regarding the length of time that the patient will need to use the brace. Recommendations run from 6 weeks to 6 months.
- Operative treatment.
  - If unrelenting pain despite active nonoperative interventions, then surgical intervention is acceptable.
  - Surgical indication for spondylolysis is rare, but bone grafting and internal fixation of the defect (pars repair) have been performed in some cases of spondylolysis that have been refractory to conservative treatment.
  - Other surgical option is spinal fusion with or without instrumentation.

Spondylolithesis

- Nonoperative treatment.
  - If asymptomatic and less than 50% (grade 1 and 2) slip, then observe.

- If symptomatic and grade 1 or 2 slip, initiate conservative interventions.
- If asymptomatic and greater than 50%, then observe carefully and if progressive slip documented then surgical intervention is indicated.
- After initial inflammatory phase may initiate back and abdominal strengthening and hamstring stretching.
- Operative treatment.
  - Surgical indications include the following:
    - If unrelenting pain despite active nonoperative interventions.
    - Evidence of progressive slip.
    - Evidence of neurologic involvement.
  - Surgical options depend on history, examination, and imaging and vary.

- Decisions include the following:
  - Levels to include in fusion.
  - Slip reduction versus *in situ* fusion.
  - Fusion with or without instrumentation.
  - Posterolateral versus interbody fusion versus circumferential fusion.
- If neurologic symptoms are present, a decompression should be included with the fusion.

References

Blume HG, Rojas CH: Unilateral lumbar interbody fusion (posterior approach) utilizing dowel grafts: experience in over 200 patients. *J Neurol Orthop Surg* 2:171-175, 1981.

Fundamental work that demonstrated a more unilateral posterior approach to interbody lumbar fusion.

Bradford DS, Boachie-Adjei O: Treatment of severe spondylolisthesis by anterior and posterior reduction and stabilization. A long-term follow-up study. *J Bone Joint Surg Am* 72:1060-1066, 1990.

This long-term follow-up study noted the efficacy of anterior and posterior operative management of high-grade spondylolisthesis. The study noted that 17 of 22 patients had restoration of their sagittal plane alignment on last follow-up evaluation.

Cloward RB: The treatment of ruptured lumbar intervertebral discs by vertebral body fusion. I. Indications, operative technique, after care. *J Neurosurg* 10:154-168, 1953.

Seminal work illustrating the operative technique and indications for posterior lumbar interbody fusion.

Harms J, Jeszenszky D, Stoltze D, Bohm H: True spondylolisthesis reduction and monosegmental fusion in spondylolisthesis. In Bridwell KH, DeWald RL, editors: *The textbook of spinal surgery,* 2nd ed. Philadelphia, 1997, Lippincott-Raven.

The work highlighted a transforaminal lumbar interbody fusion technique with posterior instrumentation for operative management of spondylolisthesis.

Iguchi T, Wakami T, Kurihara A, et al: Lumbar multilevel degenerative spondylolisthesis: radiological evaluation and factors related to anterolisthesis and retrolisthesis. *J Spinal Disord Tech* 15:93-99, 2002.

This study noted various factors that increase the risk of anterolisthesis in degenerative spondylolisthesis patients. However, no factors were found or correlated to the occurrence of retrolisthesis.

Jackson DW, Wiltse LL, Dingeman RD, Hayes M: Stress reactions involving the pars interarticularis in young athletes. *Am J Sports Med* 9:304-312, 1981.

This study stresses the importance of early diagnosis and treatment of pars interarticularis defects in the young athlete. The study noted that with early detection and treatment, the average time to return to competition is decreased.

Jenis LG, An HS: Posterior lumbar interbody fusion for spondylolisthesis. *Semin Spine Surg* 11:56-66, 1999.

This work presents a thorough discussion of the indications and contraindications of posterior lumbar interbody fusion for the treatment of spondylolisthesis.

Miller SF, Congeni J, Swanson K: Long-term functional and anatomical follow-up of early detected spondylolysis in young athletes. *Am J Sports Med* 32:928-933, 2004.

Early pars lesions are those that may be detected by nuclear scintigraphy but not by plain radiography. This study noted that despite the degree of healing determined by CT scan early after detection, almost all of these lesions can be expected to go on to good clinical results (with 7- to 11-year follow-up). Bilateral defects are much less likely to heal radiographically than unilateral defects.

Neugebauer FI: The classic: a new contribution to the history and etiology of spondylolisthesis by F. L. Neugebauer. *Clin Orthop* 117:4-22, 1976.

This work presents an interesting historical perspective as to the development of spondylolisthesis. An interesting note was that the first clinical identification of spondylolisthesis was attributed to Dr. Herbiniaux, a Belgian obstetrician, in 1782.

Nozawa S, Shimizu K, Miyamoto K, Tanaka M: Repair of pars interarticularis defect by segmental wire fixation in young athletes with spondylolysis. *Am J Sports Med* 31:359-364, 2003.

This study reported that segmental wire fixation of pars defects in an athletic population may produce good results with a high rate of fusion and return to sports. Scores of subjective symptoms show significant improvement, and although not all athletes return to their previous level of activity, most may return to some level of sports.

Wiltse LL, Newman PH, Macnab I: Classification of spondylolysis and spondylolisthesis. *Clin Orthop* 117:23-29, 1976.

This seminal work proposed a five-tier classification system of spondylolisthesis.

CHAPTER 63

Preparticipation Evaluation

Introduction

- The preparticipation examination (PPE) is a screening tool that allows physicians and other appropriate personnel to evaluate an athlete's level of fitness and potential risks prior to sport participation.
- It is used in essentially all athletics at or above high school sports.
- Primary objectives of the examination include detecting predisposing injury conditions and life-threatening conditions.
- Secondary objectives include assessment of general health and counseling on health-related issues and proper training techniques.
- When performing the examination and counseling the athlete, the examiner must have a good understanding of the most common injuries observed among specific sports (Table 63–1).
- It is suggested that a standard protocol be used, preferably with an outlined form, to achieve uniform assessment of sport participants and allow a ready medical reference to guide care and treatment of athletes before starting play and when injury occurs.
- A recommended form has been produced by the American Academy of Family Physicians, American Academy of Pediatrics, American Medical Society for Sports Medicine, American Orthopaedic Society for Sports Medicine, and American Osteopathic Academy for Sports Medicine (Figure 63–1).
- Some organizations may have preestablished forms and protocols. However, modifications to the preceding form can be made to meet the needs of the establishment and preferences of the examiner as demonstrated in the form used at West Point (Figure 63–2).
- Further research and data are still required to determine which history questions and physical examination tests and methods are best at identifying conditions that increase risk of injury and improve the PPE.
- It is advised that the examination be performed on entering a new school level or sport organization followed by yearly updated medical histories, with proper detailed evaluations of significant findings.
- The most common methods for performing the examination include using an athlete's primary care physician and an assembly line or a multistation format at the athletic institution using a single physician or team of health care providers, respectively. Each of these have their respective advantages and disadvantages, which are taken into account before deciding the method most suitable and effective to meet the objectives set up by the particular institution (Table 63–2).
- The use of a computer questionnaire followed by a single physician or multistation examination is another viable option that can possibly make the process more effective.
- The performance of the PPE also provides the health care provider the opportunity to address other medically related issues with the athletes such as nutrition, drug use, and preventive measures.
- It is recommended that the PPE be performed at least 6 weeks prior to the start of preseason practice to allow sufficient time for workup and treatment of medical problems.
- In addition to the PPE, the use of a problem list attached to the athlete's record allows easy reference to medical problems that can be transferred among medical team members and at the time the athlete moves to a new institution.

History, Physical Examination, and Imaging

- A thorough history is critical in identifying the majority of medical problems.
- A list of screening questions used on the PPE form can serve as a basic guide.
- The evaluating provider must ensure that the information is accurate and complete, often requiring parental involvement in the younger population.
- A complete documented physical examination should be supplemented with appropriate additional tests addressing conditions identified during the history (Table 63–3).

Table 63–1:	Sport-Specific Musculoskeletal Injuries*
SPORT	**MOST COMMON INJURIES**
Football	Concussions, brachial plexus injuries, ankle and knee ligament injuries, quadriceps and hamstring strains, muscle contusions, spondylolysis in football linemen, shoulder dislocations, finger injuries
Soccer	Concussions, ankle and knee ligament injuries, hip adductor strains
Basketball	Ocular and maxillofacial injuries, hand/wrist injury, patellar tendinitis, ankle sprains
Volleyball	Shoulder impingement, finger injuries, patellar tendinitis
Racquet sports	Epicondylitis, low back strains, Achilles tendon ruptures, "tennis leg"
Baseball/softball	Eye injuries, impingement syndrome and instability of the shoulder, valgus overload syndromes, hook of the hamate fractures
Running	Iliotibial band syndrome, shin splints/stress fractures, Achilles tendinitis, recurrent compartment syndrome, patellar tendinopathies, plantar fasciitis
Wrestling/judo	Ear injuries, neck/back strains, costochondral injuries, brachial plexus injuries, prepatellar bursitis, ankle sprains
Dance	Back sprains, spondylolysis and spondylolisthesis, snapping hip syndrome, patella femoral syndrome, stress fractures, cuboid syndrome, ankle impingement, flexor hallucis longus tendonitis
Gymnastics	Wrist overuse syndromes, spondylolysis and spondylolisthesis
Weightlifting	Finger crush injuries, back sprains, pectoralis major ruptures, acromioclavicular arthrosis
Swimming	Impingement and instability of the shoulder, breaststroker's knee
Skiing	Concussions, lacerations, thoracolumbar burst fractures, gamekeeper's thumb, shoulder dislocations, tibial fractures, knee ligament ruptures
Ice hockey	Concussions, facial contusions and lacerations, syndesmosis ankle sprains
Bicycling	Head, maxillofacial and dental injuries, neck and back sprains, pudendal and ulnar and median nerve palsies
Boxing	Head and ocular injuries, low back sprains
Rock climbing	Brachialis tendonitis, finger injuries

*This list is limited to injuries that are common or unique to the specific sport. Injuries may vary by age and level of sports.
From Somogyi DM, Shrier I: Customizing the preparticipation evaluation. In Fu FH, Stone DA, editors: *Sports injuries: mechanisms, prevention, treatment.* Philadelphia, 2001, Lippincott Williams & Wilkins. Modified from Caine DJ, Caine CG, Koenraad J. *Epidemiology of sports injuries.* Champaign, IL, 1996, Human Kinetics.

- Temperature and vital signs should be recorded.
  - If fever is present, appropriate workup and treatment are required.
  - One should take note that hypertension is classified according to age (Table 63–4).
  - If hypertension is present, repeat measurements should be performed with an appropriate-sized cuff, and, if still elevated, the athlete must be questioned about the use of stimulants (caffeine, nicotine, ephedrine, cocaine).
  - True hypertension requires further evaluation and treatment by the athlete's primary care physician.
- Height and weight measurements enable assessment of obesity and possible eating disorders, which demands further questioning about eating habits, body image, or growth disturbance and proper referrals if problems exist.
- Eyes should be evaluated for visual acuity and pupil size.
  - If there is a significant history of eye injury, absence of one eye, or best corrected vision poorer than 20/40 in either eye, the athlete requires proper eye protection if sport participation is considered.
  - Anisocoria may be otherwise normal but must be documented and discussed with the coaches and trainers to avoid improper evaluation in case the athlete sustains a head injury.
- The tympanic membrane should be evaluated for scarring or perforations.
  - If indicated, audiology should be performed.
  - Athletes with perforated membranes involved in water sports should be advised to wear proper fitting protective earplugs.

- Nasal polyps and a deviated septum should be documented and can be referred for correction, although they usually do not impose any sport restrictions.
- Findings in the oral cavity may suggest underlying conditions.
  - Leukoplakia is associated with the use of smokeless tobacco.
  - A high arched palate deserves further evaluation for other Marfan syndrome characteristics (see Table 63–3).
  - Oral ulcers, gingival atrophy, and tooth enamel loss are found among bulimic patients.
  - A mouth guard is recommended in contact sport athletes with corrective braces to prevent lacerations.
- In addition to blood pressure, cardiovascular evaluation requires the palpation of radial and femoral pulses and auscultation of the heart.
  - Absence of a femoral pulse suggests coarctation of the aorta.
  - Murmurs of hypertrophic cardiomyopathy are louder when standing (rather than sitting) and during Valsalva maneuvers (decreases venous return) and diminish with squatting (increases venous return).
  - Murmurs of aortic stenosis increase with squatting and decrease with Valsalva maneuvers.
  - Generally, systolic murmurs of grade 3 or higher, any diastolic murmur, and murmurs that increase with Valsalva require further evaluation.
  - Arrhythmias should be further evaluated by electrocardiography and referred to a cardiologist if multifocal premature ventricular contractions, doublets, or triplets are present.

Text Continued on p. 455

Preparticipation Physical Evaluation

| History | Date of Exam _____ |

Name _____ Sex _____ Age _____ Date of Birth _____
Grade _____ School _____ Sport(s) _____
Address _____ Phone _____
Personal physician _____
In case of emergency, contact
Name _____ Relationship _____ Phone(H) _____ (W) _____

Explain "Yes" answers below. Circle questions you don't know the answers to.

Yes No (left column) / **Yes No** (right column)

1. Have you had a medical illness or injury since your last checkup or sports physical? ☐ ☐

   Do you have an ongoing or chronic illness? ☐ ☐

2. Have you ever been hospitalized overnight? ☐ ☐

   Have you ever had surgery? ☐ ☐

3. Are you currently taking any prescription or nonprescription (over-the-counter) medication or pills or using an inhaler? ☐ ☐

   Have you ever taken any supplements or vitamins to help you gain or lose weight or improve your performance? ☐ ☐

4. Do you have any allergies (for example, to pollen, medicine, food, or stinging insects)? ☐ ☐

   Have you ever had a rash or hives develop during or after exercise? ☐ ☐

5. Have you ever passed out during or after exercise? ☐ ☐

   Have you ever been dizzy during or after exercise? ☐ ☐

   Have you ever had chest pain during or after exercise? ☐ ☐

   Do you get tired more quickly than your friends do during exercise? ☐ ☐

   Have you ever had racing of your heart or skipped heartbeats? ☐ ☐

   Have you had high blood pressure or high cholesterol? ☐ ☐

   Have you ever been told you have a heart murmur? ☐ ☐

   Has any family member or relative died of heart problems or of sudden death before age 50? ☐ ☐

   Have you had a severe viral infection (for example, myocarditis or mononucleosis) within the past month? ☐ ☐

   Has a physician ever denied or restricted your participation in sports for any heart problems? ☐ ☐

6. Do you have any current skin problems (for example, itching, rashes, acne, warts, fungus, or blisters)? ☐ ☐

7. Have you ever had a head injury or concussion? ☐ ☐

   Have you ever been knocked out, become unconscious, or lost your memory? ☐ ☐

   Have you ever had a seizure? ☐ ☐

   Do you have frequent or severe headaches? ☐ ☐

   Have you ever had numbness or tingling in your arms, hands, legs, or feet? ☐ ☐

   Have you ever had a stinger, burner, or pinched nerve? ☐ ☐

8. Have you ever become ill from exercising in the heat? ☐ ☐

9. Do you cough, wheeze, or have trouble breathing during or after activity? ☐ ☐

   Do you have asthma? ☐ ☐

Do you have seasonal allergies that require medical treatment? ☐ ☐

10. Do you use any special protective or corrective equipment or devices that aren't usually used for your sport or position (for example, knee brace, special neck roll, foot orthotics, retainer on your teeth, hearing aid)? ☐ ☐

11. Have you had any problems with your eyes or vision? ☐ ☐

    Do you wear glasses, contacts, or protective eyewear? ☐ ☐

12. Have you ever had a sprain, strain, or swelling after injury? ☐ ☐

    Have you broken or fractured any bones or dislocated any joints? ☐ ☐

    Have you had any other problems with pain or swelling in muscles, tendons, bones, or joints? ☐ ☐

    If yes, check appropriate box and explain below.

    ☐ Head ☐ Upper arm ☐ Finger ☐ Ankle
    ☐ Neck ☐ Elbow ☐ Hip ☐ Foot
    ☐ Back ☐ Forearm ☐ Thigh
    ☐ Chest ☐ Wrist ☐ Knee
    ☐ Shoulder ☐ Hand ☐ Shin/calf

13. Do you want to weigh more or less than you do now? ☐ ☐

    Do you lose weight regularly to meet weight requirements for your sport? ☐ ☐

14. Do you feel stressed out? ☐ ☐

15. Record the dates of your most recent immunizations (shots) for:

    Tetanus _____ Measles _____
    Hepatitis B _____ Chickenpox _____

FEMALES ONLY

16. When was your first menstrual period? _____

    When was your most recent menstrual period? _____

    How much time do you usually have from the start of one period to the start of another? _____

    How many periods have you had in the past year? _____

    What was the longest time between periods in the past year? _____

Explain "Yes" answers here: _____
_____
_____
_____
_____
_____

I hereby state that, to the best of my knowledge, my answers to the above questions are complete and correct.

Signature of athlete _____ Signature of parent/guardian _____ Date _____

Figure 63–1:
Recommended preparticipation physical evaluation form developed by the American Academy of Family Physicians, American Academy of Pediatrics, American Medical Society for Sports Medicine, American Orthopaedic Society for Sports Medicine, and American Osteopathic Academy for Sports Medicine. (Modified from American Academy of Family Physicians, American Academy of Pediatrics, American Medical Society for Sports Medicine, American Orthopaedic Society for Sports Medicine, Osteopathic Academy of Sports Medicine: The preparticipation physical evaluation physical examination. In Arendt EA, editor: *Orthopaedic knowledge update sports medicine 2.* Rosemont, IL, 1999, American Academy of Orthopaedic Surgeons.)

Army Corps Squad
Preparticipation Physical History

Name_____ _____ _____
　　　　(Last)　　　　　　　　　　　　　(First)　　　　　　　　　　　　　(Middle)

Age_____ Sex: ☐Male ☐Female Date of Birth_____ SSN_____

Class of_____ Academic Company_____ Company Phone_____ Personal Phone_____

Sport_____ _____ _____
　　　　Fall　　　　　　　　　　　　　　Winter　　　　　　　　　　　　　Spring

Explain "Yes" answers　　　　　　　　　　　　　　　　　　　　　　　　　　　　　　　Yes　No

1. Have you ever been hospitalized?.. ☐ ☐
   Have you ever had surgery?... ☐ ☐
2. Are you currently taking any medications or pills?... ☐ ☐
   Have you tried to control your weight through vigorous exercise, diet pills, laxatives, etc? .... ☐ ☐
3. Do you have any allergies? (medicine, bees or other stinging insects)............................ ☐ ☐
4. Have you ever passed out during or after exercise?... ☐ ☐
   Have you ever been dizzy during or after exercise?... ☐ ☐
   Have you ever had chest pain during or after exercise?... ☐ ☐
   Do you tire more quickly than your friends during exercise?.. ☐ ☐
   Have you ever had high blood pressure?.. ☐ ☐
   Do you worry or have you been told that you are not eating enough or that you exercise too much? ... ☐ ☐
   Have you ever been told you have a heart murmur?... ☐ ☐
   Have you ever had racing of your heart or skipped heartbeats?....................................... ☐ ☐
   Has anyone in your family died of heart problems or a sudden death before age 50? .... ☐ ☐
5. Do you have any skin problems? (itching, rashes, acne) .... ☐ ☐
6. Have you ever had a head injury?.. ☐ ☐
   Have you ever been knocked out or unconscious? .... ☐ ☐
   Have you ever had a seizure?.. ☐ ☐
   Have you ever had a stinger, burner, or pinched nerve?... ☐ ☐
7. Have you ever had heat or muscle cramps?... ☐ ☐
   Have you ever been dizzy or passed out in the heat?.. ☐ ☐
8. Do you have trouble breathing or do you cough during or after activity?...................... ☐ ☐
9. Do you use any special equipment? (Pads, braces, neck rolls, mouth guards, eye guards, etc) ...... ☐ ☐
10. Have you had any problems with your eyes or vision?... ☐ ☐
11. Have you ever sprained / strained, dislocated, fractured, broken or had repeated swelling, chronic pain or other injuries
    to any bones or joints?.. ☐ ☐

☐ Head　　☐ Shoulder　　☐ Thigh　　☐ Neck　　☐ Elbow　　☐ Chest　　☐ Knee
☐ Forearm　☐ Shin / Calf　☐ Back　　☐ Wrist　☐ Ankle　☐ Hand　☐ Foot

12. Have you had any other medical problems? (infectious mononucleosis, diabetes, etc.)......... ☐ ☐
13. Have you had a medical problem or injury since your last evaluation?............................ ☐ ☐
14. What do you consider your ideal weight? _____
15. When was your first menstrual period? _____
    When was your last menstrual period? _____
    What was the longest time between your periods last year? _____

Explain "Yes" answers:

_____

_____

_____

_____

_____

_____

I hereby state that, to the best of my knowledge, my answers to the above questions are correct.

Date _____

Signature of athlete _____

Figure 63–2:
Army Corps Squad preparticipation physical history and examination form. (From Miller MD, Cooper DE, Warner JJP: *Review of sports medicine and arthroscopy.* Philadelphia, 2002, Saunders; modified from Smith DM, Kovan JR, Rich BS, Tanner SM: *Preparticipation physical examination,* 2nd ed. Minneapolis, 1997, McGraw-Hill.)

(continued)

**Army Corps Squad
Preparticipation Physical Examination**

Height_____ Weight _____ BP ____ / _____ Pulse_____

Vision R 20/_____ L 20/_____ Corrected   Y   N   Pupils_____

	Normal	Abnormal Findings	Initials
Pulses			
Heart			
Lungs			
Skin			
Abdominal			
Genitalia			
HEENT			
Musculoskeletal			
Neck			
Shoulder			
Elbow			
Wrist			
Hand			
Back			
Knee			
Ankle			
Foot			
Other			

Clearance:

A. Cleared

B. Cleared after completing evaluation / rehabilitation for:

C. Not cleared for:

☐ Collision

☐ Contact

☐ Non-contact   _____Strenuous   _____Moderately Strenuous   _____Non-strenuous

Due to:_____

Recommendation:_____

_____

_____

_____

_____

Orthopedic Physician (Print) _____ Signature _____ Date _____

Medical Physician (Print) _____ Signature _____ Date _____

Figure 63–2, cont'd

Table 63–2: Advantages and Disadvantages of the Various Formats Used for the Preparticipation Evaluation

CATEGORY	PRIVATE PHYSICIAN	ASSEMBLY LINE	COMPUTERIZED MULTISTATION	QUESTIONNAIRE
Communication				
Advantages	Ongoing physician-patient relationship One-on-one questioning allows discussion of sensitive psychosocial issues May have more time per patient Prior medical history known	Good communication with school and athletic staff	More expedient Good communication with school and athletic staff	Most expedient Allows discussion of highlighted sensitive issues
Disadvantages	No contact with school or athletic staff	Noisy, hurried environment Variable experience or interest in primary psychosocial needs of students Poor communication with parents Lack of privacy	Noisy, hurried environment Variable experience or interest in primary psychosocial needs of students Poor communication with parents Lack of privacy	Lacks personal relationship for those without problems
Expertise				
Advantages	No advantages	Sports directed Increased consistency	Sports directed Specialized personnel with individual expertise in a variety of areas	N/A
Disadvantages	Variable physician interest and consistency in sports medicine decision making	No disadvantages	No disadvantages	N/A
Availability				
Advantages	Can provide long-term care	No advantages	No advantages	N/A
Disadvantages	Not always available preseason for athletes	Continuity of care may be compromised	Continuity of care may be compromised	N/A
Cost-effectiveness				
Advantages	Effectiveness varies with clinician	Effectiveness and reporting more consistent	Most complete/effective	Follow-up info easily compared with previous information
Disadvantages	More expensive than assembly-line format	Less time for clinicians than multistation format	Most expensive	Cost of setting up database program and computers
Administration				
Advantages	No system to set up	Easy to set up	No advantages	Athletes complete at own convenience Administratively easy after pilot period of 1–3 yr
Disadvantages	May have to chase after athletes to comply	No disadvantage	Requires space and significant effort Problem if not all examiners or athletes show up	Still requires other approach for physical examination

From Somogyi DM, Shrier I: Customizing the preparticipation evaluation. In Fu FH, Stone DA, editors: *Sports injuries: mechanisms, prevention, treatment.* Philadelphia, 2001, Lippincott Williams & Williams.

Table 63–3: Suggested Examination Protocol for the Physician

Musculoskeletal

Have patient:
Stand facing examiner
Look at ceiling, floor, over shoulders, touch ears to shoulders
Shrug shoulders (against resistance)
Abduct shoulders 90 degrees, hold against resistance
Externally rotate arms fully
Flex and extend elbows
Arms at sides, elbows 90 degrees flexed, pronate/suspinate wrists
Spread fingers, make fist
Contract quadriceps, relax quadriceps
"Duck walk" four steps away from examiner
Stand with back to examiner
Knees straight, touch toes
Rise up on heels, then toes

To check for:
Extremities joints, general habitus
Cervical spine motion
Trapezius strength
Deltoid strength
Shoulder motion
Elbow motion
Elbow and wrist motion
Hand and finger motion, deformities
Symmetry and knee/ankle effusion
Hip, knee, and ankle motion
Shoulder symmetry, scoliosis
Scoliosis, hip motion, hamstrings
Calf symmetry, leg strength

Murmur evaluation

Auscultation should be performed sitting, supine, and squatting in a quiet room
    using the diaphragm and bell of a stethoscope
Auscultation finding of:
S1 heard easily; not holosystolic, soft, low-pitched
Normal S2
No ejection or midsystolic click
Continuous diastolic murmur absent
No early diastolic murmur
Normal femoral pulses (equivalent to brachial pulses in strength and arrival)

Rules out:
Ventricular septal defect and mitral regurgitation
Tetralogy, atrial septal defect, and pulmonary hypertension
Aortic stenosis and pulmonary stenosis
Patent ductus arteriosus
Aortic insufficiency
Coarctation

Marfan's screen

Screen all men taller than 6'0" and all women taller than 5'10" in height with echocardiogram
    and slit lamp examination when any two of the following are found:
Family history of Marfan's syndrome (this finding alone should prompt further investigation)
Cardiac murmur or midsystolic click
Kyphoscoliosis
Anterior thoracic deformity
Arm span greater than height
Upper to lower body ratio more than 1 SD below mean
Myopia
Ectopic lens
High arched palate
Arachnodactyly

SD, Standard deviation.
From Bader RS, Goldberg L, Sahn DJ: *Ped Clin North Am* 52: 1421-25.

- Lungs are assessed for wheezing or rubs. Odor of tobacco should prompt the examiner to discuss smoking cessation.
- Masses, tenderness, rigidity, or enlargement of the liver or spleen detected on abdominal examination require further evaluation. Females should be examined for a gravid uterus.
- The male genitalia is assessed for hernias and testes that are undescended, absent, or irregular.
  - Athletes with undescended or unpaired testicles should be counseled on proper protection and follow-up.
  - The athlete should be advised that testicular cancer is the leading cause of cancer death in men 18 to 35 years and instructed on proper self-examinations and provided with a handout if available.
- A genitourinary examination of females is not a component of the PPE.
- The skin is examined for rashes, infections, or infestations that may restrict participation in close contact sport such as in wrestling, judo, and rugby (Table 63–5). Suspicious nevi or other skin anomalies should be worked up appropriately but usually do not limit sport participation.
- The musculoskeletal examination, which is generally low yield in asymptomatic patients, can be accomplished by different methods.
- The general musculoskeletal examination provides a quick assessment of range of motion, muscle strength, asymmetry, and significant abnormalities.

Table 63–4:	Classification of Hypertension	
AGE (YR)	SIGNIFICANT HYPERTENSION (MM HG)*	SEVERE HYPERTENSION (MM HG)†
6-9	Systolic 122-129 Diastolic 70-85	Systolic >129 Diastolic >85
10-12	Systolic 126-133 Diastolic 82-89	Systolic >133 Diastolic >89
13-15	Systolic 136-143 Diastolic 86-91	Systolic >143 Diastolic >91
16-18	Systolic 142-149 Diastolic 92-97	Systolic >149 Diastolic >97
>18	Systolic [140-179]‡ Diastolic [90-109]‡	Systolic [>179] Diastolic [>109]

*95th to 98th percentile for age, boys and girls combined.
†99th percentile for age, boys and girls combined.
‡Because the Second Task Force did not discuss youth older than 18 years, the values in brackets are those for mild and moderate hypertension given by the 26th Bethesda Conference.
From Miller MD, Cooper DE, Warner JJP: *Review of sports medicine and arthroscopy*, 2nd ed. Philadelphia, 2002, Saunders. Modified from Risser WL, Anderson SJ, Boulduc SP, et al: *Pediatrics* 99:637-638, 1997.

- The general screen cannot establish a specific diagnosis or severity of a musculoskeletal injury and therefore must be supplemented by joint-specific examinations if positive findings exist or are indicated by history.
- A full joint-specific examination involves inspection; palpation; range of motion; muscle strength; and maneuvers of the neck, spine, shoulders, elbows, wrists, fingers, hips, knees, elbows, and ankles.
  - Although more definitive than the general examination, it is time consuming and may be limited by the expertise of the examiner.
  - Significant findings encourage a more focused examination with diagnostic testing.

Table 63–5: Categories of Infectious Skin Condition

Impetigo
Erysipelas
Carbuncle
Staphylococcal disease
Foliculitis (generalized)
Hidradenitis suppurativa
Parasitic skin infections
  Pediculosis
  Scabies
Viral skin infections
  Herpes simplex
  Herpes zoster (chickenpox)
  Molluscum contagiosum
Fungal skin infections
  Tinea corporis (ringworm)

From Miller MD, Cooper DE, Warner JJP: *Review of sports medicine and arthroscopy.* Philadelphia, 2002, Saunders.

- Some physicians advocate sport-specific examinations that concentrate on areas placed under stress in particular sports.
  - These examinations are also time consuming and usually require in-depth knowledge of sports and orthopaedic evaluations and injuries, beyond that which is used in the joint-specific examination.
- Neurologic status is considered normal if the general musculoskeletal examination is normal. However, athletes who have suffered concussions, recurrent stingers/burners, or seizures warrant further investigation.
- Laboratory and imaging studies and other ancillary tests are not components of the PPE and are only indicated when further evaluation of specific problems is necessary.

Determination of Fitness for Participation

- More than 95% of athletes pass the PPE with no restrictions, and less than 1% are excluded from all sport participation.
- On completing the PPE, the examiner must use his or her findings to assign the athlete to one of the following categories:
  - Unrestricted clearance.
  - Clearance after completion of additional evaluation and rehabilitation.
  - Not cleared for certain types of sports or all sports.
- Sport activities can be divided into three general categories: (1) contact and collision, (2) limited contact, and (3) noncontact (Table 63–6). Sports may also be classified according to static and dynamic demands (Table 63–7). This guides the examiner to make restriction or clearance recommendations according to a group of sports.
- Factors to consider when making a determination include whether findings on the PPE place athletes or other participants at an increased risk of injury, whether they can participate with treatment, and if not cleared for particular activities, whether they can safely participate in any other activities.
- The American Academy of Pediatrics developed a medical list of conditions considered limiting or disqualifying (Table 63–8).
- It should be noted that 80% to 90% of sudden deaths occurring in athletes younger than 35 years involve cardiovascular abnormalities, particularly hypertrophic cardiomyopathy (see Boxes 63–1 and 63–2, Figure 63–3).

Text continued on p. 461

Table 63–6: Classification of Sports by Contact

CONTACT/COLLISION	LIMITED CONTACT	NONCONTACT
Basketball	Baseball	Archery
Boxing	Bicycling	Badminton
Diving	Cheerleading	Bodybuilding
Field hockey	Canoeing/kayaking	Bowling
Football	(white water)	Canoeing/
Flag	Fencing	kayaking
Tackle	Field events	(flat water)
Ice hockey	High jump	Crew/rowing
Lacrosse	Pole vault	Curling
Martial arts	Floor hockey	Dancing
Rodeo	Gymnastics	Field events
Rugby	Handball	Discus
Ski jumping	Horseback riding	Javelin
Soccer	Racquetball	Shot put
Team handball	Skating	Golf
Water polo	Ice	Orienteering
Wrestling	In-line	Powerlifting
	Roller	Racewalking
	Skiing	Riflery
	Cross-country	Rope jumping
	Downhill	Running
	Water	Sailing
	Softball	Scuba diving
	Squash	Strength training
	Ultimate frisbee	Swimming
	Volleyball	Table tennis
	Windsurfing/surfing	Tennis
		Track
		Weightlifting

From Miller MD, Cooper DE, Warner JJP: *Review of sports medicine and arthroscopy.* Philadelphia, 2002, Saunders. Modified from Risser WL, Anderson SJ, Boulduc SP, et al: *Pediatrics* 94:757-760, 1994.

Table 63–7: Classification of Sports by Strenuousness

HIGH TO MODERATE INTENSITY		
HIGH TO MODERATE DYNAMIC AND STATIC DEMANDS	HIGH TO MODERATE DYNAMIC AND LOW STATIC DEMANDS	HIGH TO MODERATE STATIC AND LOW DYNAMIC DEMANDS
Boxing	Badminton	Archery
Crew/rowing	Baseball	Auto racing
Cross-country skiing	Basketball	Diving
Cycling	Field hockey	Equestrian
Downhill skiing	Lacrosse	Field events
Fencing	Orienteering	Jumping
Football	Ping-Pong	Throwing
Ice hockey	Racewalking	Gymnastics
Rugby	Racquetball	Karate/judo
Running (sprint)	Soccer	Motorcycling
Speed skating	Squash	Rodeo
Water polo	Swimming	Sailing
Wrestling	Tennis	Ski jumping
	Volleyball	Water-skiing
		Weightlifting

LOW INTENSITY (LOW DYNAMIC AND LOW STATIC DEMANDS)

Bowling
Cricket
Curling
Golf
Riflery

From Miller MD, Cooper DE, Warner JJP: *Review of sports medicine and arthroscopy.* Philadelphia, 2002, Saunders. Modified from Risser WL, Anderson SJ, Boulduc SP, et al: *Pediatrics* 94:757-760, 1994.

Table 63–8: Medical Conditions and Sports Participation*

CONDITION	MAY PARTICIPATE?
Atlantoaxial instability (instability of the joint between C1 and C2)	Qualified
Explanation: Athlete needs evaluation to assess risk of spinal cord injury during sports participation.	Yes
Bleeding disorder	Qualified
Explanation: Athlete needs evaluation.	Yes
Cardiovascular diseases	
Carditis (inflammation of the heart)	No
Explanation: Carditis may result in sudden death with exertion.	
Hypertension (high blood pressure)	Qualified
Explanation: Those with significant essential (unexplained) hypertension should avoid weight- and powerlifting, bodybuilding, and strength training. Those with secondary hypertension (hypertension caused by a previously identified disease), or severe essential hypertension, need evaluation.	Yes
Congenital heart disease (structural heart defects present at birth)	Qualified
Explanation: Those with mild forms may participate fully; those with moderate or severe forms, or who have undergone surgery, need evaluation. Graham and colleagues define mild, moderate, and severe disease for the common cardiac lesions.	Yes
Dysrhythmia (irregular heart rhythm)	Qualified
Explanation: Athlete needs evaluation because some types require therapy or make certain sports dangerous, or both.	Yes
Mitral valve prolapse (abnormal heart valve)	Qualified
Explanation: Those with symptoms (chest pain, symptoms of possible dysrhythmia) or evidence of mitral regurgitation (leaking) on physical examination need evaluation. All others may participate fully.	Yes
Heart murmur	Qualified
Explanation: If the murmur is innocent (does not indicate heart disease), full participation is permitted. Otherwise, the athlete needs evaluation (see congenital heart disease and mitral valve prolapse above).	Yes
Cerebral palsy	Qualified
Explanation: Athlete needs evaluation.	Yes
Diabetes mellitus	Yes
Explanation: All sports can be played with proper attention to diet, hydration, and insulin therapy. Particular attention is necessary for activities that last ≥ 30 min.	
Diarrhea	Qualified
Explanation: Unless disease is mild, no participation is permitted because diarrhea may increase the risk of dehydration and heat illness. See fever below.	No
Eating disorders	Qualified
Anorexia nervosa, bulimia nervosa	Yes
Explanation: These patients need both medical and psychiatric assessment before participation.	
Eyes	
Functionally one-eyed athlete, loss of an eye, detached retina, previous eye surgery, or serious eye injury	Qualified
Explanation: A functionally one-eyed athlete has a best corrected visual acuity of < 20/40 in the worse eye. These athletes would suffer significant disability if the better eye was seriously injured as would those with loss of an eye. Some athletes who have previously undergone eye surgery or had a serious eye injury may have an increased risk of injury because of weakened eye tissue. Availability of eye guards approved by the American Society for Testing Materials (ASTM) and other protective equipment may allow participation in most sports, but this must be judged on an individual basis.	Yes
Fever	No
Explanation: Fever can increase cardiopulmonary effort, reduce maximum exercise capacity, make heat illness more likely, and increase orthostatic hypotension during exercise. Fever may rarely accompany myocarditis or other infections that may make exercise dangerous.	
Heat illness, history of	Qualified
Explanation: Because of the increased likelihood of recurrence, the athlete needs individual assessment to determine the presence of predisposing conditions and to arrange a prevention strategy.	Yes
HIV infection	Yes
Explanation: Because of the apparent minimal risk to others, all sports may be played that the state of health allows. In all athletes, skin lesions should be properly covered, and athletic personnel should use universal precautions when handling blood or body fluids with visible blood.	
Kidney, absence of one	Qualified
Explanation: Athlete needs individual assessment for contact collision and limited-contact sports.	Yes
Liver, enlarged	Qualified
Explanation: If the liver is acutely enlarged, participation should be avoided because of risk of rupture. If the liver is chronically enlarged, individual assessment is necessary before collision/contact or limited-contact sports are played.	Yes
Malignancy	Qualified
Explanation: Athlete needs individual assessment.	Yes

*This table is designed to be understood by medical and nonmedical personnel. In the *Explanation* sections "needs individual assessment" means that a physician with appropriate knowledge and experience should assess the safety of a given sport for the athlete with the listed medical condition. Unless otherwise noted, this is because of the variability of the severity of the disease or of the risk of injury among the specific sports, or both.

Graham TP, Bricken JT, James FW, Strong WB: *Congenital heart disease.* American College of Sports Medicine, American College of Cardiology, 26th Bethesda Conference. *Med Sci Sports Exerc* 26: S246-S253,1994.

Table 63–8: Medical Conditions and Sports Participation*—cont'd

CONDITION	MAY PARTICIPATE?
Musculoskeletal disorders	Qualified Yes
Explanation: Athlete needs individual assessment.	
Neurologic	
History of serious head or spine trauma, severe or repeated concussions, or craniotomy.	Qualified Yes
Explanation: Athlete needs individual assessment for collision/contact or limited-contact sports, and also for noncontact sports if there are deficits in judgment or cognition. Recent research supports a conservative approach to management of concussion.	
Convulsive disorder, well-controlled	Yes
Explanation: Risk of convulsion during participation is minimal	
Convulsive disorder, poorly controlled	Qualified Yes
Explanation: Athlete needs individual assessment for collision/contact or limited-contact sports. Avoid the following noncontact sports: archery, riflery, swimming, weight- or powerlifting, strength training, or sports involving heights. In these sports, occurrence of a convulsion may be a risk to self or others.	
Obesity	Qualified Yes
Explanation: Because of the risk of heat illness, obese persons need careful acclimatization and hydration.	
Organ transplant recipient	Qualified Yes
Explanation: Athlete needs individual assessment.	
Ovary, absence of one	Yes
Explanation: risk of severe injury to the remaining ovary is minimal.	
Respiratory disorders	
Pulmonary compromise, including cystic fibrosis	Qualified Yes
Explanation: Athlete needs individual assessment, but generally all sports may be played if oxygenation remains satisfactory during a graded exercise test. Patients with cystic fibrosis need acclimatization and good hydration to reduce the risk of heat illness.	
Asthma	Yes
Explanation: With proper medication and education, only athletes with the most severe asthma will have to modify their participation.	
Acute upper respiratory infection	Qualified Yes
Explanation: Upper respiratory obstruction may affect pulmonary function. Athlete needs individual assessment for all but mild disease. See fever.	
Sickle cell disease	Qualified Yes
Explanation: Athlete needs individual assessment. In general, if status of the illness permits, all but high-exertion, collision/contact sports may be played. Overheating, dehydration, and chilling must be avoided.	
Sickle cell trait	Yes
Explanation: It is unlikely that individuals with sickle cell trait (AS) have an increased risk of sudden death or other medical problems during athletic participation except under the most extreme conditions of heat, humidity, and possibly increased altitude. These individuals, like all athletes, should be carefully conditioned, acclimatized, and hydrated to reduce any possible risk.	
Skin: boils, herpes simplex, impetigo, scabies, molluscum contagiosum	Qualified Yes
Explanation: While the patient is contagious, participation in gymnastics with mats, martial arts, wrestling, or other collision/contact or limited-contact sports is not allowed. Herpes simplex virus probably is not transmitted via mats.	
Spleen, enlarged	Qualified Yes
Explanation: Patients with an acutely enlarged spleen should avoid all sports because of risk of rupture. Those with a chronically enlarged spleen need individual assessment before playing collision/contact or limited-contact sports.	
Testicle, absent or undescended	Yes
Explanation: Certain sports may require a protective cup.	

*This table is designed to be understood by medical and nonmedical personnel. In the *Explanation* sections "needs individual assessment" means that a physician with appropriate knowledge and experience should assess the safety of a given sport for the athlete with the listed medical condition. Unless otherwise noted, this is because of the variability of the severity of the disease or of the risk of injury among the specific sports, or both.

Modified from Miller MD, Cooper DE, Warner JJP: *Review of sports medicine and arthroscopy*, 2nd ed. Philadelphia, 2002, Saunders. Modified from Risser WL, Anderson SJ, Boulduc SP, et al: *Pediatrics* 94:757-760, 1994.

	Pediatric Syndromes and Disorders: Increased Risk for Sudden Cardiac Death in Young Athletes
Box 63–1	

- Hypertropic cardiomyopathy (HCM)
- Long QT syndromes (LQTS)
  - Congenital
  - Acquired
- Marfan syndrome
- Ehlers-Danlos syndrome
- Arrhythmogenic right ventricular cardiomyopathy
- Commotio cordis
- Dilated cardiomyopathy
- Acquired cardiac disease
  - Myocardial
  - Pericardial
  - Endocardial
- Congenital heart disease
  - Aortic stenosis
  - Coarctation of aorta
- Mitral valve prolapse
- Anomalous coronary arteries
- Postoperative congenital heart arrhythmias
  - Postoperative tetralogy of Fallot
  - Postoperative atrial switch transposition of great vessels
  - Postoperative ASD repair
- Brugada syndrome
- Wolff-Parkinson-White syndrome (preexcitation syndrome)
- Congenital heart block
  - Moebius type II
  - Third-degree (complete) heart block

ASD, atrial septal defect.
Luckstead EF: *Pediatr Clin North Am.* 49:681-707, 2002.

	Summary of the American College of Obstetricians and Gynecologists Contraindications to and Recommendations for Exercise During Pregnancy
Box 63–2	

Contraindications
  Pregnancy-induced hypertension
  Preterm rupture of membranes
  Preterm labor during the prior or current pregnancy, or both
  Incompetent cervix/cerclage
  Persistent second- or third-trimester bleeding
  Intrauterine growth retardation

1. During pregnancy, women can continue to exercise and derive health benefits even from mild-to-moderate exercise routines. Regular exercise (at least 3 times per week) is preferable to intermittent activity.
2. Women should avoid exercise in the supine position after the first trimester. Such a position is associated with decreased cardiac output in most pregnant women; because the remaining cardiac output will be preferentially distributed away from splanchnic beds (including the uterus) during vigorous exercise, such regimens are best avoided during pregnancy. Prolonged periods of motionless standing should also be avoided.
3. Women should be aware of the decreased oxygen available for aerobic exercise during pregnancy. They should be encouraged to modify the intensity of their exercise according to maternal symptoms. Pregnant women should stop exercising when fatigued and not exercise to exhaustion. Weightbearing exercises may under some circumstances be continued at intensities similar to those prior to pregnancy throughout pregnancy. Nonweightbearing exercises such as cycling or swimming will minimize the risk of injury and facilitate the continuation of exercise during pregnancy.
4. Morphologic changes in pregnancy should serve as a relative contraindication to types of exercise in which loss of balance could be detrimental to maternal or fetal well-being, especially in the third trimester. Further, any type of exercise involving the potential for even mild abdominal trauma should be avoided.
5. Pregnancy requires an additional 300 kcal/d to maintain metabolic homeostasis. Thus women who exercise during pregnancy should be particularly careful to ensure an adequate diet.
6. Pregnant women who exercise in the first trimester should augment heat dissipation by ensuring adequate hydration, appropriate clothing, and optimal environmental surroundings during exercise.
7. Many of the physiological and morphological changes of pregnancy persist 4-6 wks postpartum. Thus prepregnancy exercise routines should be resumed gradually on the basis of a woman's physical capability.

Ireland ML, Ott SM: *Clin Sport Med* 23:281-298, 2004. Modified from *Exercise during pregnancy and the postpartum period.* ACOG Technical Bulletin, 89. Washington, DC, 1994, American College of Obstetricians and Gynecologists.

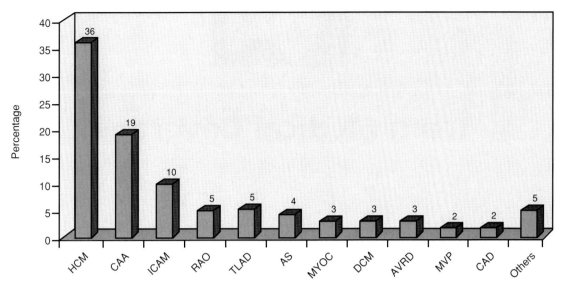

Figure 63–3:
Causes of sudden cardiac death in young competitive athletes (median age = 17 years) based on systematic tracking of 158 athletes in the United States from 1985-1995. AS, Aortic stenosis; AVRD, arrhythmogenic right ventricular dysplasia; CAA, coronary artery abnormality; CAD, coronary artery diseases; DCM, dilated cardiomyopathy; HCM, hypertrophic cardiomyopathy; ICAM, increased cardiac mass; MVP, mitral valve prolapse; MYOC, myocarditis; RAO, ruptured aorta; TLAD, intramural tunneling of the left anterior descending artery. (From Bader RS, Goldberg L, Sahn DJ: *Pediatr Clin North Am* 52:1421-1441, 2004.)

References

American Academy of Family Physicians, American Academy of Pediatrics, American Medical Society for Sports Medicine, American Orthopaedic Society for Sports Medicine, Osteopathic Academy of Sports Medicine: The preparticipation physical evaluation physical examination. In Arendt EA, editor: *Orthopaedic knowledge update sports medicine 2*. Rosemont, IL, 1999, American Academy of Orthopaedic Surgeons.

A good general review of how to perform the preparticipation physical evaluation.

Bader RS, Goldberg L, Sahn DJ: Risk of sudden cardiac death in young athletes: which screening strategies are appropriate? *Pediatr Clin North Am* 51:1421-1441, 2004.

Reviews cardiovascular causes (the most common cause) of sudden death in young athletes with typical presentations, history, and diagnostic techniques. Authors comment on the difficulties of detecting such conditions using the standard preparticipation examination protocols and stress the importance of using more sensitive tests (although costly) in suspicious or high-risk cases.

Fallon KE: Utility of hematological and iron-related screening in elite athletes. *Clin J Sport Med* 14:145-152, 2004.

Prospective cohort study evaluating the utility of hematologic screening by reviewing the results of full blood counts and iron studies in male (n = 121) and female (n = 174) athletes. In the male group, screening blood tests detected only two athletes with significant abnormalities that would otherwise not have been evaluated after a general history and physical examination. Another three male athletes with significant findings on history and physical examination were determined to have iron deficiency anemia. Of the female group, screening tests resulted in 1 athlete with a clinical disorder and 27 athletes requiring iron supplementation. Although hematologic screening is generally of low yield, the author emphasizes it is reasonable to perform among elite athletes secondary to the performance consequences of undetected, untreated anemia.

Ireland ML, Ott SM: Special concerns of the female athlete. *Clin J Sport Med* 23:281-298, 2004.

Good extensive overview examining the anatomic, hormonal, and functional differences between men and women and the different injury rates and medical conditions affecting the female athlete. It is determined that female athletes have a concerning incidence of knee injuries and those with hormonal imbalances or eating disorders are at risk for stress fractures. Issues such as the aging female athlete and exercise during and after pregnancy are also discussed.

Luckstead EF: Cardiac risk factors and participation guidelines for youth sports. *Pediatr Clin North Am* 49:681-707, 2002.

Good review of cardiac causes of sudden cardiac death. Conditions are discussed in detail including diagnostic and screening strategies.

Seto CK: Preparticipation cardiovascular screening. *Clin J Sport Med* 22:23-35, 2003.

Review of cardiovascular screening for athletes prior to participation in sports. Because the majority of sudden deaths in young athletes is caused by cardiovascular conditions, the author stresses that the American Heart Association's cardiovascular screening recommendations be uniformly adopted into all preparticipation examinations. Recommendations are discussed.

Smith DM: Pre-participation physical evaluations. *Sports Med* 18:293-300, 1994.

Review of the development, objectives, format, and performance of the preparticipation physical evaluation. The author suggests that the development of more effective examination questions and tests will require further study to produce uniform guidelines that can best ensure the safety and health of athletes.

Somogyi DM, Shrier I: Customizing the preparticipation evaluation. In Fu FH, Stone DA, editors: *Sports injuries: mechanisms, prevention, treatment*. Philadelphia, 2001, Lippincott Williams & Wilkins.

Excellent review of the components of the preparticipation evaluation include history, physical examination, and several key elements and points to focus on to avoid missing important potential conditions that can lead to morbidity.

CHAPTER 64

Team Medical Coverage

Introduction

- The concept of the sports medicine team is not a new one. However, the definition of the sports medicine team has changed and expanded over the years.
- Generally, the sports medicine team consists of the covering team physician, the athletic trainer, the coach, the athlete, and the athlete's parents if he or she is a minor.
- The sports medicine team may also be expanded to involve physician specialists, physical therapists, the school nurse, and even teachers or counselors.
- Basically, the sports medicine team involves anyone who may help to make decisions regarding the care of an athlete.
- The members of the team can change with each individual case, but the key in all cases is good communication between the members.
  - Often this responsibility lies with the athletic trainer because he or she is in a unique position to be knowledgeable about the athlete's medical condition, the athlete as an individual, and the requirements of the particular sport involved.
  - He or she acts as a coordinator and liaison for the other members of the team.

Responsibilities of the Team Physician

- The team physician is the physician responsible for the health and wellness of the sports team or teams with which he or she is working. This may be a specialist in the area of family medicine, orthopaedics, pediatrics, or any other area of medicine.
- Initial contact with the athletes typically occurs during the preparticipation physical examinations.
  - This is one of the most important ways for the team physician to get to know the athletes and screen for potential health risks.

- Chapter 63 provides more detailed information regarding preparticipation physical examinations.
- Education of the athletes is also an important part of the team physician's role.
  - This may occur on an individual basis or as a group.
  - This should include such things as proper nutrition, heat illness prevention, medication and drug use, and proper use of sports supplements.
- Practice coverage is variable depending on the amount of contact the team physician has with the athletes.
  - In many cases, the athletic trainer attends practice sessions and is able to communicate any problems that arise to the team physician.
  - Because more injuries occur during team practice than in formal competition, the team physician should make himself or herself available and confirm that all necessary medical equipment is also available.
- Game day coverage is probably the most obvious of the responsibilities.
  - Again, all necessary medical equipment should be tested and available for use if necessary.
  - On the day of the game, the physician should arrive with enough time before the event is scheduled to begin to examine any athlete with a question of ability to play that day.
  - In addition, the physician should make himself or herself available after the game to evaluate injuries from play.
  - An alternative is to establish an "injury clinic" on the day following a scheduled athletic event for athletes who sustained injury during play to be evaluated and treated.
  - Injury clinics afford the physician, trainer, and athlete a quieter and more controlled environment for examination and discussion of treatment.
- Emergency injury assessment.
  - This includes following preestablished guidelines for treating on-field emergencies including advanced cardiac life support (ACLS) and advanced trauma life support (ATLS) (Figure 64–1).
- Determination of safe environment for sports activity.

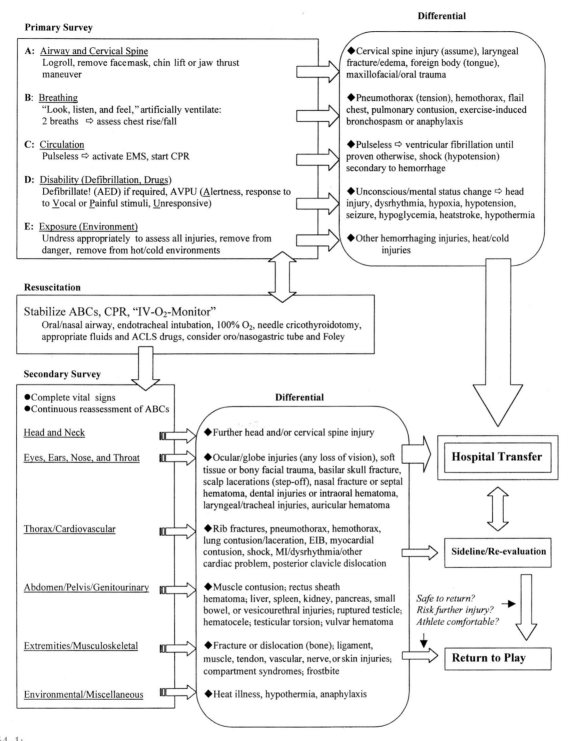

Primary Survey

A: Airway and Cervical Spine
Logroll, remove facemask, chin lift or jaw thrust maneuver

B: Breathing
"Look, listen, and feel," artificially ventilate: 2 breaths ⇒ assess chest rise/fall

C: Circulation
Pulseless ⇒ activate EMS, start CPR

D: Disability (Defibrillation, Drugs)
Defibrillate! (AED) if required, AVPU (Alertness, response to to Vocal or Painful stimuli, Unresponsive)

E: Exposure (Environment)
Undress appropriately to assess all injuries, remove from danger, remove from hot/cold environments

Differential

◆ Cervical spine injury (assume), laryngeal fracture/edema, foreign body (tongue), maxillofacial/oral trauma

◆ Pneumothorax (tension), hemothorax, flail chest, pulmonary contusion, exercise-induced bronchospasm or anaphylaxis

◆ Pulseless ⇒ ventricular fibrillation until proven otherwise, shock (hypotension) secondary to hemorrhage

◆ Unconscious/mental status change ⇒ head injury, dysrhythmia, hypoxia, hypotension, seizure, hypoglycemia, heatstroke, hypothermia

◆ Other hemorrhaging injuries, heat/cold injuries

Resuscitation

Stabilize ABCs, CPR, "IV-O$_2$-Monitor"
Oral/nasal airway, endotracheal intubation, 100% O$_2$, needle cricothyroidotomy, appropriate fluids and ACLS drugs, consider oro/nasogastric tube and Foley

Secondary Survey

● Complete vital signs
● Continuous reassessment of ABCs

Differential

Head and Neck

◆ Further head and/or cervical spine injury

Eyes, Ears, Nose, and Throat

◆ Ocular/globe injuries (any loss of vision), soft tissue or bony facial trauma, basilar skull fracture, scalp lacerations (step-off), nasal fracture or septal hematoma, dental injuries or intraoral hematoma, laryngeal/tracheal injuries, auricular hematoma

Thorax/Cardiovascular

◆ Rib fractures, pneumothorax, hemothorax, lung contusion/laceration, EIB, myocardial contusion, shock, MI/dysrhythmia/other cardiac problem, posterior clavicle dislocation

Abdomen/Pelvis/Genitourinary

◆ Muscle contusion; rectus sheath hematoma; liver, spleen, kidney, pancreas, small bowel, or vesicourethral injuries; ruptured testicle; hematocele; testicular torsion; vulvar hematoma

Extremities/Musculoskeletal

◆ Fracture or dislocation (bone); ligament, muscle, tendon, vascular, nerve, or skin injuries; compartment syndromes; frostbite

Environmental/Miscellaneous

◆ Heat illness, hypothermia, anaphylaxis

Hospital Transfer

Sideline/Re-evaluation

Safe to return?
Risk further injury?
Athlete comfortable?

Return to Play

Figure 64–1:
Emergency injury assessment. ACLS, Advanced cardiac life support; AED, automated external defibrillator; CPR, cardiopulmonary resuscitation; EIB, exercise induced bronchospasm; EMS, emergency medical system; MI, myocardial infarction. (From Madden CC, Walsh WM, Mellion MB: The team physician: the preparticipation examination and on-field emergencies. In DeLee JC, Drez Jr D, Miller MD, editors: *DeLee and Drez's orthopaedic sports medicine: principles and practice,* 2nd ed. Philadelphia, 2003, Saunders.)

- This includes awareness of the heat index (Figure 64–2).
- Cessation of play for lightning.
- Excessive temperature extremes and precipitation.
- Communication, as in all fields of medicine, is a key component of the team physician's job.
  - Education is one aspect of this.
  - In case of injury to the athlete, parents (in the case of high school and college teams), coaches, and trainers will all need to be part of the decision-making process.

Physician Bag and Equipment

- The "physician bag" refers to any equipment deemed necessary for adequate evaluation and treatment of on-field athletic injuries (Box 64–1).
- Necessary equipment should be tailored to the event being covered with thought also given to any potential emergencies involving spectators. Indoor sports, outdoor sports, and aquatic sports all will have some varying aspects to consider.
- Special consideration may be given to athletes or coaches with specific medical conditions requiring medication or other equipment. The team physician should be aware of any such special need and be prepared to act to treat any problems that may arise as a result of that medical condition.

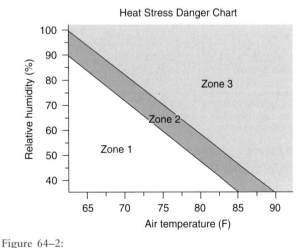

Figure 64–2:

Heat stress danger chart. Zone 1—safe for participation. Zone 2—moderate heat stress precautions. Workouts should be less intense, shorter, and with more frequent fluid breaks. Zone 3—greatest heat stress danger. Workouts should be rescheduled if possible. (Redrawn from Mellion M, Shelton G: Thermoregulation, heat illness, and safe exercise in the heat. In Mellion M, editor: *Office of sports medicine,* 2nd ed. Philadelphia, 1996, Hanley & Belfus.)

Box 64–1 The Team Physician "Bag"

BLS/ACLS Supplies

BP cuff	Stethoscope
CPR mask	AED unit
Oral airways	Endotrachial tubes
IV kits and fluids	ACLS drugs (epinephrine, lidocaine, atropine, sodium bicarbonate)

Trauma/Fracture Equipment

Spine board	Cervical collar
Extremity splints	Slings
Braces	Crutches
Transport cart	SAC test card
EMS contact number	Casting supplies (stockinette, fiberglass, padding)

Wound Care

Sterile gloves	Nonsterile gloves
Gauze	ACE wraps
Tape	Bandages
Suture kit/suture	Betadine
Alcohol	Saline for irrigation
Steri-strips	Syringes/needles
Scalpels	Sharps container
Dermabond	Biohazard bag
Sterile scissors	Nonsterile scissors

Physical Examination Equipment

Penlight	Ophthalmascope/otoscope
Eye patch	Reflex hammer

Medications

Antiinflammatories	Acetaminophen
Narcotic pain meds	Eye drops
Albuterol inhaler	Lidocaine/Marcaine
Injectable steroid	Epinephrine
Diphenhydramine	Insulin
Glucagon	Antibiotic ointment
Antibiotics	Topical steroid
Topical antifungal	Viral illness medications (antidiarrheals, antacids, cough syrup/drops, decongestant, antihistamine, etc.)

Miscellaneous

Dictaphone and tapes	Prescription pad
Copies of preparticipation physical forms and emergency information	

AED, Automated external defibrillator; BLS/ACLS, basic life support/advanced cardiac life support; BP, blood pressure; CPR, cardiopulmonary resuscitation; EMS, emergency medical services; SAC, standard assessment of concussion.

References

ACSM Position Statement: The team physician and return-to-play issues: a consensus statement. *Med Sci Sports Exerc* 34:1212-1214, 2002.
> *An expert panel suggests guidelines for return to full sports participation after injury or illness. Recommendations include maintaining good communication throughout the decision-making process, evaluating athletes in a timely manner, overseeing and evaluating the rehabilitation progress, and individualizing the plan.*

Anderson JC, Courson RW, Kleiner DM, McLoda TA: National Athletic Trainer's Association position statement: emergency planning in athletics. *J Athletic Training* 37:99-104, 2002.
> *This describes the official position of the National Athletic Trainer's Association on emergencies in athletics. It suggests that each institution have a written plan of action with which all personnel are familiar and have practiced on a regular basis. Emphasis is placed on communication between members of the sports medicine team in terms of each individual's role and the readiness of the equipment needed in case of emergency.*

Madden CC, Walsh WM, Mellion MB: The team physician: the preparticipation examination and on-field emergencies. In DeLee JC, Drez Jr D, Miller MD, editors: *DeLee and Drez's orthopaedic sports medicine: principles and practice,* 2nd ed. Philadelphia, 2003, Saunders.
> *This chapter provides good guidelines for preparticipation examinations and guidance for medical bag contents, emergency evaluation and treatment, and environmental issues affecting athletes.*

Stricker PR: The sports medicine kit: basics of the bag. *Pediatr Ann* 31:14-16, 2002.
> *This article discusses the team bag including appropriate equipment and supplies that may be necessary in the on-field management of athletic injuries.*

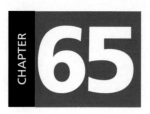

CHAPTER 65

Drug Use/Abuse/Ergogenic Aids/Supplements/Nutrition

Introduction

- A discussion of drug use, supplements, and nutrition should be incorporated into all athletic programs.
- In response to the demands placed by competition, athletes attempt to enhance their performance through ergogenic substances found in natural and synthetic compounds.
- The athletic program is responsible for instructing players on proper nutrition, dispelling myths, and advising them on policies concerning drug and supplement use.
- For proper guidance, physicians must have a firm understanding of the characteristics, effects, and complications of nutritional and drug compounds (Box 65–1).
- It is essential that the coaches be well informed because they often exert the greatest influence on athletes' behaviors and attitudes.

Drug Use and Misuse

- Drug use by athletes includes ergogenic and illicit substances, therapeutic medications, and recreational drugs such as alcohol and tobacco.
- Some therapeutic medications administered by physicians have addictive or abuse potential and are banned substances in certain sport organizations.
- The team care provider should be aware of federal and institutional protocols and regulations regarding drug use and testing and closely follow medication use by individual players.
- Athletes may use medications to mask the presence of banned substances in their urine.
- Drug testing has become commonplace among sport participants.
- Drugs remain in the urine for different lengths of time (Table 65–1).

Anabolic Steroids

- Synthetic derivative of testosterone with mainly anabolic properties.

- Medical indications include treatment of specific anemias and patients experiencing severe catabolism secondary to trauma or surgery.
- Athletes involved in activities requiring strength turn to anabolic steroids as ergogenic aids to assist them in gaining muscle mass and strength.
- Noncompetitive athletes more commonly take anabolic steroids for cosmetic reasons and are more likely to use them indefinitely to maintain their physique.
- Generally does not enhance aerobic performance.
- Anabolic steroids achieve their effects through three mechanisms.
  - Anticatabolic (most significant)—displaces cortisol (high levels during intense training) from their receptors, reversing their catabolic effects.
  - Anabolic—increases protein synthesis in muscle and release of endogenous growth hormone.
  - Motivational—placebo effect and development of aggressive personalities intensify training.
- The positive effects of anabolic steroids quickly disappear after they are discontinued, resulting in rapid loss in size and strength and encouraging the athlete to continue use to maintain their effects.
- May be taken orally or parenterally.
- Parenteral form is detectable for a longer period of time, whereas the oral form is noted for its greater adverse effects.
- Reversible side effects include impaired fertility, testicular atrophy, liver effects, decreased immunity, decreased thyroid function, tendon degeneration, acne, altered libido, cardiovascular disease (increased low-density lipoprotein, decreased high-density lipoprotein), mood swings, and psychosis.
- Gynecomastia, acceleration of male pattern baldness, and premature closure of bones are generally not reversible.
- Reversible female adverse effects include increased muscularity; clitoral enlargement; altered libido; and menstrual irregularities with hirsutism, coarsening of the skin, male pattern baldness, and deepening of the voice usually not reversible.
- Parenteral form risks transmission of AIDS and hepatitis.

Box 65–1	**Substances and Their Associated Potential Adverse Effects**

- Anabolic steroid—impaired fertility, testicular atrophy, liver damage, diminished immunity, reduced thyroid function, tendon degeneration, acne, altered libido, increased low-density lipoprotein, decreased high-density lipoprotein, mood swings, psychosis, gynecomastia, accelerated male pattern baldness, premature closure of bones, hirsutism, menstrual irregularities, and risk of AIDS and hepatitis (with parenteral form)
- Growth hormone—diabetes, osteoporosis, cardiac failure, muscle weakness, acromegaly, gigantism, and risk of AIDS and hepatitis (with shared needles)
- Cocaine/crack—tolerance, nasal septum ulceration or perforation, rhinitis, sinusitis, bronchitis, hyperthermia, agitation, restlessness, insomnia, anxiety, psychosis, ventricular arrhythmias, coronary artery vasospasms, myocardial infarction, cerebrovascular accidents (strokes), seizures, and sudden death
- Caffeine—dehydration, arrhythmias, insomnia, and withdrawal symptoms (headaches, drowsiness, lethargy, irritability)
- Amphetamine—similar profile to cocaine
- Phenylpropanolamine/ephedrine—tremors, nervousness, insomnia, seizures, transient hypertension, palpitations, arrhythmias, and myocardial infarction
- Creatine—generally safe profile, weight gain, muscle cramping, and dehydration
- Sodium bicarbonate—nausea, vomiting, diarrhea, muscle spasms, and arrhythmias
- Alcohol—decreased coordination and reaction time, reduced muscular strength and endurance, liver damage, impaired thermoregulation, dehydration, and impaired performance
- Marijuana—orthostatic hypotension, palpitations, tachycardia, impaired coordination and performance, impaired short-term memory and sweat inhibition, asthma, bronchitis, and reduced concentration
- Blood doping—hyperviscosity syndrome, thrombosis, pulmonary embolism, heart failure, myocardial infarction, infection, and death
- Erythropoietin—headaches, arthralgias, hypertension, and thrombosis
- Diuretics—dehydration, electrolyte abnormalities, fatigue, weakness, dizziness, orthostatic hypotension, impotence, muscle cramping, and impaired performance
- Narcotics—increased risk of injury (secondary to increased pain threshold), addiction, and withdrawal symptoms

- Addiction is primarily psychologic, although physiologic dependence has also been suggested.
- Cessation of anabolic steroids may result in severe depression.
- Generally banned from all athletic competition.

Growth Hormone

- Naturally found in the anterior pituitary and affects the growth of all organs and tissues in the human body.
- Low levels of the hormone result in pituitary dwarfism.
- An excess of the hormone results in gigantism in prepubertal individuals or acromegaly in skeletally mature individuals.
- Many athletes begin using biosynthetic growth hormone because it is difficult to test for and they believe it will provide them with similar results as anabolic steroids.
- The use of biosynthetic growth hormone is medically indicated only in patients with pituitary dwarfism.
- Growth hormone has been shown to have an anabolic effect through retention of nitrogen and increased amino acid transport into tissues.
- Stimulates lipolysis, sparing muscle glycogen, which may translate into improved strength during athletic training.
- Available as injections.
- High cost and use of syringes are deterrent factors.
- Side effects include the development of diabetes, osteoporosis, cardiac failure, muscle weakness, and features of acromegaly or gigantism depending on the age of the user.

- AIDS and hepatitis may be transmitted through shared needles and syringes.
- Generally banned from all athletic competition.

Clenbuterol

- A beta-2 adrenergic agonist used in asthmatic patients secondary to its potent bronchodilation effects.
- High dosages have been reported to increase muscle size in animal studies, making it desirable by athletes.
- Musculoskeletal effects include increased protein synthesis and decreased protein degradation, primarily on fast twitch fibers, resulting in muscle hypertrophy.
- Other beta-adrenoreceptor agonist action includes lipolysis and decreased lipogenesis, which has resulted in decreased body fat in animal studies.
- Use of clenbuterol by athletes does not appear to result in significant muscle hypertrophy but rather an increase in lean body mass, which can likely be explained by the use of lower doses, lipolysis, and greater effect on preventing protein degradation rather than muscle hypertrophy. (As a result, athletes may decide to additionally use growth hormone.)
- Difficult to detect in urine 48 hours after use.
- Chronic use may result in tolerance.
- Has relatively mild side effects including headaches, nervousness, and insomnia.
- Banned by the International Olympic Committee.

Table 65–1: Duration of Drug Urinary Excretion

DRUG	APPROXIMATE ELIMINATION TIME
Stimulants (amphetamines & derivatives)	1 to 7 days
Cocaine	
Occasional use	6 to 12 hr
Repeated use, within 48 hours	3 to 5 days*
Over-the-counter cold medications containing ephedrine derivatives as decongestants	48 to 72 hr
Narcotics in cough medicines	24 to 48 hr
Marijuana (tetrahydrocannabinol)	3 to 5 wk
Anabolic steroids	
Injectable types (fat soluble)	6 to 8 mo
Water-soluble types (oral)	3 to 6 wk
Corticosteroids	
Oral	1 wk
Injection	4 to 6 wk

*Possibly longer.
From the *Drug free handbook*. Colorado Springs, CO, 1993-1996, United States Olympic Committee Drug Education Program, United States Olympic Committee.

Cocaine/Crack

- Derived from the leaf of the *Erythroxylon coca* plant.
- Only medically indicated as a local anesthetic and nasal vasoconstrictor.
- Active drug is cocaine hydrochloride, a potent stimulant.
- Cocaine decomposes with heat.
- Primarily snorted.
- Stimulates release of norepinephrine and blocks its reuptake, resulting in feelings of euphoria, decreased fatigue, and grandiosity, making an athlete overly confident in his or her ability to perform.
- Tolerance may develop with this very addictive drug.
- Side effects include nasal septum ulceration or perforation, rhinitis, sinusitis, bronchitis, hyperthermia (hazardous when training in hot climates), agitation, restlessness, insomnia, anxiety, psychosis, ventricular arrhythmias, coronary artery vasospasms, myocardial infarction, strokes, seizures, and sudden death.
- Extraction of its hydrochloride produces crack, which is less expensive and usually smoked because of its heat tolerance.
- Crack is quickly absorbed through the lungs and produces an intense, short-lived cocaine effect usually followed by a "crash" encouraging frequent repeat dosing.
- Is an illicit substance.

Caffeine

- A methylxanthine.
- Frequently used by athletes as an ergogenic aid.
- Commonly obtained through consumption of coffee but available in other beverages and in tablet form.
- Prevents adenosine inhibition of neurotransmitter release by blocking adenosine receptors within the central nervous system (CNS), thus acting as a stimulant, possibly improving performance.
- Blood levels peak at approximately 30 minutes.
- Promotes lipolysis by blocking adenosine receptors on adipocytes.
- Its lipolytic effects allow the sparing of glycogen, which prevents fatigue in endurance activities.
- Also acts as a diuretic.
- Adverse effects include dehydration (especially in endurance sports), arrhythmias, and insomnia.
- Withdrawal symptoms occur after discontinuance from chronic use and consist of headaches, drowsiness, lethargy, and occasionally irritability.
- High levels are banned by the International and United States Olympic Committees.

Amphetamines

- One of the most potent sympathomimetic amines that has fallen out of fashion with the introduction of cocaine.
- Indirectly stimulate the adrenergic nervous system through the release of endogenous catecholamines.
- Produce improved concentration and alertness and decrease the sense of fatigue, enabling the athlete to perform at a higher level.
- Also serve as appetite suppressants, which may be abused by weight-conscious athletes such as gymnasts, wrestlers, figure skaters, and dancers.
- Tolerance and addiction can occur.
- The adrenergic adverse effects are similar to those of cocaine.
- Banned by the International and United States Olympic Committees.

Phenylpropanolamine/Ephedrine

- Sympathomimetic amines commonly found in many over-the-counter and prescribed medications for appetite suppression, cold medications, and nasal decongestants.

- Their ready availability makes them vulnerable for abuse.
- Athletes may abuse this drug as an ergogenic aid because of its stimulant characteristics or for its appetite suppression if they are trying to lose or maintain weight.
- Phenylpropanolamine has an additional hydroxyl group compared with amphetamine, which weakens its adrenergic effect.
- Phenylpropanolamine primarily stimulates alpha adrenergic receptors, making it an effective nasal vasoconstrictor, whereas ephedrine stimulates both alpha and beta receptors, resulting in greater CNS stimulation.
- Ephedrine functions much like epinephrine but with a longer action duration and greater CNS effects with lower potency.
- In China, herbal ephedrine is known as Ma Huang.
- Adverse effects, marked with abuse, may include tremors, nervousness, insomnia, seizures, transient hypertension, palpitations, arrhythmias, and myocardial infarctions.
- Banned by the International and United States Olympic Committees.

Creatine

- Creatine is a very popular and effective ergogenic aid that enhances energy and provides muscles with more substrate with little adverse effects.
- It is a natural compound that can be found in foods such as raw meat and fish and is also produced in the kidneys and liver.
- Creatine in the body helps with the function of cardiac and smooth muscle, but athletes are principally interested in its function in skeletal muscle.
- Creatine is phosphorylated to creatine phosphate within the body and serves as an energy source for skeletal muscle, especially during intense anaerobic activity.
- Creatine phosphate additionally serves to buffer the acidic environment produced during intense training by consuming the hydrogen byproducts of glycolysis and lactic acid during anaerobic activity. This buffering mechanism is believed to delay fatigue and improve recovery.
- Creatine has also been described as a component of the energy shuttle between mitochondria and contractile proteins, allowing muscles to generate greater energy at a faster rate.
- Does not improve aerobic activities.
- Creatine draws water into cells and may predispose athletes to dehydration and muscle cramps.
- Because of the short half-life of creatine, supplementation requires an initial loading dose (20 g/day divided in 4 doses/day for 1 week) to raise plasma concentration to approximately 500 mmol/L followed by a 1 to 3 g/day maintenance dose. It is common for athletes to take more than the recommended dose in hopes of a greater ergogenic response.
- Carbohydrates may improve uptake of creatine.

- Several studies have demonstrated the positive ergogenic effects of creatine supplementation on strength and short intense athletic activities. However, other studies have been unable to produce similar results.
- The only reported common side effect is weight gain. It is still to be determined whether this weight change is a result of added water weight or increased protein/tissue synthesis.

Beta-Hydroxy-Beta-Methylbutyrate

- A relatively new ergogenic aid with only few studies.
- It is a metabolite of leucine believed to inhibit muscle catabolism, which would allow the maintenance of greater amounts of muscle.
- Some studies have demonstrated some beneficial effects in untrained athletes beginning a resistance training program, by increasing strength and lean body mass. Similar effects were not produced among elite athletes.
- Studies have yet to show reproducible positive effects.

Sodium Bicarbonate

- It is believed that the drop in muscle and blood pH seen with high–intensity anaerobic activities may cause fatigue and decrease glycolysis.
- Sodium bicarbonate can be used to buffer the acidic environment and improve performance, endurance, and power in short intense activities.
- Studies have been unable to identify the duration of its effects.
- Overdosing may result in nausea, vomiting, diarrhea, muscle spasms, and heart arrhythmias.
- It does not produce an effect with aerobic activity.

Carnitine

- Secondary to its key role in the oxidation of fat and carbohydrates, carnitine has been proposed to improve endurance and performance.
- Many sport and nutrition businesses also sell this product for weight loss because of its ability to promote the use of body fat for oxidation.
- Studies have been unable to demonstrate positive ergogenic effects.

Glycerol

- A hyperhydration agent that can combat dehydration during sport participation and thus improve endurance.
- Lack of studies limits our understanding of its role as an ergogenic aid and its safety profile.

Alcohol

- Most commonly abused substance by adolescents, and widely used by athletes.
- Involved in approximately half of fatal automobile accidents.

- Predominantly results in depressive effects including decreased coordination, reaction time, hand coordination, and balance, which can place an athlete playing under the influence at great risk for injury.
- Diuretic effects may result in dehydration.
- May reduce muscular strength and endurance and impair thermoregulation.
- Hangovers following a night of consumption can negatively affect an athlete's aerobic and general performance aside from its psychological effects from feeling ill.
- Noted to result in a greater incidence of spinal injuries and drowning when consumed during recreational water sports.
- Athletes must be advised to drink only in moderation and educated on alcohol's adverse effects and possible legal implications if driving under the influence.
- Not banned by the International and United States Olympic Committees.

Tobacco

- The use of smoked and smokeless tobacco is commonly seen among athletes.
- Athletes may describe a sense of increased reactivity, which can be attributed to the increased heart rate and blood pressure seen with nicotine use.
- The chronic use of tobacco has been implicated as a risk factor for several serious medical conditions, including heart disease and cancer.
- The use of smokeless tobacco has been associated with periodontal disease and oropharyngeal cancers.
- It is important to discuss the harmful effects of tobacco use with athletes of all ages and provide users with options for cessation.
- Not banned by the International and United States Olympic Committees.

Marijuana

- Derived from the *Cannabis sativa* plant.
- The active ingredient is delta-9-tetrahydrocannabinol (delta-9-THC), most commonly referred to as *THC*.
- Primarily acts on the CNS after it is rapidly absorbed across the blood-brain barrier.
- As a lipid soluble substance, THC and its metabolites are slowly released into the bloodstream from fat cells, allowing detection of the substance up to a month after its use.
- Some medical indications include the treatment of asthma (bronchodilatory effect), glaucoma (reduces intraocular pressure), head injuries (decreases muscle spasticity), and chemotherapy (reduces nausea and vomiting).
- Offers no performance advantage to the athlete.
- Adverse effects include orthostatic hypotension, palpitations, tachycardia, decreased hand-eye coordination,

decline in performance of perceptual tasks, impaired short-term memory, and sweat inhibition, which may lead to a rise in core body temperature.
- Adverse effects that degrade performance can last up to 24 hours after use.
- Heavy use of marijuana has been associated with airway obstructive disease, asthma, and bronchitis.
- Long-term use may have psychological effects in which the individual loses ambition and motivation, becomes indifferent, and has difficulty with memory and concentration.
- Various contaminants of marijuana may be more harmful than marijuana itself.
- Not banned by the International and United States Olympic Committees.

Blood Doping

- Popularized as an ergogenic aid that cannot be detected by testing.
- This technique involves transfusion of blood to an athlete 1 to 2 days prior to competition in efforts to increase the red cell volume of an athlete's blood, which results in an increased endurance capacity and enhanced aerobic performance.
- Studies have demonstrated that the resulting normovolemic erythrocythemia can improve VO_2max and endurance exercise capacity and enhance performance in direct relation to the rise in hemoglobin levels.
- Autologous transfusions are preferred over homologous matching blood transfusions because it avoids the risks of immunologic reactions and blood-borne pathogen transmission.
- Fortunately, the process is made difficult logistically. The athlete recovers his or her normal hematocrit approximately 3 to 6 weeks after donating blood, which is the limit for storing blood in a refrigerated blood bank. As a result, the blood must be specially stored frozen for optimal results, which is expensive and not readily available.
- Levels of hemoglobin remain elevated for approximately 1 week and then gradually decline over a period of 15 weeks.
- Transfusing greater than two units of blood may result in a hyperviscosity syndrome (pronounced with sport-induced dehydration), which can lead to clotting, thrombosis, pulmonary embolism, heart failure, myocardial infarction, and death.
- Risks of the procedure include infection and air or clot emboli.
- Banned by most sport organizations.

Erythropoietin

- Naturally synthesized in the kidney cells, often in response to low levels of oxygen tension as seen with anemia or hypoxia.

- Mechanism of action involves inhibiting the destruction of erythroid progenitor cells, thus allowing them to mature into erythrocytes and increase red cell mass.
- Since the advent of recombinant human erythropoietin (1985), athletes have gained interest in its use as an ergogenic aid that would provide equal or greater benefits as seen with blood doping.
- In the medical field, it is effectively used to reverse anemia resulting from chronic renal disease and other medical conditions and to increase hematocrits of certain patients undergoing elective surgery who have donated autologous blood.
- Because the recombinant form is degraded in the gastrointestinal tract, it is administered intravenously or subcutaneously.
- Dosing is usually three times per week, with positive effects seen within 1 to 2 weeks.
- Adverse effects are generally benign and include headaches, arthralgias, hypertension (in anemic patients), and thrombosis.
- Excessive use may also result in a hyperviscosity syndrome, carrying the same potential risks as described previously.
- Several methods have been devised to detect the illegal use of recombinant human erythropoietin.
- Banned by most sport organizations.

Diuretics

- Athletes may turn to diuretics as a method of weight loss or diluting their urine to conceal banned substances.
- Athletes must be made aware of the risks involved including diminished performance, dehydration, electrolyte abnormalities, fatigue, weakness, dizziness, orthostatic hypotension, transient impotence, and muscle cramping.
- Because diluted urine makes the detection of certain substances more difficult, several organizations now require that the sample urine be above a certain specific gravity.

Local Anesthetics

- May be used to assist certain examinations and when performing minor procedures such as repair of lacerations.
- Local or intraarticular injections can commonly be used if medically justified but should not be used to reduce pain during sport participation because it places the athlete at increased risk of injury.

Narcotic Analgesics

- Many sport organizations ban the use of narcotic analgesics because they increase the pain threshold and produce feelings of euphoria and invincibility, which puts the athlete at risk of participating without caution and inability to recognize further injury.

- May become addictive and lead to withdrawal syndromes after cessation from long-term use.
- The use of codeine may be accepted by some organizations.

Corticosteroids

- A potent antiinflammatory medication that can be used intravenously, orally, topically, or locally by injection.
- Generally, the use of intravenous and oral steroids is banned by most sport organizations.
- The use of topical and inhalational corticosteroids is acceptable and effective in treating several skin conditions and asthma, respectively.
- Intraarticular corticosteroid injections are also allowed by many organizations but should be used cautiously.
- There are no definitive studies linking intraarticular steroid injections with the development of arthropathy.
- Local steroid injection into tendons is perilous and may risk rupture, especially if the athlete is returned to competitive activity too early. Other local injection complications include subcutaneous fat atrophy, depigmentation, ligament rupture, and possibly accelerated joint destruction.
- Systemic adverse effects include vasovagal attacks, allergic reactions, weight gain, psychological manifestations, and transient hyperglycemia in diabetics.

Nonsteroidal Antiinflammatory Drugs

- The most commonly recommended class of drugs for the initial treatment of musculoskeletal pain.
- Athletes should be advised to take nonselective nonsteroidal antiinflammatory drugs with food to avoid the potential gastrointestinal side effects.
- Other adverse effects include headaches, drowsiness, dizziness, lightheadedness, confusion, allergic reactions, increased bleeding time, and impaired renal or hepatic function.

Nutrition

- The body of knowledge surrounding nutrition and supplements is constantly growing and adding to our understanding of how different macronutrients and micronutrients play a role in maintaining or enhancing our health.
- Most people are intimidated by nutritional programs that demand certain balances of nutrients, vitamins, and calories and are unable to distinguish which foods provide the proper nutritional demands.
- Although general guidelines are used as a base for most dietary recommendations, individual adjustments are often required based on an athlete's specific needs, level of activity, training regimen, age, gender, body composition, medical conditions, and personal goals (Box 65–2).

- Many people are turned on to different diet fads that promise weight loss or weight gain or enhanced performance.
- It is critical that athletes are informed of the essentials and basic concepts regarding proper nutrition and appropriate supplement use.
- Many athletes are well disciplined and can incorporate recommendations readily.
- Education programs can involve handouts, computer programs, bulletin board posting, presentations, and, if budget allows, the involvement of a nutritionist to provide individual recommendations.
- Because schools now are incorporating a greater variety of options in their food services, it should not be difficult to attain proper nutrition.
- Nutritional deficits and poor diet practices are more common in weight-conscious athletes such as wrestlers, dancers, gymnasts, figure skaters, cheerleaders, and jockeys.

Hydration

- Water makes up approximately 60% of our body composition and is essential for proper circulation and metabolic function within organs and tissues.
- Dehydration results in reduced plasma volume, cardiac output, and blood flow to essential organs and can adversely affect performance with as little as a 2% loss of body weight due to water loss.
- Sweating is reduced with dehydration and in the face of athletic activity can predispose athletes to heat injury.
- Approximately 2.5 quarts of water is lost through urine, feces, sweat, breathing, and skin.
- Sweat rates can exceed 1.8 kg/hour with intense activities in warmer climates. In addition to water, an average of 1 g/L of sodium is also lost.

Box 65–2	General Nutritional Guidelines for Active Individuals*
Hydration	14-22 oz prior to exercise
	4-12 oz approximately every 15 minutes of play
	16 oz of replacement per pound lost during play
Calories	Approximately 2200-2900 kcal/day
	37-41 kcal/kg of body weight per day
	Strength training athletes may require 44 kcal/kg/day or more
Carbohydrates	5-10 g/kg of body weight per day
Protein	Endurance athlete: 1.2-1.4 g/kg of body weight per day
	Strength training athlete: 1.6-1.7 g/kg of body weight per day
Fat	15%-30% of caloric intake

*Adjustments may be required on an individual basis, according to a person's age, activity level, body habitus, and training goals.

- Significant sodium loss is generally not a concern unless exercise or athletic activity is of long duration (> 3 hours).
- Water is replenished by consuming liquids and foods and through energy metabolism.
- Exercise, medications, and other drugs often increase the water intake requirement to maintain proper hydration.
- Athletes should develop a hydration routine starting with a baseline that is supplemented prior to, during, and after athletic activities.
- Patients must not rely on thirst as an indicator for water consumption because it is an inaccurate measure of fluid status.
- It is encouraged that players consume 4 to 12 oz of water or sports drink approximately every 15 minutes of play.
- Beverages supplemented with 4% to 8% of carbohydrates are recommended during activities lasting longer than 1 hour.
- Athletes may also be advised to weigh themselves prior to and after competition and replace each lost pound with 16 oz of fluid.
- Sodium content must also be at normal levels to maintain proper hydration. The intake of large amounts of water alone may result in hyponatremia and a false sense of hydration. Sodium is commonly added to sports drinks.

Calories

- Calories can be considered equivalent to fuel for the body.
- Calories are derived from the consumption of macronutrients, which include carbohydrates, protein, and fat.
- The average required caloric intake is approximately 13 times the body weight of a sedentary individual. Depending on the level of exercise, activity, and training, adjustments between 15 and 20 times body weight are made.
- According to the recommended dietary allowances made in 1989, men and women between the ages of 19 and 50 who are moderately active require 2900 and 2200 kcal/day, respectively. Alternatively, calorie intake should equal 37 to 41 kcal/kg of body weight per day.
- Endurance athletes may require an intake of 3000 to 5000 kcal or greater per day to meet their additional energy needs.
- Athletes involved in intense strength training and desiring optimal muscle growth may need 44 to 50 kcal/kg body weight per day or more.

Carbohydrates

- Carbohydrate is a principal source of fuel that is readily available during the performance of all activities.
- Provides 4 calories/g.

- Anaerobic activities depend only on carbohydrate as an energy source, whereas aerobic activity can additionally draw energy from protein and fat.
- Helps maintain blood glucose levels and allows for glycogen synthesis and storage.
- Carbohydrates are necessary for the metabolism of both protein and fat.
- Recommended amounts depend on an athlete's level of conditioning and intensity and length of exercise, training, and sport activities. Generally, athletes require between 5 and 10 g/kg/day.
- Serves as the primary fuel for high-intensity, short-duration activities and used almost exclusively during the initial stages of endurance activities.
- Sacrificing carbohydrates may result in poor performance.
- Glycogen, the storage form of carbohydrate, is found in the liver, where it helps maintain blood glucose, and in the muscles, where it provides fuel during activity.
- Without adequate carbohydrate intake, glycogen stores may be depleted after an hour of athletic activity and result in early fatigue and decreased performance.
- A glycemic index (GI) describes the response a 50 g dose of carbohydrate has on blood sugar compared with 50 g of glucose. Glucose has a GI of 100. Using this index can help compare the carbohydrate component of different foods and their ability to provide fuel in the form of glucose. Several authorities recommend low GI foods prior to competition, allowing a greater dependence on free fatty acids for fuel, and high GI foods after to restore glycogen stores.
- In the face of low-carbohydrate fads, it is critical athletes understand the requirement of carbohydrate in their diets to optimize competitive performance.

Protein

- Protein is essential for the synthesis of hormones, enzymes, and red blood cells and for tissue repair. In addition, it enhances glycogen synthesis when combined with carbohydrates.
- Provides 4 calories/g.
- Athletes tend to overeat protein because it is a critical component for building muscle mass and thus usually do not suffer from protein deficiencies unless they are explicitly avoiding it or are vegetarian.
- Protein requirements are higher in athletes to repair tissues stressed during training and competition.
- Whereas sedentary individuals require 0.8 g/kg of body weight, athletes may require up to more than double as much.
- Generally, the protein requirements are higher in strength athletes than endurance athletes.
- Athletes should be advised that protein can be provided by foods other than meats such as grains, dairy products, and vegetables.

Fat

- Fat is required for the composition of cell membranes, hormones, prostaglandins, and nerve sheaths and required for proper immune function, digestion, and transport of fat-soluble vitamins.
- Dietary fat provides 9 calories/g, which is greater than double the calories of carbohydrate and protein.
- It is critical that athletes understand fat is an essential component of every diet and restricting fat can compromise normal function of cells and other systems in the body.
- There is no consensus over the optimal amount of fat intake.
- Although many experts recommend fat not exceed 30% of caloric intake, it may be more beneficial to make individual calculations on the basis of a person's size, activity, and goals.
- Emphasis should be placed on consuming the "right" or "good" type of fat by preferring monounsaturated or unsaturated fats over saturated fats.
- Athletes should be advised that a lower percentage of body fat does not translate to better performance.

Micronutrients

- Vitamins and minerals are essential components of several biochemical systems that maintain normal body function.
- They assist with metabolism of macronutrients, cell development, muscle contraction, thermoregulation, and blood pH maintenance.
- Act as antioxidants and contribute to bone strength and stability.
- Vitamin or mineral deficiencies can negatively affect overall health and athletic performance.
- A properly balanced diet can easily meet the daily requirements, which involves choosing foods that are dense in nutrients.
- Nutritional supplements should only be used when there is a specific medical or dietary reason.
- The use of a multivitamin is recommended to individuals who have difficulty maintaining a properly balanced diet.
- Megadosing of single vitamins or minerals may impair the absorption of other vitamins or minerals.
- Female athletes may require calcium or iron supplementation.

Energy Bars and Sports Drinks

- There is nothing magical about energy bars and sports drinks.
- Provide essential nutrients and electrolytes in different compositions that are convenient to implement within a dietary regimen and training program.
- Many recommend their use during training and competition to provide energy and restore nutritional balance.

- Many energy bars should be consumed with liquid.
- Athletes should be wary of bars promising fat-burning or muscle-building properties.

Competition Regimens

- Athletes should pay greater attention to their diet approximately 2 days prior to competition because it takes 24 to 48 hours to replenish muscle glycogen after intensive workouts or practices.
- Athletes must ensure adequate carbohydrate intake to restore glycogen stores.
- Consuming low-glycemic foods (pasta, oatmeal, barley, lentils, kidney beans, milk, apples, oranges) at the last meal prior to competition may benefit performance.
- The pregame meal can consist of any food that will not impair performance and provide adequate satiety and hydration.
- Athletes should stick with familiar foods that do not cause stomach upset.
- Generally, the athlete should consume approximately 1 to 4 g of carbohydrate per kg of body weight, a small amount of low-fat protein, and limited fat products 1 to 4 hours before competition, with smaller portions nearing gametime.
- It is best if the stomach is nearly empty before sport participation.
- A small amount of carbohydrate can be taken immediately before game time to boost blood sugar and delay glycogen depletion.
- During competition, consumption of 40 to 60 g of carbohydrate per hour is recommended.
- After the game, carbohydrate intake is suggested to replete glycogen stores.
- Some recommend emphasizing high-glycemic foods (potato, honey, cornflakes, white rice, white or wheat bread) after athletic events to maximize postexercise glycogen synthesis.
- The addition of protein after competition may assist in carbohydrate uptake.

Diets

- Many athletes who are required to "make weight" such as wrestlers and judoists use a dangerous weight-cycling regimen whereby they accept practices that enable them to lose significant weight in a very short period of time. This can place the athlete in great danger of malnutrition and risk of injury and result in a negative psychology affecting school, work, and social interactions.
- To establish an ideal weight, an individual's body composition, age, and development should all be taken into account.
- With any type of diet, it is important to set realistic goals and discuss expectations with the athlete.
- When weight loss is indicated, efforts should begin early enough before the start of a season to achieve the

recommended goal. Generally, 1 to 2 pounds of weight loss per week is a safe practice, which can often be achieved by cutting back 500 calories of the recommended daily intake.
- It is best to provide athletes with a listed regimen with options that they can follow and instruct them on how to properly supplement caloric intake during training.
- It is important to stay well hydrated because it may be difficult to cut weight if dehydrated.
- A higher metabolism can be maintained by eating small amounts of food frequently throughout the day.
- Consultation with a nutritionist can assist with developing a healthy and realistic diet regimen.
- For weight gain, it is recommended that 500 to 1000 calories be added to their daily intake and that resistance training be emphasized to build up muscle.

Eating Disorders

- Although these disorders usually manifest from abnormal eating habits, the underlying etiology is psychological.
- Anorexia is characterized by restricting caloric intake, distorted body image, fear of gaining weight, and being below 85% of ideal body weight.
  - Complications include gastrointestinal problems, electrolyte imbalances, impaired thermoregulation and endocrine function, bone loss, cardiovascular disturbances, and even death.
- Bulimia nervosa is defined by binge eating episodes followed by purging either by vomiting, increased exercise, diuretics, or laxative abuse.
  - These patients may appear to be of normal weight but can suffer many of the same complications as anorexics.
- The female triad consisting of disordered eating, amenorrhea, and osteoporosis is a consequence of a restrictive diet that impairs hormonal production and function that can severely weaken bones and increase the risk of stress fractures.
- The treatment of these disorders usually requires a team approach that includes evaluation and guidance from physicians, trainers, psychiatrists, and nutritionists.

References

Beard J, Tobin B: Iron status and exercise. *Am J Clin Nutr* 72(suppl):594S-597S, 2000.

Review of dietary iron, bioavailability, and consequences of iron deficiency in the athletic population. Iron deficiency anemia can significantly impair the oxygen transport capacity and VO₂max but is treatable with appropriate dietary/supplemental management.

Burke LM, Kiens B, Ivy JL: Carbohydrates and fat for training and recovery. *J Sports Sci* 22:15-30, 2004.
Comprehensive review of carbohydrate and fat requirements and recommendations in athletes involved in training and prior to, during, and following competition. Past and present views and knowledge are

discussed, and new updated recommendations by the authors are presented.

Green GA, Uryasz FD, Petr TA, Bray CD: NCAA study of substance abuse habits of college student-athletes. *Clin J Sport Med* 11:51-56, 2001.

Study assessing substance abuse patterns among college athletes for alcohol, amphetamines, anabolic steroids, cocaine/crack, ephedrine, marijuana/hashish, hallucinogens/psychedelics, and smokeless tobacco. Athletes from 30 sports in 637 institutions (of 991) involved in Division I, II, and III NCAA competition were surveyed. Alcohol was shown to be the most commonly used substance (80.5%) followed by marijuana (28.4%) and smokeless tobacco (22.5%). Substance use was significantly higher among Division III athletes and Caucasians. Anabolic steroid use was found in 1.1% of all athletes, with physicians other than their team physician as their source in 32% of cases followed by teammates or other athletes (20.8%) and friends or relatives (17%). Additional results by gender, division, and sports are described.

Manore MM: Dietary recommendations and athletic menstrual dysfunction. *Sports Med* 32:887-901, 2002.

Author reviews mechanisms, factors, health consequences, and nutritional issues associated with athletic menstrual dysfunction. Proposed mechanisms include the energy-drain and exercise-intensity hypotheses. Evaluation and treatment recommendations are comprehensively discussed.

Maughan RJ, King DS, Lea T: Dietary supplements. *J Sports Sci* 22:95-113, 2004.

Authors provide a brief review of common dietary and ergogenic supplements used among athletes. Proposed mechanism of actions and studies supporting or refuting their effects on performance are discussed. Authors describe the supplements within categories of desired effects: improving strength and power, losing weight and fat, promoting energy supply, promoting immune function, promoting joint health, and stimulating the CNS. Other considerations include the contamination and cost of supplements.

Naylor AH, Gardner D, Zaichkowsky: Drug use patterns among high school athletes and nonathletes. *Adolescence* 36:627-639, 2001.

Study comparing substance use between high school athletes and nonathletes (total n = 1515) from 15 schools in Massachusetts. Results demonstrated greater use of cocaine, psychedelics, and cigarettes among nonathletes. Athletes were more likely to use creatine. Use of anabolic steroids and alcohol were similar in both groups. Overall, the authors conclude that athletes have healthier lifestyle habits than nonathletes.

Position of the American Dietetic Association, Dietitians of Canada, and the American College of Sports Medicine: Nutrition and athletic performance. *J Am Diet Assoc* 100:1543-1556, 2000.

Excellent review of nutritional requirements for athletes. Dietary needs prior, during, and after exercise and competition, in addition to general everyday recommendations, are discussed.

Rockwell MS, Nickols-Richardson SM, Thye FW: Nutrition knowledge, opinions, and practices of coaches and athletic trainers at a division I university. *Int J Sports Nutr Exerc Metab* 11:174-185, 2001.

Investigation evaluating the nutrition knowledge among 53 coaches and athletic trainers from 21 sport teams at a Division I university, using a questionnaire format. Overall, participants answered 67% of questions correctly with participants guiding female athletes, strength and conditioning coaches, and those with greater than 15 years of experience scoring higher than other participants. When assessing nutrition opinion, body weight was believed to be of greater importance than body composition to an athlete's performance. Thirty percent of participants reported using dietitians. Fifty-three percent of participants believed that athletes were more likely to consume nutritious meals if given a higher allowance during team trips.

Siu PM, Wong SHS: Use of the glycemic index: effects on feeding patterns and exercise performance. *J Physiol Anthropol Appl Human Sci* 23:1-6, 2004.

Authors review the classification of carbohydrates on the basis of GI and how it relates to exercise performance. After evaluating several studies in the literature, the authors concluded that there is substantial evidence that consuming low GI foods prior to exercise may promote carbohydrate availability during activity, prolonging endurance, and high GI foods consumed after exercise improves glycogen storage. However, the authors caution that further research is required before definitive recommendations can be made.

Spriet LL, Gibala MJ: Nutritional strategies to influence adaptations to training. *J Sports Sci* 22:127-141, 2004.

Scientific article reviewing the evolving understanding in four areas associated with ergogenic aids and nutrition: (1) caffeine use, (2) creatine use, (3) intramuscular triacylglycerol use and response to nutrition, and (4) role of nutrition in gene expression during and following exercise. Authors conclude that small amounts caffeine appear to have a positive ergogenic effect through the stimulation of the CNS. The effects of creatine on performance are still equivocal, and the last two topics require much further study prior to assuming any recommendations.

The Female Athlete

Introduction

- The number of female athletic participants has been on the rise recently.
- Because of the higher level of sports participation by females, there has also been an increase in injury rates among players of this gender.
- Some of the injuries are sport specific, whereas others such as anterior cruciate ligament injury are felt to have some biomechanical and physiologic considerations that predispose the female athlete to injury.
- Understanding some of the special concerns related to female athletes is of utmost importance in early recognition and treatment of disorders associated with this population.

The Female Athlete Triad

- The female athlete triad refers to a term developed by the American College of Sports Medicine in 1992 to describe special concerns of female athletes.
- The female athlete triad consists of disordered eating, amenorrhea, and osteoporosis (Figure 66–1).
- Disordered eating may be as simple as skipping meals, restricting calories unnecessarily, or failing to eat balanced meals. In more severe cases, disordered eating may refer to diseases such as anorexia nervosa and bulimia nervosa (see section on eating disorders).
- Menstrual irregularities in female athletes have been reported to be as high as 27% to 37% compared with 5% in a nonathletic population (Figure 66–2).
- Common menstrual irregularities seen in athletes include delayed onset of menses, secondary amenorrhea, and oligomenorrhea.
- Disordered eating and irregular menstrual cycles are both risk factors for the development of osteoporosis, which may predispose athletes to stress fractures (see section on stress fractures). This leads to lower bone mineral density (BMD) in adulthood because almost 90% of the BMD is achieved by the end of adolescence.

- Athletes thought to have risk factors for the development of osteoporosis should have BMD screening. BMD of 1 to 2.5 standard deviations below normal for that age group is defined as osteopenia, and greater than 2.5 standard deviations below normal is defined as osteoporosis (Box 66–1).
- The most important thing in dealing with the female triad is early recognition.
- It is suggested that all physicians, coaches, trainers, and parents who work with young women be educated regarding the signs, symptoms, and consequences of the conditions associated with the female athlete triad.

Eating Disorders

Anorexia Nervosa

- Anorexia nervosa is a psychological disorder that involves distorted body image, excessive dieting, and/or excessive exercise routines.
- Risk factors for the development of this disorder include psychological issues such as low self-esteem and depression, underlying medical disorders such as diabetes, and increased emphasis on appearance and fitness.
- A multitude of medical complications may occur as a result of this form of severe disordered eating. These include electrolyte disturbances, development of

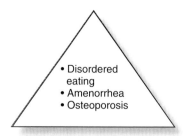

Figure 66–1:
The female athlete triad.

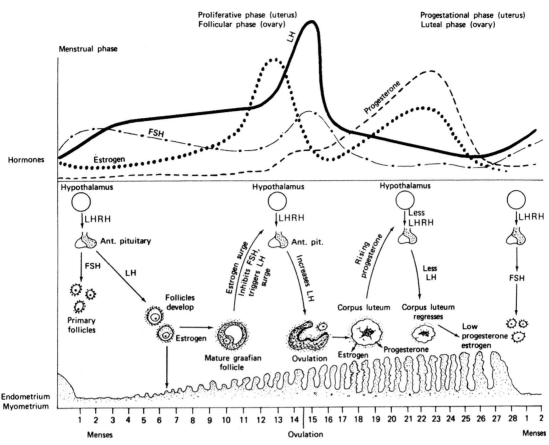

Figure 66–2:
The normal menstrual cycle. FSH, Follicle stimulating hormone; LH, luteinizing hormone; LHRH, luteinizing hormone releasing hormone. (From Sloane E: *Biology of women*. Albany, NY, 1980, Delmar.)

osteoporosis, gastrointestinal ulceration, cardiac arrhythmias, and renal dysfunction (Box 66–2).
- Mortality rates may be as high as 12% to 18% in cases of untreated anorexia nervosa.

Bulimia Nervosa

- Bulimia nervosa is a common eating disorder affecting an estimated 1% to 10% of females between the ages of 13 and 25.
- It is characterized by distorted body image and episodes of binging and purging.
- Weight loss and amenorrhea are not as striking in patients suffering from this disorder, often making it much more difficult to diagnose.
- One often subtle feature of this disorder is known as Russell's sign and consists of lesions, superficial lacerations, or calluses over the dorsum of the hand. Most often seen over the metacarpophalangeal or interphalangeal joints, these lesions are caused by repeated contact with the teeth during self-induced vomiting episodes.

- In severe cases, medical complications such as those listed previously may occur if this is not properly recognized and treated.

Stress Fractures In Female Athletes

- Stress fractures are common in all endurance athletes but have been shown to be more prevalent in females than males secondary to the female athlete triad. In fact, studies have shown that athletes with very irregular menses (0 to 5 cycles/year) have as high as a 47% risk of developing a stress fracture.
- The most common stress fractures are in the tibia and metatarsals and are the most common in running athletes.
- Stress fractures have also been shown to occur in the posterolateral aspect of the ribs in female athletes who participate in sports that involve an increased amount of scapular retraction and protraction such as rowing.

Box 66–1	Bone Density Testing

Normal

Bone density is within 1 standard deviation (SD) (±1 SD) of the young adult mean

Low Bone Mass

Bone density is 1 to 2.5 SD below the young adult mean (–1 to –2.5 SD)

Osteoporosis

Bone density is 2.5 SD or more below the young adult mean (>–2.5 SD)

Severe (Established) Osteoporosis

Bone density is more than 2.5 SD below the young adult mean and there has been one or more osteoporotic fractures

- Despite the location, the cause of stress fractures is repetitive loading across the bone greater than that which can be compensated for by the natural role of osteoblasts and osteoclasts in bone maintenance.
- In taking a history from a patient suspected of having a stress fracture, one should focus on the rate of progression of speed and distance in the training program, running surface, shoes worn, history of previous stress fracture, menstrual history, and potential for having an eating disorder (Box 66–3).
- Diagnosis includes physical examination to determine exact location of the pain and degree of tenderness. Plain radiographs should be obtained but may be normal initially. Bone scan provides information about increased activity at the site of the potential stress reaction. Magnetic resonance imaging or computed tomography scan may provide more information about the surrounding tissue and the degree of severity of the reaction (Figure 66–3).
- Treatment is predominately conservative and should include rest until the pain resolves. If weight-bearing is painful, the patient should be given crutches until the pain resolves. Surgery may be indicated if the fracture is persistent despite adequate conservative treatment or if the fracture becomes unstable (Figure 66–4).

Box 66–2	Complications of Eating Disorders in Athletes

Electrolyte disturbances
Development of osteoporosis
Gastrointestinal ulceration
Cardiac arrhythmias
Renal dysfunction

Box 66–3	History Questions to Evaluate Stress Fractures in Athletes

How rapidly have you progressed your running program (speed and distance)?
What type of surface do you run on?
What type of shoes do you wear? Do you have orthotics?
Have you ever had a previous stress reaction or fracture?
Do you have regular menstrual cycles?
How do you feel about your current weight and exercise level? (to ascertain the possibility of eating disorder)

The Pregnant Athlete

- It is generally agreed that the healthy pregnant or breast-feeding female may continue to participate in physical activity.
- The level of physical activity performed should not exceed that to which the athlete is already accustomed.
- It is important to understand that certain physiologic changes occur during a normal pregnancy that might affect athletic performance. These include weight gain, increase in total blood volume, and change in cardiac output.
- However, in low-risk pregnancies, aerobic capacity has been shown to be maintained or even improved as long as exercise is progressed slowly and not excessive for the patient's level of fitness.

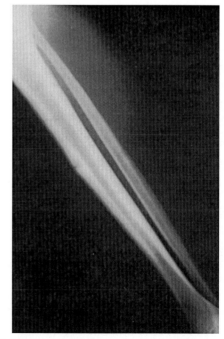

Figure 66–3:
Tibial stress fracture. (From Miller MD, Cooper DE, Warner JJP: *Review of sports medicine and arthroscopy.* Philadelphia, 2002, Saunders.)

Activity Progression

Non–weight-bearing, nonimpacting activities
(swimming and biking)

↓

Weight-bearing, nonimpacting activities
(StairMaster and cross-country machine)

↓

Weight-bearing, impacting activities (walking)

Progression within an Activity

Low intensity, short duration

↓

Low intensity, longer duration

↓

Higher intensity, shorter duration

↓

Higher intensity, longer duration

↓

Advance to the next activity level

Figure 66–4:
Return to sports participation after a tibial stress fracture in the female athlete. (From Griffin LY: The female athlete. In DeLee JC, Drez D Jr, Miller MD, editors: *DeLee and Drez's orthopaedic sports medicine: principles and practice,* 2nd ed. Philadelphia, 2003, Saunders.)

- Activities that involve any risk of impact should be avoided. This includes activities that have an increased risk of collision or fall and any activity that involves balls or projectiles that might strike the abdomen.
- In addition, after the first trimester, exercises in the supine position should be avoided secondary to increased strain on the abdominal muscles and the possibility of intraabdominal vascular compression.

Other Special Considerations

- Idiopathic scoliosis is more common in females then males but may also be more common in the athletic female group. Treatment typically consists of simple observation, but bracing and even surgery may be indicated depending on the severity of the curve.
- Spondylolysis involves a type of stress fracture through the pars interarticularis and is a common condition in female athletes, especially those involved in such sports as gymnastics, dancing, and figure skating because of the amount of lumbar extension involved in these activities.

References

Artal R, O'Toole M: Guidelines of the American College of Obstetricians and Gynecologists for exercise during pregnancy and the postpartum period. *Br J Sports Med* 37:6-12, 2003.
 A statement of the current view of the American College of Obstetricians and Gynecologists on physical activity in the prenatal and postnatal periods. Maintenance of a regular physical activity program during pregnancy is recommended to decrease the chance of excessive weight gain and complications associated with this. Aerobic exercise is the activity of choice and should be in line with the individual's level of fitness prior to pregnancy. Exercise is also recommended for patients with medical complications of pregnancy but only after clearance by the obstetrician on an individual basis.

Barrow GW, Saha S: Menstrual irregularity and stress fractures in collegiate female distance runners. *Am J Sports Med* 16:209-216, 1998.
 A study looking at the prevalence of stress fractures in college-aged endurance runners that shows rates of stress fractures as high as 49% in the group with very irregular menses. In addition, females who demonstrated no active menstrual cycle were much more likely (47%) to show signs of an eating disorder. Female runners who had never taken oral contraceptives also show a two times increase in the risk of developing a stress fracture.

Daluiski A, Rahbar B, Meals RA: Russell's signs. Subtle hand changes in patients with bulimia nervosa. *Clin Orthop Rel Res* 343:107-109, 1997.
 Bulimia nervosa affects 1% to 10% of young women, making it a disease of concern. Russell's sign involves small scrapes or calluses over the dorsum of the index finger from contact with the incisors during purging practices. Because this is an area that may be more likely to be seen by health care professionals, it may provide one of the few clues to the presence of a problem in the athlete.

Fogelholm M, Hiilloskorpi H: Weight and diet concerns in Finnish female and male athletes. *Med Sci Sports Exerc* 31(2):229-235, 1999.
 In comparing male and female populations regarding weight-reduction goals, we see that female athletes are much more likely to be unhappy with current weight. However, female controls had higher weight-loss goals than their endurance athlete counterparts.

Holda DL, Jackson DW: Stress fracture of the ribs in female rowers. *Am J Sports Med* 13:342-348, 1985.
 Seven documented cases of stress fracture of the ribs are reported in female athletes in the sports of rowing, tennis, golf, and gymnastics. All presented with periscapular pain and were initially treated for muscle strain. Diagnosis was made with plain radiography and bone scan an average of 2 to 6 months after the development of symptoms. Successful treatment for this condition involves a 4- to 8-week period of rest. These authors feel that the reason for the development of these stress reactions is an increased biomechanical force across the posterolateral rib from repetitive scapular motion. Women are thought to be at increased risk because of inadequate strength training in this area.

Kulpa PJ, White BM, Visscher R: Aerobic exercise in pregnancy. *Am J Obstet Gynecol* 156:1395-1403, 1987.
 One hundred forty-one pregnant subjects classified as low risk are randomized into control and aerobic exercise groups and tested for aerobic capacity during the first and third trimester and during the postpartum period. Results show that there is no increased morbidity associated with

aerobic activity during a normal low-risk pregnancy. In addition, we learn that aerobic capacity may be maintained or even improved during this period.

Omey ML, Micheli LJ, Gerbino PG: Idiopathic scoliosis and spondylolysis in the female athlete. Tips for treatment. *Clin Orthop Rel Res* 372:74-84, 2000.

Back pain is a common complaint in female athletes. Idiopathic scoliosis and spondylolysis are two conditions that may affect this population. Certain sports such as gymnastics, dancing, and figure skating may predispose the patient to developing such back pain. Treatment for these conditions is generally conservative. However early diagnosis and intervention may help to decrease patient morbidity.

Reeder MT, Dick BH, Atkins JK, et al: Stress fractures. Current concepts of diagnosis and treatment. *Sports Med* 22:198-212, 1996.

The stress fracture is a common athletic injury, especially in endurance athletes. It is also one of the complications of the so-called female athlete triad, making it an important consideration in this patient population. Maintaining a high level of suspicion in this group is important in early diagnosis and prevention of possible complications associated with stress fractures.

Rigotti NA, Neer SJ, Herzog DB, Nussbaum SR: The clinical course of osteoporosis in anorexia nervosa. A longitudinal study of cortical bone mass. *JAMA* 265:1133-1138, 1991.

In following 27 women with anorexia nervosa, these authors demonstrate that at the time of enrollment BMD was very low and found to be inversely proportional to degree of menstrual irregularity. Despite improvement in overall weight, exercise level, and supplementation with calcium, BMD did not rapidly improve over the course of the study (average follow-up of 25 months), which shows that the effects on BMD from anorexia are not quickly reversed with improvement of the condition.

Wiggins DL, Wiggins ME: The female athlete. *Clin Sports Med* 16:593-612, 1997.

This emphasizes the importance of understanding the female athlete as the number of female competitors continues to rise. The authors suggest that the most important aspect of caring for female athletes involves the prompt recognition of symptoms of the so-called female triad: disordered eating, amenorrhea, and osteoporosis. They also believe that most of the increased risk to female athletes is a result of selected sport rather than a gender issue.

Medical Conditions

CHAPTER **67**

Introduction

- Although physicians evaluating athletes are thought to deal predominantly with musculoskeletal injuries, they must be cognizant of other common medical conditions that require attention and can affect sport participation.
- It is more likely for an athlete to suffer from medical problems than orthopaedic injury.
- From minor colds to fatal diseases, the physician must be able to provide proper diagnosis, evaluation, and management and to advise the athlete and coaches of the ability to perform in competition.

Sudden Death

- The occurrence of sudden death among athletes often receives great attention from the media and concern from the athletic organizations.
- Sudden death in the young athlete is often secondary to underlying cardiac disorders, whereas in the middle-aged and older population is more likely to result from coronary artery disease.
- Obstructive hypertrophic cardiomyopathy is the most common cardiac condition causing sudden death in young players (Chapter 63, Figure 63–3).
  - This genetically linked condition is defined by asymmetrical hypertrophy of the interventricular septum that results in practically complete obliteration of the left ventricle and restricts blood outflow from that ventricle during systole.
  - Individuals with this condition often die before the age of 35, and thus athletes should be questioned about a possible family history of unknown or cardiac deaths.
  - A history of syncope, dizziness, shortness of breath, palpitations, or chest pain must be carefully evaluated for underlying cardiac conditions.
  - The characteristic systolic murmur that increases with Valsalva is not always present on examination.
  - Electrocardiogram is usually abnormal but may show no irregularities in up to 10% of cases.
  - Occasionally, it is difficult to distinguish from an athletic heart, which is characterized by left ventricular dilatation and subsequent concentric thickening. An echocardiogram can help make the distinction.
  - Athletes with this condition must be restricted from vigorous athletic participation.
- Coronary artery abnormalities are the second most common cause of sudden death in the young athlete.
  - Most common abnormality is an anomalous left coronary artery.
  - Anomalous right coronary arteries and single coronary arteries have also been described.
  - These are difficult to detect during a general examination but must be considered in athletes complaining of syncope or chest pain.
- Marfan's syndrome has also been associated with cases of sudden death.
  - Also genetically linked, Marfan's syndrome is associated with aortic dissection and rupture, which can be fatal.
  - Patients with Marfan's syndrome have a characteristic appearance with a tall stature, protruding jaw, and long extremities and may have skeletal chest and spine deformities (see Chapter 63, Table 63–3).
  - Cardiac abnormalities include mitral valve prolapse, aortic regurgitation, and dilatation of the ascending aorta and should be evaluated by echocardiography if Marfan's syndrome is suspected.
  - Subluxation of the lens (detected by slit lamp) with significant myopia is an additional common finding.
  - Athletes with Marfan's syndrome must be precluded from activities that raise their arterial pressure, which could risk aortic dilatation and rupture.
- Atherosclerotic coronary artery disease is the most common cause of death in the older population (older than 30 years).
  - Evaluation and workup is required in patients with positive risk factors and symptoms (Box 67–1).

481

Box 67–1	Risk Factors for Coronary Artery Disease

Family history
Smoking
Diabetes
Hypertension
Hypercholesterolemia

Hypertension

- Develops in athletes as commonly as in the general population.
- Arbitrary measurements have been established to define hypertension according to different ages (see Chapter 63, Table 63–4).
- It is important to ensure that measurements are taken with an appropriately sized blood pressure cuff.
- Other essential components of the physical examination include examination of the optic fundi, peripheral pulses, cardiac rhythm and sounds, and the presence of abdominal murmurs.
- There are no established guidelines for further workup but generally should at least include urinalysis, complete blood count, basic metabolic panel with fasting blood glucose, and an electrocardiogram.
- When pharmacologic treatment is indicated, the physician should consider agents that do not depress the myocardium, potentially cause arrhythmias, and interfere with substrate utilization and can preserve blood distribution to working muscles.
- Angiotensin-converting enzyme (ACE) inhibitors are a good choice for young and older athletes.
- Older athletes may also respond well to calcium channel blockers alone or in combination with ACE inhibitors.
- Generally beta-blockers should be avoided because they impair left ventricular function and can negatively influence lipid values and substrate mobilization.
- Diuretics may predispose an athlete to electrolyte balances and dehydration.
- Hypertension among black athletes is often volume dependent and may have a better response to small doses of diuretics or antiadrenergic agents and calcium channel blockers.

Heat Injury

- Thermal injuries can cause devastating effects.
- These injuries are predominantly preventable by taking precautions with proper fluid management and restricting or limiting training or competition under extremely high temperatures.
- Intensive activity results in generation of heat and raises core body temperatures, which are primarily dissipated by the conduction, radiation, convection, and evaporation of sweat.
- In hot environments, an athlete can lose approximately 5% of total body water per hour, which increases heart rate by approximately 30 beats per minute and core body temperature by 1°C. It is thus important to emphasize fluid maintenance during sport activity, especially under extreme temperatures.
- The inability of the body to maintain a safe core body temperature results in heat injury that can range from heat fatigue to heatstroke.
- Proper recognition of symptoms can prevent the progression of illness and subsequent manifestations.
- Heat illness in its mildest form often presents itself with heat cramps.
- Heat syncope results from arterial dilatation, as the body attempts to maintain temperature equilibrium, without the appropriate increase in cardiac output. This is a variant of a vasovagal syncope.
- The athlete with heat syncope should be placed in a Trendelenburg position and be administered fluid.
- Heat exhaustion and heatstroke can be considered a continuum of the same process and described in three phases (Box 67–2).
  - Management should consist of cooling measures such as fans and mist sprays to reduce rectal temperatures to 39°C.
  - Intravenous fluid should be administered as quickly as possible, and the patient should be transported to the nearest acute care facility for further care.
- In cases in which there is significant sweat loss, athletes may have electrolyte abnormalities that require replacement.
- Children require special attention secondary to their reduced sweat capacity, greater metabolic heat production, and larger surface area, which places them at an increased risk of heat injury.
- Apart from proper hydration, athletes should be advised to wear loose-fitting clothes promoting heat loss, recognize symptoms, and be cautious if febrile or taking certain medications such as diuretics or anticholinergics.

Exercise-Induced Asthma

- Occurs among approximately 10% of the athletic population, 90% of asthmatics, and 40% of individuals with allergic rhinitis.

Box 67–2	Stages of Heat Exhaustion/Stroke

Stage I—Rectal temperature of 40°C to 41°C, throbbing temples, and cold/shivering sensation of the trunk.
Stage II—Rectal temperature of 41°C to 42°C, muscle weakness, confusion, and loss of balance.
Stage III—Rectal temperature > 42°C, anhydrosis, loss of consciousness. In severe cases, this can result in death.

- When properly treated, athletes with exercise-induced asthma can compete at any level without restrictions. Such individuals have become successful elite athletes and won Olympic gold medals.
- Exercise-induced asthma is defined by 15% reduction in peak expiratory flow rate of forced expiratory volume in 1 second, caused by airflow obstruction after approximately 5 to 15 minutes of exercise.
- Symptoms include coughing, chest tightness, dyspnea, and wheezing during or following exercise (Box 67–3).
- Two theories, which are not necessarily mutually exclusive, have been proposed to explain the bronchoconstriction associated with exercise-induced asthma.
  - Water loss theory—increased respiratory rate during exercise leads to evaporative water loss resulting in increased pulmonary osmolarity and release of chemical mediators causing bronchial obstruction.
  - Respiratory heat exchange theory—after heat is exchanged from the tracheobronchial tree to condition the inspired air during exercise, bronchial vessels dilate in attempts to rewarm the bronchial tree, causing narrowing. This process is exaggerated under conditions of low humidity and cold temperatures.
- Diagnosis is usually made by history but can be confirmed by exercise testing with spirometric evaluation if uncertainty exists (Figure 67–1).
- Treatment primarily involves the use of a beta-2-agonist or cromolyn alone or in combination prior to exercise.
  - Because of its rapid onset and long duration, albuterol is preferred over the other available beta-agonists and should be prophylactically used 15 minutes prior to exercise and can repeatedly be administered during exercise as needed.
  - Cromolyn may be used alone or in combination with a beta-agonist (synergistic) if the beta-agonist cannot control the symptoms adequately.
- Other useful treatment recommendations include warming up before exercise and the use of an inhalation face mask in cold, dry weather or when high pollen counts are present. Athletes should attempt to avoid triggers as much as possible.
- Individuals with underlying asthma, exacerbated with exercise, may require chronic daily medication such as inhaled steroids (or leukotriene inhibitors) that can be combined with the previously mentioned recommendations.

Exercise-Induced Urticaria and Angioedema

- Exercise-induced urticaria (hives) is a histamine-mediated process characterized by the development of superficial edematous plaques (wheals), normally larger than 1 cm, which are often pruritic and usually resolve within 24 hours.
- Urticaria can progress to angioedema whereby the edematous process extends into the deeper layers of the skin and subcutaneous tissues and can last for several days.
- Occasionally this process can lead to anaphylaxis.
- When recurrences take place for greater than 6 weeks, the condition is considered chronic.
- Symptoms occur after approximately 5 minutes of exercise and can be associated with consumption of certain foods or medications.
- Exercise-induced urticaria should be distinguished from cholinergic urticaria, which produces smaller plaques

Box 67–3	Subjective and Objective Findings in Exercise-Induced Asthma

Subjective Findings with Exertion

1. Wheeze
2. Cough
3. Shortness of breath
4. Perception of poor physical conditioning
5. Lack of interest in physical activities

Objective Findings with Exertion

1. 10% to 15% fall in lung function
2. Protection against a 15% fall in FEV_1
3. Protection with bronchodilators

FEV_1, Forced expiratory volume in 1 second.
From Sheth KK: *Pediatr Clin North Am* 50: 697-716, 2003.

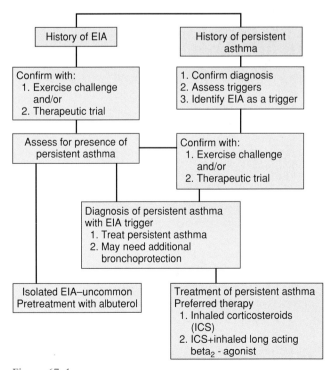

Figure 67–1:
Algorithm for evaluating a child with potential exercise-induced asthma (EIA). (From Sheth KK: *Pediatr Clin North Am* 50:697-716, 2003.)

(<5 mm) and wheezing, is considered less debilitating, rarely carries the risk of anaphylaxis, and is associated with a history of atopy and increased levels of histamines and basophils in the blood.
- Exercise-induced urticaria can be diagnosed with a detailed history and evaluation of triggers.
- Tests for cholinergic urticaria include the passive heat challenge by immersing the athlete in hot water or draping a heating blanket around the body and the methacholine challenge whereby the athlete receives an intradermal injection of acetyl methochloride chloride and is observed for the development of urticaria. These tests lack sensitivity but are very specific.
- Treatment includes the avoidance of triggers, use of antihistamines during acute attacks or prophylactically, and delay of exercise after eating.
- Cases that show progress of anaphylaxis and involve the respiratory tract should be additionally treated with epinephrine and corticosteroids.

Anemia

- Anemia is defined as a reduction in the hemoglobin concentration or number of red blood cells below normal values.
- Causes of anemia can result from physiologic changes (pregnancy and sports anemia), excess destruction (spherocytosis), blood loss [gastrointestinal (GI) bleed], or decreased production (iron or erythropoietin deficiency).
- Similar to the pseudoanemia seen in pregnancy, sports anemia is characterized by a dilutional type of anemia whereby there is an increase in plasma volume from chronic endurance exercising while the red blood cell mass remains relatively unchanged.
  - Appears to develop as an adaptive response attempting to maximize cardiac output and oxygen transportation in endurance activity.
  - Does not require restrictions or treatment.
  - Other forms of treatable anemia must be ruled out.
- Iron deficiency is the most common form of anemia.
  - It is more frequently seen in the female population.
  - Usually results from inadequate iron intake or bleeding (menstruation, GI blood loss).
  - Workup includes a careful history of dietary intake, complete blood count, peripheral blood smear, and iron studies and an evaluation for blood loss.
  - Iron deficiency anemia is characterized by a microcytic anemia with a low mean corpuscular volume and a low ferritin level (the most sensitive test).
  - Treatment consists of taking 325 mg of ferrous sulfate three times a day, preferably between meals with juice (enhancing GI absorption).
  - Replacement of iron stores usually takes at least 6 months.

- Anemias may result from GI or genitourinary (GU) bleeding or menstruating women.
  - Exercise-related GI or GU bleeds, associated with long races or trauma, are usually self-limiting and do not cause anemia.
  - GI bleeding often results from nonsteroidal antiinflammatory drug use and responds to cessation of the medication and treatment with histamine-2 blockers.
  - Fecal occult blood samples should be performed to diagnose suspected GI blood loss, and thorough evaluation for colon pathology is indicated in patients older than 30 with positive findings.
  - Macroscopic or microscopic hematuria seldom results in anemia but requires thorough evaluation using laboratory tests, imaging, and possibly cystoscopy.
- Exertion hemolysis, believed to result from rupture of red blood cells during heavy impact (as seen with repetitive heel strike in long distance runners), is generally a diagnosis of exclusion.
  - Nonimpact exertion hemolysis has also been described and thought to result from the accumulation of factors that destroy red blood cells during intense exercise.
  - Anemia is usually mild and can be reversed by stopping the inciting activity.
  - Prophylactic recommendations include cushioning the heel in runners and encouraging proper hydration.

Sickle Cell Trait

- Present in approximately 6% to 10% of the black population.
- An autosomal recessive trait characterized by the replacement of glutamic acid with valine on the hemoglobin beta chain that forms abnormal sickle-shaped red blood cells under hypoxic conditions that can occlude capillaries and cause ischemia.
- Individuals with sickle cell trait, the heterozygous form of sickle cell anemia, are usually asymptomatic and are able to perform at all levels of athletic activity.
- Severe dehydration, heat, and exercising at high altitudes may predispose individuals to sickling crisis.
- Fatalities in athletes secondary to sickling crisis have been documented.
- Individuals affected with the disease should be attentive to early symptoms of a sickling crisis and seek proper immediate medical care.
- Physicians must advise sickle cell athletes to avoid exercising at high altitudes and maintain adequate hydration.
- When required, treatment usually involves hydration and urine alkalization with sodium bicarbonate.

Diabetes Mellitus

- Type I diabetes mellitus, also known as insulin-dependent diabetes, typically occurs during childhood and is believed to be caused by an autoimmune disorder that limits the production of insulin by pancreatic cells and can result in hyperglycemia, ketosis, and acidemia starting at a young age if not treated with exogenous insulin. Affected individuals are usually thin in appearance.
- Type II diabetes, known as non–insulin-dependent diabetes, comprises 85% to 90% of diabetics and is characterized by an insensitivity to insulin that is produced by the individual. This form is often genetically linked and can be associated with obesity, hypertension, and hyperlipidemia.
- Diabetics have altered metabolic responses when participating in athletic activities.
- Exercise is believed to be beneficial among diabetics, providing non–insulin-dependent diabetics with improved glucose control and weight maintenance and countering the risk factors of hypertension and atherosclerosis in all diabetics. Exercise is often included among the treatment recommendations.
- In well-controlled diabetics, especially in type I diabetics, excessive insulin availability during exercise results in glucose uptake and inadequate glucose production by the liver that can produce a state of hypoglycemia.
- Type II diabetics are less likely to develop hypoglycemia unless they are taking sulfonylureas or exogenous insulin. Although other medications such as metformin and the metiglinides have less of a risk, careful monitoring is required and evidence of hypoglycemia usually demands withholding these medications prior to exercise.
- Diabetics under poor control that participate in athletics with increased levels of blood glucose are unable to provide the muscle with adequate glucose (secondary to the lack of insulin), and regulatory hormones increase the demand of the liver to produce more available glucose, further increasing the level of hyperglycemia, which risks the development of ketoacidosis.
- Examination of the diabetic must include evaluation of kidney function, cardiovascular status, neuropathy, and retinopathy, which may restrict them from certain athletic activities.
- All diabetics require proper treatment with medication and/or glucose that must be tailored to their individual diet needs and lifestyles, including their frequency and intensity in sport participation, and should be closely monitored by their caring physician until a stable regimen has been established.
- Adjusting doses of therapeutic medications is performed according to recorded glucose levels that should be maintained in a log by the patient during several times of the day including before, during, and after typical athletic activity.

- In general, less insulin is necessary during exercise, requiring smaller doses or withholding medications prior to sport participation.
- Diabetics should be aware of symptoms of hypoglycemia such as lightheadedness, dizziness, and disorientation that require the consumption of carbohydrates to recover blood glucose levels.
- Diabetics must be advised not to exercise during peak insulin levels, drink plenty of fluids, and carry supplemental carbohydrates at all times in case of severe hypoglycemic episodes.
- Individuals on insulin should avoid injections into muscle that will be extremely active during exercise.
- MedicAlert bracelets are recommended for all diabetics.
- Diabetics should exercise with a companion aware of their condition and potential complications and who knows how to respond in an emergency situation.
- When properly treated, diabetes does not affect the overall performance of the athlete.

Proteinuria

- Proteinuria, detected on urinalysis, is commonly seen in athletes after intense exercise.
- Exercise-induced proteinuria, also referred to as pseudonephritis, is usually idiopathic and benign.
- The proteinuria detected after exercise should return to normal values after 24 to 48 hours of rest. If the proteinuria does not resolve, other causes must be excluded.
- Another common diagnosis is orthostatic proteinuria whereby protein in the urine appears after periods of standing and resolves with recumbency. This condition is usually benign.
- Orthostatic proteinuria can be diagnosed by collecting urine samples on waking in the morning and comparing them with urine collected later in the day. The absence of protein in the morning samples and appearance of protein in the urine later in the day confirms the diagnosis.
- If proteinuria cannot be explained by either of the previous two disorders, further evaluation is required.

Overtraining

- A successful training program includes periods of overload training that produce stress on the body and adequate periods of recovery to allow muscles to replace glycogen and increase in mass.
- When athletes do not allow sufficient recovery time repeatedly, muscles begin to fatigue and performance is impaired.
- Frequently, athletes are unaware that they are overtraining and in response to their decreased performance continue

to increase their efforts in training, perpetuating the cycle of chronic fatigue.

- Chronic fatigue and worsening performance can negatively affect an athlete psychologically and cause depressive-like symptoms including altered mood and sleep disturbances, producing a chronic fatigue-depression syndrome.
- This syndrome is most common among endurance athletes such as runners and swimmers.
- The chronic fatigue-depression syndrome has been reproduced in a study of 12 male swimmers whereby training was significantly increased and decreased performance and depressive symptoms were observed and appeared to correlate in a linear fashion. Furthermore, levels of muscle glycogen stores were found to be inversely related to psychological complaints.
- Symptoms of fatigue, muscle soreness, and psychological symptoms should alert the examiner that the athlete may be overtraining. However, other conditions such as anemia, viral illness, hypothyroidism, and psychological disorders should be entertained and ruled out with appropriate workup on an individual basis.
- Because recovery from overtraining can take weeks to months, prevention of this phenomenon is important to avoid stopping an athlete's training or participation in competition.
- Athletes should be counseled on proper nutrition, including the increased carbohydrate requirements prior to and after training, and the consequences of overtraining.
- When treatment is required, a period of rest and proper nutrition (a high carbohydrate diet) followed by a graduated training regimen is often successful. In addition, the coach should be informed and advised to reduce training frequency or intensity, or both.

Exertional Rhabdomyolysis

- Intense exercise may produce significant muscle damage that can lead to rhabdomyolysis and myoglobinuria.
- More commonly affects the untrained athlete with associated risk factors such as dehydration, drug use, illness, or training under hot environments.
- The athlete may present with specific muscle soreness, weakness, tenderness, and swelling.
- Laboratory values characteristically demonstrate elevated creatine kinase and creatinine and urinalysis may reveal dark urine with casts and myoglobin.
- Increased myoglobin can damage the nephrotubules and cause acute renal failure.
- Treatment requires hydration and alkalinization of the urine if myoglobin is present. Mannitol for diuresis may occasionally be indicated.

Amenorrhea

- Many female athletes involved in vigorous training and competition may experience amenorrhea.
- Primary amenorrhea is defined as the absence of menstruation by age 14, whereas secondary amenorrhea is characterized by loss of menstruation for three or more consecutive cycles in females who have already undergone menarche.
- Athletes are commonly affected by secondary amenorrhea as a result of alterations in the hypothalamic-pituitary-ovarian axis producing a hypothalamic state, which prevents the normal production of luteinizing hormone and follicle-stimulating hormone (FSH) required for ovulation.
- Amenorrhea has been associated with irreversible decreased bone mineral density that predisposes the individual to premature osteoporosis and an increased risk of stress fractures.
- Evaluation should include a thorough history, review of dietary intake, complete physical examination and laboratory workup, and other ancillary studies as needed to rule our other etiologies.
- Athletes should also be evaluated for anorexia because it is also frequently associated with amenorrhea and can form the devastating "female triad" if osteoporosis develops.
- Laboratory studies should include a pregnancy test, thyroid-stimulating hormone (TSH), FSH, and prolactin.
- A dual-energy x-ray absorptiometry scan to assess bone density is indicated if osteoporosis is suspected or the athlete has experienced prolonged amenorrhea.
- If the patient is negative for human chorionic gonadotropin, progestin and estrogen progestin challenges can be performed and confirm the diagnosis of hypothalamic amenorrhea if the return of a normal menstrual cycle is observed.
- Although normal menstrual cycles usually return after decreased activity, this may not be an option for the competitive athlete.
- Treatment involves proper dietary counseling to ensure adequate caloric intake and calcium supplementation of 1500 mg per day.
- Supplemental estrogen, such as in the form of oral contraceptives, can help improve bone mineral density.

Mononucleosis

- Mononucleosis is caused by the Epstein-Barr virus (EBV).
- Approximately 90% of individuals have antibodies to EBV by their third decade of life.
- Individuals may complain of general symptoms such as fatigue, malaise, headaches, and loss of appetite and can

progress to involve fever, chills, sore throat, and lymphadenitis.

- Cytomegalovirus, early human immunodeficiency virus infection, toxoplasmosis, and streptococcal pharyngitis and other less serious viruses may have similar presentations.
- Typical incubation period is 30 to 50 days and transmission is often through saliva directly or aerosolized.
- Posterior palate petechiae and cervical node lymphadenopathy are suggestive but not specific for the diagnosis of mononucleosis.
- Most concerning manifestation of mononucleosis is spleen enlargement, occurring in 50% of patients, that predisposes the individual to a higher risk of rupture, which occurs in approximately 0.06% of cases, most commonly between the first and third weeks.
- Because physical examination is unreliable in detecting spleen enlargement, ultrasound (test of choice) should be performed if the physician considers returning the athlete to play prior to 4 weeks.
- The mono spot test is 90% sensitive.
- A blood smear may reveal atypical lymphocytes.
- Testing for EBV antibodies is 100% sensitive by 3 weeks of infection.
- Treatment is primarily supportive with analgesics and encouraging hydration.
- Patients with pharyngitis may also benefit from throat lozenges and salt water gargles.
- All patients should initially be restricted from exercise.
- An enlarged spleen, fever greater than 100°F, dehydration, inability to maintain adequate food intake, or extreme fatigue or malaise are other indications restricting sport participation.
- Patients without an enlarged spleen may return to noncontact sports by 3 weeks and participate in contact activity by 4 weeks.
- Athletes affected with spleen enlargement may only return to contact sports when the spleen returns to normal size as demonstrated by ultrasound.

Colds

- Upper respiratory infections are one of the most common diseases affecting both athletes and the general population.
- Causative agents include an exhaustive list of viruses, with rhinovirus highlighted as the most common. Occasionally, bacterial infections may be present.
- Symptoms include myalgia; malaise; rhinorrhea; sore throat; headaches; nasal congestion; and, occasionally, mild difficulty breathing.
- Colds can frequently impair athletic performance and are a frequent reason athletes miss practice or are unable to participate in competition.
- Symptoms usually last between 2 days and 2 weeks.

- Treatment is conservative with the use of analgesics, antihistamines, and decongestants.
- Antibiotics must be used sparingly because they may cause unwanted side effects and often do not shorten the period of illness.
- Physician must ensure the medications do not include banned substances and will not significantly affect performance.
- Athletes with fevers above 101°F, bronchospasm, or excessive fatigue should be withheld from competition.
- Athletes should be advised of proper precautions such as handwashing and not sharing water bottles to prevent spread and exposure to other contagious individuals.

Diarrhea

- Etiologies include viral or bacterial infections and other GI disorders (irritable bowel syndrome).
- Diarrhea may also result after intensive exercise, thought to be produced from decreased blood supply to the intestine, which increases intestinal mobility.
- Diarrhea is defined by passing three or more unformed stools in a 24-hour period.
- This condition is usually self-limited.
- Disease is usually contracted from contaminated water or foods, especially when traveling to another country.
- Prevention is the best treatment. Athletes should be instructed on possible sources of infection and proper selection of foods and methods of cooking.
- When visiting a foreign country, the athlete should be advised to avoid tap water (including ice cubes and when brushing teeth), salads, raw fish, or meats and to only consume fruits that can be washed and peeled.
- Treatment is supportive and includes proper hydration and occasionally the use of antiemetics and antidiarrheal agents.
- When bacteria etiology is suspected and antibiotic use considered, stool cultures should be performed.
- Antibiotics should be used sparingly. When indicated, fluoroquinolones are preferred except in adolescents and pregnant women because of their potential effects on open growth plates.
- Antibiotics are not recommended in patients with bloody diarrhea.
- The decision to use prophylactic antibiotics when traveling is determined by the level of competition, necessity to participate, immune status, and medical history of the individual or team.
- The athlete may participate in competition when he or she is afebrile and well hydrated and the diarrhea is under control.

Blood-Borne Pathogens

- Human immunodeficiency virus (HIV) and hepatitis B virus (HBV) are the most prominent blood-borne pathogens transmitted via sexual contact, perinatally, and by direct contact with infected blood such as in needle sharing or blood transfusions.

- HBV is considered more contagious than HIV and is therefore more readily transmitted.
- The risk of transmission during athletic competition is close to nonexistent with only one reported case of HBV transmission among Sumo wrestlers in Japan in which there was exposure to a competitor with dermatitis who was a chronic HBV carrier.
- Individuals at greater risk include those involved in high-risk sexual activity and needle sharing. Male athletes are significantly more likely to participate in high-risk behavior than female athletes.
- Because these viruses can present insidiously with few or no symptoms, many athletes may be unaware of their infection.
- It is essential to test individuals involved in high-risk behavior or those who desire testing.
- Currently, there are no guidelines restricting HIV- or HBV-infected athletes from sport participation. However, because of the higher risk of HBV transmission, some recommend restricting athletes who are HBV carriers from close contact sports such as wrestling, martial arts, and rugby.
- As with any other medical illness, the decision to restrict the athlete from play depends on health status, nature of infection, and signs and symptoms.
- Educating athletes, coaches, and caregivers on preventive measures and universal precautions both on and off the field is an important component in reducing the risk of transmission.

Dermatologic Conditions

- Dermatologic conditions are commonly seen among athletic participants.
- The examiner should have a general knowledge of common skin manifestations, their etiologies, proper treatment, and ability to spread during contact sports.
- In general, athletes should be restricted from participating in close contact sports (e.g., wrestling) if they are affected with a skin condition that risks transmission to another athlete.
- Impetigo is a highly infectious bacterial infection characterized by honey-colored crusted lesions with an erythematous base. Treatment involves antibiotics (topical or systemic) and preclusion from close contact sports until the athlete is free of any new lesions.
- Erysipelas is a type of bacterial cellulitis producing warm erythematous patches usually affecting the face and occasionally involving the extremities. Treatment involves systemic antibiotics and the athlete should be precluded from close contact sports.
- Furuncles and carbuncles are painful abscess-like lesions that frequently occur along the anterior thigh, buttocks,

groin, and axilla. Treatment consists of warm compresses, incision, and drainage and the use of systemic antibiotics if surrounding cellulitis is present.

- Hidradenitis suppurativa describes an acneform eruption, usually involving the groin or axilla. Treatment includes oral antibiotics and drainage or excision for recalcitrant lesions. Athletes are excluded from close contact sports until they receive proper treatment and are free from purulent lesions.
- Folliculitis describes a bacterial infection of hair follicles that produces pruritic, urticarial papules or pustules. Pseudomonas folliculitis (associated with hot-tub use) is usually self-limited, but staphylococcal folliculitis (most common) requires antibiotic treatment.
- Herpes simplex infection produces uniform grouped vesicles that can appear anywhere on the body and can result in herpes gladiatorum that is transmitted through close contact sports and affects the face, trunk, or extremities. Recurrence is common. Acyclovir is the treatment of choice. Athletes are restricted from close contact sports.
- Molluscum contagiosum, a highly infectious disorder caused by a poxvirus, is characterized by white or flesh-colored papules with central umbilication that is predominantly seen in the genital area but can be spread to other locations. Treatment options include curettage, cryotherapy, or the use of cantharidin solution. Athletes should be restricted from contact sports until the lesions resolve or can be adequately covered.
- Plantar warts are caused by the human papillomavirus and typically produce rough indurated lesions that can easily be mistaken for corns but are distinguished by central black dots when pared down that can bleed. Treatment is only recommended when symptomatic and can include cryotherapy; salicylic acid solution; curettage; laser therapy; and, rarely with recalcitrant cases, injections of bleomycin sulfate.
- Tinea cruris ("jock itch") is a fungal infection of the groin producing erythematous patches with scaly or vesicular edges that initially appear along the crural folds and can extend outward. The use of topical antifungals usually provides effective therapy. Athletes unable to properly cover the lesion should be restricted from contact sports.
- Tinea pedis ("athlete's foot") is a fungal infection that involves the feet resulting in pruritic, scaly lesions that can lead to fissures between the toes. Treatment involves the use of topical antifungals. If lesions cannot be appropriately covered, athletes should refrain from participating in contact sports.
- Calluses and corns are hyperkeratotic lesions that appear on pressure points. Symptomatic lesions can be treated with debridement using a pumice stone, paring with a blade, using topical keratolytic agents, and using padded, properly fitting equipment and footwear.

- Blisters result from repetitive friction, producing fluid-filled lesions, commonly on the hands and feet. They generally should be left to resolve on their own. However, they may require drainage with a needle or use of occlusive dressings, especially if the roof of the lesion is torn.
- Jogger's nipples describes painful erosions occurring around the areola and nipples from repetitive friction with overlying sportswear. In women, sport bras provide adequate protection and adhesive bandages or other types of tape can be used over the affected area in men.
- Acne mechanica describes an acneform eruption that is seen among athletes who wear irritating occlusive clothing and gear. Symptoms can be reduced by wearing cotton shirts that absorb moisture and ensuring good hygiene. Treatments include benzoyl peroxide, tretinoin, topical antibiotics, and oral antibiotics in severe persistent cases.
- Contact dermatitis is a broad term for conditions caused by allergic reactions (e.g., poison ivy, rubber straps, leather shoes, nickel) or irritants (e.g., adhesive tape, tight clothing) that result in several different presentations ranging from mild erythema to weeping vesicles and bullae. It is recommended that the athlete undergo patch testing to detect allergic compounds that they should avoid. Treatment includes cold compresses, antihistamines, topical corticosteroids, and systemic corticosteroids in extensive cases.

References

Albright A, Franz M, Hornsby G, Kriska A, Marrero D, Ullrich I, Verity LS. American College of Medicine Sports position stand. *Med Sci Sports Exerc* 32(7):1345-1360.

Position stand article discussing the importance of regular exercise activity as a treatment modality in patients with type II diabetes. Authors review and make recommendations regarding the use of physical activity for prevention and management of type II diabetes.

American Medical Society for Sports Medicine, American Academy of Sports Medicine: Human immunodeficiency virus and other blood-borne pathogens in sports. Joint position statement. The American Medical Society for Sports Medicine (AMSSM) and the American Academy of Sports Medicine (AASM). *Am J Sports Med* (4):510-514.

A joint position statement providing general guidelines for health care providers involved with athletes to reduce the possible risk of transmission of blood-borne pathogens.

Barrow MW, Clark KA: Heat-related illnesses. *Am Family Physician* 58:749-756, 1998.

General overview of the etiology, risk factors, presentation, evaluation, and treatment of the various types of heat-related illnesses.

Braverman AC: Exercise and the Marfan syndrome. *Med Sci Sports Exerc* 30:S387-S395, 1998.

Extensive review of the genetics, evaluation, diagnosis, and management of Marfan's syndrome. Secondary to its association with cardiovascular

conditions and sudden death among athletes, guidelines for exercise and sport participation are discussed.

Butcher JD: Runner's diarrhea and other intestinal problems of athletes. *Am Family Physician* 48:623-627, 1993.

Review of bloody and nonbloody diarrhea and other common intestinal conditions affecting athletes, particularly runners. Presentation, evaluation, and treatment are discussed.

Clerico A, Giammattei C, Cecchini L, et al: Exercise-induced proteinuria in well-trained athletes. *Clin Chem* 36:562-564, 1990.

Study evaluating the effect of exercise on urinary excretion of protein. Authors evaluated the excretion of albumin, microglobulin, sodium, potassium, and creatinine in the basal state (overnight samples) and after exercise in 10 professional cyclists. Basal rates were found to be similar to those of healthy nonathletes. The mean excretion of albumin (from 4.2 to 18.1 µg/minute) and microglobulin (from 0.3 to 6.6 mg/L) significantly increased after exercise but were found to be reversible. Sodium and potassium also significantly increased. The authors concluded that albuminuria provides the greatest contribution of exercise-induced proteinuria, which is both glomerular and tubular in origin and quickly reversible to normal levels.

Committee on Sports Medicine and Fitness: Human immunodeficiency virus and other blood-borne viral pathogens in the athletic setting. *Pediatrics* 104:1400-1403, 1999.

Reviews issues surrounding participation of athletes infected with blood-borne pathogens and precautions that should be implemented to reduce the risk of transmission during play. The committee notes that the rate of transmission during sport activity is low and therefore should not preclude an athlete from participation. Legal issues and recommendations are discussed.

Dice JP: Physical urticaria. *Immunol Allergy Clin North Am* 24:225-246, 2004.

Extensive review of several types of physical urticarias including dermatographism, cholinergic urticaria, local heat urticaria, exercise-induced anaphylaxis, vibratory angioedema, solar urticaria, and aquagenic urticaria. Pathogenesis, diagnosis, and treatment are discussed for each of the conditions.

Helm TN, Bergfeld WF: Sports dermatology. *Clin Dermatol* 16:159-165, 1998.

Authors review several common dermatologic conditions encountered in athletes and provide diagnostic and treatment recommendations.

Maki DG, Reich RM: Infectious mononucleosis in the athlete. *Am J Sports Med* 10:162-173, 1982.

Review of the pathophysiology, epidemiology, clinical evaluation, diagnosis, complications, and treatment of mononucleosis. Authors address how this condition can affect athletes and offer management recommendations regarding athletic training and participation.

Marron BJ: Medical progress: sudden death in young athletes. *N Engl J Med* 349:1064-1075, 2003.

Good review of the epidemiology and causes of sudden death in young athletes. Although cardiovascular conditions (most common cause) are emphasized, noncardiac etiologies are also discussed. Screening protocols and criteria for sport participation are also examined.

Mast EE, Goodman RA, Bond WW, et al: Transmission of blood-borne pathogens during sports: risk and prevention. *Ann Intern Med* 122:283-285, 1995.

General overview of HIV and HBV transmission among athletes. Authors stress that transmission during sport activity is extremely rare and preventive measures should aim at educating athletes in risky off-the-field behavior. Preventive recommendations for athletes are provided.

Moghtader J, Brady WJ, Bonadio W: Exertional rhabdomyolysis in an adolescent athlete. *Pediatr Emerg Care* 13:382–385, 1997.
Case presentation and discussion of exertional rhabdomyolysis. Authors state that this rare condition should be considered in the differential of athletes presenting with a history of muscle weakness or pain. The classical triad of myalgias, muscle weakness, and dark urine is not always present and a high index of suspicion is necessary to make the diagnosis.

Niedfeldt MW: Managing hypertension in athletes and physically active patients. *Am Family Physician* 66:445–452, 2002.
Review of the evaluation and treatment of hypertension among athletes. Nonpharmacologic and pharmacologic management and recommendations on exercise restrictions are discussed.

Perkins DN, Keith PK: Food- and exercise-induced anaphylaxis: importance of history in diagnosis. *Ann Allergy Asthma Immun* 89:15–23, 2002.
Authors provide a case review followed by a detailed discussion regarding food and exercise-induced anaphylaxis. Authors discuss differential, diagnostic, and treatment considerations of this condition.

Sheth KK: Activity-induced asthma. *Pediatr Clin North Am* 50:697–716, 2003.
Extensive review of exercise-induced asthma. Epidemiology, pathophysiology, evaluation, diagnosis, and management are well covered. The author stresses the importance of proper identification of children with exercise-induced asthma (with or without underlying persistent asthma) and treatment to return athletes to normal sport activity without restriction.

Storms WW: Review of exercise-induced asthma. *Med Sci Sport Med* 35:1464–1470, 2003.
A review of exercise-induced asthma using recent literature to describe the pathophysiology, diagnosis, and treatment of this condition that may affect many athletes.

Warren MP: Health issues for women athletes: exercise-induced amenorrhea. *J Clin Endocrinol Metab* 84:1892–1896, 1999.
Author reviews the pathophysiology, diagnosis, health consequences, and management of exercise-induced amenorrhea. The author notes that detection is difficult unless active efforts are implemented. The psychological, skeletal, and reproductive disorders resulting from this condition can often be reversed with proper medical attention.

Zinker BA: Nutritional aspects of exercise: nutrition and exercise in individuals with diabetes. *Clin Sport Med* 18:585–606, 1999.
Discussion of the effects and importance of exercise and diet in the management of both type I and type II diabetics. Author reviews management strategies and stresses the importance of establishing tight glucose control and tailoring therapy according to individual needs. Author also comments on the need for further research in certain areas to provide improved guidelines to health care providers treating patients with diabetes.

CHAPTER 68

Ethical and Legal Issues

Ethics

- Definition: although closely related, law is defined as a set of enforceable social rules, and ethics refers to moral rules.
- Priorities.
  - Do no harm (as in the Hippocratic oath).
  - Make the athlete a priority.
  - Give the athlete the right to participate in decisions regarding his or her care.
    - Informed consent.
      - Four criteria.
        1. Person making decision must be competent.
        2. Full discussion of procedure and risk.
        3. Patient must understand.
        4. Voluntary.
    - In public and school settings, athletes have a right to participate if there is no valid medical contraindication.
      - They may also insist on participation by waiving the institution's liability if they are injured or have a medical condition that increases their risk.
- Team physician responsibilities.
  - Know the sport you are covering.
  - Know the athletes you are taking care of.
    - Preparticipation physicals.
    - Rosters/press releases.
  - Protect the individual athlete in the context of the team.
    - Remain objective.
  - Develop and maintain mutual trust and respect between athletes, trainers, parents, coaches, and management.
  - Protect the athlete from injury, reinjury, and permanent disability.
    - Council athletes regarding risks and dangers of participation.
- Record keeping.
  - This should be kept to the same standard as office-based medicine.

- Records should include a preparticipation physical examination, current office notes, surgery notes, and appropriate arthroscopic images.
- Privacy issues.
  - Health Information Portability and Accountability Act (HIPAA) requires careful screening of medical information that can be released.
  - Care with dealing with the media—consult with athletic trainers, coaching staff, and consultants.
- Weighing short-term gain versus long-term risk.
  - Efficacious use of injections and analgesics.
  - Return to play decisions.
- Ergogenic drug use.
  - Providing, encouraging, or tolerating banned substances is unethical.
  - Nutritional supplements more controversial.
- Standard of care—higher for athletes?
  - Magnetic resonance imaging required for every injury?
- Advertising.
  - Must avoid misleading the public.
  - Avoid auctioning team care to the "highest bidder."

Legal Considerations

- If a physician is compensated for his or her duties, the normal rules of medical liability apply.
  - If the physician is a volunteer, "good Samaritan" laws apply.
- Difficult issues occur when the physician travels outside the area in which he or she is licensed.
  - Generally temporary licenses may be granted.
  - Usually the host team or physician can help with injuries at individual events.
- Athletes who are minors require written permission from their adult caregiver.
  - These forms should travel with the team to away events.
- Guidelines for return to play.
  - Definitive diagnosis made.
  - Injury cannot be worsened.
  - The athlete can protect himself or herself.

References

Bunch WH, Dvonch VM: Informed consent in sports medicine. *Clin Sports Med* 23:183-194, 2004.

> *This article serves as an overview of the process of informed consent in sports medicine. The authors review the basic components of informed consent, discussing procedures with athletes, and answering questions.*

Johnson R: The unique ethics of sports medicine. *Clin Sports Med* 23:175-182, 2004.

> *This is a review of some of the more unusual circumstances in which a team physician may find himself or herself. This includes issues of traveling, care of minor athletes, surrogate consent, and payment of services.*

Johnson R: Ethics and the team physician. *Clin Sports Med* 23:215-226, 2004.

> *This is a review article that discusses ethical consideration of the team physician including responsibilities, practice consideration, and documentation.*

Madden CC, Walsh WM, Mellion MB: The team physician: the preparticipation examination and on-field emergencies. In DeLee JC, Drez D Jr, Miller MD, editors: *Delee and Drez's orthopaedic sports medicine: principles and practice.* Philadelphia, 2003, Saunders.

> *This article provides an in-depth discussion of the components of the preparticipation physical examination and emergency management.*

Research Principles

Introduction

- Research is an integral part of the practice of orthopaedic surgery and sports medicine.
- Without research, we would be unable to review the outcomes of our surgical interventions, determine the natural history of the various disease and injury processes, and determine optimal methods of treating our patients.
- With the recent emphasis on evidence-based practice and medicine, we are continuing to improve the ways we approach and treat orthopaedic disease and injury through the highest level of evidence (Table 69–1).

Statistical Analysis

- Basic terminology.
  - Specific aims—purpose or purposes of the study.
  - Hypothesis—a provable or testable theory can be proved or disproved. The null hypothesis is the opposite of the hypothesis. The goal of any study is to reject the null hypothesis or prove the hypothesis to be true.
  - Population—the whole group from which to draw from to test a hypothesis.
  - Sample—a subset of the population to be tested. Samples should be randomized to avoid bias. Two samples that are being compared should also have similar characteristics and be representative of the entire population.
  - Bias—several types of bias including selection, informational, and observational. Methods to avoid bias include randomization and blinding.
  - Intention to treat—a technique to minimize bias by keeping the analysis in the same group that they were initially randomized to. Example: A patient is randomized to the nonoperative group and eventually desires surgery. The patient will be analyzed in the nonoperative group even though he or she received surgery to reduce the risk of selection bias.
  - Sensitivity—the ability of a test to detect the condition if it truly exists (Figure 69–1).

- Specificity—the ability of a test to detect the absence of the condition if it truly does not exist (see Figure 69–1).
  - Positive predictive value—the chance that the condition is truly present if the test is positive.
  - Negative predictive value—the chance that the condition is truly absent if the test is negative.
- Descriptive statistics.
  - Mean—the average value.
  - Median—the middle point of the values.
  - Mode—the most frequently occurring observation.
  - Standard deviation—a measure of variation.
  - Range—the highest to the lowest value.
  - Variance—the average of the squares of each observation's deviation from the mean.
  - Standard error of the mean—standard deviation of multiple samples' means when comparing different samples.
- Two group comparisons.
  - Hypothesis testing—analytic studies are designed to test hypothesis.
    - Type I error—the risk of false-positive results. Also termed alpha error or p value. Typical p values are set as 0.05 or 5%. If a difference is found with a p value of less than 0.05, then the risk of a difference existing by chance only is less than 5%.
    - Type II error—the risk of false-negative results. Also termed beta error or power. Typical power values are set at 0.80 or 80%. If no difference is found with a power of greater than 0.80, then it is usually assumed that sufficient power exists to find a difference if one truly exists. If the power is less than 0.80, then a difference may exist, but there is not enough of a sample to detect a difference if one truly exists.
  - Unpaired t-test—used to compare the means of two independent samples with continuous data that follow a normal distribution.
  - Paired t-test—Used to test the means of two paired samples with continuous data that follow a normal distribution. Paired samples would include a before and after analysis of the same sample or a matched case-control study.

Table 69–1: Levels of Evidence for Primary Research

	THERAPEUTIC STUDIES— INVESTIGATING THE RESULTS OF TREATMENT	PROGNOSTIC STUDIES— INVESTIGATING THE OUTCOME OF DISEASE	DIAGNOSTIC STUDIES— INVESTIGATING A DIAGNOSTIC TEST	ECONOMIC AND DECISION ANALYSES—DEVELOPING AN ECONOMIC OR DECISION MODEL

Level I	1. Randomized controlled trial
	   a. Significant difference
	   b. No significant difference but narrow confidence intervals
	2. Systematic review[†] of level I randomized controlled trials (studies were homogeneous)
		1. Prospective study[*]
		
		2. Systematic review[†] of level I studies
			1. Testing of previously developed diagnostic criteria in series of consecutive patients (with universally applied reference "gold" standard)
			2. Systematic review[†] of level I studies
				1. Clinically sensible costs and alternatives: values obtained from many studies: multiway sensitivity analyses
				2. Systematic review[†] of Level I studies

Level II	1. Prospective cohort study[‡]
	
	2. Poor-quality randomized controlled trial (e.g., <80% follow-up)
	3. Systematic review[†]
	   a. level II studies
	   b. Nonhomogeneous level I studies
		1. Retrospective study[§]
		
		2. Study of untreated controls from a previous randomized controlled trial
		3. Systematic review[†] of level II studies
			1. Development of diagnostic criteria on basis of consecutive patients (with universally applied reference "gold" standard)
			2. Systematic review[†] of level II studies
				1. Clinically sensible costs and alternatives: values obtained from limited studies: multiway sensitivity analyses
				2. Systematic review[†] of level II studies

Level III	1. Case-control study[‖] 2. Restrospective cohort study[§] 3. Systematic review[†] of level III studies		1. Study of nonconsecutive patients (no consistently applied reference "gold" standard) 2. Systematic review[†] of level III studies	1. Limited alternatives and costs: poor estimates 2. Systematic review[†] of level III studies
Level IV	Case series (no. or historical, control group)	Case series	1. Case-control study 2. Poor reference standard	No sensitivity analyses
Level V	Expert opinion	Expert opinion	Expert opinion	Expert opinion

[*]All patients were enrolled at the same point in their disease course (inception cohort) with ≥80% follow-up of enrolled patients.
[†]A study of results from two or more previous studies.
[‡]Patients were compared with a control group of patients treated at the same time and institution.
[§]The study was initiated after treatment was performed.
[‖]Patients with a particular outcome ("cases" with, for example, a failed total arthroplasty) were compared with those who did not have the outcome ("controls" with, for example, a total hip arthroplasty that did not fail).
From Wright JG, Swiontkowski MF, Heckman JD: *J Bone Joint Surg Am* 85A:1-3, 2003.

- Analysis of variance (ANOVA)—Used to compare the means of more than two independent samples with continuous data that follow a normal distribution.
- Nonparametric tests—used to compare means of samples with data that do not follow a normal distribution. An example of this would be a comparison of workers' missed days—the data would be skewed toward the left.
- Chi-square test—used to compared proportions (instead of means) of two groups. This test is better for larger groups of data because accuracy of determining the *p* value decreases for lower numbers (<5).
- Fisher's exact test—can also be used to compare proportions as with the chi-square test. Better for smaller numbers (<5) because accurate values are always

produced. Larger values are still accurate; however, the multiple calculations with larger numbers are computationally prohibitive.
- Determining association.
  - Correlation—the correlation coefficient ranges from −1 to +1 with positive being direct correlation and negative representing inverse correlation. A correlation coefficient of 0 indicates no correlation.
  - Linear regression—a test to determine the best fit curve that represents the data points.
- Sample size calculation—determining sample size of a study population is performed during the planning phases of a study. This is done to ensure that if difference does truly exist between the groups being studied, there are sufficient data to find that difference statistically. Common values are

	TEST +	TEST −
DISEASE +	TP	FN
DISEASE −	FP	TN

Sensitivity: TP/TP + FN
Specificity: TN/FP + TN
Positive predictive value: TP/TP + FP
Negative predictive value: TN/FN + TN

Figure 69–1:
Sensitivity, specificity, positive predictive value, negative predictive value. FN, False negative; FP, false positive; TN, true negative; TP, true positive.

set at a *p* value of <0.05 and a power of 0.80. Determining sample size requires an estimate from previous studies/pilot data of means and variation to calculate an effect size.

Types of Studies and Levels of Evidence

- Levels of evidence (Table 69–1).
- Study design.
  - Case reports—uncontrolled, descriptive study involving a single patient. Usually involves an intervention and outcome of clinical interest. Often rare conditions or conditions or interventions that have not been previously described.
  - Case series—similar to a case report but with more than one case being described.
  - Case-control studies—observational study comparing one group of patients with a particular outcome and comparing then to a suitable control group without the outcome. Example: comparing a group of patients with stable shoulder following surgery with a group with recurrent instability. The finding may include a higher incidence of bony defects of the humeral head or glenoid in the failed instability group. This study design is useful to determine prognostic variables.
  - Cohort studies—a large group of individuals are followed over time to see if a specific outcome develops. Cohorts are carefully designed with inclusion criteria of interest and well-designed outcome variables.
  - Randomized controlled trial—subjects are randomized to a treatment and a control group and compared in terms of carefully planned outcome variables. The highest level of evidence to which all other study designs should be compared.

Institutional Review Board

- Studies that involve human subjects require prior review and approval through an institutional review board (IRB).
- Recent importance and emphasis highlighted by several orthopaedic journals and societies requiring proof of IRB approval for human research.
- History.
- The Nuremberg Code (1948)—created from the Nuremberg trials in which Nazi physicians were tried for their crimes of performing medical experiments on prisoners. The code includes the right to voluntary informed consent, a favorable risk/benefit analysis, and the right to withdraw from the study without penalty.
- The Thalidomide Experience (1962)—investigational drug used in pregnant patients that caused severe growth deformities in infants. Led to the Food, Drug, and Cosmetic Act and to required informed consent of the use of investigational drugs.
- The World Medical Association Declaration of Helsinki (1964)—supports the statements of the Nuremberg Code and that the interests of the subject should always take priority over those of society and that every subject in clinical research should get the best known treatment.
- Congressional Hearings on the Quality of Health Care and Human Experimentation (1973)—response to public concern over ethical issues and the way medical research was being conducted in this country.
  - Willowbrook Hepatitis Studies—intentionally infecting healthy children with hepatitis.
  - Jewish Chronic Disease Hospital Studies—live cancer cells were injected into the bloodstream of chronically ill, demented patients.
  - Tuskegee Syphilis Study—study of a vulnerable population of approximately 300 uneducated, indigent, African-American sharecroppers with syphilis. Informed consent was not obtained and the subjects were followed without treatment for many years, even after penicillin became widely available and was known to be beneficial in the treatment of syphilis.
- The National Research Act and the IRB System (1974)—established the modern IRB system for regulating research involving human subjects and the National Commission for Protection of Human Subjects of Biomedical and Behavioral Research.
- Belmont Report.
  - Principle 1—Respect for Persons.
    - Right to individual autonomy and self-determination.
    - Protecting vulnerable subjects.
    - Avoid coercion or undue influence versus voluntary actions.
    - Informed consent.

○ Protect privacy and confidentiality.
- Principle 2—Beneficence.
  ○ Risks of research are justified by the potential benefits to the individual and/or society.
  ○ Study design minimizes risks and potential benefits are maximized.
- Principle 3—Justice.
  ○ Potential risks of research should be borne equally by the members of our society that are likely to benefit from it.
  ○ The research project does not systematically exclude a specific class or type of person who is likely to benefit from research participation or in whom the results of a specific kind of research are likely to be applied.

Research Support

- Several means of funding both clinical and basic science research are available at various levels including the institution, professional organizations, federal, and private sources.
- Often institutions provide seed money for young investigators or physicians in training to obtain funding for pilot studies. These can be from industry support, larger grants, or from clinical productivity dollars.
- Professional organizations such as the Orthopaedic Research and Education Foundation provide various level grants to residents and staff in hopes of stimulating research and funding to higher levels, that is, from the National Institutes of Health.
- The National Institutes of Health has several institutes that support orthopaedic research, most commonly the National Institute of Arthritis, Musculoskeletal and Skin Diseases; the National Institute of Aging; and the National Cancer Institute.
- Private sources include corporations and business that support research relevant to their particular financial interests. Care must be taken in these instances to avoid bias in research study design that favors the company that is funding or providing funds to the study.

Reading the Literature

- *Evidence-based medicine* is a term used to tailor your clinical practice on the basis of the best available scientific data to guide your decisions. There is a current move in orthopaedic surgery and sports medicine to head toward this end. It is highlighted by several of our peer-reviewed journals (*Journal of Bone and Joint Surgery, American Journal of Sports Medicine,* and *Arthroscopy*) to include an analysis of the level of evidence with each scientific article.
- Systematic reviews—an overview of studies with specific statements of objectives, materials, and methods and has been conducted according to explicit and reproducible methodology. Advantages include the limitations of bias

for inclusion and exclusion criteria for studies, and therefore conclusions are more reliable and accurate.
- Meta-analysis—statistical synthesis of the numerical results of several trials that all address the same question, that is, a quantitative systematic review.

References

Amdur R, editor: *Institutional review board: member handbook.* Sudbury, MA, 2003, Jones & Bartlett Publishers.
  Informational book concerning the IRB and how to interpret laws concerning the protection of human subjects research. Useful knowledge for designing human subjects clinical research.

Bernstein J: Evidence-based medicine. *J Am Acad Orthop Surg* 12:80-88, 2004.
  Review on the recent focus of evidence-based medicine in the orthopaedic surgery literature and how to evaluate the current literature and incorporate this information into clinical practice.

Brighton B, Bhandari M, Tornetta P, Felson DT: Hierarchy of evidence: from case reports to randomized controlled trials. *Clin Orthop* 413:19-24, 2003.
  Review describing various types of study design including case reports, case series, case-control studies, cohort studies, and randomized controlled trials, the highest level of evidence.

Devereaux PJ, McKee MD, Yusuf S: Methodologic issues in randomized controlled trials of surgical interventions. *Clin Orthop* 413:25-32, 2003.
  A specialized discussion is described in this explanation of the randomized controlled trial and how this study design relates to surgical interventions. Although randomization limits bias, which can alter the outcomes of the study, other issues are also discussed including technical considerations with surgery including learning curves with techniques, blinding, differing rehabilitation considerations, and intention to treat analysis.

Freedman KB, Bernstein J: Current concepts review: Sample size and statistical power in clinical orthopaedic research. *J Bone Joint Surg Am* 81A:1454-1460, 1999.
  Review detailing the importance of study design and statistical analysis in making conclusions regarding prospectively controlled clinical studies.

Greenhalgh T, editor: *How to read a paper: the basics of evidence based medicine,* 2nd ed. London, 2001, BMJ Books.
  A guide to the critical review of evidence-based medical literature including systematic reviews. Also describes different types of studies, statistics, and how to implement research into clinical practice.

Griffin D, Audige L: Common statistical methods in orthopaedic clinical studies. *Clin Orthop* 413:70-79, 2003.
  Various statistical methods are discussed including descriptive statistics, comparison of two groups with various t-tests, and analysis of variance when three or more means are compared; nonparametric testing; chi-square, and Fisher's exact tests. In addition, sample size calculations and correlation by various methods are discussed.

Keller RB: Outcomes research in orthopaedics. *J Am Acad Orthop Surg* 1:122-129, 1993.
  Review of clinical research methods and describes study design. Also gives instruction on how to design prospective clinical studies and conduct a meta-analysis of existing literature.

Myers ER: Elements of research: study design and data analysis. In Buckwalter JA, Einhorn TA, Simon SR, editors: *Orthopaedic basic science: biology and biomechanics of the musculoskeletal system,* 2nd ed. Rosemont, IL, 2000, American Academy of Orthopaedic Surgeons.

A basic review of different types of study design and statistical methods of analyzing data.

Wright JG, Swiontkowski MF, Heckman JD: Introducing levels of evidence to the journal. *J Bone Joint Surg Am* 85A:1-3, 2003.

Editorial introducing an evidence-based medicine approach to the Journal of Bone and Joint Surgery. This widely used rating scale evaluates study design and classifies the study from Level I to V in decreasing order of evidence level.

Index

Page numbers followed by "b" indicate boxes; "f," figures; "t," tables.

A

Abrasion chondroplasty, for focal osteochondral defects, 46, 46b

Abuse
  drug, 466–468, 467f, 468t. *See also* Drug abuse
  tobacco, 470

Achilles peritendinitis, 188, 190f

Achilles tendinitis, 188, 190f

Achilles tendon rupture, 188–191, 190f–193f, 190t, 191b
  evaluation of, Thompson test in, 189, 190f
  treatment of, 189–191, 190t, 191b, 191f–193f
    surgical reconstruction in
      Bosworth technique in, 192f
      fascia lata strips in, 193f
      fascial turn-down flap using proximal segment in, 193f
      indications for, 189, 191b
      peroneus brevis tendon transfer in, 192f
      suture techniques, 190, 191f
      V-Y gastroplasty in, 193f

ACL injuries. *See* Anterior cruciate ligament (ACL) injuries

Acne mechanica, 489

Acromioclavicular (AC) arthritis, 344, 346f, 347

Acromioclavicular (AC) joint, 241f, 246–247
  disrupted, anatomy of, 342, 343f
  injuries of, classification for, 343f–344f

Acromioclavicular (AC) separations, 342, 343f–345f, 344b, 346f
  classification of, 342, 344b
  primary repair of, 345f

Acromion, classification of, 295, 298b
  morphologic, 295, 297f

Acute calcific tendinitis, of flexor carpi ulnaris, 405

Adhesion(s), arthroscopic lysis of, 110, 111f

Adhesive capsulitis, 319–327
  arthrography of, 320
  complications of, 326
  factors associated with, 319, 319b
  imaging of, 320, 320f, 322f–323f
  MRI of, 320, 322f–323f
  pathogenic mechanisms of, 319, 321t

Adhesive capsulitis *(Continued)*
  patient history in, 319–320, 319b, 320b, 321t
  physical examination of, 319–320, 319b, 320b, 324t
  radiography of, 320, 320f
  rehabilitation for, 325
  stages of, 319, 319b, 320b
  treatment of, 321, 323, 325b, 325f, 326f
  types of, 320–321, 321t, 324t

Adult osteochondritis dissecans (AOCD), 43

Age, as factor in disc disease, 431

Alcohol, 467b, 468t, 469–470

Allograft(s), for focal osteochondral defects, 47, 48f, 49f, 49t

Amenorrhea, 486

American Spine Injury Association
  impairment scale of, 425t
  spinal cord injury classification of, 424f

Amphetamine(s), abuse of, 467b, 468

Anabolic steroids, abuse of, 466–467, 467b, 468t

Analgesia/analgesics, narcotic, abuse of, 467b, 468t, 471

Analysis of variance (ANOVA), 494

Anemia, 484

Anesthesia/anesthetics
  abuse of, 471
  injections, in low back pain, 439

Angioedema, 483–484

Ankle(s)
  arthroscopy of, 181–186
    complications of, 185, 186b
    diagnostic, 183, 184f, 185f
    indications for, 181
    patient positioning in, 181, 182f
    portal placement in, 181–183, 182f
    treatment-related, 183, 185f
  fractures of, 223, 223b, 223f–224f
  instability of, 209–219. *See also* Ankle(s), sprains of
    medial, classification of, 210, 215t
  joints of, anatomy of, 168–169
  ligaments of, 169, 172b, 173f

Ankle(s) *(Continued)*
  nerve entrapment syndromes of, 226–233. *See also specific nerve*
  overuse syndromes of, 187–205. *See also* Overuse syndromes, of leg, ankle, and foot
  sports-associated injuries of, 162b
  sprains of, 209–219
    classification system for, 213t
    complications of, 214
    imaging of, 209–210, 212f
    ligaments damaged in, incidence of, 209, 209b
    patient history in, 209
    rehabilitation for, 214, 218b
    treatment of, 210–214, 215t, 216f–218f
      augmentation procedures in, 212, 216f
      Brostrom procedure in, 214, 216f
      immobilization methods in, 212–213, 215t
    types of, 210, 213, 210b, 213t, 215t

Anorexia nervosa, in female athletes, 476–477, 478b

ANOVA. *See* Analysis of variance (ANOVA)

Anterior cruciate ligament (ACL), 1, 2f, 4f

Anterior cruciate ligament (ACL) avulsion/tibial eminence fractures, 113, 116f–117f

Anterior cruciate ligament (ACL) graft, placement of, problems associated with, 109, 110t

Anterior cruciate ligament (ACL) injuries, 55–61
  in children, 113
    treatment of, overuse injuries and, 115, 117–118, 118b, 119f
  described, 55
  history of, 55
  imaging of, 55, 56f, 57f
  physical examination of, 55, 55f, 56b, 56f
  prevention of, 59–60, 60f
  transphyseal, treatment of, 113, 115f
  treatment of, 55–58, 58f, 59f
    complications of, 58–59, 59f

Anterior cruciate ligament (ACL)
  injuries *(Continued)*
    graft choices in, 57–58, 58f
    rehabilitation after, 58
    tunnel placement in, 58, 59f
Anterior drawer test, 209, 211f
  in knee evaluation, 11, 15f
Anterior fat pad syndrome, 98–99, 98b
Anterior impingement syndrome, 183, 185f
Anterior interosseus nerve (AIN) palsy, 375
Anterior interosseus nerve (AIN) syndrome, 375
Anterior shoulder instability, 270–275. *See also*
    Shoulder instability, anterior
Anterior tibial artery, 167, 171f
Anterior tibialis tendon injury, 195–196
Antiinflammatory drugs, nonsteroidal, 471
AOCD. *See* Adult osteochondritis dissecans
    (AOCD)
Apophyseal ring fractures, low back pain due to,
    441, 443
Apophysitis, hip, 140
Apprehension test, in shoulder evaluation, 254,
    256f
Army Corps Squad Preparticipation Physical
    History form, 452f–453f
Artery(ies)
  coronary, abnormalities of, sudden death due
    to, 481
  dorsalis pedis, 168
  of elbow, 355–356, 358f
  fibular, 168, 171f
  of leg, 167–168, 171f
    distribution of, 171f
  popliteal, 167, 171f
  of shoulder, 248, 249f
  tibial
    anterior, 167, 171f
    posterior, 168, 171f
  of wrist and hand, anatomy and biomechanics
    of, 388, 388f
Arthritis
  acromioclavicular, 344, 346f, 347
  pisotriquetral, ulnar-sided wrist pain in, 402
Arthrofibrosis
  of knee, 109–112
    postoperative considerations in, 109–110
    prevention of, 109, 110b, 110t
    treatment of, 110–111, 110f–112f
  risk factors for, 110b
Arthrography
  in adhesive capsulitis, 320
  of elbow injuries, 366
  of ulnar-sided wrist pain, 399
Arthrometry, of ACL injuries, 55
Arthroscope(s), defined, 22
Arthroscopic synovectomy, 53, 54b
Arthroscopy. *See also specific sites, e.g.,* Ankle(s),
    arthroscopy of
  of ankle, 181–186
  diagnostic, of ulnar-sided wrist pain, 399
  of displaced glenoid fracture, 335f
  elbow, 367–369
  hip, 127–133
  knee, 22–26
  of meniscal tears, 27, 28f
  for rotator cuff injuries, 302b, 303f–310f

Arthroscopy *(Continued)*
  of shoulder, 263–269
  of SLAP tears, 286, 287f–288f
  of wrist, 393–395
Arthroscopy tower, 23f
Articular cartilage injuries
  classification of, 107b
  decision making in, 49t
Articular cartilage lesions, treatment algorithm
    for, 49f
Asthma, exercise-induced, 482–483, 483b, 483f
Atherosclerotic coronary artery disease, sudden
    death due to, 481, 482b
Athlete(s), young, sudden cardiac death in, risk
    factors for, 460b, 461f
Athlete's foot, 488
Athletic pubalgia, 134–135, 135f
Atlantoaxial rotatory subluxation, 426
Atlanto-occipital dislocation, 426, 426f
Atlas fracture, 426
Atraumatic osteonecrosis, 44
Axis isthmus fracture, 427

B

Back pain, low. *See* Low back pain
Bankart lesion, 270, 270f–272f, 271
Baseball finger, 408
Belly-press test, in rotator cuff injury evaluation,
    295, 296f
Belly-push test, 254, 256f
Belmont Report, 495–496
Beta-hydroxy-beta-methylbutyrate, 467b, 469
Bias, defined, 493
Biceps tendon
  distal, rupture of, 372, 373f
  in shoulder evaluation, 254, 256, 258f
Bigliani classification, of acromion morphology,
    295, 297f
Blackburne-Peel index, 18, 18f
Blic, Joseph, *see* Blumensaat line, 18
Blisters, 489
Blood doping, 467b, 470
Blood-borne pathogens, 487–488
Blumensaat line, 18
Bone(s), carpal, anatomy and biomechanics of,
    383, 384b, 384f, 385f
Bone density testing, 476, 478b
Bone scan, technetium-99m, in knee
    evaluation, 19
Bosworth technique, in Achilles tendon
    reconstruction, 192f
Boutonniere deformity, 389, 390f
Brace(s)
  for ankle sprains, 212–213, 214t
  extension, 110, 110f
Brachial plexus, 248, 250f
Broden's stress view, 212, 213f
Brostrom procedure, for ankle sprains, 212, 216f
Bucket handle tears, resection of, procedure
    for, 32f
Bulimia nervosa, in female athletes, 477
"Burners," 423f, 427–428
Bursa(ae)
  elbow, 354–355
  shoulder, 241f, 247, 249b, 249f
  subacromial, 241f, 247
  subscapular, 241f, 247

Bursitis, 99, 101f
  hip, 140, 141f
  retrocalcaneal, 199, 199b, 199f
Bursography, iliopsoas, 144, 146f

C

Caffeine, abuse of, 467b, 468
Calcaneus, fractures of, 223
Calluses, 488
Calories, 472, 472b
Capitellum, OCD of, 379
Capsulitis, adhesive, 319–327. *See also* Adhesive
    capsulitis
Capsulorrhaphy, thermal, in anterior shoulder
    instability management, 273
Carbohydrates, 472–473, 472b
Carbuncles, 488
Cardiomyopathy, obstructive hypertrophic,
    sudden death due to, 481
Carnitine, 469
Carpal bones, anatomy and biomechanics of,
    383, 384b, 384f, 385f
Carpal instability, 396–398
  classification of, 396, 396f
Carpal instability combined (CIC), 398, 398f
Carpal instability dissociative (CID), 396,
    396f, 397f
Carpal instability longitudinal (CIL), 398
Carpal instability nondissociative (CIND),
    397–398
Carpal tunnel, anatomy of, 383, 385f
Carpal tunnel syndrome, 375–376
Carpometacarpal joints, anatomy and
    biomechanics of, 385
Cast(s)
  for ankle sprains, 213, 215t
  extension drop-out, 110, 111f
Central slip injury, 408
Cervical disc disease, 432–433
Cervical disc herniation, 428
Cervical spine, anatomy of, 419, 419f, 420f
Cervical spine injuries, 423–430
  atlantoaxial rotatory subluxation, 426
  atlanto-occipital dislocations, 426, 426f
  atlas fracture, 426
  axis isthmus fracture, 427
  cervical disc herniation, 428
  compression-extension fractures, 427
  compression-flexion fractures, 427
  distraction injuries, 427
  hangman's fracture, 427
  imaging of, 425
  lateral flexion injuries, 427
  lower cervical injuries, 427–428, 428f
  neurapraxia, 423f, 427–428
  occipital condyle fractures, 425–426
  odontoid fracture, 426–427
  patient history in, 423
  physical examination of, 423, 424f
  rehabilitation after, 429
  return to play after, 429, 429b
  spear tackler's spine, 428
  spinal cord injuries, 425, 425t
  sports-related, 423
  sprains, 428
  strains, 428

Cervical spine injuries *(Continued)*
transient quadriplegia, 428, 428f
types of, 423, 423f, 425–428, 425t, 426f, 428f
upper cervical injuries, 425–427, 426f
Children, knee injuries in, 113–120
complications of, 120
extensor mechanism disorders, 114–115, 117–118, 118b, 118f, 117b, 119f
ligament injuries, 113–114, 115b, 115f–117f
physeal injuries, 113, 114f
rehabilitation for, 120
Chi-square test, 494
Chondral injury, treatment algorithm for, 44f
Chondral lesions, evaluation of, factors in, 45t
Chondrocyte transplantation/implantation, for focal osteochondral defects, 46–47, 48f
Chondromalacia, 104, 107b, 107f
Outerbridge classification of, 42b, 42f, 107f
Chondromatosis, synovial, 51, 52b, 52f
phases of, 52b
Chondroplasty, abrasion, for focal osteochondral defects, 46, 46b
CIC. *See* Carpal instability combined (CIC)
CID. *See* Carpal instability dissociative (CID)
CIL. *See* Carpal instability longitudinal (CIL)
CIND. *See* Carpal instability nondissociative (CIND)
Clavicle, 239, 239f, 240f
fractures of, 331–332, 331b, 332f, 333f, 347–348, 348f
Clenbuterol, abuse of, 467
Colds, 487
Collagen, in intervertebral disc disease, composition of, 431, 432t
Collateral ligament injuries, 91
lateral, 370–371
medial, 370
of PIP and MCP joints, 408–409
Common peroneal nerve, 166, 170f
anatomy of, 228f
entrapment of, 159, 226–227, 226b, 227t, 228f
Competition regimens, diet in, 474
Complex regional pain syndrome
classic stages of, 98, 98b
signs and symptoms of, 110b
Compression-extension fractures, 427
Compression-flexion fractures, 427
Computed tomography (CT)
of concussion, 414
in elbow injuries, 366
in knee evaluation, 19
in low back pain, 439
of posterior shoulder instability, 280
in shoulder evaluation, 262
of ulnar-sided wrist pain, 399
of upper extremity fractures, 331, 334f
in wrist and hand evaluation, 391, 392f
Concussion, 413–418
classification/grading of, 414–415, 416t
cranial nerve evaluation after, 413, 415t
defined, 413
head injury evaluation after, 414, 415t
imaging of, 414
management of, 416, 417t
pathophysiology of, 413
patient history in, 413

Concussion *(Continued)*
physical examination of, 413–414, 414b–416b, 415t
postconcussional syndrome, 416
return to play decision after, 416, 417t
signs and symptoms of, 413, 414b
SIS, 416–417
sports associated with, 413
standardized assessment of, 415b–416b
Congressional Hearings on the Quality of Health Care and Human Experimentation (1973), 495
Congruence angle, 18, 19f
Contact dermatitis, 489
Contusion(s)
of hip, 150–156. *See also* Hip(s), muscle strains and contusions of
of thigh, 150–156. *See also* Thigh(s), muscle strains and contusions of
Corns, 488
Coronary artery, abnormalities of, sudden death due to, 481
Coronary artery disease, atherosclerotic, sudden death due to, 481, 482b
Corticosteroid(s), abuse of, 468t, 471
Cranial nerves, 415t
Creatine, 467b, 469
Cross–body abduction test, in shoulder evaluation, 256
Cruciate ligament injuries, 91
CT. *See* Computed tomography (CT)
Cubital fossa, anatomy of, 353, 357f
Cubital tunnel syndrome, 376–377
Cyst(s)
ganglion, ulnar-sided wrist pain with, 402, 402f
meniscal, 30f

D

Danis-Weber classification, of ankle fractures, 223, 223f
de Quervain's disease, 404
Deep peroneal nerve, 167, 168f, 171f
entrapment of, 226b, 227–228, 228f, 227t
Degenerative disease, of hip, 141
Deltoid rupture, 314
Dermatitis, contact, 489
Dermatologic conditions, 488–489
Dermatome(s), lumbosacral, 433, 434f
Diabetes mellitus, 485
Diarrhea, 487
Diet(s), 474
Digit(s). *See* Finger(s); Finger injuries; Phalange(s)
Disc disease, 431–436
age as factor in, 431
cervical, 432–433
described, 431
lumbar, 433–435, 433f, 433t, 434f, 435t
thoracic, 433
Discitis, vertebral, low back pain due to, 443
Discography, in low back pain, 439
Discoid menisci
classification of, 28, 31f
saucerization of, 34f

Dislocation(s)
atlanto-occipital, 426, 426f
dorsal PIP, 409–410
elbow, 371
knee. *See* Knee dislocations
lunate, radiography of, 391, 391f
metacarpophalangeal joint, 410
of peroneal tendon, 194f
posterior shoulder, classification of, 280, 280f
proximal tib-fib, 91
thumb, 410
toe, 234
volar PIP, 410
Distal biceps tendon, rupture of, 372, 373f
Distal clavicle osteolysis, 343, 346f
Distal femoral epiphyseal fractures, Salter-Harris classification of, 113, 114f
Distal femur, right, 1, 2f
Distal humerus, anatomy of, 350, 351f, 352t, 353t
Distal triceps tendon, rupture of, 372–373, 374f
Distraction injuries, 427
Diuretics, abuse of, 467b, 468t, 471
Dorsal PIP dislocation, 409–410
Dorsalis pedis artery, 168
Double crush phenomenon, 375
"Dreaded black line," of anterior tibial stress fracture, 188, 190f
Drilling/microfracture, for focal osteochondral defects, 46, 46f
Drinks, sports, 413–414
Drop arm test, in shoulder evaluation, 254
Drop finger, 408
Drug abuse, 466–468, 467b, 468t
anabolic steroids, 466–467, 467b, 468t
clenbuterol, 467
cocaine/crack, 467b, 468, 468t
growth hormone, 467, 467b
marijuana, 467b, 468t, 470
Drug use, 466–468, 467b, 468t
Dynamic peel-back test, 286, 287f

E

Eating disorders, 474
in female athletes, 476–477, 478b
anorexia nervosa, 476–477, 478b
bulimia nervosa, 477
Effusion(s), intraarticular, assessment of, in knee evaluation, 10, 13f
Elbow
anatomy of, 350–362
arteries of, 355–356, 358f
biomechanics of, 350–362
bursae of, 354–355
golfer's, 378–379
loss of motion of, 381–382
causes of, 381, 381b
described, 381
examination of, 381
imaging of, 381
treatment of, 381–382
muscles of, 353
nerve entrapment about, 375–377
nerve(s) of, 356, 359f–361f
tendon injuries about, 372–374, 373f, 374f
complications of, 373–374

Elbow (Continued)
    distal biceps tendon rupture, 372, 373t
    distal triceps tendon rupture, 372, 373t
    rehabilitation of, 373
  tennis, 378, 379f
  vessels of, 355–356, 358f
Elbow arthroscopy, 367–369
  complications of, 369
  contraindications for, 367
  described, 367
  indications for, 367
  patient positioning for, 367
  portals in, 367–369, 368f
  rehabilitation after, 369
  technique of, 367–369, 368f
Elbow injuries
  arthrography of, 366
  CT in, 366
  dislocation, 371
  elbow motion after, strength testing of, 364
  imaging of, 365–366, 365f
  MRI of, 366
  overuse injuries, 378–380
    lateral epicondylitis, 378, 379f
    medial epicondylitis, 378–379
    OCD of capitellum, 379
    triceps tendinitis, 379
    valgus extension overload posteromedial
      impingement, 379, 380f
  patient history in, 363
  physical examination of, 363–365, 364f, 365f
  pivot–shift test after, 365, 365f
  provocative testing after, 364–365, 364f
  radiography of, 365–366, 365f
  ROM after, 363
Elbow instability, 370–371
Elbow joint, 350–353, 355f, 356f, 356t
Electromyography (EMG)
  of nerve entrapment syndromes of lower
    extremity, 226
  of ulnar-sided wrist pain, 399
Emergency injury assessment, 462, 463f
Energy bars, 473–474
Epicondylitis
  lateral, 378, 379f
  medial, 378–379
Ergogenic aids, 467b, 468–469
  amphetamines, 467b, 468
  beta-hydroxy-beta-methylbutyrate, 467b, 469
  caffeine, 467b, 468
  creatine, 467b, 469
  phenylpropanolamine/ephedrine, 467b,
    468–469
Erysipelas, 488
Erythropoietin, 467b, 470–471
Ethics, defined, 491
Evidence-based medicine, defined, 496
Exercise, during pregnancy, recommendations
  for, 460b
Exercise-induced asthma, 482–483, 483b, 483f
Exercise-induced urticaria, 483–484
Exertional compartment syndrome, 206–208
  anatomy of, 207
  causes of, 207b
  defined, 206
  diagnostic testing in, 207, 207f

Exertional compartment syndrome (Continued)
  differential diagnosis of, 207
  treatment of, 207–208, 208f
Exertional rhabdomyolysis, 486
Extension brace, 110, 110f
Extension drop-out cast, 110, 111f
Extensor carpi ulnaris tendinitis/subluxation, 404
  ulnar-sided wrist pain in, 401–402
Extensor forearm, muscles of, 353t
Extensor mechanism disorders, in children,
    114–115, 117–118, 118b, 118f, 117b, 119f
  acute, 114–115, 117b, 118f
Extensor mechanism rupture, 408
Extensor pollicis longus tenosynovitis, 404
External rotation dial test, in knee evaluation,
  13, 16f
External rotation recurvatum test, in knee
  evaluation, 13
External rotation splint, 270, 271f

F

Fascia lata strips, in Achilles tendon
  reconstruction, 193f
Fascial turn-down flap, using proximal segment,
  in Achilles tendon reconstruction, 193f
Fasciitis, plantar, 199–200, 200b, 201f
Fats, 472b, 473
Female athlete(s), 476–480
  anorexia nervosa in, 476–477, 478b
  bulimia nervosa in, 477
  eating disorders in, 476–477, 478b
  menstrual irregularities in, 476, 477f
  pregnant, 478–479
  stress fractures in, 477–478, 478b, 478f, 479f
Female athlete triad, 476, 476f, 477f, 478b
Femoral nerve, entrapment of, 157
Femur, 1, 2f
  distal, right, 1, 2f
  fractures of, 220
Fibula, 162, 163f
Fibular artery, 168, 171f
Fifth metatarsal base, fractures of, 224–225f
Finger(s). See also Finger injuries; Phalange(s);
    Thumb(s)
  baseball, 408
  Jersey, 406–407, 407t
  mallet, 408
  trigger, 405
Finger injuries, 406–412. See also Thumb injuries
  causes of, 406
  collateral ligament injuries of PIP and MCP
    joints, 408–409
  extensor mechanism rupture, 408
  flexor tendon injury, 407, 407f
  fractures, 411–412
  imaging of, 406
  Jersey finger, 406–407, 407t
  mallet finger, 408
  metacarpal fractures, 410–411
  metacarpophalangeal joint dislocation, 410
  patient history of, 406
  phalangeal fractures, 411–412
  physical examination of, 406
  sagittal band rupture, 408
  tendon-related, zones of, 407f
  volar PIP dislocation, 410

Fisher's exact test, 494
Flexor carpi radialis, 405
Flexor carpi ulnaris, acute calcific tendinitis
  of, 405
Flexor digitorum profundus, avulsions of,
  406, 407t
  Leddy classification of, 406, 407f
Flexor forearm, muscles of, 352t
Flexor hallucis longus injury, 194–195, 199b
Flexor pulleys, 388, 388f
Flexor tendon injury, 407, 407f
Flexor tendon sheath, anatomy and
  biomechanics of, 388, 388f
Focal osteochondral defects, treatment of, 45–47,
    45t, 46b, 46f–49f, 49t
  abrasion chondroplasty in, 46, 46b
  allografts in, 47, 48f, 49f, 49t
  chondrocyte transplantation/implantation in,
    46–47, 48f
  drilling/microfracture in, 46, 46f
  OATS in, 46, 46b, 47f
Folliculitis, 488
Foot (feet)
  athlete's, 488
  "jogger's," 229
  joints of, 172
  muscles of, 172, 175b, 176f–178f
  nerve entrapment syndromes of, 226–233. See
    also specific nerve
  osteology of, 170–172, 174f
  overuse syndromes of, 187–205. See also
    Overuse syndromes, of leg, ankle,
    and foot
  sport-associated injuries of, 162b
  sprains of, treatment of, immobilization
    methods in, 212–213, 214t
  tendons of, 172, 175b, 176f–178f
Forearm
  extensor, muscles of, 353t
  flexor, muscles of, 352t
Fracture(s)
  ACL avulsion/tibial eminence, 113, 116f–117f
  ankle, 223, 223b, 223f–224f
  apophyseal ring, low back pain due to,
    441, 443
  atlas, 426
  axis isthmus, 427
  bony avulsion about knee, 221, 221f
  calcaneus, 223–224
  compression-extension, 427
  compression-flexion, 427
  distal femoral epiphyseal, Salter-Harris
    classification of, 113, 114f
  femur, 220
  fifth metatarsal base, 224–225f
  hamate, CT of, 391, 392f
  hangman's, 427
  hip, 220
    stress-related, 220, 220f
  Jones, 224–225f
  of lower extremities, 220–225. See also Lower
    extremity(ies), fractures of
  metacarpal, 410–411
  occipital condyle, 425–426
  odontoid, 426–427
  patellar, 97, 97f, 98b, 98f, 114, 118f, 221

Fracture(s) *(Continued)*
  phalangeal, 411–412
  sesamoid, 235
  sleeve, of patella, 114, 118f
  stress. *See* Stress fractures
  talus, lateral process of, 223, 224f
  thumb metacarpal base, 411, 411f
  tibial, 222–223, 222f
  tibial eminence, Meyers and McKeever
    classification of, 115b
  tibial tuberosity, Watson-Jones classification of,
    117b, 118f
  toe, 234, 235
  trapezium, CT of, 391, 392f
  upper extremity, 331–341. *See also specific sites
    and* Upper extremity(ies), fractures of
Frankel scale, 425t
Frozen shoulder, 319–327. *See also* Adhesive
  capsulitis
Furuncles, 488

G

Gait, in knee evaluation, 9, 10f
Gait cycle, 172, 178, 179f
Gamekeeper's thumb, 409, 409f
Ganglion(a), suprascapular notch, MRI of, 328,
  329f
Ganglion cyst, ulnar-sided wrist pain with, 402,
  402f
Gastrocnemius-soleus strains, 196
Gastroplasty, V-Y, in Achilles tendon
  reconstruction, 193f
GIRD. *See* Glenohumeral internal rotation
  deficit (GIRD)
Glenohumeral internal rotation deficit (GIRD),
  285, 285f
Glenohumeral joint, 241–246, 242f–246f, 243b
  anatomy of, 245f
  static and dynamic restraints of, 243b
Glenohumeral ligaments, 243f
  tightening of, 244f
Glenoid, humeral head and, relationship
  between, 243f
Gluteal region, muscles of, 155b
Golfer's elbow, 378–379
Groin, contusions of, 150
Groin pain, 134–139
  athletic pubalgia, 134–135, 135f
  differential diagnosis of, 134, 135b
  hernias and, 135, 136f
  osteitis pubis, 135–136, 137f
  piriformis syndrome, 136–139, 137f, 138f
  stress fracture of hip and, 139
Growth hormone, abuse of, 467, 467b
Guhl arthroscopic classification, of
  osteochondritis dissecans, 43b
Guyon's canal, 377
Glycerol, 469

H

Haglund's deformity, 199, 199b, 199f
Hamate, fracture of, CT of, 391, 392f
Hamstring, strain of, 150
Hand(s)
  anatomy and biomechanics of, 383–388
    carpal bones, 383, 384b, 384f, 385f

Hand(s) *(Continued)*
    carpometacarpal joints, 385
    interphalangeal joints, 385
    metacarpals, 383, 384f, 385b
    metacarpophalangeal joints, 385
    muscles, 386–387, 386b, 386f, 387f
    nerves, 388
    phalanges, 383, 384f
    vasculature, 388
  evaluation of
    imaging in, 391–392, 391f, 392f
    patient history in, 389
    physical examination in, 389–391, 389f, 390f
      inspection in, 389, 389f, 390f
      neurovascular system in, 390–391
      palpation in, 389–390
      provocative testing in, 391
      range of motion in, 390
  kinematics of, 383
  osteology of, 384f
Hand, overuse injuries of, 404–405
Hangman's fracture, 427
Hawkin's impingement sign, 253, 254f, 295, 297f
HBV. *See* Hepatitis B virus (HBV)
Head injury, evaluation of, after concussion,
  414, 415t
Heat exhaustion/stroke, stages of, 482, 482b
Heat injury, 482, 482b
Heat stress danger chart, 463–464, 464f
Hepatitis B virus (HBV), 487–488
Hernia(s), groin pain due to, 135, 136f
Herniated disc
  cervical, 428
  low back pain due to, 439–441, 439t
Herpes simplex virus (HSV), 488
Hidradenitis, 488
Hill-Sachs lesions, 271, 271f
Hip(s)
  anatomy of, 121, 122f–125f
  biomechanics of, 121, 126
  fractures of, 220
    stress-related, 220, 220f
  joints of, 121, 122f, 123f
  ligamentous constraints of, 127, 127f
  muscle(s) of, 121, 123f, 124f
  muscle strains and contusions of, 150–156
    complications of, 153
    groin contusion, 150
    iliac crest contusion, 150
    imaging of, 150
    patient history in, 150
    physical examination of, 150, 151f–153f,
      154b, 155b
    rehabilitation for, 152, 156b
    treatment of, 151–152
    types of, 150–151
  nerve entrapment syndromes of, 157–161. *See
    also* Nerve entrapment syndromes, of hip
    and knee
  neurovascular structures of, 121, 125f
  overuse syndromes of, 140–142
    apophysitis, 140
    bursitis, 140, 141f
    complications of, 141
    degenerative disease, 141
    imaging of, 140

Hip(s) *(Continued)*
    osteitis pubis, 140–141
    patient history in, 140
    physical examination of, 140
    rehabilitation for, 141
    stress fractures, 140, 141f
    treatment of, 141
    types of, 140–141, 141f
  snapping, 143–149
    diagnosis of, 143–144, 145f, 146f
    treatment of
      conservative, 144
      surgical, 144–146, 147f, 148f
    types of, 143, 143f, 144f
  stress fracture of, groin pain due to, 139
Hip arthroscopy, 127–133
  complications of, 129–130, 132f, 132t
  mini-open technique in, 129, 132f
  patient positioning for, 127, 129f
  rehabilitation after, 129
  surgical contraindications to, 127b
  surgical indications for, 127b
  surgical technique in, 127–129, 129f–132f
Hormone(s), growth, abuse of, 467, 467b
Housemaid's knee, 99, 101f
Human immunodeficiency virus (HIV),
  487–488
Humeral head, 240, 242f
  glenoid and, relationship between, 243f
Humeral shaft, fractures of, 338–339, 339b,
  338f–340f
Humerus
  distal, anatomy of, 350, 351f, 352t, 353t
  proximal, fractures of, 335–337, 336f–337f
Hydration, 472, 472b
Hypertension, 482
  classification of, 450, 456t
Hypothesis, defined, 493

I

Iliac crest, contusion of, 150
Ilioinguinal nerve, entrapment of, 157
Iliopsoas, strains of, 151
Iliopsoas bursography, 144, 146f
Iliotibial band, 99–100, 102f
Imaging. *See also* Ultrasound; *specific site or
  modality, e.g.,* Knee(s), imaging of
Immobilization
  in anterior shoulder instability management,
    272
  for foot and ankle injuries, 212–213, 214t
Impetigo, 488
Impingement
  defined, 293
  subacromial, 299–300, 300t
Impingement testing, in shoulder evaluation,
  253, 253f
Insall-Salvati index, 18, 18f
Instability
  ankle, 209–219. *See also* Ankle(s), instability of;
    Ankle(s), sprains of
  carpal, 396–398
  elbow, 370–371
  patellar, 101–102, 104b, 104f–106f
  shoulder. *See* Shoulder instability
  spinal, three-column classification of, 419, 420f

Institutional review board (IRB), in research studies, 495–496
Intention to treat, defined, 493
Intercarpal joint, anatomy and biomechanics of, 385
Interdigital nerve, entrapment of, 226b, 227t, 230, 231f
Internal impingement, 288, 291, 291f
Interphalangeal joints, anatomy and biomechanics of, 385
Intersection syndrome, 404
Intervertebral disc, 431–432, 431f, 432t
    collagen composition of, 431, 432t
Intraarticular effusion, assessment of, in knee evaluation, 10, 13f
Inverted pear concept, 273, 273f
IRB. See Institutional review board (IRB)
Itch, jock, 488

J

Jerk test
    in posterior shoulder instability evaluation, 277–278, 279f
    in shoulder evaluation, 254, 257f
Jersey finger, 406–407, 407t
Jobe's test, in rotator cuff injury evaluation, 295, 295b, 295f
JOCD. See Juvenile osteochondritis dissecans (JOCD)
Jock itch, 488
"Jogger's foot," 229
Jogger's nipples, 489
Joint(s)
    AC. See Acromioclavicular (AC) joint
    ankle, 168–169
    carpometacarpal, anatomy and biomechanics of, 385
    elbow, 350–353, 355f, 356f, 356t
    foot, 172
    hip, 121, 122f, 123f
    intercarpal, anatomy and biomechanics of, 385
    interphalangeal, anatomy and biomechanics of, 385
    midcarpal, anatomy and biomechanics of, 385
    patellofemoral, 1, 5, 5f
    radiocarpal/ulnocarpal, anatomy and biomechanics of, 383–384, 385b, 385f
    scapulothoracic, 247
    shoulder, 241–247, 242f–246f, 243b. See also specific joint, e.g., Glenohumeral joint
    sternoclavicular, 247, 247f
Jones fracture, 224–225f
Juvenile osteochondritis dissecans (JOCD), 43

K

Knee(s)
    anatomy of, 1–7
    arthrofibrosis of, 109–112. See also Arthrofibrosis, of knee
    arthroscopy of. See Knee arthroscopy
    biomechanics of, 1–7
    bony avulsion fractures about, 221, 221f
    injuries of. See Knee injuries
    lateral
        anatomy of, 76f
        layers of, structures of, 77b

Knee(s) (Continued)
    ligaments of, 1, 2f–4f
    medial
        cross sectional view of, 64f
        layers of, anatomy of, 63f
        medial joint line opening with valgus stress of, classification of, 64b
    meniscectomized, 31, 37, 38f–40f
    menisci of, 5, 6f
    nerve entrapment syndromes of, 157–161. See also Nerve entrapment syndromes, of hip and knee
    osteochondral injuries to, 42–50
    patellofemoral joint of, 1, 5, 5f
    physical examination of, 9–13, 9t, 10f–16f
    plicae of, 52b
    spontaneous osteonecrosis of, 44–45, 45f, 45t
Knee arthroscopy, 22–26
    anatomy in, 25f
    complications of, 25–26, 26b
    diagnostic, 23, 25, 25f, 26f
    indications for, 22
    instrumentation in, 22, 23f
    irrigation setup for, 22, 23f
    patient positioning for, 22, 24f
    portal placement in, 22–23, 24f
    setup for, 24f
Knee dislocations
    classification of, 90, 90f
    diagnostic studies of, 92, 92f, 93f
    imaging of, 92, 92f, 93f
    surgical reconstruction of, 93
Knee, housemaid's, 99, 101f
Knee injuries
    in children, 113–120. See also Children, knee injuries in
    evaluation of
        patient history in, 8, 8b
        reverse pivot shift test in, 13
        stress radiography in, 19, 20f
    imaging of, 13, 17f–21f, 17t, 18–21
        CT in, 19
        MRI in, 19, 21, 21f
        radiography in, 13, 17f–20f, 17t, 18–19
        stress radiography in, 19, 20f
        technetium-99m bone scanning, 19
        ultrasound in, 21
    osteochondral. See also Osteochondral injuries, of knee

L

Lachman's test, in knee evaluation, 11, 15f
Lateral collateral ligament (LCL), 1, 4f
Lateral collateral ligament (LCL) injuries, 76–89, 91
    complications of, 85
    history of, 77
    imaging of, 77–79, 78f–81f
    physical examination of, 77, 77b
    treatment of, 79, 82f–84f, 83, 85, 86f, 87f, 88b
        algorithm for, 82f
        rehabilitation after, 85
Lateral epicondylitis, 378, 379f
Lateral femoral cutaneous nerve, entrapment of, 159, 160f
Lateral flexion injuries, 427

Lateral patellar compression syndrome, 100–101, 101f–104f, 104b
Lateral plantar nerve, 166, 169f
    entrapment of, 226b, 227t, 228–229
Latissimus dorsi rupture, 314, 316
Laurin's angle, 18, 19f
Law, defined, 491
LCL injuries. See Lateral collateral ligament (LCL) injuries
Leg(s)
    anatomy of, 162–168, 163f, 164b, 165b, 165f–171f, 167b
    anterior compartment of, muscles in, 164b, 165f
    arteries of, 167–168, 171f
    lateral compartment of, muscles in, 164b, 166f
    lower
        compartments in, 206, 206f
            cross-sectional anatomy of, 206f
            motor and sensory distribution of nerves of, 227t
        muscles of, 162–166, 164b, 165b, 165f–167f
        nerve entrapment syndromes of, 226–233. See also specific nerve, e.g., Saphenous nerve, entrapment of
        nerve(s) of, 166–167, 169f–171f
        overuse syndromes of, 187–205. See also Overuse syndromes, of leg, ankle, and foot
    posterior compartment of
        deep, muscles in, 165b, 167f
        superficial, muscles in, 164b, 166f
    sport-associated injuries of, 162b
    tibia, 162, 163f
    vessels of, 167–168, 171f
Legal considerations, 491
Lesion(s)
    Bankart, 270, 270f–272f, 271
    chondral, evaluation of, factors in, 45t
    Hill-Sachs, 271, 271f
    reverse Hill-Sachs, 278–280
    synovial, 51–54
Lift-off test
    in rotator cuff injury evaluation, 295, 296f
    in shoulder evaluation, 254, 255f–256f
Ligament(s)
    of ankle, 169, 172b, 173f
    glenohumeral, 243f
        tightening of, 244f
    injuries of, in children, 113–114, 115b, 115f–117f
    of knee, 1, 2f–4f
    testing of, in knee evaluation, 11, 15f
Load and shift test, in shoulder evaluation, 254, 256f
Local anesthetics, abuse of, 471
Long thoracic nerve, neuropathy of, 330
Low back pain, 437–444
    apophyseal ring fractures and, 441, 443
    differential diagnosis of, 439, 440t
        algorithm for, 438f
    herniated disc and, 439–441, 439t
    imaging of, 439, 440f
    patient history in, 437, 438f, 439t
    physical examination of, 437, 439, 439t
    prevalence of, 437

Low back pain *(Continued)*
  red flag symptoms of, 439t
  rehabilitation for, 443–444
  risk factors for, 435t, 437
  spondylolisthesis and, 441, 442f
  spondylolysis and, 440f, 441
  spondylosis and, 441
  treatment of, 443
  vertebral discitis and, 443
  vertebral osteomyelitis and, 443
Lower extremity(ies)
  dermatomes of, 157, 158f
  fractures of, 220–225
    ankle, 223, 223b, 223f–224f
    bony avulsion about knee, 221, 221f
    calcaneus, 223–224
    femur, 220
    fifth metatarsal base, 224–225f
    hip, 220, 220f
    patella, 221
    talus, lateral process of, 223, 224f
    tibia, 222–223, 222f
  neurologic signs and symptoms of, causes of,
    157b
Lumbar degenerative disease, low back pain due
    to, 441
Lumbar disc(s), herniated, clinical features of,
    433, 433f
Lumbar disc disease, 433–435, 433f, 433t, 434f,
    435t
  findings in, 439, 439f
Lumbar disc pressure, 433, 433f
Lumbar spine, anatomy of, 419f, 420–421
Lumbosacral dermatomes, 433, 434f
Lunate dislocation, radiography of, 391, 391f
Lunotriquetral ligament injury, ulnar-sided wrist
    pain in, 402

M

Magnetic resonance imaging (MRI)
  of ACL injuries, 55, 56f, 57f
  in adhesive capsulitis, 320, 322f–323f
  of anterior shoulder instability, 271–272, 272f
  of concussion, 414
  of elbow injuries, 366
  of hip overuse syndromes, 140
  in knee evaluation, 19, 21, 21f
  of LCL and PLC injuries, 79, 80f–81f
  in low back pain, 439
  of MCL injuries, 62, 65b, 65f
  of meniscal tears, 27, 28f
  of muscle strains and contusions of hip and
    thigh, 150
  of nerve entrapment syndromes of lower
    extremity, 226
  of PCL injuries, 69, 70f
  of pectoral muscle rupture, 313, 314f
  of peroneal tendon injury, 191, 195f
  of PLC avulsion, 221, 221f
  of posterior shoulder instability, 276, 277f,
    278f, 280
  of rotator cuff injuries, 298, 299f
  in shoulder evaluation, 260, 261f
  of SLAP tears, 286, 286f
  of stress fracture of hip, 220, 220f
  of suprascapular notch ganglion, 328, 329f

Magnetic resonance imaging (MRI) *(Continued)*
  of ulnar-sided wrist pain, 399
  of upper extremity fractures, 331
  in wrist and hand evaluation, 392
Mallet finger, 408
Marfan's syndrome, sudden death due to, 481
Marijuana, abuse of, 467b, 468t, 470
Mason-Allen stitch, modified, 308f
MCL injuries. *See* Medial collateral ligament
    (MCL) injuries
McMurray's testing, in knee evaluation, 9, 12f
Medial collateral ligament (MCL), 1
Medial collateral ligament (MCL) injuries,
    62–68, 91
  complications of, 65, 67
  history of, 62
  imaging of, 62, 65b, 65f
  physical examination of, 62
  treatment of, 62–64, 66f, 67f
    algorithm for, 66f
    rehabilitation after, 64–65
Medial epicondylitis, 378–379
Medial patellofemoral ligament (MPFL), 5, 5f
Medial plantar nerve, 166, 169f
  entrapment of, 226b, 227t, 229
Medial plica, Lino classification of, 53b
Medial plica syndrome, arthroscopic view of, 53f
Medial tibial stress syndrome, 196–197
Median nerve
  anatomy and biomechanics of, 388
  distribution of, 356, 359f
Medical conditions, 481–490
  amenorrhea, 486
  anemia, 484
  angioedema, 483–484
  blood-borne pathogens, 487–488
  colds, 487
  dermatologic conditions, 488–489
  diabetes mellitus, 485
  diarrhea, 487
  exercise-induced asthma, 482–483, 483b, 483f
  exercise-induced urticaria, 483–484
  exertional rhabdomyolysis, 486
  as factor in sports participation, 458t–459t
  HBV infection, 487–488
  heat injury, 482, 482b
  HIV infection, 487–488
  hypertension, 482
  mononucleosis, 486–487
  overtraining, 485–486
  proteinuria, 485
  sudden death, 481
Medical coverage, for team, 462–465
Meniscal cyst, 30f
Meniscal tears, 27–41
  arthroscopy of, 27, 28f
  bucket handle, resection of, 32f
  classification of, 30f
  imaging of, 27
  MRI of, 27, 28f
  patient history in, 27, 27b
  patterns of, not amenable to repair–related,
    34b
  physical examination of, 27, 27b
  repair of
    complications of, 40

Meniscal tears *(Continued)*
    procedures, 31–31, 32f–34f
    rehabilitation after, 37, 40
  techniques for, 31, 34b, 34f–37f
  types of, 28, 29f–31f
Meniscal transplantation, 31, 37, 38f–40f
Meniscus(i), 5, 6f
  described, 27
  discoid
    classification of, 28, 31f
    saucerization of, 34f
  pathology of, 27–41. *See also* Meniscal tears
Menstrual cycle
  irregularities of, in female athletes, 476, 477f
  normal, 476, 477f
Meralgia paresthetica, 159, 160f
Merchant view, 18, 19f
Metacarpal(s), anatomy and biomechanics of,
    383, 384f, 385b
Metacarpal fractures, 410–411
Metacarpophalangeal joint
  anatomy and biomechanics of, 385
  dislocation of, 410
Meyerding's classification, for degree of slip, 445,
    446f
Meyers and McKeever classification, of tibial
    eminence fractures, 115b
Micronutrients, 473
Midcarpal joint, anatomy and biomechanics
    of, 385
Molluscum contagiosum, 488
Mononucleosis, 486–487
Motion, shoulder, loss of, 319–327. *See also*
    Adhesive capsulitis
MPFL. *See* Medial patellofemoral ligament
    (MPFL)
MRI. *See* Magnetic resonance imaging (MRI)
Multiple ligament injuries, 90–95
  complications of, 93–94
  Schenck classification of, 90t
Muscle(s)
  abductor group of, 154b
  elbow, 353
  foot, 172, 175b, 176f–178f
  forearm, 352t, 353t
  hip, 121, 123f, 124f
  leg, 162–166, 164b, 165b, 165f–167f
  rotator cuff, 243f
  shoulder, 247, 248b, 248t
  wrist and hand, anatomy and biomechanics
    of, 386–387, 386b, 386f, 387f
Muscle injuries, in elite athletes, rehabilitation,
    156b
Muscle ruptures, of shoulder, 313–318. *See also*
    Shoulder(s), muscle ruptures of
Muscle strains
  of hip, 150–156. *See also* Hip(s), muscle strains
    and contusions of
  of thigh, 150–156. *See also* Thigh(s), muscle
    strains and contusions of
Musculoskeletal injuries, sport-specific, 450t

N

Nail bed, disorders of, toe-related, 235–236,
    236f–238f
Narcotic analgesics, abuse of, 467b, 468t, 471

National Institutes of Health, 496
National Research Act and the IRB System (1974), The, 495
Neer classification, of proximal humerus fractures, 335, 336f
Neer's impingement sign, 253, 253f, 295, 296f
Neer's impingement test, in rotator cuff injury evaluation, 295, 296f
Negative predictive value, defined, 493
Nerve(s). *See also* Median nerve; *specific nerve, e.g.,* Deep peroneal nerve
  of elbow, 356, 359f–361f
  of leg, 166–167, 169f–171f
    distribution of, 171f
    lower, motor and sensory distribution of nerves of, 227t
  of shoulder, 248, 250f
  spinal, 421
  of wrist and hand, anatomy and biomechanics of, 388
Nerve conduction studies
  of nerve entrapment syndromes of lower extremity, 226
  of ulnar-sided wrist pain, 399
Nerve entrapment
  elbow-related, 375–377
  at shoulder, 328–330
  sites of, 226b
Nerve entrapment syndromes
  of hip and knee, 157–161
    common peroneal nerve, 159
    femoral nerve, 157
    ilioinguinal nerve, 157
    lateral femoral cutaneous nerve, 159, 160f
    obturator nerve, 157
    pudendal nerve, 157
    saphenous nerve, 159–161, 160f
    sciatic nerve, 157, 159f
  of leg, ankle, and foot, 226–233
    common peroneal nerve, 226–227, 226b, 227t, 228f
    complications of, 231
    deep peroneal nerve, 226b, 227–228, 228f, 227t
    imaging of, 226
    interdigital nerve, 226b, 227t, 230, 231f
    lateral plantar nerve, 226b, 227t, 228–229
    medial plantar nerve, 226b, 227t, 229
    patient history in, 226
    physical examination of, 226, 227t
    rehabilitation for, 231
    saphenous nerve, 226
    superficial peroneal nerve, 226b, 227, 227t, 229f
    sural nerve, 226b, 227t, 228, 229f
    tibial nerve, 226b, 227t, 228, 229f
    treatment of, 230–231, 231f, 232f
    types of, 226–230, 228f–231f
  sites of, 226b
Neurapraxia, 423f, 427–428
Neuropathy(ies), suprascapular, 328, 328f, 329f
Neurovascular system, evaluation of, in wrist and hand evaluation, 390–391
Nick and spread method, 181, 183
Nipples, jogger's, 489
Nonparametric tests, 494

NSAIDs. *See* Antiinflammatory drugs, nonsteroidal
Nutrition, 471–474, 472b
  calories, 472, 472b
  carbohydrates, 472–473, 472b
  competition regimens, 474
  diets, 474
  eating disorders, 474
  energy bars, 473–474
  fats, 472b, 473
  guidelines for active persons, 471, 472b
  hydration in, 472, 472b
  micronutrients, 473
  protein, 472b, 473
  sports drinks, 473–474
Nuremberg Code (1948), The, 495

O

OATS. *See* OsteoArticular Transfer System (OATS)
O'Brien's test, in shoulder evaluation, 254, 256, 258f
Obstructive hypertrophic cardiomyopathy, sudden death due to, 481
Obturator nerve, entrapment of, 157
Occipital condyle fractures, 425–426
OCD. *See* Osteochondritis dissecans (OCD)
Odontoid fracture, 426–427
Open capsular shift, 272, 272f
Open reduction and internal fixation (ORIF), for lower extremity fractures, 220–225
ORIF. *See* Open reduction and internal fixation (ORIF)
Orthopaedic Research and Education Foundation, 496
Osgood-Schlatter disease, 119f
Osteitis pubis, 135–136, 137f
  of hip, 140–141
OsteoArticular Transfer System (OATS), 46, 46b, 47f
Osteochondral injuries, of knee, 42–50
  atraumatic osteonecrosis, 44
  focal osteochondral defects, 45–47, 45t, 46b, 46f–49f, 49t
  imaging of, 43, 43f
  osteochondritis dissecans, 43–44, 43b, 43f, 44f
  patient history in, 43
  physical examination of, 43
  SONK, 44–45, 45f, 45t
Osteochondral plug transfer, for focal osteochondral defects, 46, 46b, 47f
Osteochondritis dissecans, 43–44, 43b, 43f, 44f
  adult, 43
  of capitellum, 379
  Guhl arthroscopic classification of, 43b
  juvenile, 43
Osteology, 350
Osteolysis, distal clavicle, 343, 346f
Osteomyelitis, vertebral, low back pain due to, 443
Osteonecrosis, atraumatic, 44
Ottawa ankle rules, 223, 223b
Outerbridge classification, of chondromalacia, 42b, 42f
Overtraining, 485–486

Overuse injuries
  in children, 115, 117–118, 118b, 119f
  of elbow, 378–380
  of wrist and hand, 404–405
Overuse syndromes
  of hip, 140–142. *See also* Hip(s), overuse syndromes of
  of leg, ankle, and foot, 187–205. *See also specific injuries*
    Achilles tendon injury, 188–193, 190f–193f, 190t, 191b
    anterior tibialis tendon injury, 195–196
    complications of, 200, 202
    flexor hallucis longus injury, 194–195, 199b
    gastrocnemius-soleus strains, 196
    imaging of, 187
    medial tibial stress syndrome, 196–197
    patient history in, 187
    peroneal tendon injury, 191–192, 194b, 194f–197f
    physical examination in, 187
    plantar fasciitis, 199–200, 200b, 201f
    posterior tibialis tendon injury, 192–194, 197b, 197f, 198f
    rehabilitation for, 200
    retrocalcaneal bursitis, 199, 199b, 199f
    stress fractures, 187–188, 187t, 188t, 189f, 190f
    turf toe, 200, 202f, 202t, 203f
    types of, 187–200

P

Pain
  back, low. *See* Low back pain
  groin, 134–139. *See also* Groin pain
  wrist, ulnar-sided, 399–403. *See also* Wrist pain, ulnar-sided
Patella
  fractures of, 97, 97f, 98b, 98f, 221
  sleeve of, fractures of, 114, 118f
Patella alta/infera, 102, 104, 107f
Patellar instability, 101–102, 104b, 104f–106f
Patellofemoral disorders, 96–108
  anterior fat pad syndrome, 98–99, 98b
  bursitis, 99, 101f
  chondromalacia, 104, 107b, 107f
  classification of, 96b
  complications of, 105, 107
  iliotibial band, 97–100, 101f, 102f
  lateral patellar compression syndrome, 100–101, 101f–104f, 104b
  patella alta/infera, 102, 104, 107f
  patellar fracture, 97, 97f, 98b, 98f
  patellar instability, 101–102, 104b, 104f–106f
  rehabilitation after, 104–105
  tendinitis, 99
  tendon ruptures, 99, 100f, 101f
  treatment of, 104
  types of, 97–104, 98b, 98f, 97f, 100f–107f, 102b, 104b, 107b
Patellofemoral examination, in knee evaluation, 10, 14f
Patellofemoral joint, 1, 5, 5f
PCL injuries. *See* Posterior cruciate ligament (PCL) injuries
Pectoralis major rupture, 313, 313f–315f

Peel-back test, 286, 287f
Pelvis, bursae about, 140, 141f
Peritendinitis, Achilles, 188, 190f
Peroneal nerve
  common
    anatomy of, 228f
    entrapment of, 159, 226–227, 226b,
      227t, 228f
    deep, entrapment of, 226b, 227–228,
      228f, 227t
    superficial, entrapment of, 226b, 227,
      227t, 229f
Peroneal tendon(s)
  dislocations of, 194f
  normal relationship of, 194f
Peroneal tendon injury, 191–192, 194b,
  194f–197f
  diagnosis of, 191, 194b, 195f
  findings associated with, 194b
  MRI of, 191, 195f
  treatment of, 191–192, 196f, 197f
Peroneal tunnel, anatomy of, 228f
Peroneus brevis tendon transfer, in Achilles
  tendon reconstruction, 192f
Phalange(s). See also Finger(s)
  anatomy and biomechanics of, 383, 384f
  extensor apparatus of, 387, 387f
  fractures of, 411–412
Phenylpropanolamine/ephedrine, abuse of, 467b,
  468–469
Physeal injuries, in children, 113, 114f
Physical therapy, in anterior shoulder instability
  management, 272
Physicians, team
  bag and equipment of, 464, 464b
  responsibilities of, 462f, 462–463, 463f
Pigmented villonodular synovitis (PVNS),
  51, 51f
Piriformis syndrome, 136–139, 137f, 138f,
  157, 159f
Pisotriquetral arthritis, ulnar-sided wrist pain
  in, 402
Pivot jerk test, in knee evaluation, 11
Pivot shift test, 55, 56f
  in elbow evaluation, 365, 365f
  grading of, 56b
  in knee evaluation, 11, 15f
Plantar fasciitis, 199–200, 200b, 201f
Plantar nerve, lateral, entrapment of, 226b, 227t,
  228–229
Plantar warts, 488
PLC injuries. See Posterolateral corner (PLC)
  injuries
Plicae, synovial, 51–53, 52b, 53b, 53f
Plyometric training, for ACL injury prevention,
  59, 60f
Popliteal artery, 167, 171f
Port of Wilmington, 290f
Portal(s)
  in ankle arthroscopy, 181–183, 182f
  arthroscopic, 181–183, 182f
  in elbow arthroscopy, 367–369, 368f
  in wrist arthroscopy, 393–395, 394f
Positive predictive value, defined, 493
Postconcussional syndrome, 416
Posterior cruciate ligament (PCL), 1, 2f, 4f

Posterior cruciate ligament (PCL) injuries,
  69–75
  acute, treatment of, algorithm for, 71f
  chronic, treatment of, algorithm for, 72f
  diagnosis of, 69–70, 70f
  grades of, 69, 69t
  mechanism of, 69, 69f, 69t, 70f
  MRI of, 69, 70f
  stress radiography of, 69, 70f
  treatment of, 70–73, 71f–74f
    double-bundle technique in, 72–73,
      73f, 74f
    rehabilitation after, 73–74
    surgical reconstruction in, 71–73, 73f, 74f
    tibial inlay technique in, 72, 73f
    transtibial technique in, 71–72, 73f
Posterior drawer testing, in knee evaluation, 11
Posterior interosseus nerve (PIN) syndrome, 376
Posterior shoulder instability, 276–284. See also
  Shoulder instability, posterior
Posterior tibial artery, 168, 171f
Posterior tibial tendon injury, 192–194, 197b,
  197f, 198f
  clinical findings associated with, 193, 197b
  deformity associated with, 193, 197f
  treatment of, 193–194, 198f
Posterolateral corner (PLC) injuries, 76–89, 91,
  91b, 91f, 92f
  complications of, 85
  history of, 77
  imaging of, 77–79, 78f–81f
  physical examination of, 77, 77b
    maneuvers testing in, 77, 78f
  structures of, 77b
  treatment of, 79, 82f–84f, 83, 85, 86f, 87f, 88b
    rehabilitation after, 85
PPE. See Preparticipation evaluation (PPE)
Predictive value
  negative, defined, 493
  positive, defined, 493
Pregnancy
  exercise during, recommendations for, 460b
  in female athletes, 478–479
Preparticipation evaluation (PPE), 449–461
  Army Corps Squad Preparticipation Physical
    History form, 452f–453f
  described, 449
  determination of fitness for participation, 456,
    457t–459t, 460b, 461f
  formats used in, advantages and disadvantages
    of, 454t
  patient history in, 449
  physical examination in, 449–450, 455–456,
    455t, 456t
    recommended form for, 449, 451f
  protocol for, 455t
Pronator syndrome, 375
Protein, 472b, 473
Proteinuria, 485
Provocative testing
  in elbow evaluation, 364–365, 364f
  in wrist and hand evaluation, 391
Proximal humerus, fractures of, 335–337,
  336f–337f
Proximal tib-fib dislocations, 91
Pudendal nerve, entrapment of, 157

Pulleys, flexor, 388, 388f
PVNS. See Pigmented villonodular synovitis
  (PVNS)

Q

Quadriceps, contusions of, 150
Quadriceps (Q) angle, in knee evaluation, 10
Quadrilateral space syndrome, 330
Quadriplegia, transient, 428, 428f

R

Radial collateral ligament injury, of thumb MCP
  joint, 409
Radial nerve
  anatomy and biomechanics of, 388
  distribution of, 356, 361f
Radial tunnel syndrome, 376
Radiocarpal/ulnocarpal joint, anatomy and
  biomechanics of, 383–384, 385b, 385f
Radiography
  of ACL injuries, 55, 56f
  in adhesive capsulitis, 320, 320f
  in distal clavicle osteolysis, 346f
  of elbow injuries, 365–366, 365f
  of finger injuries, 406
  in hip overuse syndromes, 140
  imaging of, 13, 17f–20f, 17t, 18–19
  in low back pain, 439, 440f
  of meniscal tears, 27
  of nerve entrapment syndromes of lower
    extremity, 226
  in osteochondritis dissecans, 43, 43f
  plain, in LCL and PLC injuries, 77, 79f
  of posterior shoulder instability, 278, 280f
  of rotator cuff injuries, 295, 298, 299f
  in shoulder evaluation, 256, 258–259,
    259f–261f
  of SLAP tears, 285
  of SONK, 45f
  stress
    in knee evaluation, 19, 20f
    of PCL injuries, 69, 70f
    of ulnar-sided wrist pain, 399
    of upper extremity fractures, 331, 333f, 334f,
      337f–340f
  in wrist and hand evaluation, 391, 391f
Radius, anatomy of, 350, 354f
Range of motion
  in elbow evaluation, 363
  after lysis of adhesions and manipulation
    under anesthesia, 110, 112f
Range-of-motion testing
  in knee evaluation, 9, 11f
  in rotator cuff injury evaluation, 295
  in shoulder evaluation, 253, 253b
  in wrist and hand evaluation, 390
Rehabilitation
  ACL, 58
  for adhesive capsulitis, 325
  after ankle injuries, 214, 218b
  after cervical spine injuries, 429
  after elbow arthroscopy, 369
  after hip arthroscopy, 129
  after knee injuries in children, 120
  after meniscal repair, 37, 40
  after rotator cuff injury repair, 306–309, 311t

Rehabilitation *(Continued)*
  after shoulder arthroscopy, 266, 268
  after SLAP tears repair, 288
  after upper extremity fractures, 340
  LCL, 85
  for low back pain, 443–444
  MCL, 64–65
  for muscle strains and contusions of hip and
      thigh, 152, 156b
  for nerve entrapment syndromes of lower
      extremity, 231
  for overuse syndromes, 200
    of hip, 141
  PCL, 73–74
  PLC, 85
  for posterior shoulder instability,
      282–283, 283b
Relocation test, in shoulder evaluation, 254, 256f
Research, 493–497
  levels of evidence, 494t, 495
  reading literature in, 496
  statistical analysis, 493–495, 495f
  support for, 496
  types of studies, 494t, 495
Retrocalcaneal bursitis, 199, 199b, 199f
Return to play
  after cervical spine injuries, 429, 429b
  after concussion, 416, 417t
  after tibial stress fracture in female athletes,
      478, 479f
Reverse Hill-Sachs lesions, 278
Reverse pivot shift test, in knee evaluation, 13
Rhabdomyolysis, exertional, 486
ROM. *See* Range of motion (ROM)
Rotator cuff
  functions of, 293
  in shoulder evaluation, 253–254, 255f–256f
Rotator cuff complex, described, 293
Rotator cuff injuries, 293–313
  causes of, 293, 294b
  described, 293, 293f
  evaluation of
    Jobe's test in, 295, 295b, 295f
    lift-off test in, 295, 296f
    Neer's impingement test in, 295, 296f
    physical examination in, 295, 295b,
        295f–298f, 298b
    range-of-motion testing in, 295
    Sperling's test in, 295, 297f
  imaging of, 295, 298, 299f
  MRI of, 298, 299f
  patient history in, 294–295, 294t
  radiography of, 295, 298, 299f
  in rotator cuff injury evaluation, Hawkins
      impingement sign in, 295, 297f
  rotator cuff tears. *See* Rotator cuff tears
  rotator cuff tendinitis/tendinosis, 300, 300f
  subacromial impingement, 299–300, 300t
  treatment of, 301–306, 302b, 303f–310f
    arthroscopic, 302b, 303f–310f
    complications of, 311
    rehabilitation after, 306–309, 311t
  types of, 299–300, 300f, 300t, 301f
Rotator cuff muscles, 243f
Rotator cuff tears, 300, 301f
  conditions associated with, 294, 294t

Rotator cuff tears *(Continued)*
  conditions confused with, 294, 294t
  configuration of, arthroscopic repair according
      to, 302, 305t
  mini-open repair of, 304f
  patterns of, 301f
  treatment of, 301–306, 302b, 303f–310f
    according to tear pattern, 305f
Rotator cuff tendinitis/tendinosis, 300, 300f
Rotator interval, anatomy of, 244f
Rupture(s)
  extensor mechanism, 408
  muscle, of shoulder, 313–318. *See also*
      Shoulder(s), muscle ruptures of
  sagittal band, 408
  tendon, 99, 100f, 101f
    elbow-related, 372–374, 373f, 374f

S

Sagittal band rupture, 408
Salter-Harris classification, of distal femoral
      epiphyseal fractures, 113, 114f
Sample, defined, 493
Sand toe injuries, 202t
Saphenous nerve, 167
  entrapment of, 159–161, 160f, 226
Saupe's classification, of accessory ossification
      centers of patella, 118b, 119f
Scapholunate advanced collapse (SLAC), stages
      of, 397f
Scapula, 239–240, 241f–242f
  bursae around, 249b
  fractures of, 332–335, 333b, 334f, 335b, 335f
Scapulothoracic joint, 247
Schenck classification, of multiple ligament
      injuries, 90t
Sciatic nerve, entrapment of, 157, 159f
Sciatic notch, anatomy of, 137f
Sciatica, risk factors for, 435t
Second impact syndrome (SIS), 413, 414f,
      416–417
Sensitivity, defined, 493, 495f
Separations, acromioclavicular, 342,
      343f–345f, 344b
Sesamoid fractures, 235
Sesamoiditis, 234–234
Shoulder(s)
  anatomy of, 239–251
  arteries of, 248, 249f
  arthroscopy of, 263–269
    complications of, 268
    contraindications for, 264b
    indications for, 263b, 264f–267f
    rehabilitation after, 266, 268
    in shoulder stabilization, 265–266, 268f
    technique of, 263–264, 265f
  biomechanics of, 239–251
  bursae of, 241f, 247, 249b, 249f
  evaluation of, 252–262
    arthrogram in, 260
    biceps tendon, 254, 256, 258f
    CT in, 262
    imaging studies in, 256, 258–262, 259f–261f
    impingement testing in, 253, 253f
    inspection/palpation in, 252
    instability testing in, 254, 256f–257f

Shoulder(s) *(Continued)*
    MRI in, 260, 261f
    patient history in, 252
    physical examination in, 252–256, 253b,
        252f–258f
    radiography in, 256, 258–259, 259f–261f
    range of motion in, 253, 253b
    rotator cuff, 253–254, 255f–256f
    special testing in, 253–256, 253f–258f
    strength testing in, 253, 253b
    ultrasound in, 262
  frozen, 319–327. *See also* Adhesive capsulitis
  infraspinatus muscle atrophy of, 328, 329f
  instability of. *See* Shoulder instability
  joints of, 241–247, 242f–246f, 243b. *See also*
      specific joint, e.g., Glenohumeral joint
  layers of, 239, 239b, 239f
  ligaments about, 241f
  loss of motion of, 319–327. *See also* Adhesive
      capsulitis
  muscle(s) of, 247, 248b, 248t
  muscle ruptures of, 313–318
    deltoid, 314
    latissimus dorsi, 314, 316
    pectoralis major, 313, 313f–315f
    subscapularis tendon, 316, 316f, 317
    triceps, 316
  musculature of, 245f
  nerve entrapment at, 328–330
  nerve(s) of, 248, 250f
  range of motion of, normal, 253b
  stabilization of, arthroscopic, 265–266, 268f
  stiffness of, differential diagnosis of, 324t
  veins of, 248, 249f
  vessels of, 248, 249f
Shoulder girdle, anatomy of, 239, 239f
Shoulder instability
  anterior, 270–275
    atraumatic, 270–271
    classification of, 270–271, 270f, 271f
    imaging of, 271–272, 271f–272f
    MRI of, 271–272, 272f
    pathology associated with, 270, 271f
    physical examination of, 271
    traumatic, 270, 270f, 271f
    treatment of, 272–273, 272f–274f,
        272t, 273t
      anatomic considerations in, 272t
      immobilization in, 272
      physical therapy in, 272
      reduction in, 272
      surgical, 272–273, 272f–274f, 272t, 273t
      techniques of, 272–273, 273t
  evaluation of, 254, 256f–257f
  posterior, 276–284
    clinical findings in, 278b
    CT of, 280
    dislocations and
      classification of, 280, 280b
      management of, 280–282, 280b,
          281f, 282f
    imaging of, 276, 277f, 278, 278b, 278f, 280
    management of, 280–282, 280b, 281f, 282f
      complications of, 283
    MRI of, 276, 277f, 278f, 280
    patient history in, 276–278, 278b

Shoulder instability (Continued)
   physical examination of, 276–278, 278b,
      278f, 279b, 279f
   radiography of, 278, 280f
   rehabilitation of, 282–283, 283b
   types of, 280, 280b
Shoulder translation, grading of, 279b
Sickle cell trait, 484
Sinding-Larsen-Johansson disease,
   117–118, 119f
SIS. See Second impact syndrome (SIS)
Skier's thumb, 409, 409f
Skin, infectious conditions of, categories
   of, 455, 456t
SLAC. See Scapholunate advanced collapse
   (CLAC)
SLAP tears, 285–292
   arthroscopy of, 286, 287f–288f
   classification of, 286, 289f, 290f
   imaging of, 285–286, 286f
   mechanism of, 285
   MRI of, 286, 286f
   patient history in, 285
   physical examination of, 285, 285f
   radiography of, 285
   treatment of, 288, 290f
      rehabilitation after, 288
Sleeve fracture, of patella, 114, 118f
Snapping hip, 143–149. See also Hip(s),
   snapping
Sodium bicarbonate, 469
SONK. See Spontaneous osteonecrosis of knee
   (SONK)
Spear tackler's spine, 428
Specific aims, defined, 493
Specificity, defined, 493, 495f
Speed's test, in shoulder evaluation, 256
Sperling's test, for cervical nerve root
   impingement in rotator cuff injury
   evaluation, 295, 297f
Spinal column
   anatomy of, 419–422
      cervical spine, 419, 419f, 420f
      lumbar spine, 419f, 420–421
      spinal cord, 421, 421f
      spinal nerves, 421
      thoracic spine, 419–420, 419f
   described, 419, 419f, 420f, 420t
   kinematics of, 419, 420f
Spinal cord, 421, 421f
   cross-section of, 421, 421f
Spinal cord injuries, 425, 425t
   American Spine Injury Association standard
      neurologic classification of, 424f
Spinal instability, three-column classification of,
   419, 420f
Spinal nerves, 421
Spine
   cervical
      anatomy of, 419, 419f, 420f
      injuries of, 423–430. See also Cervical spine
         injuries
   lumbar, anatomy of, 419f, 420–421
   spear tackler's, 428
   thoracic, anatomy of, 419–420, 419f
Splint, external rotation, 270, 271f

Spondylolisthesis, 445–448
   causes of, 445
   classification of, 445, 446t
   described, 445, 446f
   low back pain due to, 441, 442f
   Marchetti and Bartolozzi classification of, 445,
      446t
   measurement of
      sacral inclination in, 447f
      slip angle in, 447f
   progression of, risk factors for, 445, 446f
   treatment of, 447–448
   Wiltse classification of, 445, 446f
Spondylolysis, 445–447
   causes of, 445
   classification of, 445
   described, 445
   diagnosis of, 445–446, 447f
   low back pain due to, 440f, 441
   treatment of, 446–447
Spondylosis, low back pain due to, 441
Spontaneous osteonecrosis of knee (SONK),
   44–45, 45f, 45t
Sports
   classification of
      by contact, 457t
      by strenuousness, 457t
   participation in, medical conditions and,
      458t–459t
Sports drinks, 473–474
Sprain(s)
   ankle, 209–210
   cervical, 428
Squatting, in knee evaluation, 9, 10f
Standing alignment, assessment of, in knee
   evaluation, 9, 10f
Statistical analysis, 493–495, 495f
   ANOVA in, 494
   chi-square test, 494
   descriptive statistics, 493
   determining association, 494
   Fisher's exact test, 494
   nonparametric tests, 494
   paired t-test, 493
   sample size calculation, 494–495
   terminology related to, 493
   two group comparisons, 493
   unpaired t-test, 493
Sternoclavicular injuries, 347, 347f, 348f
Sternoclavicular joint, 247, 247f
Steroid(s), anabolic, abuse of, 466–467, 467b, 468t
"Stingers," 423f, 427–428
Strain(s)
   cervical, 428
   gastrocnemius-soleus, 196
   muscle. See Muscle strains
Strength testing
   after elbow injury, 364
   in shoulder evaluation, 253, 253b
Stress fracture, of hip, 139
Stress fractures
   in female athletes, 477–478, 478b, 478f, 479f
   of hip, groin pain due to, 140, 141f, 220, 220f
   radiologic grading system for, 188t
   sport-specific, 187–188, 187t, 188t, 189f, 190f
      location of, 187t

Stress fractures (Continued)
   tibial, anterior, "dreaded black line," 188, 190f
      treatment of, 188, 189f
         algorithm for, 189f
Stress radiography
   in knee evaluation, 19, 20f
   of PCL injuries, 69, 70f
Subacromial bursa, 241f, 247
Subacromial impingement, 299–300, 300t
Subacromial impingement syndrome, stages
   of, 300t
Subluxation(s)
   atlantoaxial rotatory, 426
   extensor carpi ulnaris, 404
Subscapular bursa, 241f, 247
Subscapularis tendon rupture, 316, 316f, 317
Sudden cardiac death, in young athletes,
   460b, 461f
Sudden death, 481
   causes of, 481
Sulcus angle, 18, 19f
Sulcus sign, in shoulder evaluation, 254, 257f
Superficial peroneal nerve, 167, 168f
   entrapment of, 226b, 227, 227t, 229f
Superficial radial nerve compression
   syndrome, 376
Superior labrum anterior to posterior (SLAP)
   tears. See SLAP tears
Supplements, 467b, 468t, 469
   alcohol, 467b, 468t, 469–470
   carnitine, 469
   corticosteroids, 468t, 471
   diuretics, 467b, 468t, 471
   erythropoietin, 467b, 470–471
   glycerol, 469
   local anesthetics, 471
   NSAIDs, 471
   sickle cell trait, 484
   sodium bicarbonate, 469
   tobacco, 470
Suprascapular nerve, anatomy surrounding,
   328, 328f
Suprascapular neuropathy, 328, 328f, 329f
Suprascapular notch ganglion, MRI of, 328, 329f
Supraspinatus stress test, in shoulder evaluation,
   253–254, 255f
Sural nerve, 167
   entrapment of, 226b, 227t, 228, 229f
Suture techniques, in Achilles tendon rupture
   repair, 190, 191f
Syndesmotic injuries, 213–214
   classification of, 210, 214b
Synovectomy
   arthroscopic, 53, 54b
   complete, 54b
Synovial chondromatosis, 51, 52b, 52f
   phases of, 52b
Synovial lesions, 51–54
Synovial plicae, 51–53, 52b, 53b, 53f
Synovitis, pigmented, villonodular, 51, 51f

T
Talus, fractures of, lateral process of, 223, 224f
Tarsal tunnel
   anatomy of, 230f
   anterior, anatomy of, 229t

Tarsal tunnel syndrome, diagnosis of, dorsiflexion–eversion test in, 230f
Team medical coverage, 462–465
Team physician
  bag and equipment of, 464, 464b
  responsibilities of, 462f, 462–463, 463f
Tear(s)
  bucket handle, resection of, procedure for, 32f
  meniscal, 27–41. See also Meniscal tears
  rotator cuff. See Rotator cuff tears
  SLAP, 285–292. See also SLAP tears
Technetium-99m bone scanning, in knee evaluation, 19
Telos device, for performing stress radiographs in PCL injuries, 69, 70f
Tendinitis, 99
  Achilles, 188, 190f
  acute calcific, of flexor carpi ulnaris, 405
  extensor carpi ulnaris, 404
  triceps, 379
Tendon(s). See specific types, e.g., Achilles tendon
Tendon ruptures, 99, 100f, 101f
  distal biceps, 372, 373f
  elbow-related, 372–374, 373f, 374f
Tennis elbow, 378, 379f
Tenosynovitis, extensor pollicis longus, 404
TFCC. See Triangular fibrocartilage complex (TFCC)
Thalidomide Experience (1962), The, 495
Thermal capsulorrhaphy, in anterior shoulder instability management, 273
Thigh(s)
  muscle(s) of
    anterior, 154b
    posterior, 155b
  muscle strains and contusions of, 150–156
    complications of, 153
    hamstring strain, 150
    iliopsoas strain, 151
    imaging of, 150
    patient history in, 150
    physical examination of, 150, 151f–153f, 154b, 155b
    quadriceps contusion, 150
    rehabilitation for, 152, 156b
    treatment of, 151–152
    types of, 150–151
Thompson test, in Achilles tendon evaluation, 189, 190f
Thoracic disc disease, 433
Thoracic nerve, long, neuropathy of, 330
Thoracic outlet syndrome, 328–329, 330f, 377
Thoracic spine, anatomy of, 419–420, 419f
Thumb(s)
  gamekeeper's, 409, 409f
  skier's, 409, 409f
Thumb injuries
  dislocations, 410
  metacarpal base fractures, 411, 411f
  radial collateral ligament injury of MCP joint, 409
  ulnar collateral ligament injury of MCP joint, 409, 409f
Tibia, 162, 163f
  fractures of, 222–223, 222f
  stress fracture of, in female athletes, 478, 478f, 479f

Tibial eminence fractures, Meyers and McKeever classification of, 115b
Tibial nerve, 166, 169f–171f
  entrapment of, 226b, 227t, 228, 229f
Tibial stress reactions/fractures, 223
Tibial tuberosity fractures, Watson-Jones classification of, 117b, 118f
Tinea cruris, 488
Tinea pedis, 488
Tobacco abuse, 470
Toe(s). See also Toe injuries/disorders
  sand, 200, 202f, 202t, 203f
  turf, 200, 202f, 202t, 203f, 234, 234f, 235f, 235t, 236b
Toe injuries/disorders, 234–238
  dislocations, 234
  fractures, 234, 235
  nail bed disorders, 235–236, 236f–238f
  sesamoid fractures, 235
  turf toe, 202, 202f, 202t, 203f, 234, 234f, 235f, 235t, 236b
Torg ratio, 428, 428f
Traction tower, 393, 394f
Transient quadriplegia, 428, 428f
Transplantation, meniscal, 31, 37, 38f–40f
Trapezium, fracture of, CT of, 391, 392f
Triangular fibrocartilage complex (TFCC), 383–384, 385f
  anatomy of, 400f
Triangular fibrocartilage complex (TFCC) injuries
  arthroscopy for, 393
  classification of, 400, 401t
  ulnar-sided wrist pain in, 399–401, 400f, 401t
Triceps rupture, 316
Triceps tendinitis, 379
Trigger finger, 405
Turf toe, 200, 202f, 202t, 203f, 234, 234f, 235f, 235t, 236b

U

Ulna, anatomy of, 350, 354f
Ulnar collateral ligament injury, of thumb MCP joint, 409, 409f
Ulnar nerve
  anatomy and biomechanics of, 388
  distribution of, 356, 360f
Ulnar tunnel syndrome, 377
Ulnar-sided wrist pain, 399–403. See also Wrist pain, ulnar-sided
Ulnocarpal impaction syndrome, ulnar-sided wrist pain in, 401
Ultrasound
  in knee evaluation, 21
  in shoulder evaluation, 262
Upper extremity(ies), fractures of, 331–341, 333b, 334f, 335b, 335f
  arthroscopy of, 335f
  clavicle, 331–332, 331b, 332f, 333f
  complications of, 340
  CT of, 331, 334f
  humeral shaft, 338–339, 339b, 338f–340f
  imaging of, 331
  MRI of, 331
  patient history in, 331
  physical examination of, 331
  proximal humerus, 335–337, 336f–337f

Upper extremity(ies), fractures of (Continued)
  radiography of, 331, 333f, 334f, 337f–340f
  rehabilitation after, 340
Urticaria, exercise-induced, 483–484

V

Valgus extension overload posteromedial impingement, 379, 380f
Varus/valgus testing, in knee evaluation, 13, 16f
Vasculature, of wrist and hand, anatomy and biomechanics of, 388
Vein(s), shoulder, 247, 249f
Velpeau view, technique for, 278, 280f
Vertebral discitis, low back pain due to, 443
Vertebral osteomyelitis, low back pain due to, 443
Vessel(s), of elbow, 355–356, 358f
Vessels. See also Artery(ies); Vein(s)
  of leg, 167–168, 171f
Volar PIP dislocation, 410
Volar plate injury, 409–410
V-Y gastroplasty, in Achilles tendon reconstruction, 193f

W

Wart(s), plantar, 488
Wartenberg's syndrome, 376
Watson-Jones classification, of tibial tuberosity fractures, 117b, 118f
Weaver-Dunn procedure, 345f
Weber classification, of ankle fractures, 223, 223f–224f
World Medical Association Declaration of Helsinki (1964), The, 495
Wrist(s)
  anatomy and biomechanics of, 383–388
    carpal bones, 383, 384b, 384f, 385f
    flexor tendon sheath, 388, 388f
    intercarpal joint, 385
    midcarpal joint, 385
    muscles, 386–387, 386b, 386f, 387f
    nerves, 388
    radiocarpal/ulnocarpal joint, 383–384, 385b, 385f
    vasculature, 388
  arthroscopy of, 393–395
    complications of, 395
    indications for, 393
    portals in, 393–395, 394f
    postoperative care, 395
    technique of, 393, 394f
  evaluation of
    imaging in, 391–392, 391f, 392f
    patient history in, 389
    physical examination in, 389–391, 389f, 390f
      inspection in, 389
      neurovascular system in, 390–391
      palpation in, 389–390
      provocative testing in, 391
      range of motion in, 390
  extensor compartments of, 386, 386b, 386f
  instability of, 396–398. See also Carpal instability
  kinematics of, 383
  osteology of, 384f
  overuse injuries of, 404–405

Wrist joint
  anatomy and biomechanics of, 383–384,
    385b, 385f
  ligamentous structures about, 385b
Wrist pain, ulnar-sided, 399–403
  extensor carpi ulnaris tendinitis/subluxation
    and, 401–402

Wrist pain, ulnar-sided *(Continued)*
  ganglion cyst and, 402, 402f
  injury of, 399
  lunotriquetral ligament injury and, 402
  patient history in, 399
  physical examination of, 399
  pisotriquetral arthritis and, 402

Wrist pain, ulnar-sided *(Continued)*
  TFCC injury and, 399–401, 400f, 401t
  ulnocarpal impaction syndrome
    and, 401

Y

Yergason's test, in shoulder evaluation, 256